Children with Neurodevelopmental Disabilities

© 2013 Mac Keith Press

6 Market Road, London N7 9PW

Editors: Arnab Seal, Gillian Robinson, Anne M Kelly and Jane Williams
Managing Director: Ann-Marie Halligan
Production Manager: Udoka Ohuonu
Project Management: Prepress Projects Ltd

First published in this edition 2013

British Library Cataloguing-in-Publication data
A catalogue record for this book is available from the British Library

Front cover shows Ben and Rachel Dixon. Photograph reproduced with kind permission of Elspeth and Peter Dixon.

ISBN: 978-1-908316-62-2

Typeset by Prepress Projects Ltd, Perth, UK

Printed by Charlesworth Press, Wakefield, UK
Mac Keith Press is supported by Scope

Children with Neurodevelopmental Disabilities

The Essential Guide to Assessment and Management

Edited by

ARNAB SEAL, GILLIAN ROBINSON,
ANNE M KELLY, JANE WILLIAMS

2013
Mac Keith Press

Dedication

To the children and families we work with and look after.

To our teachers and colleagues who inspired us.

To the caring professionals and volunteers working alone or in teams with children, the world over.

To our own children and spouses who tolerated our absence and supported us while we worked to complete this book. Our thanks and love.

Contents

Authors' Appointments

Amanda Allard — Principal Officer, Council for Disabled Children, London, UK

Anne-Marie Childs — Consultant Paediatric Neurologist, The General Infirmary at Leeds, Leeds, UK

David Cundall — Retired Community Paediatrician, Leeds, UK

Val Harpin — Consultant Neurodevelopmental Paediatrician, Ryegate Children's Centre, Sheffield, UK

Helen Harrison — Senior Paediatric Dietitian, The Leeds Children's Hospital, Leeds, UK

Lorna Highet — Consultant in Community Paediatrics, Leeds Community Healthcare, Leeds, UK

Donna Hilton — Youth Service Manager; NUH Youth Service; Nottingham Children's Hospital, Nottingham, UK

Karen Horridge — Neurodisability Paediatrician, City Hospitals Sunderland NHS Foundation Trust, Sunderland, UK

Anne M Kelly — Consultant Paediatrician and Senior Lecturer in Child Health, NHS Leeds Community Healthcare Trust and University of Leeds, Leeds, UK

Christine Lenehan — Director, Council for Disabled Children, London, UK

Jeremy Parr — Clinical Senior Lecturer and Consultant, Paediatric Neurodisability, Newcastle University, Newcastle, UK

Benita Powrie — Occupational Therapist, Leeds Community Healthcare NHS Trust, Leeds, UK; Doctoral Candidate, School of Health and Rehabilitation Science, University of Queensland, Brisbane, Queensland, Australia

Shiela Puri — Consultant Paediatrician in Community Child Health, NHS Leeds Community Healthcare; Honorary Senior Lecturer, University of Leeds, Leeds, UK

Gillian Robinson — Consultant Community Paediatrician, St George's Centre, Leeds, UK

Alison Salt — Consultant Paediatrician (Neurodisability), Great Ormond Street Hospital for Children; Honorary Senior Lecturer, University College London, Institute of Child Health, London, UK

Joanne Sandiford — Highly Specialist Speech and Language Therapist/Section Leader, Children's Speech and Language Therapy Service, Leeds Community Healthcare NHS Trust, Leeds West/North West Child Development Team, Wortley Beck Health Centre, Leeds, UK

Arnab Seal — Consultant Paediatrician, Leeds Community Healthcare NHS Trust; Leeds Teaching Hospitals Trust; Honorary Senior Lecturer in Paediatrics and Child Health, University of Leeds, Leeds, UK

Mohnish Suri — Consultant Clinical Geneticist, Nottingham Clinical Genetics Service, Nottingham University Hospitals NHS Trust, Nottingham, UK

Gail Treml — Special Educational Needs Independent Consultant and Adviser, UK. Formerly SEN Professional Advisor, Department for Education, London, UK

Martina Waring — Principal Clinical Psychologist, Leeds Child and Adolescent Mental Health Services, Leeds, UK

Jane Williams — Consultant Paediatrician (Neurodisability and Community Child Health), Nottingham University Hospitals NHS Trust, Nottingham, UK

Toni Wolff — Consultant Paediatrician in Neurodisability, Child Development Centre, Nottingham University Hospitals, Nottingham, UK

Foreword

When I was a medical student in the 1960s, some paediatricians were still advising the parents of a newborn with Down syndrome to 'put him in an institution and forget about him'. With my fellow students I visited one such institution and, although the nurses were kind and caring, the environment was utterly sterile because the children were regarded as uneducable. Some children were misdiagnosed as 'severely mentally handicapped' when they were in fact profoundly deaf.

Many individuals and organizations have contributed to the changes in the ways in which professionals, parents and politicians today respond to the challenges presented by people with disabilities. For example, Dr Winthrop Phelps, an orthopaedic surgeon in Baltimore, founded the first treatment programme for cerebral palsy in the USA, in 1937. Four parents who were dissatisfied with the information and care available in the UK for their children with cerebral palsy set up the Spastics Society, in 1951. Alf Morris, MP for Manchester Wythenshawe, introduced the pioneering Chronically Sick and Disabled Persons Act in 1970 and in 1974 became Britain's first minister for disabled people.

Although there have been paediatricians with a special interest in child development and assessment for at least 40 years, only a small minority were able to devote most of their time to this work and even fewer had opportunities to keep abreast of research, let alone undertake any studies themselves. The dramatic advances in many areas of research including genetics, neuroscience, linguistics, acoustics and bioengineering have presented new challenges. Children with multiple complex problems who previously would have died in infancy now survive into adult life. As paediatricians are naturally more familiar with rare childhood disorders than their adult physician counterparts, they increasingly recognize a need to continue their involvement beyond adolescence. All these changes have focused public and professional interest and debate on the many ethical dilemmas that arise.

Now that the specialty has come of age, there is a clear need for comprehensive texts that cover the whole field of childhood disability, yet, somewhat surprisingly, there have been very few available. It is a mammoth task to cover such a wide range of disorders that present not only complex medical and scientific questions about causation but also changing problems in management, education and care. This book is an important and invaluable contribution to the subject. As one would expect, it offers a comprehensive overview of the scientific and technical aspects of childhood disability with excellent sections on the disorders that account for most of the clientele of a disability service. But the paediatrician must also coordinate the specialist advice and skills of colleagues and act as an advocate for the holistic care of the child and family.

Too often the advice offered by professionals can be dismissive, irrelevant or impractical. What I particularly like about this text is the discussion of the complex social and care topics that arise in a high-quality paediatric disability service and the authors' detailed guidance on how to manage the many practical problems faced by the parents and teachers of children with disabilities.

I predict that this book will become the preferred foundation text for UK paediatricians and other health professionals who wish to make paediatric disability their area of special expertise.

David Hall
Emeritus Professor of Community Paediatrics, University of Sheffield
Honorary Professor of Paediatrics, University of Cape Town
and Red Cross War Memorial Children's Hospital, Cape Town
December 2012

Preface

Around 10 years ago, we realized that there was no single current textbook available to recommend to colleagues or students who wanted to learn about up-to-date best practice for children and young people with a neurodisability. Evidence for various treatments could be found by trawling the Internet for scholarly articles, or by comparing different websites that provided information for parents and professionals; however, a single source of information about all the essential topics, educational or practical, involved in working in paediatric neurodisability in the twenty-first century was not accessible. A comprehensive book that could be reached for when starting a topic was lacking. The last authoritative book on the subject, by David Hall, was out of print and out of date. The seeds of this book were laid then, and it has taken a few years for the fruits to reach your plate!

The journey for people with disabilities, children in particular, has been a rapidly evolving and largely positive one over the last few decades. While medical science has brought many investigative and treatment possibilities, the advances in technology have made many things previously thought impossible into a reality. The Internet has fostered an information revolution whereby individuals and families are no longer dependent on professionals or organizations for information and advice.

This book aims to bring together the necessary knowledge and advice on the practical aspects of caring for children with disabilities, as required in the current era. Whether you are sitting in a busy clinic trying to work out the next step in managing a child with a complex disability or in your office writing up a report for education authorities on a child with complex needs, or possibly mulling over an ethical dilemma affecting a child with multiple needs, having this book to hand will give you a framework and some tools. This book provides practical information and advice based on best practice written by practitioners in the field. It will be useful to paediatricians in training as well as therapists and professionals who work with disabled children. It will also be of relevance to general paediatric consultants who have responsibilities for children with neurodisability.

We will be delighted if this book serves its purpose. If you read it and feel something in it needs to change, tell us. If you read this book, found it useful and enjoyed it, please tell others!

Arnab Seal, Gillian Robinson, Anne M Kelly, Jane Williams
Leeds and Nottingham, UK
December 2012

Section 1

Health and disability

1
Health, disability and functioning

Arnab Seal

From early civilization humans have revered and pursued perfection. This preoccupation has often moulded negative societal attitudes towards people with any form of impairment or disability. The impact of this can be most devastating in childhood, when the psychological consequence of being different from one's peers is most pronounced. Supporting children and families to discover, enjoy and maximize their different abilities enables them to live fulfilled lives.

Children with a disability and their families need to be able to live a 'normal life', and this can be challenging. Not only do families have to deal with the consequences of the impairment but they also have to overcome social, environmental and psychological barriers that are often 'a consequence of' the disability. Over the last few decades there has been a welcome positive change in social attitudes towards disability and an increasing respect for the rights of every individual to fully participate in society.

Defining childhood disability is complex because the perception of who is disabled varies between and within individuals, communities and society as a whole. For the purpose of this book a child with a disability may be defined as anyone below 18 years of age with a medically determined physical or mental impairment that results in a marked, pervasive and significant activity limitation, and is expected to last for a continuous period of at least 12 months, or result in death. In the UK, 7.3% of children are reported to experience disability (Blackburn et al. 2010). The prevalence of conditions affecting physical coordination, communication, memory, concentration and learning is higher in males. These difficulties are compounded as a child with a disability is more likely to live in a household with a single parent, living on a low income in poor housing. The Children's Society reports that 40% of children with a disability in the UK live in poverty (www.chidrenssociety.org.uk).

Concept of disability

From the middle of the twentieth century, the prevailing notion of disability was based on the medical model, which focused predominantly on disease and disability. In the medical model the 'problem' lay with the individual with a disability. The interventions were aimed at correcting the impairment and achieving 'normality'. During the 1960s this notion was robustly challenged by sociologists and disability rights champions, who argued that it is society and its institutions that are oppressive, discriminatory and disabling. This concept suggested that the 'problem' lay not with the disabled individual but with society. Society was deemed to be playing a greater role in putting up barriers to the participation of disabled people in mainstream life. It was therefore the responsibility of society to change, in order to uphold the rights of the individual. It was argued that the then prevailing notion of disability was a construct of able-bodied people, who saw disability as a tragedy and developed services to be compensatory in nature. As a result, these services were often more disabling than enabling. Thus evolved the 'social model' of disability, which focused attention on the need to remove barriers and effect change in institutions and regulations. Its proponents argued that the removal of environmental barriers, economic barriers and cultural stigma would result in the process of inclusion, equal opportunities, and equal rights for all people with disabilities.

The current construct is of a 'biopsychosocial model' that acknowledges the role of individual biological and psychological factors alongside the social, personal and environmental factors that influence function. This model recognizes that all individuals and their circumstances are unique.

International Classification of Functioning, Disability and Health

The International Classification of Functioning, Disability and Health (ICF) was constructed to reflect the changing social attitudes to disability, and was adopted by the World Health Organization (WHO) in 2001 (WHO 2001). This was followed in 2007 by a children and young people's version (ICF-CY). It has changed the focus from a negative perception of 'inability to perform' to a positive perception of functioning. The ICF acknowledges that every human being can experience a decrement in health and thereby experience some degree of disability. Disability is not something that happens to a minority of humanity. The ICF therefore mainstreams the experience of disability and recognizes it as a universal human experience. By shifting the focus from the diagnosis to the impact of the diagnosis it places all health conditions on an equal footing, allowing them to be compared using a common scale. This takes into account the individual, personal, social and environmental factors which influence the effects of health, disability and functioning.

Alongside the development of the ICF there were changes in health care in the twentieth century because of the changing patterns of disease prevalence. There was a need to shift focus from managing acute illness to the management of chronic illness and/or disability. There has also been a shift from mere management of symptoms to having specific goals and outcomes, which can potentially be used as standards for measuring healthcare effectiveness. This theme continues into the twenty-first century and its effects are most palpable in the field of child disability.

Framework of the International Classification of Functioning, Disability and Health

The ICF is structured around three broad components (Fig. 1.1):

- body function (b) and body structure (s)
- activity and participation (d)
- environmental factors (e).

This synthesis of different health perspectives – biological, individual and social – enables a person's difficulties to be viewed as a whole and is called a biopsychosocial model.

Alterations of body function and/or body structure lead to activity limitation, which in turn affects the participation of the individual in everyday life situations and in society. In the ICF framework, functioning and disability are viewed as a complex interaction between the health condition, environmental factors, as well as personal factors which influence the capacity of the individual. The scale is dynamic in nature to reflect the variability which can affect each component.

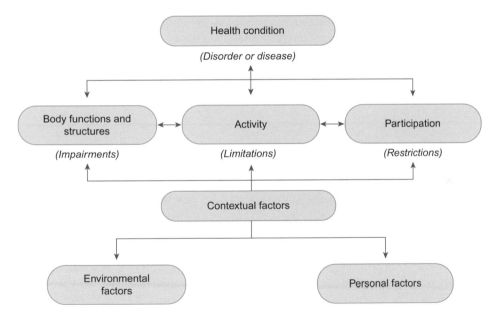

Figure 1.1 Framework of the International Classification of Functioning, Disability and Health (WHO 2001).

Applying the International Classification of Functioning,
Disability and Health to a child with a disability

The following case vignettes illustrate how a common medical diagnosis can still result in extremely variable levels of participation and outcomes.

Case vignette 1

Five-year-old Adam was given a diagnosis of hemiplegia at 15 months of age, when investigations revealed an antenatal middle cerebral artery infarction. He lives on the outskirts of Manchester with his parents, one of whom is a teacher and the other an accountant. Adam's parents have a good understanding of his difficulties from their involvement with health services and voluntary agencies, in particular 'HemiHelp' (www.hemihelp.org.uk).

Adam's parents and therapists from the local child development team have set realistic goals for Adam and helped him achieve them by providing programmes of intervention ('constraint-induced movement therapy'), equipment (hand and leg splints) and interventions (botulinum toxin injections to the calf muscles). They have also worked closely with professionals from education authorities and social care to support Adam, both in school and in out-of-school activities. Currently, Adam is a happy child who attends his local primary school. He is a popular child who is keen on playing football with his friends and is learning to ride a bike. He finds it difficult to cut his own food and has to use some special cutlery to help with his grip. His teachers describe him as no different from any other child in the class in spite of his difficulties. His parents are delighted with his progress.

Case vignette 2

Adnan is 5 years old and has a diagnosis of hemiplegia. He lives in a village in India and his parents are farmers. When Adnan started walking it was noticed that he had a limp, and he was also unable to use his right hand. His parents took him to a doctor in the city, who performed tests and told them that Adnan's condition was permanent and was caused by brain damage. Adnan's parents were shown some exercises to perform at home. Adnan's parents were frustrated as the exercises did not cure Adnan's weakness. They took him to many doctors and faith healers hoping for a cure; nothing really helped. Adnan now can walk only a small distance with a stick. His parents have enrolled him in the village school, where he has made friends. He loves football and watches his friends play from the sidelines. Adnan's teacher loves Adnan but knows that his life outcomes will be very different from those of his classmates.

> ## Case vignette 3
>
> Adeel is 5 years old and has a diagnosis of hemiplegia. His mother used crack cocaine during the pregnancy. He lives in inner-city London. Adeel's parents are very young and separated soon after the diagnosis was confirmed, when he was 18 months old. Adeel's mother is a known drug user and also has mental health needs. She struggles to meet Adeel's needs. The child development team try to support Adeel and his mother, but they struggle to establish relationships because of irregular attendance. He is discussed at the team's child protection supervision meeting.
>
> Adeel has splints but does not like wearing them. He has been referred to the botulinum toxin clinic and has missed the first appointment. He is quite limited with the use of the hand on the hemiplegic side and has quite a marked limp when trying to run. He enjoys going to his local primary school, but he regularly has angry outbursts and his attendance is erratic. His teachers, therapists and other professionals meet regularly to set goals and provide family support. Adeel's mother's engagement with the process is sporadic. Adeel would like to play football but isn't always included in games as he finds them tiring and he often resorts to outbursts of aggressive behaviour.

The case vignettes show three children with identical diagnoses but, coming from different social, environmental and cultural backgrounds, three very different levels of participation and outcome. It is worth noting that a child may have good functional capacity but can function at a significantly lower level than this capacity if he or she is in an inappropriate environment or adverse circumstance.

A specific medical diagnosis provides medical information but says little about functional abilities. A diagnosis can be important in defining the cause of any illness and the likely course it may take. However, identifying the limitations of function and participation informs us of the capacity of the individual child and helps in planning and implementing interventions which can enhance the child's participation. The ICF allows an assessment of the degree of ability. It removes the focus from the diagnosis and highlights all aspects of a child's life, including development, participation and environmental factors.

The ICF-CY is a derived portion of the ICF and is designed to record characteristics of the developing child. The nature and form of functioning is different in children and adults and varies at different developmental ages. Child development and childhood disability are parallel processes. The nature of any disability and its impact on function is dependent on the developmental stage of the child, for example the presence of severe talipes equinovarus will have a different effect on the functioning of a 6-month-old infant compared with a 2-year-old because of the variation of motor ability at different ages. The ICF-CY has additional codes to the adult ICF to allow this changing pattern of childhood to be recognized.

The coding system in the ICF identifies domains within body function (b), body structure (s), activity/participation (d) and environment (e). The user must identify the appropriate code within any individual domain which fits in closest to a particular area of a child's functioning. This code is then further qualified on a scale of 0 to 4, grading the severity of the impairment. The activity/participation codes can be used for framing interventions to maximize the capacity of the child and can be used to set goals and monitor outcomes.

Key messages

- Disability in a child impacts on the child's siblings and family.
- Many children with a disability live in poverty.
- Clinicians need to look at the impact of the diagnosis and beyond.
- Environmental, cultural and psychological factors influence a child's functioning and participation.
- Function and participation are key in facilitating positive outcomes.

References

Blackburn C, Spencer N, Read J (2010) Prevalence of childhood disability and the characteristics and circumstances of disabled children in the UK: secondary analysis of the Family Resources Survey. *BMC Paediatrics*, 10 (21). http://dx.doi.org/10.1186/1471-2431-10-21

WHO (World Health Organization) (2001) The International Classification of Functioning, Disability and Health. Available at: www.who.int/classifications/icf/en/ (accessed 5 October 2012).

Further reading

World Health Organization (2007) *International Classification of Functioning, Disability and Health, Children and Youth Version* (ICF-CY). Geneva: WHO.

2
Quality of life

David Cundall

Learning objectives

- To understand the concept of quality of life (QoL).
- To reflect on the implications for practice of recent QoL research.

Case vignette

Dr Adele, a trainee paediatrician, was being shown round a school by the headteacher. Adele was introduced to Matilda, who was described as 'one of our star pupils'. 'How are you?' asked Adele, smiling down at Matilda, who was seated in her powered chair. Matilda smiled back and started knocking her head irregularly against her headrest.

'I do wonder about her quality of life, though,' sighed Adele, not waiting for a reply and turning back to the headteacher, who raised his eyebrows and said nothing.

'I'm fine, thank you,' replied Matilda via her communication aid, 'Who were you talking about?'

The study of the QoL of children with disabilities has developed in the context of the rights of children in general, encapsulated in the United Nations Convention on the Rights of the Child, and the social model of disability, which underpins the International Classification of Functioning, Disability and Health. There are major difficulties in trying to define what is meant by QoL. It is defined by the World Health Organization as 'an individual's perception of their position in life in the context of the culture and value systems in which they live, and in relation to their goals, expectations, standards and concerns' (WHO 1995). This definition is subjective and avoids any attempt to impose absolute values independent of the context in which a person lives.

The understanding of the QoL of children with disabilities has two additional layers of difficulty:

- Can we devise measures of QoL that are not confounded by factors related to the child's disability?
- Are children able to articulate their views about their QoL, particularly if they have communication and/or learning difficulties?

Very significant progress has been made on both these issues as a result of a European study (SPARCLE), which has looked at QoL of children with cerebral palsy aged 8 to 12 years across eight European nations (Dickinson et al. 2007). The researchers make the helpful distinction between subjective measures of QoL and objective measures of participation. They chose KIDSCREEN (KIDSCREEN Group Europe 2006) as their measure of self-reported QoL (Table 2.1).

Table 2.1 Description of each 'KIDSCREEN' domain of quality of life

Theme of questions	Measured perceptions of these aspects of life
Physical well-being	Physical activity, energy and fitness
Psychological well-being	Positive emotions and satisfaction with life
Moods and emotions	Negative moods, boredom and stress
Self-perception	Self, bodily appearance and body image
Autonomy	Freedom of choice and self-determination; autonomy in leisure time
Relationships with parents	Interactions with parents and the socio-emotional atmosphere at home
Social support and peers	Social support available from friends and peers
School environment	Learning and feelings about school and teachers
Financial resources	Adequacy of pocket money relative to peers
Social acceptance	Social acceptance or rejection by peers; bullying

The major findings on QoL were

- Children with cerebral palsy had similar QoL to their peers in the general population in all domains except schooling, in which evidence was equivocal, and physical well-being, where it was not possible to make a comparison.
- The type and severity of cerebral palsy did not affect QoL in six domains.
- Pain was a significant contributor to lower QoL in all domains.

The finding that, in general, children with cerebral palsy have as good a QoL of life as other children should encourage everyone to ensure that children with disabilities have as much opportunity to participate in society as possible. Comparisons across countries confirmed that cultural factors and government policy do affect QoL. The impact of pain on QoL has reminded clinicians to ask about pain and discomfort and treat its causes and symptoms.

Not surprisingly, only just over 60% of the children studied were able to self-report their QoL. There were many children for whom parental and/or professional reports were the only source of information (White-Koning et al. 2008). Non-verbal children may be able to communicate their wishes and feelings in other ways, which often requires time as well as technology. It is likely that children who are unable to self-report have a greater level of disability, which may affect their actual QoL but may not be accurately reflected in proxy reports. SPARCLE selected children with cerebral palsy and there may be a difference in children with other types of disability, especially if there is increasing pain with the severity of the condition, for example chronic arthritis. The results may be different for teenagers and a follow-up study of the same children into adolescence is under way.

Key messages

- Try to ensure effective communication by all methods available.
- Always ask children with disabilities and their caregivers about pain and discomfort.
- Do all that you can to enhance the QoL of children with disabilities.

References

Dickinson HO, Parkinson KN, Ravens-Sieberer U et al. (2007) Self-reported quality of life of 8–12-year-old children with cerebral palsy: a cross-sectional European study. *Lancet* 369: 2171–8. http://dx.doi.org/10.1016/S0140-6736(07)61013-7

KIDSCREEN Group Europe (2006) *The KIDSCREEN Questionnaires. Quality of Life Questionnaires for Children and Adolescents – Handbook*. Lengerich: Papst Science Publisher.

White-Koning M, Grandjean H, Colver A, Arnaud C (2008) Parent and professional reports of the quality of life of children with cerebral palsy and associated intellectual impairment. *Dev Med Child Neurol* 50: 618–24. http://dx.doi.org/10.1111/j.1469–8749.2008.03026.x

WHO (1995) The World Health Organization Quality of Life assessment (WHOQOL): position paper from the World Health Organization. *Soc Sci Med* 41: 1403–9. http://dx.doi.org/10.1016/0277-9536(95)00112-K

3

Prevention of disability and health promotion

Arnab Seal

Learning objectives

- To understand the principles of prevention of developmental disabilities.
- To know the difference between screening and diagnostic tests.
- To appreciate the difference in causes of preventable developmental disability between developed and developing countries.

Case vignette

Alice, aged 34 years, is 13 weeks pregnant. She has two healthy children aged 8 and 3 years. She and her partner Sam, aged 36 years, have attended antenatal appointments and undergone all screening tests offered. They have been recalled to the clinic as the screening test has identified a 'high risk' of Down syndrome of 1 in 250. During the consultation they have been offered a diagnostic test, which would carry a 1% chance of miscarriage.

Neither Alice nor Sam had thought too much about consenting to the screening investigations during their previous antenatal visit. After returning home from the risk counselling visit they realized that they did not really know much about Down syndrome apart from what Sam recalled about the brother of a friend who he studied with in school. Sam recalled that he had problems with learning. They searched the Internet and accessed the Down Syndrome Association site to get more information. They weigh up the information regarding Down syndrome, the risk of their infant being affected and the risk of miscarriage from the diagnostic test and decide that they do not want to proceed with the test. They agree that they want this child and would be happy to continue the pregnancy. Having had the discussion they find that their commitment to their family and to each other has strengthened and wonder in retrospect if they should have consented to the screening procedure.

Learning points

- Good-quality counselling and information is important for any screening programme.
- There are a range of options after a positive screen.

The gestational age at which the various screening and diagnostic tests are carried out and the type of procedure involved are described in Tables 3.1 and 3.2.

Table 3.1 Antenatal screening tests

Diagnosis tested for	Procedure	Gestation
Down and Edward syndrome	Blood (integrated test or quadruple test) and USG	9–20wk
Fragile X syndrome, SMA, CF	Parental gene test	Any time/pre-pregnancy
NTD and AWD	Blood (AFP)	15–20wk

USG, ultrasonography; SMA, spinal muscular atrophy; CF, cystic fibrosis; NTD, neural tube defects; AWD, abdominal wall defect; AFP, alpha-fetoprotein.

Table 3.2 Diagnostic tests

Diagnosis tested for	Procedure	Gestation
Chromosomal conditions, e.g. Down syndrome, fragile X syndrome, SMA, CF	Choriomic villous sampling	11–14wk
	Amniocentesis	14wk or later
Spina bifida	Specialist USG/MRI	18wk or later
Anencephaly	Specialist USG/MRI	13wk or later
AWDs	Specialist USG/MRI	18wk or later

SMA, spinal muscular atrophy; CF, cystic fibrosis; USG, ultrasonography; MRI, magnetic resonance imaging; AWD, abdominal wall defect.

Neonatal screening

Neonatal screening is offered to identify congenital disorders as soon as possible after birth, and treatment is offered as early as possible. Neonatal screening aims to ameliorate disabling conditions that impair a child's quality of life. The timeliness of screening ensures that appropriate treatment may begin and lead to the maximum possible reduction in the adverse effects of the condition.

Neonatal bloodspot screen (Guthrie test) is a whole-population screening test. The UK National Screening Committee recommends that the screen includes phenylketonuria (PKU), congenital hypothyroidism, cystic fibrosis, sickle cell disorders and MCADD (medium-chain acyl-CoA dehydrogenase deficiency). Untreated PKU, MCADD and congenital hypothyroidism usually result in significant physical and developmental difficulties. The current screening programme in Wales is slightly different from that in the rest of the UK. There is ongoing consultation on expanding the neonatal bloodspot screen across the UK.

A **neonatal clinical examination** is performed within 72 hours after birth to check for visible malformations, cataracts, hip dysplasia, heart disease and undescended testes.

In the UK the **Newborn Hearing Screening** programme offers testing of all newborn infants in the first few weeks of life to identify congenital moderate, severe or profound hearing impairment.

Childhood screening for developmental disabilities

Early identification of developmental disorders is important for better outcomes. Early identification leads to intervention, which lessens the impact on the functioning of the child and family. There is evidence to suggest that the biology of a number of developmental disorders may be altered by early intervention at critical periods of development. Developmental surveillance is an important method of detecting delays and should be an integral part of any review by a healthcare professional. Any concerns raised by parents, other professionals or through routine screening questions should be assessed. Further, this can be done by using a developmental screening tool, for example the Checklist for Autism in Toddlers (CHAT) for autism spectrum disorders (Baron-Cohen et al. 1992).

The use of standardized, practical and easy-to-use developmental screening tools at periodic intervals will increase identification. Successful early identification of developmental disabilities requires the paediatrician to be skilled in the use of screening techniques, to be an active listener and to seek parental concerns about development, so that early diagnosis and treatment can be achieved.

Prevention of developmental disabilities

There is a great need and huge potential for the prevention of developmental disabilities. In developed countries the most readily preventable conditions include

* fetal alcohol syndrome
* other conditions caused by exposure to drugs or medications during pregnancy
* genetic disorders for which testing can be carried out
* conditions related to preterm birth
* conditions related to intrauterine and postnatal infections
* conditions related to preventable injuries
* disabling conditions related to psychosocial disadvantage.

Antenatal screening programmes such as the UK National Infectious Diseases in Pregnancy screening, targeted counselling and testing of carriers have reduced the incidence of some genetic disorders. Using folic acid during planned conceptions has contributed to reducing the incidence of neural tube defects. The use of antenatal steroids to improve lung maturity in preterm births and stopping the use of high-dose steroids in the neonatal period for treatment of chronic lung disease have been effective strategies to prevent developmental disorders in later life.

Psychosocial disadvantage and poverty are associated with a higher risk of general developmental, cognitive and communication delay. Lack of stimulation and inadequate parenting can result in poorer life chances, which is often transgenerational. Early identification and intervention can be particularly effective. The Child Health and Disability Prevention (CHDP) programme in California, USA, is an example of how a state-sponsored public health programme can address some of the preventative disabling consequences of poverty (www.dhcs.ca.gov/services/chdp/).

Table 3.3 Preventable causes of developmental disorders in developing countries

Prenatal
* Poor maternal health and education
* Nutritional deficiencies (calories, protein, iron, folic acid, iodine)
* Lack of immunization, e.g. rubella, tetanus
* Intrauterine infections (TORCHS, HIV)
* Exposure to drugs and environmental toxins, e.g. alcohol, lead, mercury, arsenic
* Lack of access to antenatal screening for genetic conditions

Perinatal
* Lack of good obstetric care
* Unclean delivery causing sepsis, meningitis
* Asphyxia
* Birth injuries
* Maternal mortality
* Lack of good neonatal care
* Improper feeding, hypoglycaemia
* Bilirubin encephalopathy causing hearing impairment and cerebral palsy
* HIV transmission
* Lack of good facilities for preterm and sick newborn infant care

Postnatal
* Improper feeding, poor nutrition
* Infections from preventable diseases, e.g. HIB meningitis
* Conditions not screened for, e.g. congenital hypothyroidism, congenital hearing impairment
* Exposure to toxins, e.g. lead
* Preventable injuries and accidents
* Psychosocial and economic factors, e.g. lack of stimulation from poor maternal education

TORCHS, *Toxoplasma*, rubella, cytomegalovirus, herpes/hepatitis, syphilis; HIV, human immunodeficiency virus; HIB, *Haemophilus influenzae* type B.

In developing countries access to good obstetric and neonatal care, immunization programmes, good nutrition, developmental screening and antenatal screening programmes is limited. A much larger number of developmental disorders are preventable, but resources to tackle these are limited. Well-resourced public health programmes can reduce a significant proportion of these disorders (Table 3.3).

Reference

Baron-Cohen S, Wheelwright S, Cox A et al. (2000) Early identification of autism by the Checklist for Autism in Toddlers (CHAT). *J R Soc Med* 93: 521–5.

Further reading

Raffle AE and Muir Gray JA (2007) *Screening: Evidence and Practice*. Oxford: Oxford University Press.

Websites

UK Screening Portal: www.screening.nhs.uk
UK Newborn Screening Programme Centre: www.newbornbloodspot.screening.nhs.uk/

Section 2

Development

4
Child development

Anne M Kelly

Learning objectives

- To understand the relevance of child development in paediatric practice.
- To learn how to assess development.
- To know the normal sequence of development, benign variants and red flags indicating the need for further assessment.

It is important for all paediatricians to have some knowledge of healthy child development and to understand that

- developmental concerns are common; 5% to 15% of all children have some developmental delay
- developmental delay may indicate an underlying diagnosis such as a congenital central nervous system abnormality, genetic syndrome, metabolic disorder or environmental problem such as neglect or abuse that can impede a child's progress
- developmental delay is common amongst children with chronic multisystem illnesses
- early recognition of delay and provision of appropriate input should improve the outcome for the child and family.

Disordered development has many causes and presentations affecting one or more areas of development. In order to improve outcomes for children, all paediatricians involved with seeing children need to be competent in assessing development. When development is delayed, this may be associated with long-term problems affecting metal health, learning and behaviour. This is even more so for children with complex needs, who are now surviving thanks to improved medical care, which has led to the emergence of neurodisability as a specialty.

Definition of development

Development in its broadest sense encompasses physical and mental growth that leads to the anatomical, physiological and behavioural changes that occur throughout childhood. For most paediatricians, child development relates to the changes in children's ability to move, perform fine movements with their hands, communicate, learn new knowledge, self-care and interact with others. Assessing development is about observing the usually stepwise acquisition of skills in different areas (domains) of function and detecting delays or deviation in the normal process, while trying to understand why this has occurred and provide input that may improve outcomes for the child.

Factors affecting development

Development is a dynamic process that is determined by the interaction of genetic, biological and environmental factors (Fig. 4.1).

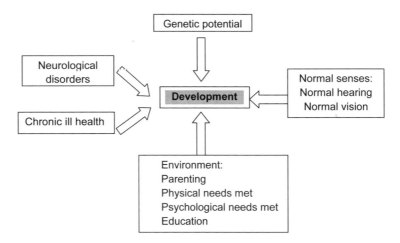

Figure 4.1 Factors affecting development.

Development usually follows a defined series of stages that are the same for all children. This process

- follows a predictable route beginning with the acquisition of control of posture and movement that begins with the head (cephalo) and moves to the toes, from proximal (truncal) to distal (limbs, hands and feet)
- involves maturation of the central nervous system (myelination continues into adolescence but maturity continues beyond adolescence, as development of behaviour is a lifelong process)

- includes increase in physical size, although this is not proportionate, for example head growth is rapid in the first 1 to 2 years
- involves psychological growth that is reflected in a visibly increasing ability to think, understand and relate to others.

Although children usually follow the same sequence of steps reflecting neurological maturation, not all children develop in the same way. The process is shaped positively or negatively by influences that may include

- familial characteristics such as intelligence and temperament
- antenatal and perinatal factors
- parenting styles
- cultural practices
- chronic illness or congenital sensory impairment, e.g. blindness
- environmental factors such as lack of opportunity or child abuse
- access to education.

There is a high degree of variability in the process, but also in children's outcomes, because of the interaction and varying contribution of the above factors affecting development: genetics, biology and environment.

Learning about the sequences is necessary for understanding developmental problems but also when planning interventions to help. The context of the child's family, parenting styles and environment must all be considered alongside the child's achievements as compared against population developmental norms.

Key stages in healthy child development

Having an overview of the key stages in a child's development (see Table 4.1), moving from the completely dependent infant towards independence in later adolescence, helps when considering specific areas.

Domains of child development

Although development is subdivided, it is essential to remember that the assessment of a child's development should be a holistic process. Development has been arbitrarily divided into discrete fields because it makes observation and assessment easier to record. Progress in one field is usually dependent on progress in another. So it is important to look at the whole child to gain an impression of developmental status in all the fields, even if the focus of the assessment is on only one or two areas.

Table 4.1 Key stages of child development

Age	Stage	Illustration	Key skills
Birth–6mo	Newborn infant		Head control; loss of primitive reflexes Looking – particularly at faces Communicating – smile
6–12mo	Sitting child		Sitting Holding – Palmar grasp and transfer Early communication – turn taking, wave goodbye
12–18mo	Mobile child		Standing and later walking Exploring – toys and environment Communicating – single words
18mo–2y	Walking child		Walking – increasingly stable gait Shaking – range of grasps include pincer Playing – symbolic play, e.g. tea party Communicating – 20+ words
2–3y	Communicating child		Movers – running and jumping Talking – two- or three-part sentences Pretending – pretend games, e.g. cooking
3–4y	Preschool child		Pedalling – bikes Talking – short sentences understood by others Playing Pretending – small world play
4–11y	Primary school child		Grouping Reading Writing Mathematical processes
11y+	Teenager		Who am I Independence

Developmental milestones are a convenient short-hand way of assessing an individual child's level, or rate of progress if assessed over a period of time.

Key message

- If a child has not reached a milestone by the upper age limit by which it is normally achieved, then the child can be said to have delay in that developmental domain.

Gross motor development

Learning points

- Motor development is related to the rate of myelination and synapse formation.
- Children need opportunities to practise motor skills in order to be able to develop them at a normal rate.
- Racial and familial patterns affect motor development.

Factors involved in motor development

The movement patterns of healthy infants are remarkably consistent, which suggests that some neural pathways are 'pre-programmed'. Initially, the infant presents in a predominantly flexed posture and has primitive spinal reflexes that have developed before birth and are easy to elicit clinically. The various reflexes that infants are born with and the ages at which these are lost are shown in Table 4.2.

These reflexes gradually disappear during the first 6 months as the infant matures and higher cortical centres assume control of movement. The movements of the infant that initially appear random and purposeless change quickly to become more spontaneous and purposeful. The flexed posture of the infant gradually becomes more extended. This enables control of the head and trunk, enabling the infant to prop him/herself up. The postural righting or protective reflexes develop so that the infant can sit independently and play. These protective reflexes appear at age 5 to 9 months (see Table 4.3). At the same time secondary reflexes develop, including jaw jerk and crossed adductor jerk.

Table 4.2 Primitive reflexes

Reflex	Illustration	Action	Age when lost
Placing		Top of foot gently dragged across surface leads to step	Birth–8wk
Walking		Sole of feet placed on surface leads to step	Birth–8wk
Grasp		Object pushed against palm of hand leads to fingers grasping	Birth–5mo
Moro		Support infant's head; allow head to drop backwards and 1–2cm lower; catch head in palm of hand; observe movement of limbs – should see symmetrical abduction of arms	Birth–5mo
Asymmetrical tonic neck reflex		Turn infant's head to one side when still – this leads to arm extension in direction of gaze and arm flexion in opposite arm	1–5mo

Red flag

Primitive spinal reflexes should disappear and be replaced by protective reflexes by age 6 to 9 months. If this does not occur, it suggests the presence of a significant neurological problem such as cerebral palsy.

Table 4.3 Protective reflexes

Reflex	Age		Action
Downwards parachute	5–6mo		Hold infant upright in vertical suspension, about 30cm from table, and rapidly lower the infant to land on the surface. Lower limbs extend and abduct as the infant lands
Sideways protective (lateral saving)	6mo		Puts arms out to save if tilted
Forward parachute	9mo		Arms and hands abduct and extend on sudden forward tilting towards the floor. Absence indicates a neurological disorder. Asymmetry is seen in hemiplegia

Traditionally, there has been a reliance on using motor milestones to monitor overall developmental progress (see Tables 4.4–4.9). However, this is of only limited value, as motor delay does not always indicate underlying difficulties affecting learning or communication that may be present. There is now much more emphasis on observing and recording the following features:

- the development of static posture and balance
- the presence of associated movements
- neurological and other markers of abnormalities
- motor development in detail.

Table 4.4 Phases of motor development

	Position	Head control	Mean age (mo)
Head control	Supine	Turns head sideways	1
	Sitting	Holds head steady	3–4
	Pull to sit	Slight head lag	4
Trunk posture	Sitting	Straight spine	7
Hands	Supine	Hands open mostly	2

Table 4.5 Development of static posture and balance

Age	Phase of motor development
Birth–4mo	Passive reflexive movements
4mo–1y	Inhibition of primitive reflexes by 6mo
	Improving postural control and balance
	Differentiated movements, e.g. reaching, sitting, standing
1–2y	More precise movements
	Improved power
2–7y	Maturing functional movements, e.g. running, jumping, writing, throwing, cutting, etc.
	Improving coordination and sequencing of actions
>7y	Applying motor skills to specialized activities of work and sport, e.g. learning to play football, tennis, etc.

Table 4.6 Benign variations in modes of locomotion and age of attainment of early motor milestones

	Mean age (mo)/age (mo) at which 97% of children have acquired this milestone		
Modes	Sit	Crawl	Walk
Crawl	7/9	9/13	13/18
Bottom shuffle	12/15		17/28
Stand and walk	7/11		11/14
Creeping/rolling	9/12	12/17	18/27

Table 4.7 Normal range for sitting, standing and walking

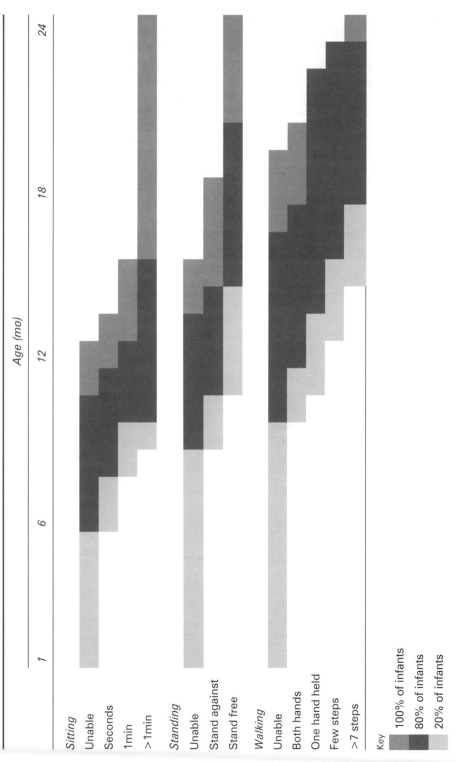

Key

■ 100% of infants
■ 80% of infants
■ 20% of infants

Table 4.8 Influences on motor development

Biologically dependent neural maturation	Experience: ongoing action–perception cycle
• Maturing muscle tone and strength • Improving balance and coordination • Information processing abilities • Ethnicity: African children walk earlier (can be as early as 7mo) • Familial patterns of development, e.g. bottom shuffling	• Interaction with other domains, e.g. cognitive, which affects the child's ability to plan • Poor vision • Specific learning difficulty • Developmental coordination disorder Experiential: • Placing infants on their back to sleep has led to reduction in practice of being placed prone; can lead to delay in crawling in some infants • Immobility – being strapped in buggies • Use of baby walkers

Case vignettes

Mel

You are referred a 2-year-old female because she is not yet walking. There is a positive family history of delayed walking. On examination she is bottom shuffling. She can rise from a squat and climb onto a chair. She obeys simple commands and produces two- to three-word phrases. She has low tone but normal reflexes in her lower limbs. Her hips can be fully abducted. You reassure the family that she is likely to walk soon; ensure that the health visitor follows up to check.

Learning points

• You need to consider all areas of development.
• Check hips carefully in all late walkers for limited abduction and arrange pelvic radiograph if any doubt.
• For a late walking male child arrange serum creatinine kinase and follow-up.

Molly

Molly was born at term + 10 days following a Ventouse extraction for fetal distress. She was intubated briefly and spent 3 days in the special baby care unit before discharge home. No follow-up was arranged. She was referred at 6 months with poor head control, head lag and lack of reaching out. She had persistent feeding difficulties and had been treated for gastro-oesophageal reflux. On examination she had truncal hypotonia with variable but increased tone in all four limbs. Her hands were fisted. Head growth had decreased. Brain MRI showed subtle changes in the basal ganglia.

> *Learning point*
>
> The neonatal history of hypoxia and early feeding difficulties raises concern, and therefore these infants require careful follow-up.

Table 4.9 Useful assessments of motor development

Age	Stage	Skills and assessment
Birth–6mo	Newborn infant	Examine in supine, prone, ventral suspension, pull to sit, supported sitting and supported standing for: • Posture – predominantly flexed or extended in supine? • Spontaneous movements – tone and symmetry • Reflexes – primitive
6–12mo	Sitting child	Examine in supine, prone, ventral suspension, pull to sit, supported sitting and supported standing for: • Posture – predominantly flexed or extended in supine? • Spontaneous movements – tone and symmetry • Reflexes – primitive and saving
12–18mo	Mobile child	• Sitting • Method of mobility
18 mo–2y	Walking child	• Gait – broad base with flexed knees, feet externally rotated and arms held high initially • Can they avoid obstacles in path? • Can they stoop and retrieve?
2–3y	Communicating child	• Gait – narrow base with reciprocal arm movements; if not present look further for hemiplegia • Look for heel strike • In-toe and out-toe gaits are common and normal • Running • Jumping • Throw ball overarm • Kicking a ball • Ability to climb stairs – two feet to a step
3–4y	Preschool child	• Runs fast and can change direction • Ability to climb stairs – reciprocal up and two feet/step down • Rises from supine to standing without support (Gower's sign) • Pedals tricycle
4–11y	Primary school child	• Stands on one foot – increasing duration • Hopping (4–6y) • Increasing ball skills (50% catch ball at 5y) • Riding a bike • Starts to be able to play team sports (9y)
11y+	Teenager	• Level of sporting ability

Motor red flags

All ages

- Abnormal tone
- Weakness

0 to 4 months

- Irritability
- Feeding/respiratory problems
- Floppiness or stiffness
- Poor head control

5 to 8 months

- Persisting primitive reflexes
- Hypotonia
- Asymmetry of movements

9 to 12 months

- Not sitting by 10 months
- Poor truncal control
- Absence/poor protective reflexes
- Hypo/hypertonia
- Scissoring when held supported

13 months to 5 years

- Not walking by 18 months
- Poor balance
- Toe walking
- Poor coordination

Visual perception and fine motor development

Learning points

- Impaired vision will profoundly affect motor development.
- Difficulties with fine motor skills will affect activities of daily living, for example feeding, dressing and practical school activities.

Factors affecting fine motor development

Children gain information from their senses: vision, hearing, touch, taste, smell and sensation of movement (kinaesthesia). Sensations become perception when they are related to previously stored information from experience, and perception is used to guide thinking and further actions. Further movements create more information that keeps the action–perception loop going (see Fig. 4.2).

Infants respond to light from birth, moving from recognition of mother's face to recognizing other people. This process develops alongside the emerging ability of the infant to reach out, find and grasp an object, combining visual perception with fine motor development (see Fig. 4.3).

Infants develop a sense of object unity, that is that visible parts of objects are connected. They look for partially hidden objects from 6 months, and by 9 months can find a completely covered object. The emergence of this concept depends on the understanding that the object still exists when it is hidden from view. This is known as *object permanence*, which is a key cognitive

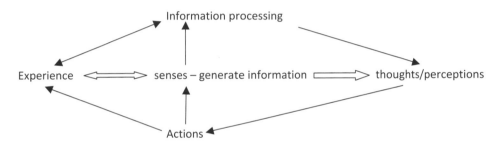

Figure 4.2 Perceptual feedback loops.

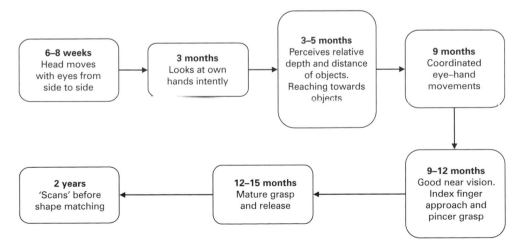

Figure 4.3 Development of vision and hand function. Based upon Sheridan (2008).

milestone. From 1 year of age, the child will anticipate the reappearance of a toy that he has followed from the point it disappeared from his view.

From 12 months onwards the child gains increasing skill in hand tasks in both placing objects and also in mark making and drawing sills. As a result, the child becomes increasingly able in daily living skills such as eating and dressing. These movements become increasingly automatic so that by 4 years a child can eat and have a conversation.

Associated movements

Children may show associated movements such as moving their tongue in and out while cutting paper. Such movements in the upper limbs can be elicited by asking the child to walk in an unusual pattern such as heel–toe walking, or walking on inverted or everted feet in a test which is known as Fogs' test. In a 4-year-old, the upper limbs usually mirror the pattern of movement of the lower limbs. These movements are signs of neurological immaturity, most of which disappear in time. Fogs' test should be negative by the age of 7 years.

Assessing fine motor development

Case vignette

You are asked to see Joe, aged 18 months, as he has been noted to be left handed, which runs in the family. He is also struggling with his feeding skills. You notice that his right hand is fisted and he is reluctant to use this, although he is able to use his left hand.

Learning points

- Handedness usually develops between 2 and 4 years of age. If hand dominance appears earlier it may indicate a neurological problem such as a hemiplegia.
- Ten per cent of the population is left handed. It is a myth that difficulty with fine motor movements is due to left handedness. Left-handed children learn to use implements that have mostly been designed for right-hand use, but this is not enough to cause significant difficulty.

Under 1 year

Assessing the fine motor development of children under the age of 1 year is done by observing how the child reaches, grasps and handles objects: initially a medium-sized object, for example a 1-inch brick, and after 10 months a smaller object such as a raisin.

One year onwards

From the age of 1 year, observation about how a child tackles a task continues to be important. Specific tasks can be used to assess skills in this domain, including tower building with 1-inch bricks, progressing to the child copying patterns to produce simple representations of a bridge or steps (see Table 4.10). Drawing and writing skills can be assessed quickly with pencil and paper. Performance in these tasks is helpful in gaining information about the child's cognitive skills (over 2 years) as these tasks can be assessed even if the child has poor language skills.

Asking a child over 3 years to draw a man (Fig. 4.4) is a simple test known as the Goodenough draw a person test (Goodenough 1926). This test is useful as it has been validated and can be scored to give a child's approximate developmental age that can be compared with his actual age.

Table 4.10 Useful assessments of children's hand function

| Age | Stage | Skills and assessment | | |
		Hand skill	Blocks	Drawing
Birth–6mo	Newborn infant	Hand regard (2mo) Hold object (3–4mo) One hand to grasp (6mo)	Grasp one block 4–6mo	
6–12mo	Sitting child	Transfer object Pick up small object, e.g. raisin	One-block transfer Two blocks in each hand Drop one block to get another	
12–18mo	Mobile child	Neat pincer grasp	Two-block tower	Marks on paper
18mo–2y	Walking child	Crayon held in palmar grasp	Three-block tower at 18mo	To-and-fro scribble
2–3y	Communicating child		Five-block tower at 2y	Circular scribble 2y 6mo: copy circle
3–4y	Preschool child	Tripod grasp – 50% at 3y	Bridge Train	Copy cross Simple face
4–11y	Primary school child	Tripod grasp – 80% at 4y	Steps at 4–5y	4y: copy square 5y: copy triangle Write first name 6y: copy diamond Write both names 7y: copy parallelogram Draw clock face Write short sentence
11y+	Teenager	Increasing fluidity and rapidity of movements Learn to play musical instruments		

Goodenough draw a person test

The scoring system: 1 point is given for each detail drawn (i.e. eyes score 1 point, as do arms, etc.), with 4 points equating to 1 year of age. As children draw circles at the age of 3 years, the basic score is 3 and the formula is: $3 + n/4$, which equates to the child's approximate cognitive age (n=the number of parts drawn).

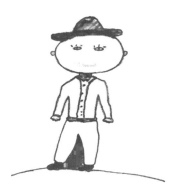

Draw a person test score

Age (y)	Males	Females
3	4	4
4	7	7
5	11	12
6	13	14
7	16	17
8	18	20

Figure 4.4 Goodenough draw a person test

Red flags

3 months

- Persistent fisting

6 months

- Not reaching with two hands
- Lack of coordinate eye gaze

9 months

- Persistent hand regard

12 months

- Lack of index finger exploration
- Difficulty with control and/or release of object
- Abnormal posturing or fingers – splaying during task

Communication

Learning points

- Language is the most complex of human skills. It is necessary for thought as well as to describe ideas.
- Human communication includes gestures, signs, speech and social behaviour.
- Both comprehension and expression must be assessed as well as speech and language.
- Understanding the terminology used by speech and language therapists is useful in order to make sense of a child's profile.
- Language development is a fairly reliable indicator of future educational progress.

Abnormalities of speech and language development are the most common single reason for referral to a child development centre. The peak age at presentation is between the child's second and third birthday, but many children are still not referred until they are about to move into reception class (4–5y). Unclear or inadequate speech may be the only problem in many of these children, whose intelligence and hearing is normal. However, the failure to develop speech may also be the presenting feature of a more serious disorder such as a learning disability or autism. Conversely, the failure to develop speech may be the predominant complaint by parents of children with a known major disability such as cerebral palsy.

Normal speech and language development

There is wide variation in the age at which children acquire specific speech and language milestones. However, there are similarities in the overall sequence, even across different languages. Language development is a cognitive process that develops through the interaction between the child and his or her carer and other responsive adults. The rate of learning and usage is influenced by the interaction between the child's biological and cognitive abilities and his or her environment.

Skills required for early communication skills

- Understanding of cause and effect (cognitive stage).
- Reciprocity (interactive social).
- Symbolic understanding (small toy represents real object).
- Memory.

Skills required for non-verbal communication

Despite the emphasis on attaining speech, it is in fact possible to communicate at the very least one's needs and wishes without the benefit of spoken language (see Table 4.11). A preverbal 1-year-old child can obtain and direct his carer's attention, make requests for objects and anticipate the response using a whole range of non-verbal communication strategies such as

- eye contact
- gesture (e.g. pointing)
- facial expression
- eye pointing
- sounds
- body posture.

Table 4.11 Early communication

Age	Developmental milestone
Birth	Mothers learn very quickly to distinguish the cries of their infant from other infants and to know what each cry is likely to mean
6wk	Social smile
2mo	The infant will 'coo' in response to overtures. 'Conversations' take place between mother and infant in a process known as 'turn taking'
6mo	The infant can copy facial expressions; he or she develops a range of sounds including laughs, grunts and chuckles. The infant imitates sounds produced by adults and practises them when babbling. Vowel sounds are the first to develop Around 5–6mo, interest shifts from people to objects or events After 6mo infants start to enjoy early games such as peekaboo and anticipation of games
>9mo	The infant uses gesture such as proto imperative pointing with his or her index finger, eye contact and sounds to request an object (proto-declarative pointing) The infant will start to copy gestures, e.g. wave bye bye The infant becomes stranger aware
>12mo	The child begins to comment on the same objects to his or her carer, i.e. saying and showing the object. The child learns to follow an adult's eyes/finger pointing and to direct the attention of others to things of interest. This allows the child to learn connections between the language heard and objects being pointed out. This key stage in communication is known as joint attention

Skills required for spoken language

- Hearing: to listen to others, to monitor one's own voice.
- Auditory discrimination: recognize the difference between sounds.
- Phonology: the ability to produce these sounds.
- Semantics: the ability to ascribe meaning to patterns of sound that are remembered (vocabulary).
- Grammar: the ability to use words within a framework of knowledge (syntax) and modify the word according to use (e.g. tenses/plurals).
- Encoding: translating objects, actions, into the words that symbolize them.
- Decoding: the ability to relate the spoken word to the object or action for which it is a symbol.
- Motivation to communicate.
- Opportunity to communicate (i.e. all needs not pre-empted).

Skills required for comprehension

The following additional influences are needed for comprehension:

- Inference.
- Context and prior knowledge.
- Start to decode before hearing the whole utterance.
- Social cognition.

Assessing language

An assessment of language needs to take account of the extent of the child's language performance (receptive and expressive) as well as an awareness of the environment in which the child is learning. This requires knowledge of the usual sequence of milestones and the benign and more significant deviations that may occur in this process.

Development of speech

Comprehension

Comprehension of words must develop before meaningful expressive language can develop. The child begins with understanding the word in context, for example 'bath' when his bath is being run. Visually impaired children will have language delay partly because they cannot see the object that is related to the spoken word.

In order to understand language acquisition it is helpful to understand some basic language concepts, as follows.

KEYWORDS

We all use sentences in which only a small number of words are key, for example 'Can I have an *ice cream*?' The keywords carry the relevant information. By asking the child to perform tasks with increasing numbers of keywords we gain an understanding into his or her comprehension level. For a word to be a keyword, the child needs to demonstrate differentiation from an alternative.

One part: Give me the *spoon* (need to have a range of items, e.g. spoon, cup, ball).
Two part: Give the *brick* to *Mummy* (range of items to chose from, and also to give to, e.g. Mummy, Daddy, teddy).
Three part: Give the *red ball* to Daddy (for this to work you need to have a range of objects of different colours in a consulting room; bricks and crayons are usually available).

SIMPLE GRAMMAR

- Noun: the name of something.
- Verb: an action word.

- Adjective: a descriptive word (this includes colours and counting).
- Preposition: describes the position of one thing relative to another, for example on, in, under.
- Personal pronoun: me, you, him.

Expression

The child has acquired a proper meaning of the word as soon as that word is internalized. Initially these words are nouns. The age at gaining the first word is around the child's first birthday, but the age range considered normal is wide (see Table 4.12).

Table 4.12 Development of children's communication skills

Age	Comprehension	Expression
12–18mo	Situational, e.g. 'Get me your shoes,' when adult getting ready to go out Common single keywords, e.g. Daddy, juice	One or two words at 12mo 6+ words at 18mo
18–24mo	Wide range of single keywords (nouns)	10–20 words Learned phrases, e.g. all gone
2y	Two-part commands Verbs, e.g. 'Which child is sleeping?' Functional use, e.g. 'Which one do you eat with?'	50 words+ Two words together
3y	Three-part commands Adjectives, e.g. colour, count by rote Prepositions	Three words together Personal pronouns, e.g. I, mine Asks what and why Mother understands Enjoys nursery rhymes and stories Can tell you their name
4–5y	Two tasks in succession, e.g. 'Get me your shoes and the car keys'	Other adults can understand speech Able to tell simple story Able to sing nursery rhyme Able to name colours Able to count to 5 Vocabulary of 2000 words
6–7y	Understands increasing complexity of verbal instructions	Able to describe complicated events Uses appropriate tense, e.g. past, future Likes to tell jokes Vocabulary of 13 000 words
8–11y	Sequence days of the week and months of the year	Clear speech which can communicate a range of ideas Able to express ideas in writing

Unfortunately, in some parts of the UK up to 50% of children start school lacking the necessary communication skills for an effective start to their learning. The delay is often specific to language and is linked to socio-economic deprivation. Most of these children will catch up with their peers in time given the necessary support. However, 10% of children are described as having a communication disability and 6% of children have a specific and persistent communication disability.

Case vignette

Jordan is a 3-year-old whose parents are concerned about his communication. He has a 4-year-old sister who 'speaks for him'. When you assess him he is interested in playing and joins in well with the assessment. He plays well with the dolls' house in your room. He often refers back to his parents for praise. He demonstrates three-part understanding and can correctly identify verbs. He colour matches four colours correctly. He has 20 single words that are unclear.

Learning points

- Jordan's language is developing normally but is delayed.
- Jordan's comprehension is appropriate, as are symbolic play skills, which are good prognostic markers.
- It is important to check that Jordan does not have a hearing impairment.

Assessing speech and language

When assessing speech and laguage (Table 4.13) there should be a range of common toys and objects available, for example a ball, bricks of different colours, cup, spoon, doll, teddy, and also some books including pictures of children involved in different activities. During the assessment consider

- non-verbal communication (e.g. eye contact, facial expression, pointing, shared interest)
- what the child can understand
- speech clarity and fluency
- sentence construction, including sentence length and the use of prepositions and personal pronouns
- whether there is shared interest or a repetitive quality to the communication.

Table 4.13 Useful assessments of children's communication skills

Age	Stage	Comprehension	Expression
Birth–6mo	Newborn infant		Smile Copy facial expression
6–12mo	Sitting child	One	Turn taking
12–18mo	Mobile child	One keyword, e.g. look or point to Daddy	How does the child let you know what he or she wants? Does he or she have any clear words – if so, how many?
18mo–2y	Walking child	One keyword, e.g. point to body parts Two keywords, e.g. give the *brick* to *teddy*	How does the child let you know what he or she wants? Does he or she have any clear words – if so, how many? Does the child put two words together?
2–3y	Communicating child	Verbs, e.g. 'Which child is sleeping?' Two keywords, e.g. 'Give cup to mummy' Identify by functional use, e.g. 'Which one do you drink from?' Prepositions, e.g. 'Put the brick in/on'	Does the child put two or three words together?
3–4y	Preschool child	Adjectives, e.g. colour matching Three keywords, e.g. 'Give blue pen to teddy' Prepositions, e.g. behind/under	Can the child tell you his or her name? Does the child put two to four words together? Can the mother understand the child? Can the child name colours and count by rote? Does the child use personal pronouns? Does the child ask 'what?' and 'why?' questions?
4–11y	Primary school child	Two tasks in succession, e.g. get your shoes and then give me a pencil	Can the child tell you about an event or story from pictures in a book in simple sentences? (4y) Can you understand? (4y) Can the child offer an explanation? (4–5y) Does the child like jokes? (6–7y)
11y+	Teenager		Sarcasm

Red flags

12 months

- No pointing or other gesture

18 months

- No single words
- No joint attention
- No pretend play

2 years

- Unable to follow simple requests
- Repetitive play
- Limited imaginary play

3 years

- Single words and learned phrases only
- Language is incomprehensible to carers
- No social interest in playing with other children

4 years

- Language is incomprehensible to adults, e.g. teacher
- Limited interest in peers

Speech and language therapy assessments

All children with delayed or disordered language and social skills will benefit from an assessment by a speech and language therapist.

Speech and language therapy terminology

The complex terminology that is used by speech and language therapists to describe children's abilities in the various aspects of communication is explained below.

- Speech: the production and combination of individual speech sounds to make words.
- Language: the system of symbols (spoken words) used to communicate ideas, wishes, and so on.
- Phonology: how speech sounds are organized.
- Articulation: the physical production of speech sounds.
- Comprehension: the ability to make sense of information from a range of possible sources.
- Expression: the ability to convey information through gesture, sign, speech, and so on.

- Communicative intent: motivation to communicate with another person.
- Social communication: understanding the thoughts and intentions of others and using appropriate behaviours to fit the circumstance and intention.
- Syntax: the ways in which words are related grammatically.
- Echolalia: repeating language; immediate or delayed.
- Jargon: fluent but unintelligible speech.
- Morphology: the form and structure of words.
- Semantics: the meaning of sentences, words and parts of words.
- Pragmatics: how language is used in social situations; non-verbal skills.
- Prosody: the rhythm (stress) and music (intonation) of speech.

Speech and language assessment tools

The Derbyshire Language Scheme (Knowles and Masidlover 1982) is a tool used to assess the number of information carrying words that a child needs in order to understand a given instruction.

Give me the *car*: one-word level.
Put the *sock* in the *box*: two-word level.
Put the *big brick* in the *bag*: three-word level.

The child would be expected to perform at the appropriate level for their age, for example two words at age 2 years as an absolute minimum.

The Reynell Developmental Language Scale (Reynell and Huntley 1985) is a scale that covers children from the age of 6 months to 6 years. It is a score for comprehension and expression that can be recorded as an age-equivalent score.

Social development (Tables 4.14 and 4.15)

Children are born into a complex social world with the innate ability to initiate social attachments. Infants are socially responsive from birth. They show a strong preference for looking at people's faces intently when awake. They quickly recognize their mother's face and voice. Carers should be aware that infants can see, hear and communicate from birth. The attention given and reactions to their infant develop into a 'dance' of social communication that continues throughout infancy. These early communications help to form the special and affectionate bond that leads to the child feeling secure and comforted; this is essential for attachment.

Attachment

Attachment is defined as a special form of affection bond between two people within which one person experiences security and comfort from the other (see Fig. 4.5). When a child is distressed and is comforted by the parent it means that the child feels understood. Over time this leads to a child who recognizes that he or she is an individual and the child will learn to understand his or her emotions and how to deal with them. In later childhood this leads to a child with positive self-esteem. This in turn leads to the ability to recognize emotions in others. This can

Table 4.14 Useful assessments of social development

Age	Stage	Social milestones
Birth–6mo	Newborn infant	Infant looks intently at faces (6wk) Smiles and imitates facial expression Smiles synchronously with caregiver (3mo)
6–12mo	Sitting child	Infant can direct carer's gaze to objects he or she is looking at – *joint attention* Wary of strangers
12–18mo	Mobile child	The child will want to be with carer in new situations. This reaction can be reduced by reassurance from his carer. The parent can 'model' appropriate behaviour and in doing so set boundaries
18mo–2y	Walking child	The child is able to walk independently for a good distance with a stable base and without repeated falls
2–3y	Communicating child	The child tests out these boundaries and will have tantrums when his wishes are denied, hence the term 'terrible twos' The child is aware of other children's distress
3–4y	Preschool child	The child learns about other people's feelings (inner state) and the rules of behaviour. Supervising play and talking to children about rules and behaviour will help them to understand Reading and talking about stories is also helpful The child starts to be able to take turn with peers
4–11y	Primary school child	The child makes links between people's feelings and their actions; this is known as *theory of mind* Children start to have friends and peers Able to play cooperatively with peers There is rigid adherence to rules, which can lead to disagreements between children which adults need to help to resolve. It also leads them to 'tell tales 'on their friends
	Juniors	The child has an increasing ability to relate to the outside world at school and with friends. Children like to fit in and be accepted by their peers and this enhances their self-esteem Children like to play games with same-sex friends By 8–9y children start to be able to understand what it is like to be in other peoples shoes, and therefore true friendships form
11y+	Teenager	Start to become independent from family

help the child to understand the behaviours of others and to start to develop coping strategies and learn how to resolve his or her own difficulties and distress. These skills together enable the child to form relationships with others.

In a healthy parent–child relationship, if the child misbehaves the parent will show disapproval, which will lead to the child feeling distress. A secure parent will help the child to manage this distress and then give opportunities to repair the relationship. This process allows the child to develop the capacity for impulse control and to develop socially appropriate behaviour (Howe 2005, McLeod 2007).

Table 4.15 Useful assessments of self-help skills

Age	Stage	Skills
Birth–6mo	Newborn infant	Dependent Learns to take solids from spoon (4–6mo)
6–12mo	Sitting child	Starts to finger feed Will grab at spoon, but cannot use it
12–18mo	Mobile child	Drinks well from feeder cup Holds a spoon and attempts to feed but very messy Puts out arm or leg to help with dressing
18mo–2y	Walking child	Can hold own cup and drink More accurate self-feeding with spoon
2–3y	Communicating child	Can feed self competently, but easily distracted Indicating and verbalizing toileting needs – but unreliable toilet use Puts on shoes and hat
3–4y	Preschool child	Eats with a fork and a spoon Washes hands but needs adult's help with drying Can use toilet (variable) and pull pants down
4–11y	Infants	Independent toileting Competent with knife and fork Washes and dries hands but needs help with bathing Can brush teeth Dresses and undresses – initially can struggle with fastenings Attempts to butter bread and make a bowl of cereal
	Juniors	Can tie shoelaces Independent with bathing Can make a simple meal Gradually becomes safe at crossing road Develops an understanding of value of money and knows how to handle money
11y+	Teenager	Travels independently Learns to prepare meals Can do laundry

Key message

- Early experiences with the child's caregiver can have a profound bearing on how children and later adults understand themselves and their interaction with others. To an extent, all later relationships have the foundations built on this first relationship.

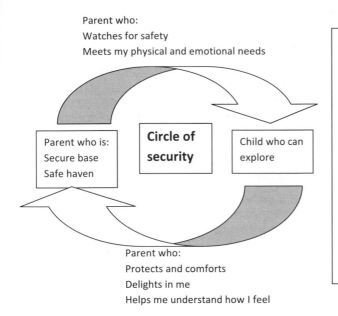

Parent who:
Watches for safety
Meets my physical and emotional needs

Parent who is:
Secure base
Safe haven

Circle of security

Child who can explore

Parent who:
Protects and comforts
Delights in me
Helps me understand how I feel

Attachment comes from an instinctive biological drive to stay close to the primary caregiver. Being close means that the child can quickly seek help if needed.

Once the child is confident and his/her needs for security and safety are met, the child becomes less anxious. This means that the child can confidently explore and play. This is called secure attachment and happens in 55% of parent–child relationships.

Figure 4.5 Factors needed for successful attachment.

Self-help skills key questions:

- Does the child understand about daily routines – meal times, bath and bedtime?
- Can the child hold his or her bottle or cup/finger feed/use a spoon?
- Does the child undress, for example can he or she remove socks or need help with dressing (e.g. put arms in sleeves)?
- Can the child wash his or her face and hands, with or without help?
- Can the child help with chores in home, for example setting the table and tidying up?
- Toileting – is the child trained? If not, does he or she indicate when in a wet or soiled nappy?

Cognitive skills

Cognition is a complex process and in order to try to understand the acquisition of cognition different clinicians have devised different hypothetical frameworks. In practice, skills are gained alongside language, play and social skills in an integrated manner and no theoretical framework can really describe this. Cognitive processes include a range of skills including attention, thinking skills and emotional skills.

Attention

Attention (Table 4.16) is a core skill for learning language, cognitive and emotional skills. Attention is linked to motivation and the ability to practise skills in order to learn.

Table 4.16 Normal development of attention

Age	Level of attention
First year	Fleeting attention, extremely distracted Attention 'captured' by stimuli
1–2y	Single channelled: fixed on one task and difficult to shift focus Can concentrate on concrete task of own choosing, ignoring other stimuli 5min
2–3y	Single channelled: cannot attend to competing auditory and visual stimuli With support can shift attention to speaker 7min
3–4y	Attention under voluntary control Can alternate full attention between task and speaker without support 9min
4–5y	Two-channelled attention: can understand verbal instruction and continue with task Group instruction possible Able to focus on one aspect of complex situation 13min
5–6y	Integrated attention: can voluntarily establish and maintain concentration, shutting out irrelevant information 15min
6y +	45–60min

Thinking or cognitive skills

Cognitive skills (Table 4.17) are important to assess as they are likely to link to a child's longer term learning trajectory, and this is particularly helpful for children with language difficulties.

As with all development, there are elements of 'nature and nurture'. The development of cognitive and emotional skills is hugely affected by the child's parenting and early relationship (see section on Attachment).

Table 4.17 Useful assessment of cognitive skills

Age	Skill	Example
Birth	Reflex activity	Sucking and grasping
3–6mo	Able to regard object	Hand regard, interest in mirrors later
6–9mo	Recognizes carer Manipulates objects Looks at pictures	Happier with carer than stranger Shakes rattle
9–12mo	Actions take on an intentional purpose Object permanence	Banging two bricks together when shown Searching for the hidden or fallen object Peekaboo
12–18mo	More than one way to do things Starts to understand objects' function: cause and effect Starts to understand pictures and symbols	Move to get, or pull the string Will use simple pretend play, e.g. phone, drink Cause and effect toys towards 18mo Looks at pictures in books
18–24mo	Starts to be able to solve simple problems	Cause and effect toys Simple insert puzzles
2–3y	Starts to be able to solve more complex problems, but the object needs to be present Progression of imaginative sills	Simple puzzles Colour match Cardboard box is a house Small-world play
3–4y	Gains basic understanding of concepts	Groups by colour, size, etc. Counts by rote Likes being read stories
4–5y	Develops early language and maths skills	Starts to know phonic letter sounds Can read some early words Can write name Counts with meaning Knows shapes
5–7y	Develops logical thought Develops the principle of conservation Understands reversal of operations Able to group things	Simple addition and later subtraction By 7y counts in 10s, 2s and 5s Amount of liquid same even in different containers e.g. 3+4=7 and therefore 7−4=3 Classifies in different groups, e.g. animal and plant
8–11y	Able to start to solve the problems they can see Read and write fluently	How to make a bridge from planks and blocks Ask to read and write, e.g. name and address or 'The quick brown fox jumps over the lazy dog'.
11y+	Logical sequences Abstract solutions and hypotheses Abstract thought	Predict next in more complex sequence, e.g. 2, 4, 8, 16 More dissolved as the solution is warmer What should your friend buy for the disco? Algebra

Play (Table 4.18)

Children have an innate motivation to explore and learn. Toys and play are not synonymous. Children can develop elaborate games without toys being present. Play is not dependent on language skills although the child may be developing their inner language through play. Carers can encourage children to learn through play so that they experience the pleasure that learning brings, but equally children can be self-motivated enough to do this for themselves.

The development of the child's play skills reflects the level of his cognitive, social and comprehension abilities. By observing the child playing, one can gain an idea about the child's abilities in these areas of development before going onto assess them more in detail. Observation of play therefore forms a major part of the preschool assessment.

Table 4.18 Development of play skills

Age	Developmental milestone
3mo	Hand regard evolving into finger play
6mo	Exploratory play: infant reaches out, grasps and mouths objects Delighted by rough and tumble play
9–12mo	Enjoys peekaboo and copying hand clapping
12mo	Functional play, e.g. pretending to use mobile phone or hair brush Likes to put objects in and out of box or cup Manipulates toys that make a noise Starts to push along wheeled toys Cause-and-effect play: pressing buttons on pop-up toys
18mo	Early pretend play, e.g. feeding dolly, imitating household chores
2y	Follows parent around house, demanding attention Non-literal use of objects in play, e.g. brick becomes a biscuit Developing play alongside other children (parallel play)
3y	Imaginative play sequences which they will allow other children to join in
4y	Narrative play: uses miniature toys to make up own story Shows a sense of humour Enjoys making 'camps' outside Likes to play with other children Can sing several nursery rhymes
5y	Group make-believe play Plans and builds constructively

Case vignette

Philip is a 2-year-old who is very active and enjoys climbing over the furniture in the consultation room. He enjoys emptying out the toys but does not settle to play with any of them. He is interested when an adult starts to play with a cause-and-effect toy and takes the adult's hand to get them to push the buttons again. He has no interest in pretend play. Philip has some single words and likes to count by rote.

Learning points

- Language, attention and social difficulties tend to go together. Autistic spectrum disorders or significant learning difficulties need to be considered as possible diagnoses.
- Children with disordered attachment and significant neglect can present with a similar picture.
- Need to ensure that hearing is normal.

Checklist for Autism in Toddlers

Autism is often not diagnosed until the child is at least 3 years of age. However, parents may suspect that their child is not developing normally at 18 months because of an absence or limitation of joint attention and pretend play, which are key behaviours seen in typically developing children at this age.

- Joint attention refers to the child's ability to establish a shared focus of attention via pointing, showing or gaze monitoring (i.e. glancing back and forth between the adult's face and the object of interest). It is the earliest indication of mind reading, which indicates that the child has a sensitivity towards another person's interests.
- Pretend play involves the attribution of imaginary features to people, objects or events. It involves an object being treated as if it represents something different, for example a twig whirled through the air is seen as an aeroplane by the child.
- Proto-declarative pointing is pointing to share interest rather than just to request an item, as is the case with imperative pointing.

The Checklist for Autism in Toddlers (CHAT; Baron-Cohen et al. 1992) is a screening tool that was devised to test the prediction that those children not exhibiting these behaviours at all at 18 months might be at risk of receiving a later diagnosis of autism. The screen takes 5 to 10 minutes to administer and is easy to score. There are nine questions for the carer and five direct observations of the child in total, of which five key items, shown below, are the most useful in predicting the risk of autism (see Baron-Cohen et al. 1992 for full version of the CHAT).

1 Ask the parent if their child ever pretends to make a cup of tea using a toy cup and teapot (pretend play).
2 Does the child ever use his or her index finger to point to indicate interest in something (proto-declarative pointing).

3   Observe: get the child's attention and then point across the room at an interesting toy and say 'Oh look, there's an aeroplane!' Does the child look across to see what you are pointing at (following a point)?

4   Say to the child 'Where's the light?' or 'Show me the light'. Does the child point at the light with his or her index finger (producing a point)?

5   Give the child a toy teapot and cup. Ask the child to make a cup of tea. Does he or she pretend to make, pour and drink from cup, etc. (pretend play)?

The child who fails all five of these items on repeated testing 1 month apart should be referred on for a comprehensive diagnostic assessment.

Sensitivity is the probability of being screen positive and having the condition. The CHAT has a sensitivity of only 18% but a specificity of 100%, which means that those who are screen negative will reliably not have the condition. It has a positive predictive value of 78%, which means that most of those who fail will ultimately go on to to receive a diagnosis of autism. The high false negativity rate is regarded as less important than the specificity as autism is obviously not a life-threatening diagnosis, but a later diagnosis is disadvantageous because the potential gains from earlier intervention will be lost.

Children who fail several items of the CHAT may have other developmental delays that require follow-up and intervention including communication and cognitive delay, but the CHAT has not been devised to screen for such delays.

A more recent version of the CHAT, the Quantitative CHAT, contains 25 items scored on a 5-point scale (0–4) and has shown improved sensitivity when used to screen 18- to 24-month-old children at risk of autism, but it is yet to be fully validated.

Assessing play skills (Table 4.19)

Provide a range of play materials suitable for children of a variety of ages/developmental stages in your clinic room. This should include a small desk and chair with puzzles, paper, pencils, 1-inch bricks, pop-up toys, toy kitchen, buggy and baby, crockery, cutlery, books, and so on. Ask the child for examples of their behaviour at home and in other settings, such as at nursery or parties. Ask, specifically, the preschool child about the following.

• How does he or she spend his or her time at home? Is he or she curious, looking for things to do and play?
• Does he or she have a favourite play activity/toy?
• Does he or she put items in and out of containers?
• Does he or she have any bricks and what does he or she construct with them?
• Does he or she scribble on paper? Scribbles, lines, shapes?
• Does he or she have favourite puzzles/jigsaws? Can he or she complete them?
• Does he or she have a favourite television programme or DVD? Can he or she operate the remote control? Does he or she play computer games (indicates not high intelligence but early exposure to such items)?
• How does he or she relate to his siblings and peers? Do they play together and what do they play at?

- Does he or she show joint attention behaviours: showing and sharing and joint interactive play?

While talking to parents observe the child's play on his or her own (free play) with suitable toys such as a pop-up toy, a doll with a bottle or a hairbrush and cot, and for older children small-world toys. Then engage the child in order to look at other areas of development and make note of the following:

- Interactive play: will the child let you take a turn, for example with cause-and-effect toy or a ball?
- Choosing: encourage the child to chose an activity.
- Imaginative play: initially feeding the dolly and becoming more abstract as the play progresses.

Table 4.19 Useful assessments of play skills

Age	Stage	Skills
Birth–6mo	Newborn infant	Hand regard
6–12mo	Sitting child	Starts to grasp and explore toys, e.g. shake rattle, bell
12–18mo	Mobile child	Does the child put things in and out of containers? Interested in cause and effect toys (pop-up toys)? Push-along toys
18mo–2y	Walking child	Does the child copy household chores, e.g. sweeping up? Does the child scribble on paper? Can the child attempt a simple inset puzzle? Does the child engage in early pretend play, e.g. give doll a drink? Can the child build a tower of bricks?
2–3y	Communicating child	How does the child relate to siblings and peers? Can the child draw lines and a circle? Can the child play inset puzzles and complete simple jigsaws? Does the child enjoy pretend play, e.g. use brick as biscuit to feed dolly? Can the child use a remote control for the television/electronic games?
3–4y	Preschool child	Can the child play alongside or with peers? Does the child have a friend? Can the child complete a jigsaw – 4, 6, 12 pieces? Does the child engage in small-world play?
4–11y	Primary school key stage 1	Can the child name a friend? Does the child play imaginative games collaboratively with other children – or does it need to be on his or her rules?
4–11y	Primary school key stage 2	Can the child play card and board games?

Red flags in play skills

1 year

- Persistence of hand regard.

18 months

- Persistent mouthing of toys.
- Shaking of toy.
- Lack of early imaginative play.

2 years

- Persistent casting of toys.

2 years 6 months

- Flitting between toys, fiddling with objects, persistent overactivity.

Process for identifying developmental impairments

- **Universal surveillance for all children** This process relies on parents reporting concerns about their child to their general practitioner (GP), health visitor (HV) or other health practitioner at routine contacts. The personal child health record (or 'red book') may be used as a prompt.
- **Developmental examination** This is a clinical evaluation usually arranged with the GP/ paediatrician to verify concerns once raised and refer the child on for more detailed assessment and/or investigations. Experience and use of developmental tools is variable at this stage, for example a **Schedule of Growing Skills II** (SOGS II; Bellman et al. 1997) may be used to indicate delays and which domains are affected.
- **Developmental assessment** This is a more detailed assessment of a child's strengths and weaknesses for planning management, and standardized assessment tools, such as the Griffiths Mental Development Scale (Griffiths 2006), the Bayley Scales of Infant Development (Bayley 2005) and the Wechsler Intelligence Scale for Children-IV (WISC-IV; Wechsler 2003), are used at this stage.
- **Diagnostic assessment** The Autism Diagnostic Observation Schedule (ADOS; Lord et al. 1989) and Autism Diagnostic Inventory (ADI; Rutter et al. 2003), validated and quantitative diagnostic tools, are used to decide whether or not the child should have a diagnostic label. A gross motor function measure such as the Gross Motor Function Classification System (GMFCS; Palisano et al. 1997) may also be used.

Formal developmental assessment tools

Case vignette

You are asked to see Jodie because of concerns about her development. In order to gain a fuller understanding you complete a SOGS II.

Profile

When completing the profile a horizontal line is drawn across as the child's chronological age. After completing the assessment the child's skills are scored and this result is then transferred to the Profile Form. This provides a visual representation of the child's strengths and weaknesses and this in itself is useful when providing an explanation to parents about the child's developmental performance.

The profile shows that Jodie's locomotor and manipulative skills are delayed as she performed at a 30 month level whilst her visual, hearing and language skills are in keeping with her age. Her speech and language, social and cognitive skills are slightly below the expected level for her age, but still within the range accepted as normal.

Using SOGS II, significant delay is said to be present if the developmental age is more than one age interval below the age block representing chronological age.

A formal record of development between birth and the age of 5 years can be obtained by using structured assessment tools such as the SOGS II, the Denver Development Screening Test, the Griffiths test and the Bayley Scales of Infant and Toddler Development.

The **SOGS II** takes around 30 minutes to administer and is a useful screening tool to determine if more detailed assessment is needed. In the SOGS II, development is divided into nine subdomains. It provides a cognitive score for children aged 2 years and above. Below this age any estimates of cognitive ability are likely to be unreliable. The areas making up the cognitive skill area are incorporated in the existing nine skill areas and so no extra testing is required. The items selected for compiling this score are dependent on the child having the thinking (cognitive) as well as the physical function to complete the item.

The **Denver Developmental Screening Test** (Frankenberg et al. 1992) is a screening tool that takes approximately 20 minutes to administer. It can help to decide if a more detailed assessment is needed.

The **Griffiths test** (Griffiths 2006) was the developmental assessment tool most commonly used by doctors until briefer assessments such as the **SOGS II** were developed. It has recently been revised to bring it up to date, but it still takes 1 to 2 hours to administer. It is because of this time demand that Griffith's assessments are not routinely undertaken in neurodisability clinics. They may still be used where detailed and precise records of a child's progress are required for specific purposes such as court reports.

The **Bayley Scales of Infant and Toddler Development**, Third Edition (Bayley-III; Bayley 2005), is an individually administered assessment that examines developmental functioning of infants and young children between 1 month and 42 months of age. It is used to identify children with developmental delay and it is set out to examine the three main developmental areas of language, cognition and motor skills. The assessment is designed so that each of these scales can be used independently. The language scale is split into receptive and expressive communication subtests and the motor scale is split between fine motor and gross motor subtests. As an adjunct to this main assessment, the Bayley-III also provides a social–emotional assessment and an adaptive behaviour assessment using a questionnaire format that is completed by the parent/caregiver and the professional involved.

Within many child development teams the most commonly used aspect of the Bayley-III is the cognitive subscale. The cognitive scale includes items that assess sensorimotor development, exploration and manipulation, object relatedness, concept formation, memory and other aspects of cognitive processing. The assessment was designed to be relatively non-reliant on a child's receptive language skills and it has been redesigned (from a previous assessment tool, the BSID-II mental scale; Black and Matula 1999) to decrease the impact of motor ability on performance, thus making it suitable for a relatively large age range of 0- to 4-year-old children with developmental delay.

The Bayley-III assessment is useful for gaining a baseline of developmental ability and can be repeated to assess a child's progress, although the recommended minimum waiting period before reassessment is 12 months.

Top tip

Practise using one developmental tool to become familiar with the methods of assessing a child's development in the various domains and become confident in setting up the relevant tasks for the child and asking appropriate questions of the carer and recording observations whilst this is being done. When you have done this often enough you can then reproduce parts of the screen in the clinic or ward to assess a child without having to find a kit and laboriously follow the instructions.

Methods of assessment for school-aged children

Overall ability

- Observation in clinic.
- Reports from school – children are assessed on at least an annual basis.
- Formal developmental assessments, which could include the following:
  - The Griffiths test (Griffiths 2006) for an overall assessment giving a developmental quotient (DQ).
  - The Wechsler Preschool and Primary Scale of Intelligence (WPPSI; Wechsler 2012) to give a cognitive assessment and IQ score for children up to the age of 7 years or the WISC for older children. A WISC assessment can be difficult to obtain on request from educational psychologists as IQ scores are not readily provided as education services do not set store in the score alone. In defence, most psychologists say that the child's performance is more

dependent on other factors such as personality, motivation, organization and support than intelligence alone. Clinical psychologists, such as those who work in neuropsychology, may be more amenable to undertaking similar cognitive assessments, for example in a child with a neurological disorder for a baseline assessment prior to an intervention such as surgery or the institution of a ketogenic diet.

Specific areas of function

- Movement: Movement Assessment Battery for Children (Henderson et al. 2007), Peabody (Rhonda Folio and Fewell 2000).
- Speech and language: Derbyshire Language Scheme (Knowles and Masidlover 1982).
- Tests of reception of grammar (TROG) (Bishop 2003).

Key messages

- The majority of children develop normally, following the same sequence of steps with minor varients.
- Delay may occur because of genetic, biological or environmental factors, or the inter-action between them.
- Children with significant delay in one area or delay in a number of areas may require input and follow-up from the local child development team.

Refer to Appendices I to IV for further information on child development.

References

Bellman M, Lingham S, Aukett, A (1997) *Schedule of Growing Skills II*. London: GL Assessment.

Bayley N (2005) *Bayley Scales of Infant Development Third Edition*. Oxford: Pearson Clinical Assessments.

Bishop D (2003) *Test for Reception of Grammar (TROG-2)*. Oxford: Pearson Clinical Assessments.

Black M M, Matula K (1999) *Essentials of Bayley Scales of Infant Development II Assessment*. New York: John Wiley.

Frankenburg WK, Dodds J, Archer P et al. (1992) The Denver II: a major revision and restandardization of the Denver Developmental Screening Test. *Pediatrics* 89: 91–7.

Goodenough F (1926) *The Measurement of Intelligence by Drawings*. New York: Harcourt Brace.

Griffiths R (2006) *Griffiths Mental Development Scale – Revised: Birth to 2 years and 2 to 8 years*. Boston: Hogrefe.

Henderson SE, Sugden DA, Branett A (2007) *Movement Assessment Battery for Children – Second Edition (Movement ABC-2)*. Oxford: Pearson Clinical Assessments.

Howe D (2005) *Child Abuse and Neglect: Attachment, Development and Intervention*. Basingstoke: Palgrave.

Knowles W, Masidlover, M (1982) *The Derbyshire Language Scheme*. Matlock: Derbyshire County Council.

Lord C, Rutter M, Goode S et al. (1989) Autism diagnostic observational schedule: a standardized observation of communication and social behaviour. *J Autism Dev Disord* 19: 185–212. http://dx.doi.org/10.1007/BF02211841

McLeod S (2007) Bowlby's Attachment Theory. Available at: http://www.simplypsychology.pwp.blueyonder.co.uk/bowlby.html (accessed 15 October 2012).

Palisano R, Rosenbaum P, Walter S, Russell D, Wood E, Galuppi B (1997) Development and validation of a gross motor function classification system for children with cerebral palsy. *Dev Med Child Neurol* 39: 214–23. http://dx.doi.org/10.1111/j.1469-8749.1997.tb07414.x

Rhonda Folio M, Fewell RR (2000) *Peabody Developmental Motor Scales, Second Edition (PDMS–2)*. Oxford: Pearson Clinical Assessments.

Rutter R, LeCouteur A, Lord C (2003) *ADI-R Autism Diagnostic Interview Revised*. Torrence, CA: Western Psychological Services.

Baron-Cohen S, Wheelwright S, Cox A et al. (2000) Early identification of autism by the Checklist for Autism in Toddlers (CHAT). *J R Soc Med* 93: 521–5.

Reynell J, Huntley MD (1985) *Developmental Language Scales: Second Revision*. Windsor: NFER-Nelson.

Sheridan MD (2008) *From Birth to Five Years: Children's Developmental Progress*, Third Edition. Revised and updated by Ajay Sharma and Helen Cockerill. New York: Routledge.

Wechsler, D (2003) *Wechsler Intelligence Scale for Children® – Fourth Edition (WISC®-IV)*. Oxford: Pearson Clinical Assessments.

Wechsler, D (2012) *Wechsler Preschool and Primary Scale of Intelligence™ – Fourth Edition (WPPSI™–IV)*. Oxford: Pearson Clinical Assessments.

Further reading

Lindon J (2010) *Understanding Child Development Linking Theory and Practice*. New York: Phillip Alan Updates.

Rees CA (2005) Thinking about children's attachments. *Arch Dis Child* 90: 1058–65. http://dx.doi.org/10.1136/adc.2004.068650

Section 3

Assessment

5
Assessment and formulation

Anne M Kelly, Arnab Seal and Gillian Robinson

Aims of assessment

Assessment is the systematic collection, organization and interpretation of information about a person and his or her situation. The aim of this process is to produce a statement of the main difficulties and in doing so provide a formulation that should help to provide a picture of the following:

- the nature of the child's difficulties
- any associated medical problems including hearing and visual impairment
- an understanding of possible aetiological factors: genetic, biological, environmental
- an indication of the child's current level of function
- an understanding of the child's social and educational situation and how this will impact on his or her ability to participate.

Current developmental status can be used as a proxy to indicate a child's functional level. Developmental status can be described using an approximate estimate or a more precise set of measurements supplemented with the results of psychometric testing and reports with objective measurements or scales from a physiotherapist, occupational therapist and speech and language therapist (SLT). This should highlight the child's strengths as well as his or her difficulties. The aim of this assessment is to enable a comprehensive management plan to be written.

The aim of this process is to help parents gain an understanding of their child's function, including strengths and difficulties, and how the advice and interventions that are being offered may influence their child's rate of progress. This may be the point at which some parents realize and accept that their child will be different. Some may have reached this point before this and find it a relief that their suspicions have been confirmed. A small number may not agree with the findings from the assessment and may struggle to work with the team. They may seek additional opinions and input. This should be facilitated at the family's request as long as it is not harmful to the child. Funding for additional assessments and input may be difficult to obtain and may be possible only if financed by private means.

Although an assessment may indicate that a problem is present, it will not necessarily identify the cause of the problem. This may require investigation and a review of the child's progress. An opinion from specialists in neurology and/or genetics may be required later. This is particularly important if there are relevant pointers in the past history or family history and/or physical findings that suggest a possible syndrome or neurological diagnosis. A small number of children may eventually be seen by a plethora of specialists but in spite of this a definite aetiology for their difficulties may still not be agreed. Parents may find it harder to explain their child's problems to friends and family without a label; it can also be more difficult to gain access to additional support. Some families find uncertainty around prognosis hard to deal with. It can be particularly concerning for those planning to have more children, although it should still be possible for a geneticist colleague to give an empirical estimate of recurrence risks.

Case vignette

Paul, aged 5 years, is asked to draw a man but produces only marks on the page.

Learning points

There are a variety of reasons for this functional difficulty. The child may have

- difficulty comprehending verbal instructions due to impaired hearing, listening or attention or receptive language difficulties
- processing difficulties or generalized learning difficulties
- severe hypermetropia impairing near vision
- poor grasp and coordination of hand movements due to dyspraxia
- difficulty grasping and manipulating the pencil due to a hemiplegia
- lack of experience of the task due to neglect or poverty.

The clinic area

In the clinic area it is important to have accurate facilities for weighing and measuring the height and weight of children of all ages and sizes. This should include wheelchair scales and hoisting equipment.

The clinic room should ideally be large enough to accommodate a child in a wheelchair, and possibly several adults and children. A range of washable toys suitable for various ages should be available. It is helpful to have lockable cupboards, as many children would like to explore them, as well as an examination couch and sink. It is best if these are in an adjoining area as again they can be a source of distraction to some children. Finally, standard medical examination equipment needs to be available but kept out of reach.

The referral

When you receive the referral letter it is useful to review the information that is already available, including investigations arranged by other doctors, as these may not always be filed. Research and print out appropriate information for the child's notes if the child has a recognized condition that you are not familiar with.

It can be helpful to have information from other sources such as inpatient notes and information from the health visitor or school, where relevant. Clearly, you need consent from the family to ask for information from other services, and the easiest way to ensure that they are happy for this to happen is to ask them to obtain the information prior to their first appointment. For example, it can be very time effective to send a copy of a questionnaire that asks for information on the child's progress at school (see Appendix VII). Send a copy to the family with a note requesting that they ask the child's teacher to complete it and to bring it along to the appointment. If there are ongoing child protection concerns, you do not need parental permission to have a conversation with the child's social worker before the child attends. Ensure that you have an appointment of appropriate length: usually 40 to 60 minutes. Check if an interpreter is needed and, if so, ask the clinic clerk to book one for you.

Talking to children and families

- Have clear introductions
  - If it is possible, ask the parents/carers questions about how they communicate with the child beforehand or obtain this information from a professional who knows the child well.
  - Greet each child by name, no matter how apparently severe the child's disability and regardless of age (unless a very young infant).
  - Always introduce yourself and describe your role to the child and carer.
  - Communicate with the child on his or her physical level: sit/kneel or bend down to do this.
  - Communicate by using eye contact, speech, gesture and touching appropriately, only on upper limbs.
- Listen to and interact with the child
  - Seek responses to questions if the child is able to communicate by speech or gesture, for example nodding, eye pointing or via his or her communication aid.
  - The parent/carer will be best placed to comprehend and interpret responses from the child to your questions and examination, for example his or her vocalizations or motor responses, if more specific responses are not possible.
  - In the case of a signing child, ask the parent/carer to convey messages via Makaton or British Sign Language, if that is their usual method of communication
  - If the child is a more cognitively able child and can respond verbally, ask him or her directly and await a response, even though this may take some time. Do not talk over the child's head in a 'Does he take sugar?' mode. There are many intellectually able children in wheelchairs, some of whom could be significantly dysarthric.
  - You should attempt to interact with the child in some way – engage the child in simple play with a toy or stimulation such as peekaboo or music.

- Be thoughtful about how to conduct the clinical examination
  - Ask permission to perform the examination. Look for consent from the child and/or carer. Say what you are going to do before doing it, for example examine a limb, abdomen, and so on.
  - Perform actions gently and at same time explain your actions to reassure the child and carer.
- Acknowledge that parents are the real expert about their child
  - Always consider parental opinion when formulating an opinion about the cause of symptoms and deciding what to do next. The parents know their child best and most are strong advocates for their child.
  - It is all the more difficult to make a diagnosis in children who are severely disabled, particularly those with very limited communication, as diagnosis is largely dependent on information obtained from the history. Every piece of the jigsaw is important when making a diagnosis but we have to rely on parents more in this scenario than we do when assessing children who can communicate independently.
  - Do not conduct sensitive discussions about treatment or end of life care in the presence of the child, who will be able to hear but may or may not cognitively be able to make sense of information and/or be able to take part in the discussion. Likewise, if the parent becomes upset, do not continue with the discussion, particularly if this seems to be upsetting the child too. Arrange to do this at another time with suitable support available for the parent/carer, in the absence of the child.

Top tips for encouraging engagement with the child – where developmentally appropriate

- Have a 'good toy' ready that may appeal to the child.
- Ask the child his or her name and age (if verbal skills are sufficient).
- You could also ask the child
  - Who is in your family?
  - Who is your teacher and which class are you in at school?
  - Who is your friend?
  - What do you like and dislike in your school day?
  - What do you like to do at home or on a special day such as on your birthday or at Christmas?
  - What makes you worried, happy or sad?
  - What do you think makes your mother or father worried, happy or sad?
  - If you had three wishes, what would you ask for?

The appointment

Re-read the referral letter. Will there be other non-health staff present with the child? If so, see these members of staff first with parental permission in order to gain background information. In the case of a school-aged child, it may be better to first meet alone with the parents to hear their concerns. Afterwards, see the child to make an assessment; usually with the parents present but, if not, a chaperone is required.

In the case of the school-age child, it may be better to first meet alone with the parents, to hear their concerns. Afterwards, see the child to make an assessment; usually with the parents present but, if not, a chaperone is required.

History

There is no substitute for good history taking as it should be possible to ascertain the most likely cause of the child's difficulties by means of history and examination. In fact, the cause of most children's difficulties can be ascertained from the history alone in 70% to 80% of cases, as is the case in most medical conditions.

Present concerns

It is helpful to follow the following points.

- Start with when the parents first became concerned.
- List the parental concerns verbatim and use this list to answer their specific concerns at the end of the consultation.
- Verify the information provided by parents by contacting the nursery or school later, if required.
- Clarify if parents feel that their child is progressing, albeit slowly, of if they think there is any loss of skills.
- What are the parents' thoughts about the nature and cause of their child's difficulties?

At this stage you are trying to answer the following questions:

- Is there a problem or is this a problem with perceptions or expectations?
- If it is developmental, is the development delayed (i.e. following a normal pattern but behind that expected for chronological age) or disordered (i.e. not following a typical pattern of development)?
- Is the quality of this delayed skill different from that displayed by peers?
- Has there been any loss of skills (regression)? A neurological opinion is needed unless it appears to be the pattern of regression seen in autism at around the age of 18 months, seen in one-third of affected children.

Examples of disordered developmental sequence

- A child who is talking but not yet walking at 2 years.
- A child who finds it easier to stand than sit because of increased extensor tone in whole-body cerebral palsy.
- Superior expressive language compared with receptive language skills, i.e. 'cocktail party speech', in a child with Williams syndrome.

Examples of qualitative abnormality of the developmental skill

- A child with a slowness in completing a cognitive task.
- A child with a tremor affecting hand movements but who can insert shapes into a form board.

Examples of regression: loss of a previously acquired skill

- The loss of purposeful hand movements seen in Rett syndrome.
- The loss of previously acquired words in some children with an autism spectrum disorder in their second year of life.
- The loss of language skills in Landau–Kleffner syndrome.

It is important to consider if the physical health of the child is affecting his or her learning, for example as in chronic lung disease of preterm birth; severe gastro-oesophageal reflux in cerebral palsy; or severe constipation in a child with a learning disability and epilepsy.

Birth history

- Were there any difficulties with conception, including infertility treatments?
- Health in pregnancy: any illnesses, especially any associated with high fever?
- Drugs: prescribed/non-prescribed/alcohol?
- Antenatal scans: were there any abnormalities?
- Intrauterine and postnatal growth.
- Gestation, delivery, resuscitation, neonatal care and follow-up.

Past medical history and current general health

- Congenital abnormalities in other systems.
- Other health problems – particularly seizures.
- Any medications.
- Immunization status.

At this stage you are trying to answer the following questions:

- Are there any possible aetiological factors?
- Are there other abnormalities that make a systemic diagnosis such as a genetic syndrome or metabolic disorder more likely?
- Is the child's physical health affecting their development?

Developmental history

This involves taking a history of developmental progress and particular milestones attained so far. Using a structured approach is essential, as parents are more likely to volunteer required information if prompted; key milestones include smiling, reaching out, sitting independently, first word, walking independently.

When asking about a child's current abilities, again, it is helpful to break this down for parents and ask specifically about

- sitting and walking
- the child's ability to use his or her hands
- understanding of what you say – in context only?
- talking and speech sounds
- self-care, for example using bottle, finger feeding, use of cup, use of spoon/fork, toileting, hygiene
- hearing and vision
- child's ability to play and get along with others
- learning
- behaviour.

Parents tend to be overoptimistic about their child's achievements and underplay difficulties on the whole. Written records of specific milestones aid memory and it is always worth examining a parent-held record book if available, in case milestones have been recorded there. This becomes less likely with each successive child as most parents become less fascinated in their child's progress and are generally busier in their lives. Information consolidating parents' concerns from records from children's centres or nurseries where the child may be attending is helpful.

At this stage you are trying to answer the following questions:

- What is the child's functional ability?

Family history/genetics

This information is best gathered by drawing a family tree (Fig. 5.1). This should include three generations. Include information about grandparents and aunts and uncles.

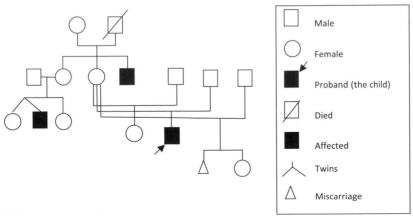

Figure 5.1 Drawing a family tree.

It is important to specifically ask about

- consanguinity
- recurrent miscarriages
- family history of learning difficulties, language disorders and autism spectrum disorder.

At this stage you are trying to find out

- Should a genetic or metabolic condition be considered?

Social factors

- Who does the child live with?
- Are the child's parents in employment?
- Who owns the housing and is it suitable for the family?
- What is the family's financial situation?
- Are there difficulties at home including drugs, alcohol, and mental health?
- Is there support from the extended family?

At this stage you are trying to answer the following questions:

- Does the home environment help or contribute to the child's difficulties?
- What practical difficulties do the family face?

Examination

This will consist of informal observation of the child's behaviour and play before setting some more formal developmental tasks. The physical examination should consist of a general systems examination with particular attention being paid to the neurological system. It may need to be done in a piecemeal fashion after the initial observation of the child in free play.

Clinic observation

Useful information can be initially obtained by collecting families from the waiting room as this provides an opportunity to watch the child being brought into the clinic room. Note the child's appearance, method of locomotion (carried, walking with or without aids, wheelchair user), interaction with carer and method of communication.

More can be obtained from watching the child in free play once in the clinic room. Suitable toys should be provided and the child and parent made comfortable so that the consultation can proceed. The toys should be appropriate for the estimated developmental age of the child, although this may have to be revised quickly depending on how the child presents. The selection of toys available should include

- rattles and bricks for infants to grasp and mouth

- simple cause-and-effect toys (e.g. pop-up farm)
- posting toys (e.g. shape sorters, stacking rings, inset boards)
- exploration and imitation toys (e.g. pull-along toys, baby and buggy, kitchen area with pots, cups, etc.)
- functional toys (e.g. cup and spoon, doll and brush)
- toys for pretend play (e.g. teddy and tea set)
- toys requiring fine motor coordination (e.g. 1-inch cubes, paper and pencils, inset boards, puzzles)
- toys that encourage language and play (e.g. books at different levels, miniature toys).

The child can be observed once he or she is safely positioned on a mat on the floor, or if mobile but contained within the room. The child should be left to play with encouragement when needed from his or her parent. This scenario can be informative, as it will give some indication of the child's interests and curiosity in his or her surroundings as well as the child's attention to task, problem solving and social interest in the examiner. Eye contact, response to name and verbal instructions should be specifically elicited if concerns have been raised about the child's communication and social skills. These informal observations together with information from the history should indicate an approximate developmental level in the various domains. It is important to note not only that the child performs a task but also the quality of his or her performance, for example the child's dexterity in matching shapes in inset boards, how the child makes a request, the clarity and length of utterances and the speed of the child's response to verbal requests, and so on.

General examination

- How is the child growing?
  - You should plot the child's weight, height and head circumference on the appropriate chart.
- Are there any dysmorphic features? Look carefully at the child's
  - face: in particular the eyes, ears, nose, palate, profile, chin
  - scalp: fontanelles and sutures in infant, hairline and hair texture, scalp defects, and neck
  - teeth and palate: palpate soft palate if necessary with clean finger
  - limbs: hands including fingers and nails and feet
  - skin: look for any pigmented or de-pigmented areas. Use Woods light if available.
- Are there signs of systemic or orthopaedic disorders?
  - Carry out a systems examination.
  - Check spine for scoliosis and sacral dimples.
  - In the non-walking child, check for leg length discrepancy and hip range of movement.

Neurological examination

INFANT

The most rapid phase of motor development occurs in the first year of life. The infant should be examined in the supine, then pulled to sit, supported sitting, standing, then ventral suspension and finally prone. You are assessing posture, tone, symmetry and range of movements. Check to see if primitive reflexes have disappeared and have been replaced by protective reflexes (described in Chapter 4).

FUNCTIONAL EXAMINATION

During the functional examination you should observe the following:

- level of alertness and eye movements
- vocalization, smiles and responsiveness to social cues
- posture: predominantly flexed or extended in supine
- spontaneous movements: lack of these is concerning
- asymmetry in posture, tone or movements
- posture in sitting, prone and ventral suspension.

FORMAL EXAMINATION

- **Fundoscopy:** Again, this is a more challenging test, but that does not mean you should not try, and again practice helps. Try to give the child a clear object to focus on so he or she is looking slightly upwards. Approach from the side and with luck the fundus should be the first, and probably the only, thing you see. If there are any doubts a formal assessment by ophthalmology is appropriate.
- **Cranial nerves:** These are difficult to assess but you can note if the child has strabismus. It is important to see if the child can track a small toy and with this you can get a crude assessment of eye movements. Look specifically for symmetry of the child's facial expression during smiling and crying. Feeding difficulties, if present, may be due to underlying pathology affecting IX to XII cranial nerves.
- **Limbs:** During the inspection look for muscle bulk noting wasting, asymmetry and if fasciculation is present.
- **Tone:** Tone is assessed by passively moving joints through a range of movement. This needs to be done slowly and also more rapidly. Spasticity is noted more commonly during more repeated rapid movements. You feel that the muscle tone suddenly increases and with ongoing steady pressure can be overcome. Tone needs to be assessed both centrally (axial) and peripherally (limb).
  - Examine the child sitting with both knees flexed and straight (in long sitting) to assess the contribution made by gastrocnemius and hamstrings. Resistance may increase as a result of stretching, leading to a dynamic increase in tone.
  - Examine ankle dorsiflexion: it should go beyond 90 degrees. Wait and gently dorsiflex the ankles several times. Clonus may occur but is regarded as being significant only if several beats occur.
- **Assess deep tendon reflexes:** This requires a little patience, as the child must be relaxed when the tendon is tapped. In principle, it is the same as in an adult examination, but it is important to remember that children's tendons are shorter than adults' and therefore accuracy is more important. This is particularly true of the triceps jerk as that tendon is very short and should be elicited just above the olecranon. Extensor plantar responses require careful interpretation in young children as they can be normal up to 18 months of age.

Abnormal findings to note

- Hypotonia due to neuromuscular disorders usually affects the trunk and limbs. In central nervous system hypotonia, axial tone is reduced, leading to head lag on pull to sit. However, limb tone may feel normal. Reduced axial tone may be noted in an infant with evolving spastic cerebral palsy, but the infant may show increased extensor tone in ventral suspension.
- The bottom shuffler may sit in a 'W' position, but so may the child with tight hamstrings due to spasticity. The bottom shuffler will have easily abducted hips and adopts a 'sitting on air' position if held, supported under his or her arms. It is not desirable to leave the child sitting in this position, in either case.
- The child with tight hamstrings due to cerebral palsy will sacral sit in long sitting, with knees flexed to compensate for shortening of tendons and muscles.
- If the child is commando crawling, look at the legs. If they are extended and stiff and the child is propelled only by the strength of his or her upper limbs, this is abnormal and may be due to spasticity in the child's lower limbs.

IN THE OLDER CHILD (TODDLER TO 3 YEARS)

FUNCTIONAL EXAMINATION

- While looking at the child's movements, think about posture, asymmetry (including the upper limbs) and the quality of the movement. During the functional examination you should observe the following:
  - Walking: including stooping to retrieve, stopping and turning around, and avoiding objects in path. Look for heel strike, in-toeing or out-toeing.
  - Running: check if the feet lose contact with the floor.
  - Rising from lying supine to standing: look at the need for support such as pushing up from the floor or using furniture. Note that turning prone initially to rise from supine is not abnormal in children less than 2 years old.
  - Climbing stairs or on to furniture: look for pelvic weakness – struggle to stand from squatting, sitting or lying.
  - Throwing and kicking a ball.
  - Jumping on the spot and off a small step.

FORMAL EXAMINATION

- Perform this as you would for an infant (described above).

OLDER CHILD

A more formal examination of the central nervous system should be possible from the age of 3 to 4 years onwards.

CRANIAL NERVES

- **Visual fields by confrontation:** Children quite enjoy this game where you both close an eye and then place your fingers just within your visual field and ask the child which finger is moving. Remember to have your hands at the mid-point and check each quadrant. Whilst this is a crude test it does identify significant visual field problems such as hemianopia.
- **Fundoscopy:** With increasing age and cooperation the success rate of this test increases. Again, encourage the child to focus on an object so he or she is looking slightly upwards. For younger children it is helpful if this is another adult who pulls faces to continue to attract the child's attention. Tell older children to keep looking in that direction and not at the light. Still approach the child from the side as the fundus remains the most important component of the examination. If there are any doubts a formal assessment by ophthalmology is appropriate.
- **Eye movements:** Observe if the child has a strabismus and then ask the child to track your finger using an H shape, followed by checking that the child has conjugate upwards gaze.
- **Facial nerves:** Facial movements are observed in smiling and crying; if the child has an upper motor neurone lesion then the forehead is spared whilst with a lower motor neurone lesion it is the whole side that is affected. Abnormalities of IX to XII cranial nerves cause bulbar difficulties and require assessment by a speech and language therapist. You can check the gag reflex, tongue and palatal movements but they rarely lead to a clinical diagnosis without further assessment.

Abnormalities of eye gaze

III cranial nerve: ptosis, immobile except outward gaze, pupil fixed and dilated

IV cranial nerve: diplopia on downwards gaze, particularly if adducted (rare)

VI cranial nerve: unable to abduct eye, leading to apparent inward gaze strabismus

EXAMINATION OF LIMBS

Functional examination

During the functional examination you should observe the following:

- Moving from supine to standing: look for Gower's sign where the child turns prone and then 'climbs up their legs' to stand: a sign of muscle weakness.
- Sitting and standing.
- Walking and running: think about movement at the trunk, hip, knee and ankle. Beware of 'best walk': children may try to walk in a manner their parents have encouraged as being appropriate, rather than their natural gait. Observing the child as he or she comes into your clinic room may be your best chance!
- Jumping on the spot.
- Standing for 5 seconds on either foot and hopping on either foot.

- Heel–toe gait.
- Walking on the outer borders of feet (Fogs' test). In young children, hand movements will mirror feet position. This is abnormal after a child's 7th birthday.

Observation

- Length, asymmetry, muscle bulk and distribution.
- Quality of the movements at rest and also during active movement.

Tone

- Tone is assessed by passively moving joints through a range of movement. This needs to be done slowly and also more rapidly. In the upper limbs, this is usually assessed by means of extending and flexing the elbow whilst pronating and supinating at the wrist.
- In the legs it should be checked with the knee flexed and the foot flexed and extended. This is then repeated with the knee extended – look out for clonus.

Power

- Power is best assessed by a 'trial of strength game'. In the younger child this may still be by functional observation or trying to pull a toy away. In the older child it can be completed as per adult examination.

Reflexes

- Deep tendon.
- Persistence of primitive reflexes.
- Saving reflexes.

COORDINATION

Functional assessment (often the most helpful)

During the functional assessment you should observe the following:

- Grasping a brick while building a tower.
- Picking up two piles of coins simultaneously.
- Putting the lid on a pen.
- Threading beads on a piece of string.

Formal examination includes

- Tapping the dorsum of one hand rapidly with the other.
- Alternately pronating and supinating the child's hand.
- Apposing little finger and thumb, and then moving on to apposing other fingers in sequence.

- Finger nose testing is when you ask a child to touch their nose and then your finger. This is more likely to show a problem if the child has to approach maximal reach, so he or she cannot splint his or her arm against the side of his or her body.

ORTHOPAEDIC EXAMINATION

You should already have noticed any limb asymmetry during the neurological examination but remember to also look at the spine for scoliosis or sacral dimples. If a scoliosis is present, see if gentle traction under the arms corrects this (positional scoliosis). In the older and more mobile child, ask the child to bend forward and touch their toes while you look both at the spine and for a rib hump.

- Assess the range of movement at all joints.
- Remember to include internal and external rotation at shoulder and hip joints, as well as flexion and extension.

Abnormal findings to note

Soleus tightness: limited dorsiflexion of ankle with knee bent.

Gastrocnemius tightness: limited dorsiflexion of ankle with knee extended.

Rectus femoris tightness: in a child lying prone with the knee flexed the opposite buttock lifts.

Abnormal findings with orthopaedic abnormalities

Femoral anteversion: leg appears internally rotated with limited hip external rotation. Patellae point inwards.

Tibial torsion: when the legs are placed in neutral the patellae point forwards but feet are internally rotated.

Metatarsus adductus: when legs are straight hips and knees are normal but feet point inwards from the junction of hind and forefoot.

At the end of the consultation

Provide the parents with a formulation

- Summarize the child's greatest strengths and difficulties and ensure that you have a common understanding with the parents.
- Say why you think the child may have these problems.
- If unsure, decide if the child needs a review or if discussion with a colleague may be helpful.
- Say if you are concerned about any possible associated problems. In particular consider if the child could have sensory difficulties.

Devise a management plan

This can include

- further assessment (it is not always possible to complete a full assessment in one clinic visit and information from other sources can be very helpful, for example information from the school or health visitor)
- therapy input
- educational input
- hearing and vision screening if indicated
- medical investigations
- medications (if appropriate)
- consideration of whether a feeding plan is needed (e.g. poor growth or difficulties with feeding).

Feedback to parents

An appointment about a child's development is very concerning for parents and it is important to come to a joint understanding of the child's strengths and difficulties. If the child's development is significantly disordered or delayed in more than one area, a multidisciplinary assessment is a method that will establish more information. It is not intrinsically therapeutic but it is important to do it in a timely manner to inform parents and start the process of securing therapy input and additional support.

The next area parents often wish to address is the underlying cause. The aetiology for the child's difficulties may already be known at the time of the first appointment (e.g. extreme preterm birth, a syndrome, neglect), or it may remain obscure, in which case appropriate investigations should be arranged. This may often lead to questions about prognosis: will it affect the child in the long term? Sometimes you can be clear after one appointment about the long-term outlook, but it is often wise to gather further information and understand the child's difficulties in greater depth before starting to answer this question. This is particularly true for children under the age of 2 years, where there is good research to show that predictions regarding cognitive potential are often inaccurate.

As a large amount of information is discussed at this appointment, it is helpful for parents to have a copy of the clinic letter. It is also important to say to parents that this could well be the start of a series of appointments. The parents are likely to go away and think about other questions they would like to ask, and you should be prepared to go over what has already been covered and answer their new questions at their next appointment.

Key areas to cover in a new patient clinic letter

SUMMARY

- The child's difficulties.
- The underlying cause (if known).
- Any secondary difficulties.
- Growth parameters.

MANAGEMENT PLAN
- Therapy or educational input planned.
- Medications.
- Investigations.
- Follow-up arranged.

Top tips: what to do if it is all going wrong during a consultation!

You should acknowledge that this is difficult and seek help from nursing staff and also parents. If the child is destructive

- Talk to the parents on their own and ask other staff to occupy the child in a waiting room until you are ready to examine him/her.
- Remove as many toys and pieces of equipment as possible prior to entry; lock the cupboards and turn off the tap at the stopcock if necessary!
- Have a task ready to the engage child.
- If all else fails, ask the parents 'What would you normally do?'
- Consider a home or nursery visit.
- Use information from other sources.

Neurodisability review

Once children have received a diagnosis there are often ongoing difficulties that mean they require ongoing paediatric care. In these situations an alternative consultation outline is needed, as often the focus has shifted from aetiology to management.

It is sensible to have an 'agenda' for the appointment, which should include the child's or parents' current concerns, and also the issues you wish to address. It is helpful to write problem-based letters. These should have a summary at the top, and then, in the body of the letter highlight the different problems discussed. This enables you to quickly identify the areas for discussion.

Preparation prior to the appointment

Read the last clinic letter and from this deduce which issues should be discussed at this appointment. Try to answer the following questions.

- Are there any outstanding investigations and if so do you have the results?
- Does the child have a specific condition that requires specific monitoring and if so is a protocol available in the notes?
- Have you received information from other people and if so have you read and digested this?
- Would it be sensible to 'batten down the hatches': remove certain toys, lock cupboards, and so on?

The appointment

Agree with the family what are the most important issues to discuss – you may not manage them all.

- Medical
  - Medical difficulties such as
    - epilepsy
    - a ventriculoperitoneal shunt
    - gastro-oesophageal reflux disease
    - constipation.
  - Review the child's general health, including pain.
  - Check if there is any specific monitoring, including hip surveillance in cerebral palsy and thyroid function in Down syndrome.
  - Check that medications are correct and doses are increased in line with weight, if indicated.
  - Check immunization status, particularly flu immunization.
  - If the patient is an adolescent, are there difficulties relating to puberty, menstruation and sexual health?
- Feeding and growth (including plotting growth parameters)
- Sensory problems
  - Vision
  - Hearing
- Therapy/education plan
- Aids and appliances
- Behaviour
  - Sleep and day-time issues
- Current functional abilities
  - Self-help and independence skills including continence
- Social support
  - Housing adaptations/environmental controls
  - Access to leisure and respite support
  - Appropriate benefits (disability living allowance, carers allowance, family fund and blue badge)
  - Access to information and voluntary organizations
- Examination – particularly for child with cerebral palsy
  - Spine
  - Pressure points
  - Hips
  - Contractures

Summarize this consultation for the family, discussing with them the areas they would most wish to address. Then write an appropriate management plan. Again, it is helpful to send the family a copy of the clinic letter to ensure you have a common understanding.

It is always worth asking yourself 'Is the underlying diagnosis correct?' If the child is not following the expected trajectory then you should reconsider this.

Neurodisability review clinic letter outline

The letter should cover the following points:

- the child's difficulties
- the underlying cause (if known)
- any secondary difficulties
- medications including emergency management plan
- growth parameters.

In the body of the letter, use subtitles for the different sections with the problems discussed. It is often easier to write a management plan for each section rather than summarizing this at the end. In addition to ensuring you act on all the difficulties identified it also enables you to identify those issues that will need to be addressed at the next consultation. You should send a copy of the letter to all professionals involved; you need to make sure that you are up to date with the names of the other professionals, as they do often change and you are not always made aware.

Reports

Clear written, as well as verbal, communication is key to meeting children's needs. Having an outline can help to ensure that all important areas are covered. In the appendices you will find outlines for

- gathering information from schools (Appendix VII)
- problem-orientated medical record (Appendix V)
- child development team report (Appendix VI)
- medical component of statement of special educational needs (Appendix VIII)
- emergency management plans (Appendix IX and Appendix XV).

Key messages

Assessment should provide an understanding of the following.

- The child's disability and ability.
- The secondary or associated medical problems including hearing and vision.
- An understanding of possible aetiological factors: genetic, biological and environmental.
- The child's family, social and educational situation and how that is impacting on their ability to participate.

Further reading

Davie M (2012) Developmental assessment in the over 5s. *Arch Dis Child Educ Pract Ed* 97: 2–8. http://dx.doi.org/10.1136/adc.2010.208140

Sharma A (2011) Developmental examination: birth to 5 years. *Arch Dis Child Educ Pract Ed* 96: 162–75. http://dx.doi.org/10.1136/adc.2009.175901

Sheridan MD (2008) *From Birth to Five Years: Children's Developmental Progress, Third Edition*. Revised and updated by Ajay Sharma and Helen Cockerill. New York: Routledge.

Section 4

Impairment of motor function

6
The infant with hypotonia

Gillian Robinson

Learning objectives

- To differentiate between normal and disordered motor development.
- To have a clinical approach to examine a child with a motor concern.
- To look for and treat associated and secondary skeletal problems.
- To have a structured approach to plan further assessment and investigation.

Case vignette

A 10-week-old infant, Pradip, presents with poor feeding and symptoms related to a chest infection. On examination he is floppy, but alert. You note that he has mild contractures at his ankles, knees and elbows and no reflexes. He is unable to feed well. There is no family history of note and this is the first child of healthy, unrelated parents.

Learning points

- Pradip has a concerning presentation as he is young, and has difficulties with feeding and motor development. Assessment of infants is not easy and a neurological opinion may prevent many unnecessary tests being ordered.
- Eighty per cent of children with low tone will have a central problem.
- In infants who are alert, muscles disorders need to be considered.
- Chest difficulties can be the first presentation of a neuromuscular disorder.

Key initial considerations

To try to identify any possible underlying cause (see Table 6.1 and Fig. 6.1). Ask the following questions:

- Is this an acute deterioration (consider sepsis or metabolic disorders) or an ongoing difficulty?
- If an ongoing difficulty, is it improving or deteriorating?
- Does the infant have dysmorphic features?

To assess the health status of the infant ask

- Are there signs of respiratory distress?
- Is the child growing well?
- Are other systems affected?

Table 6.1 Differential diagnosis for hypotonia

	Example	Clinical clues
Metabolic disorder	Paroxysomal disorders Zellweger syndromw or Refsum disease	Consanguinity Family history Hepatosplenomegaly
Genetic	Down syndrome Prader–Willi syndrome	Dysmorphic features Other systems affected, e.g. heart
Central neurological disorder	Holoprosencephaly Cerebral palsy	No other system affected History of preterm birth or birth asphyxia
Spinal cord	Spinal muscular atrophy	Bright and alert Smile Muscle fasiculation Absent reflexes
Neuromuscular junction	Congenital myaesthenia	Mother has myasthenia gravis
Muscle disorder	Congential myopathies Congential muscular dystrophies	Myopathic facies Normal reflexes

Clinical assessment

- Present problems
  - Movement difficulties
  - Chest difficulties
  - Feeding difficulties
- Past history
  - History of miscarriage or neonatal death
  - Abnormalities on ultrasonography

- Gestation at delivery and evidence of asphyxia or infection
- Birth growth parameters including head circumference
- Neonatal difficulties
- Family history – should be three generations
  - Consanguinity
  - Specifically muscle disease, birth defects and learning difficulties

Examination

- General examination
  - Growth parameters: weight, height and head circumference, which are plotted
  - Dysmorphic features
  - Look for any cutaneous signs such as café-au-lait patches or depigmented areas, which may suggest a diagnosis of a neurocutaneous syndrome such as neurofibromatosis or tuberous sclerosis. Remember, such skin signs may not have developed in the very young child (i.e. <6mo)
- Central nervous system
  - Does the child have a myopathic facies?
  - Is there any fasciculation?
  - Observe the infant's movements:
    - are they weak and if so where?
    - face – can the child smile?
    - limbs – are the upper or lower limbs affected?
    - proximal or distal?
  - Assess tone
  - Assess deep tendon reflexes
  - Assess range of movement for contractures or increased range of movement

---

Clinical features of low tone

- Frog posture in lying
- Marked head lag in pull to sit and in sitting
- Unable to support weight when held under arms
- C shaped ('rag doll') in ventral suspension

- Sensory examination
  - Look at the eyes, perform fundoscopy and examine the child for a bilateral red reflex to exclude a cataract
  - Look to see if there is any nystagmus or ptosis and normal eye movements
  - Has the infant passed the neonatal hearing screen?
- Respiratory system

Clinical features of respiratory compromise

- Respiratory rate
- Bell-shaped chest
- Paradoxical breathing (abdominal excursion leads to chest indrawing)
- Other systems
  - Abnormalities would imply a genetic or metabolic disorder

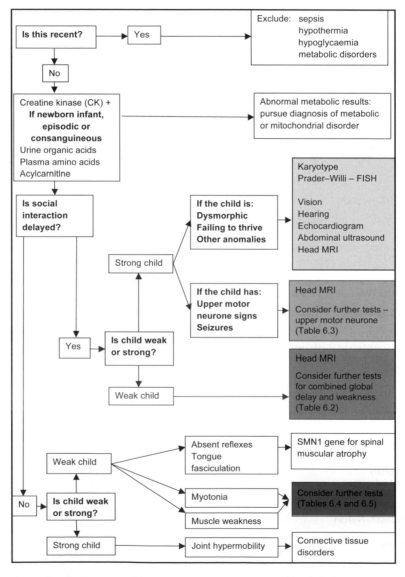

Figure 6.1 Investigations to consider when assessing a hypotonic infant. FISH, fluorescence in situ hybridization test; MRI, magnetic resonance imaging.

Table 6.2 Hypotonia and global delay: investigations to consider

Additional feature	Possible diagnosis	Test
Upslanting palpebral fissure Epicanthic folds Single transverse palmar crease Sandal toe gap Cardiac abnormalities – AVSD	Down syndrome	Karyotype
Epicanthic folds Stellate iris Upturned nose Aortic stenosis	Williams syndrome	MLPA
Unusual fat pads Inverted nipples	CDG	Glycosylation state of transferrin by isoelectric focusing
Liver abnormalities Seizures Cataracts/retinal dystrophy Hearing loss Abnormal anterior fontanelle	Peroxisomal disorders- Zellweger sndrome Refsum disease Adrenoleukodystrophy	VLCFA
Short stature Gondal hypoplasia Hyperphagia from around 1y	PWS	FISH *UBE3A* gene PWS/AS methylation
Severe speech impairment Ataxic gait Acquired mircrocephaly	AS	FISH *UBE3A* gene PWS/AS methylation
2/3 toe syndactyly or polydactyly Cataracts Cleft palate Cardiac abnormalities	Smith–Lemi–Opitz syndrome	7-Dehydrocholesterol

AVSD, atrioventricular septal defect; MLPA, multiplex ligation-dependent probe amplification; CDG, congenital disorders of glycosylation; VLCFA, very long-chain fatty acids; PWS, Prader–Willi syndrome; AS, Angelman syndrome.

Table 6.3 Hypotonia with upper motor neurone signs: investigations to consider

Additional feature	Possible diagnosis	Test
None	Structural abnormality	Brain MRI
History of preterm birth	Preterm birth in own right Intraventricular haemorrhage	Cranial ultrasound +/– MRI
Birth asphyxia	Cerebral palsy	Brain MRI

Males
  Microcephaly
  Frequent infections
	Rett syndrome or MECP2 spectrum disorder	MECP2

Seizures	Creatine deficiency disorders	MRI – delayed myelination
Self-harm (Lesch–Nyhan syndrome) Kidney stones Deafness	Disorders of purine and pyrimidine metabolism	Serum urate

MRI, magnetic resonance imaging; MECP2, M-methyl-CpG binding protein 2.

Table 6.4 Hypotonia with combined weakness and global delay: investigations to consider

Additional feature	Possible diagnosis	Test
Dysglycanopathies		
Lissenencephaly Hydrocephalus Eye abnormalities	Walker–Walburg syndrome	Creatine kinase raised Genetic testing
Neuronal migration defect Eye abnormalities	Muscle–eye–brain disease	Creatine kinase raised Genetic testing
Severe neuronal migration defect Seizures Eye abnormalities Cardiomyopathy	Fukuyama muscular dystrophy	Creatine kinase raised Genetic testing
Onset 1–40 years Dilated cardiomyopathy	Limb-girdle muscular dystrophy	Creatine kinase raised Genetic testing
Metabolic disorders		
Abnormal fat distribution Inverted nipples	Congenital disorders of glycosylation	Transferrin gycosylation by isoelectric focusing
Macrocephaly Optic atrophy Seizures	Canavan disease	*N*-acetyl aspartic acid raised in urine, blood and CSF
Excercise intolerance Seizures Encephalopathy Cardiomyopathy External ophthalmoplegia	Mitochondrial encephalopathies	Lactate – blood and CSF
Male 　Spasticity/ataxia 　Progressive loss of skills	Pelizaeus–Merzbacher disease	*PLP1* gene

CSF, cerebrospinal fluid.

Table 6.5 Hypotonia and weakness: investigations to consider

Additional feature	Possible diagnosis	Test
Congenital myotonia		
Myotonia Poor cry and facial weakness Family history Cataracts	Congenital myotonic dystrophy	*DMPK* gene repeat
Congenital muscular dystrophy		
Joint contractures Kyphoscoliosis Respiratory insufficiency	Congenital muscular dystrophy 1A	Muscle biopsy
Proximal joint contracture Distal joint hypermobility	Ullrich congenital muscular dystrophy	Creatine kinase (normal to five times normal)
Torticollis Kyphoscoliosis	Ullrich congenital muscular dystrophy	Genetic testing Muscle biopsy

Additional feature	Possible diagnosis	Test
Axial hypotonia Progressive spinal rigidity Scoliosis Respiratory difficulties	Rigid spine	Creatine kinase (normal or mild raise) Muscle biopsy
Congenital myopathy		
Congenital hip dislocation Scoliosis Non-progressive course Malignant hyperthermia	Central core or multi-minicore disease	Creatine kinase (mildly raised) Muscle biopsy
Peripheral hypotonia Facial weakness High arched palate Scoliosis Joint contractures	Nemaline myopathy	Muscle biopsy

Males
   Macrocephaly
   Archnodactyly
   Respiratory insufficiency
	Myotubular myopathy	Genetic testing *MTM1* deletion

Congenital myaesthenia		
Poor suck Weak cry Ptosis and facial weakness Fatiguablilty	Congenital myasthenia	EMG
Metabolic myopathy		
Liver failure and calcification Cardiomyopathy Neuronal migration defect Exercise-induced weakness	Carnitine palmitoyltransferase deficiency	pH Ammonia Acylcarnitine
Hepatomegaly Cardiomyopathy Macroglossia	Pompe disease	ECG – short PR interval

Males
   Cardiomyopathy
   Neutropenia
	Barth syndrome	Urine organic acids

Peripheral neuropathy		
Usually 10+ Loss of sensation and reflexes	Hereditary sensory motor neuropathy	EMG Nerve biopsy
Connective tissue disorders		
Joint hypermobility Scoliosis Pectus excavatum Archnodactyly Dilated aortic root	Marfan syndrome	Clinical – Ghent criteria
Hypertelorism Bifid uvula or cleft palate Aortic root enlargement	Loeys–Dietz sydrome	

DMPK, dystrophia myotonica protein kinase; EMG, electromyography; ECG, electrocardiography.

Management issues

RESPIRATORY COMPROMISE

If there are signs of respiratory compromise then consider whether the infant should be admitted for further respiratory evaluation including saturation monitoring, capillary gas monitoring analysis and if indicated, chest radiography.

FEEDING DIFFICULTIES

If there is a history or any sign of feeding difficulty such as coughing and choking on feeding, then you should arrange an assessment by a paediatric speech and language therapist who specializes in assessing feeding skills.

THERAPY AND PRACTICAL CARE

Handling an infant with hypotonia can be very difficult. Physiotherapy and occupational therapy advice about positioning and the supply of appropriate equipment, for example seating and bathing, if needed. In the longer term advice on standing frames to aid bone mineralization and acetabular formation is appropriate.

Key messages

- Always exclude metabolic decompensation, especially if acute, or the child is of a consanguineous relationship.
- Always test creatine kinase.
- Other investigations are as indicated by history and examination.
- Absent reflexes should lead to urgent discussion with paediatric neurology.
- Consider issues around the chest and feeding.
- If you are uncertain on how to proceed, obtain a neurological opinion.

7
The child with delayed walking or abnormal gait

Gillian Robinson

Case vignette

Paul is the first child born to two healthy parents. He has been referred because of late walking and when you meet him at 20 months of age he can take three independent steps. He was a bottom shuffler and his parents are concerned that he has flat feet.

Learning points

- All male infants not walking by age 18 months should have creatine kinase checked to exclude Duchenne muscular dystrophy. Classically, children with Duchenne present with difficulties running and climbing as toddlers. They may also present with a speech and language delay.
- The mean age at walking for a bottom shuffler is 17 months, with 98% walking by 28 months. Often there is a family history of bottom shuffling, which appears to have an autosomal dominant pattern.
- Significant ligamentous laxity delays walking.
- Consider the child's overall development: delayed walking may be a marker of learning difficulties.

Whilst this section is written about a child with delayed walking, the approach would also be useful for children who present with other motor difficulties such as

- abnormal gait
- motor delay

- falls
- muscle pain/cramps
- problems with the feet (e.g. crossed toes or unusual shaped toes and feet)
- family history of muscle problems.

Differential diagnosis of late walking (Table 7.1)

Table 7.1 Differential diagnosis of late walking

Physiological	Pathological
Familial	Part of global developmental delay
Bottom shuffling	Cerebral palsy: hemiplegia or diplegia
Failure to correct for preterm birth	Spinal dysraphism
Ligamentous laxity	Duchenne muscular dystrophy
	Developmental dysplasia of hip
	Other causes of hypotonia

Key questions for clinical assessment

- Are the child's movement skills progressive, static or regressing?
  - Assess the child's present motor skills.
  - Is there muscle pain or cramps, and, if so, when do they occur: at night or with exercise?
  - What is the child's exercise tolerance? This will give an idea of the severity of the problem.
  - What does the child find hard to do? This will give some idea about how the child's life is affected.
- Is the problem focal or general?
  - General health:
    - Are there any chest or cardiac symptoms?
    - Are there any feeding and swallowing difficulties?
  - General development:
    - Are there any difficulties in other areas?
    - Is this a generalized or specific developmental concern?
- Could the difficulties be related to a brain injury and, if so, when?
  - During pregnancy or birth, or postnatal?
- Is there any genetic predisposition?
  - Muscle or heart problems
  - Consanguinity
  - Bottom shuffling
- On examination are there any neurological or musculoskeletal abnormalities?

Observation

- Is this a bright and alert child?
- Are there signs of wasting or hypertrophy?
- Where is the child most affected?
  - Face (look for drooling)
  - Limbs
    - Is it proximal (shoulder or pelvic girdle) or distal?
    - Is there an asymmetry or hand preference?
- Is there a scoliosis?

Neurological examination

- Is the tone normal, increased or decreased? Is there a pattern to this, for example four limbs, hemiplegia or diplegia?
- Is the power normal and, if not, how severely is it affected? Which parts are affected most (for young children this is determined by observation and through play)?
- Are the deep tendon reflexes present? Are they normal?

Musculoskeletal examination

- Are there any spinal abnormalities?
- Are the child's legs of the same length and symmetrical?
- Are there deformity, contractures or ligamentous laxity?
- Is there normal and symmetrical hip movement?

Functional assessment of walking child

- What is the child's gait?
- Can he or she toe walk and heel walk?
- How does the child get up from the floor or out from a chair?
- If mobile, can the child jump and hop? Can the child climb up stairs?

Systems examination

- Examine the child's heart and chest in particular.

Table 7.2 Useful investigations for children with motor delay

	Findings on examination	Possible investigations
Upper motor neurone signs	Increased or variable tone Brisk reflexes	Head MRI – see 'The stiff child' (Chapter 8)
Lower motor neurone signs	Low tone Weak fasciculation Absent reflexes	SMN deletions for SMA (98% genetic testing positive) EMG Spine MRI Tensilon test
Muscle disorder	Weak muscle hypertrophy	Creatine kinase (if normal then dystrophinopathy is unlikely) If raised creatine kinase refer to neuromuscular team and arrange DNA for dystrophin Lactate (mitochondrial) Carnitine (fatty acid disorders) Muscle ultrasound/MRI Muscle biopsy
Hip dysplasia	Abnormal range of hip movement Leg shortening Limited abduction	Hip radiography
Normal examination	Normal or increased range of joint mobility	Creatine kinase if male not walking at 18 months

MRI, magnetic resonance imaging; SMN, survival motor neurone; SMA, spinal muscular atrophy; EMG, electromyography.

Initial management

If the child is using a baby walker, encourage the family to stop using this – it does not teach useful motor patterns that enable walking.

Arrange for a physiotherapy assessment

Physiotherapists are excellent at assessing tone and power, and their assessment can help to clarify your thoughts. Children need to learn balance in sit, high kneel and stand (with hips in alignment with trunk) before they will progress to walking. Physiotherapists will support families with encouraging the appropriate skills. Supportive footwear will help some children, and the physiotherapist will arrange an appointment with an orthoptist.

8
The 'stiff' child or the child with increased muscle tone

Gillian Robinson

Case vignette

Maisy is 7 months old and she has been referred because of concerns about growth. It is also commented that she 'prefers to stand but cannot sit'. When you meet the family they describe Maisy as a very unsettled child who has been very difficult to feed and has frequent vomiting. When you examine Maisy she has increased tone and persistent primitive reflexes.

Learning points

- Maisy has an emerging abnormality of tone and posture and this is probably best described as an evolving motor disorder at this stage. It also reminds the clinician that there are causes for this apart from cerebral palsy.
- A detailed history and examination will help to identify the appropriate investigations into the underlying cause.
- Maisy may also have significant gastro-oesophageal reflux and could have an unsafe swallow, which will require further assessment and treatment. Treating the gastro-oesophageal reflux could help with feeding. Pain increases muscle tone, so treating the reflux may also help reduce Maisy's tone.

Table 8.1 Causes of increased muscle tone

Cause	Example	Investigation
Cerebral palsy	Non-progressive lesion of the brain	Brain MRI
Tumour	Slow-growing tumours of the brain or spine	Brain MRI and spinal cord MRI
Genetic		
Abnormalities of DNA repair	Cockayne syndrome Ataxia telangiectasia	Chromosome fragilitiy studies
Gene defects	Rett syndrome Dopa-sensitive dystonia Glucose transport 1 deficiency (GLUT1)	MLPA Trial of levodopa Fasting serum and CSF glucose
Metabolic		
Mitochondrial disorders	Leigh syndrome Pyruvate dehydrogenase deficiency MERFF	Lactate Pyruvate
Peroxisomal disorders (disorders of fatty acid metabolism)	Adrenoleukodystrophy Refsum disease Zellweger syndrome	Very long-chain fatty acids
Lysosomal storage disorders		
Sphingolipidoses	Niemann–Pick disease Gaucher disease	Urine metabolic screen glycosaminoglycans
Gangliosidosis	Tay–Sachs disease	White cell enzymes
Mucopolysaccharidoses	Hunter and Hurler syndromes	
Leukodystrophy	Metachromatic leukodystrophy Krabbe leukodystrophy	Urine for oligosaccharides GALC gene defect
Neuronal ceroid lipofucinosis		Skin biopsy Lysosomal enzyme assay
Other		
Hyperekplexia		EEG
Sandifer syndrome		Barium swallow
Normal variation	Toe walking	Physical examination

MRI, magnetic resonance imaging; MLPA, multiplex ligation-dependent probe amplification; CSF, cerebrospinal fluid; MERFF, myoclonic epilepsy and ragged red fibres; EEG, electroencephalography.

Key questions

The following questions should help in understanding the nature of the problem and its course. The answers to the questions should help to focus the direction of investigations and management (Table 8.1)

- What are the present difficulties?
- What are the motor difficulties?

- Is this an intermittent, static or progressive disorder?
  - Are there are difficulties with gross and fine motor development (beware of child showing hand preference under the age of 1 year)?
- Are there difficulties in other areas of development (including feeding)?
  - Are there problems with communication and social interest?
  - Feeding:
    - Any difficulties with present feeding such as with consistency of foods or dribbling?
    - Are there any signs of aspiration such as a cough or altered respiratory rate when being fed?
    - Are there any signs of gastro-oesophageal reflux such as vomiting and/or pain?
- Is vision or hearing affected?
- Are there any difficulties with general health?
  - Constipation
  - Seizures
  - Present medication
  - Pain
  - Sleep
- Are there any clues to the underlying cause?
  - Obtain a detailed obstetric history and a history of the pregnancy and labour (reading maternal notes may help).
  - Intrapartum asphyxia: obtain delivery details including Apgar scores, cord pH and whether resuscitation was needed.
  - Neonatal course: was any intensive care required? Note the birth head circumference. Any neonatal encephalopathy?
  - Was there any postnatal illness: meningitis or head injury?
  - Family history:
    - genetic disorders
    - movement or walking difficulties
    - consanguinity.

Examination

- General:
  - Is growth, including head circumference, normal?
  - Are there any dysmorphic features?
  - Is the child bright and alert?
- Neurological examination
  - First, observe the quality of the child's movements. If the movement is abnormal, which limbs are the most affected?
  - Is the tone normal?
  - Testing power may be difficult to do formally, and if this is the case a gross motor developmental assessment will give a useful indicator of power.
  - Are the deep tendon reflexes present? Are they normal?
  - Are primitive reflexes still present?
  - Has the child developed protective/saving reflexes (Table 8.2)?
- Musculoskeletal examination

- Is there any deformity or contractures?
- Is there normal and symmetrical hip, knee and ankle movement?
- Systems examination
  - Examine the child's heart and chest in particular.

Table 8.2 Protective reflexes

Reflex	Age at onset	Description
Head righting	4mo	In vertical suspension the child is gently swayed from side to side and the head remains vertical
Trunk righting	8mo	In sitting, the child is gently pushed from side to side and the opposite arm is extended
Parachute response	10mo	In prone the child is moved head downwards which leads to arms and legs extending

Developmental assessment

Investigations

This will depend on your findings above.

Assessment of a stiff child (Fig. 8.1)

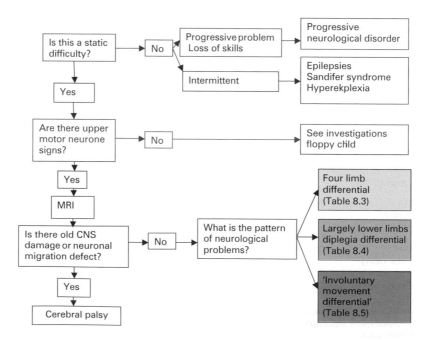

Figure 8.1 Assessment of a stiff child.

Table 8.3 Movement difficulty in all four limbs: investigations to consider

Additional problems	Possible diagnosis	Test
Vomiting, growth problems	Sandifer syndrome	Barium meal
Very irritable from birth Head retracts when nose tapped	Hyperekplexia	Mutation GLRA1 or GlyT2
Spasticity from 5 to 10y Visual impairment Loss of skills Adrenal failure	Adrenoleukodystrophy	Abnormal white matter MRI VLCFA
Flexion posturing Generalized myokymia Male	Hereditary myokymia	Channelopathy – refer to neurology
Truncal hypotonia with limb dystonia Initial feeding problems Almond-shaped eyes	Prader–Willi syndrome	MLPA
Initial hypotonia later spasticity Absent speech Severe learning difficulties Recurrent chest problems	MECP2 duplication	MLPA
Truncal hypotonia and limb spasticity Drooling Oculogyric crises	Autosomal recessive GTP cyclohydrolase deficiency	CSF monamine neurotransmitters (pterins low)
Speech and cognitive difficulties Oculogyric crises	Sepiapterin reductase deficiency	Levodopa therapeutic trial (CSF monamine neurotransmitters needed to confirm)
Spasticity, dystonia and ataxia Epilepsy – myoclonic or absence Male	Glucose transporter 1 deficiency	Fasting serum and CSF glucose
Myopathic face Thin quadriceps Paroxysmal dyskinesia	MTC8 mutation	MRI delayed myelination Increased free triiodoithyronine, lower free thyroxine
Microcephaly Failure to thrive Enlarged lymph glands	Congenital HIV infection	HIV antibody test (interpret with care in first 18 months)
Microcephaly Encephalopathy Profound delay	Aicardi–Goutieres syndrome	MRI – calcified basal ganglia CSF interferon alpha increased Gene testing
Erythematous scaly skin Developmental delay	Holocarbonase synthetase deficiency	Lactate raised Urine organic acids Respond to biotin

GLRA1, glycine receptor, alpha 1; GlyT2, glycine transporter 2; MRI, magnetic resonance imaging; VLCFA, very long-chain fatty acid; MLPA, multiplex ligation-dependent probe amplification; MECP2, M-methyl-CpG binding protein 2; GTP, guanosine triphosphate; CSF, cerebrospinal fluid; MTC8, medullary thyroid cancer 8; HIV, human immunodeficiency virus.

Table 8.4 Diplegia investigations to consider

Additional problems	Possible diagnosis	Test
Normal examination	Idiopathic toe walker	Male: creatine kinase
Early in disease weakness not picked up	Duchenne muscular dystrophy	Creatine kinase MLPA
Social and communication problems	Part of autistic spectrum disorder	Speech and language therapy to assess communication
Loss of skills Communication problems Unusual hand movements	Rett syndrome	MECP2
Toe-walking toddler Gets worse during the day	Segawa type dopa-responsive dystonia	Levodopa therapeutic trial (CSF monamine neurotransmitters needed to confirm)
Progression Pain Scoliosis	Spinal cord tumour	Consider imaging the spine – including cervical spine
Down or Hunter syndrome	Foramen magnum disorders	MRI head and cervical spine
Family history	Genetic spastic paraplegia	Mutations of SPG4 gene
Truncal unsteadiness Later overwhelming infections	Purine nucleoside phosphorylase deficiency	Low uric acid PNP deficiency in red blood cells
Progressive diplegia Abnormal hair Learning difficulties Seizures	Arginase deficiency	Plasma amino acids Ammonia may be raised

MLPA, multiplex ligation-dependent probe amplification; MECP2, M-methyl-CpG binding protein 2; CSF, cerebrospinal fluid; MRI, magnetic resonance imaging; SPG4, spastic paraplegia type 4; PNP, purine nucleoside phosphorylase deficiency.

Table 8.5 Investigations to consider for involuntary movements

Ataxia	'Ataxic cerebral palsy' is a diagnosis of exclusion. In these children thorough investigation into other possible causes is required. See Table 9.3
Involuntary movements	See Chapter 9 regarding the child with involuntary movements. See Tables 9.2 and 9.5

Initial manangement

PHYSIOTHERAPY WITH OR WITHOUT OCCUPATIONAL THERAPY ASSESSMENT

Physiotherapists are superb at assessing tone and movement difficulties and their assessment can help to clarify your thoughts. In addition, they will support the family with advice on positioning and play to help with the next stage of development.

FEEDING ASSESSMENT

If the child has a history of feeding difficulties, then an assessment by a speech and language therapist is needed. If this is the case, an assessment by the full child development team would be the appropriate way forward.

Key messages

- Not all increase in tone is caused by cerebral palsy.
- If the problem is cerebral palsy then motor development *must always* have been disordered and delayed.
- History and examination will help to identify appropriate investigations.
- Actively question if this could be a progressive disorder.
- Actively consider if feeding difficulties or gastro-oesophageal reflux are present.

9
The child with ongoing involuntary movements

Gillian Robinson

Case vignette

Paul is a 2-year-old male who was born at term, after a very traumatic vaginal delivery in Africa. His mother reports him to have been very bruised after birth. He then developed jaundice and seizures. Paul moved to the United Kingdom with his mother, but has only just begun to sit with support. In the first year of life he had had marked difficulties, with an increase in tone and feeding problems. Paul still cannot sit unaided in clinic but you notice on review that he has developed continual writhing movements which appear involuntary. Paul has good eye contact and will take turns, but his speech and language are markedly delayed

Learning points

- MR imaging of Paul's brain showed damage to basal ganglia.
- Paul also had a sensorineural hearing loss.
- Paul's difficulties could have been due to hypoxia, but the combination of difficulties together with the story of significant bruising and poor neonatal care led to kernicterus being the most likely diagnosis.

Involuntary movement disorders (Table 9.1)

There are a number of patterns of movement disorders which relate to the area of brain damage. One of the first steps in diagnosing and supporting these children is to be able to recognize and use the appropriate terminology. Observing the child in clinic is the most appropriate start. The movement disorder may fluctuate in intensity, in which case observing a video (even on someone's phone) can help to clarify the diagnosis. *Dyskinesia* is a term used to describe diminished voluntary movements and the presence of involuntary movements.

Table 9.1 Involuntary movement disorders

Cerebellum

Ataxia (Tables 9.3 and 9.4)	Broad-based gait Intention tremor (worse on approaching object) (Table 9.5) Dysmetria (loss of accuracy) Horizontal nystagmus Attention, communication and visual spatial problems

Basal ganglia

Athetosis (Table 9.2)	Convoluted, writhing movements Affects fingers, arms, legs and neck
Dystonia (Table 9.2)	Sustained muscle contractions cause twisting and abnormal postures
Ballismus	Flinging motions of the extremities Worse when active, better with rest
Parkinsonism	Difficulty initiating movements, associated with a tremor at rest

Corpus striatum

Chorea (Table 9.2)	Brief, quasi-purposeful, irregular movements Appear to flow from one muscle to the next Not repetitive or rhythmic

Substantia nigra

Restless legs syndrome	An urge to move legs because of uncomfortable sensations. Helped by movement and worsened by rest Genetic component Association with iron deficiency

Cortex or subcortex

Myoclonus	Brief, involuntary twitching of a muscle or muscle group
Stereotypy	Repetitive or ritualistic movement, posture, or utterance, e.g. rocking, head banging, hand flapping Often starts before 3 years
Tics	Sudden, repetitive, non-rhythmic, stereotyped motor movement or vocalization involving discrete muscle groups. These are increased by stress

Key questions for clinical assessment (see Fig. 9.1)

- What is the movement disorder?
  - Has the problem always been present or is it new?
  - Is the problem continuous or intermittent?
  - Is it generalized or does it affect one body part?
  - What is the nature of the movement?
  - Is the problem worse at any particular time of the day?
  - Are there any precipitants or any factors that help?
- Are there associated difficulties?
  - Development: particularly motor skills
  - Vision: including nystagmus
  - Hearing
- Are there any clues to the underlying cause?
  - History
    - Birth history and neonatal course: any features of encephalopathy or jaundice?
    - Present medications, particularly antiepileptics
    - Family history: consanguinity, movement problems
  - Examination
    - Examine the child's growth including head circumference.
    - Observe the child at rest and during active movements.
    - Ask the child to gently rest his or her hands on yours (this will make any abnormal movement more obvious).
    - Carry out a formal central nervous system examination.
- How does the disorder affect the child's function?
  - Fine motor tasks: can the child pick up a brick, toss a coin, put a pen lid onto a pen, draw or write his or her name and address?
  - Gait: is the child's gait affected including toe/heel walking?

Investigations

- Family video can be very useful, particularly for intermittent disorders.
- Other investigations relate to the neurological findings. Unless a clear diagnosis is confirmed these children should see a paediatric neurologist.

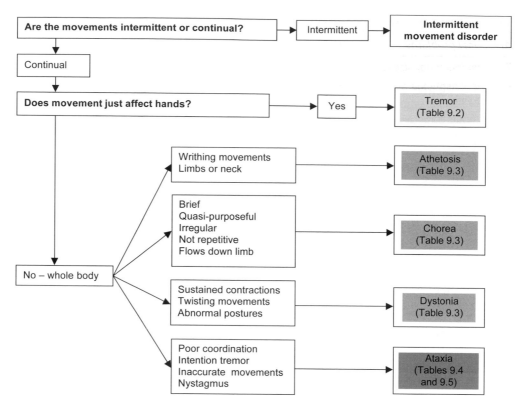

Figure 9.1 Flow chart for children with continual movement disorders.

Table 9.2 Differential diagnosis of tremor

Type of tremor	Cause	Nature of tremor
Essential tremor	Physiological Anxiety disorders Hyperthyroidism Drugs – salbutamol, theophylline Neuroblastoma Phaeochromocytoma	On active movement (6–8Hz) Often a family history
Basal ganglia	Parkinson disease Drugs – neuroleptics, metoclopramide	At rest (6–8Hz) Decreases with movement Often family history
Cerebellar	See Table 9.4 Wilson disease can present with tremor	Intention tremor (4–6Hz) Increases as approach desired goal

A tremor is an oscillation of one or more body parts (e.g. hands, arms, face).

Table 9.3 Useful investigations in long-standing choreoathetosis or dystonia

Additional problems	Possible diagnosis	Test
Trauma, infection, stroke		
History of asphyxia or encephalitis	Damage to basal ganglia	Head MRI
Genetic		
Onset 5y Family history Intially intermittent Progressive	Torsion dystonia	Mutation of *DYT1* gene
Early childhood Often starts with walking Fluctuates during the day	Dopa-responsive dystonia (Segawa disease)	Trial of levodopa (CSF monamine neurotransmitters needed to confirm)
Female Choreoathetosis/spasticity Autistic traits Seizures Abnormal respiratory pattern	Rett syndrome	DNA for *MECP2* gene
Family history Onset at age 3–9y Loss of skills	Huntington chorea	Huntingtin (HTT) gene
Slow early development Degenerative disorder Choreoathetosis with or without rigidity	Hallervorden–Spatz disease	MRI – lesion of the globus pallidus
Male Pendular nystagmus Optic atrophy Choreoathetosis Relative intellectual sparing Stridor	Pelizaeus–Merzbacher disease	MRI – various white matter abnormalities Visual evoked potentials diminished Mutation of the PLP gene
Growth retardation Profound learning difficulties Quadriplegia Opisthotonic dystonia GOR	3-methyl crotonyl CoA carboxylase deficiency	White cell enzymes
Metabolic		
Tremor Parkinsonism Liver disease	Wilson disease	Ceruloplasmin
Loss of skills Seizures Cherry red spot	GM1 and 2 gangliosidosis	Ophthalmology White cell enzymes

Table 9.3 (Continued)

Additional problems	Possible diagnosis	Test
Loss of skills Difficulty walking, muscle rigidity Seizures	Metachromatic leukodystrophy	Urine – oligosaccharides White cell enzymes
Normal until 6mo, then spasticity or athetosis Learning difficulties Severe irritability Loss of skills Self-mutilation	Lesch–Nyhan syndrome	Uric acid
Encephalopathy in newborn period	Methylmalonic and proprionic acidaemia	Serum ammonia
Macrocephaly Developmental delay With/without episodes of encephalopathy Increasing dystonia	Glutaric aciduria type I	Urine organic acids MRI – subdural collections, basal ganglia changes Definitive genetic tests
Episodes of acidosis Microcephaly Dystonia, quadriplegia	Pyruvate kinase dehydrognease deficiency Leigh syndrome	Lactate – blood and CSF MRI – altered basal ganglia Mitochondrial DNA deletions
Ataxia Involuntary movements Optic atrophy	Methylglutaconic aciduria	Metabolic acidosis Urinary organic acids

MRI, magnetic resonance imaging; MECP2, M-methyl-CpG binding protein 2; CSF, cerebrospinal fluid; PLP, proteolipid protein; GOR, gastro-oesophageal reflux.

Table 9.4 Investigations to consider in long-standing ataxia

Additional problems	Possible diagnosis	Test
Structural abnormality cerebellum or tumour		
Head tilt Increasing head circumference	Posterior fossa tumour Arnold–Chiari malformation Cerebellar malformations	Brain MRI
Genetic		
Ataxia around 10 years Explosive dysarthric speech Loss of deep tendon reflexes, extensor plantars Weak with pes cavus Loss of vibration sensation Spinal deformity	Friedreich ataxia	Mutation of *FXN* gene – chromosome 9
Spasticity – 3y Dysarthria Telangiectasia – 4y+ Immunodeficiency	Ataxia telangiectasia	Alpha fetoprotein Immunoglobulins Chromosome fragility
Failure to thrive Steatorrhoea Ataxia later childhood Retinitis pigmentosa	Abetalipoproteinaemia	Blood film – acanthocytes Low cholesterol and triglycerides Vitamin E very low
Profound language delay Dysmorphic facial features	Angelman syndrome	Angelman syndrome methylation
Gait but no other problems Champagne calves, pes cavus Family history	Hereditary sensory motor neuropathy	Nerve conduction study Genetics – complex
Nystagmus Dysarthria Ataxia, pyramidal signs Learning difficulties	X-linked spinocerebellar ataxia	Family history Genetic testing
Adolescence/adulthood	Autosomal dominant cerebellar ataxia	Genetics – complex SCA deletions
Episodes of ataxia	Hereditary paroxysmal cerebellar ataxia	Abnormal calcium channel (CACNA1A)
Metabolic		
Adolescence Liver disease Parkinsonism	Wilson disease	Ceruloplasmin
Cystic fibrosis	Vitamin E deficiency	Vitamin E very low

SCA, sickle cell anaemia; CACNA1A, calcium channel, voltage-dependent, P/Q type, alpha 1A subunit.

Table 9.5 Investigations to consider in ataxia with loss of skills

Other features	Diagnosis	Investigation
Genetic		
Normal development in infancy 1–3y loss of skills Microcephaly Hand stereotypies Hyperventilation	Rett syndrome	MLPA – MECP2 deletion
Seizures Unusual fat pads Inverted nipples Failure to thrive	Congenital disorders of glycosylation	Isoelectric focusing MRI – cerebellar hypoplasia
Failure to thrive Heptosplenomegaly Tremor Supranuclear opthalmoplegia, dysarthria Seizures	Neimann–Pick disease	Full blood count – foam cells White cell enzymes
Loss of skills Seizures Cherry red spot	GM2 gangliosidosis	Ophthalmology White cell enzymes
Metabolic		
Muscle weakness Retinitis pigmentosa	Mitochondrial disease – NARP	Lactate – blood and CSF MRI – altered basal ganglia Mitochondrial DNA deletions
Regression Abnormal eye movements Unusual breathing	Mitochondrial disease Leigh syndrome	Lactate – blood and CSF MRI – altered basal ganglia Mitochondrial DNA deletions
Infancy Failure to thrive	Hartnup disease	Urine organic acids
Seizures Optic atrophy Skin rashes	Biotinidase deficiency	Plasma biotinidase
Ichthyosis Night blindness and cataracts Hearing impairment	Refsum disease	Phytanic acid
Difficulty with eye saccades Severe sensorimotor neuropathy Chorea (80%)	Ataxia–oculomotor apraxia	MRI – cerebellar atrophy Hypoalbuminaemia Hypercholesterolaemia
Myoclonic epilepsy	Ramsay Hunt syndrome	

Other features	Diagnosis	Investigation
Infant – nystagmus and hyptonia Develop spasticity later	Pelizaeus–Merzbacher disease	MRI – abnormal white matter changes Visual evoked potentials diminished Mutation *PLP* gene
Ataxia Involuntary movements Optic atrophy	Methylglutaconic aciduria	Metabolic acidosis Urinary organic acids

MLPA, multiplex ligation-dependent probe amplification; MECP2, M-methyl-CpG binding protein 2; MRI, magnetic resonance imaging; NARP, neuropathy, ataxia and retinitis pigmentosa; CSF, cerebrospinal fluid; PLP, proteolipid protein.

Initial management

- Assessment by the child development team is usually indicated if more than two areas of development are affected. Consider feeding issues as part of this.
- Appropriate positioning and seating may improve function significantly.
- Working with the child and family around communication to enable participation will improve the quality of life of both child and family.

> **Key messages**
>
> - Being clear about the movement disorder will help you to arrange appropriate investigations.
> - If you are not clear about the diagnosis or do not have a diagnosis, consider referral to a paediatric neurologist.

10
The child with paroxysmal movement disorder

Gillian Robinson

Case vignette

Adam is a 2-year-old male who suffered significant birth asphyxia and has subsequently developed a four-limb spastic cerebral palsy. His mother is concerned that he may have developed epilepsy as he has episodes when he has an opisthotonic posture, which have become more frequent during a recent upper respiratory tract infection.

Learning points

- While epilepsy is more common in children with cerebral palsy than in typically developing children so are non-epileptic paroxysmal movement disorders.
- Tone in cerebral palsy is increased during intercurrent illness and this may be contributing to Adam's difficulties.
- It is important to take a careful history including precipitants. Adam's episodes were associated with eating, and therefore Sandifer syndrome should be considered.

There are a number of reasons why children with paroxysmal movement disorders are seen by a community paediatrician.

- Children are referred because of concern that they may have a seizure disorder or that this is a marker of a neurological disorder.
- Children are referred because of concerns about their development and associated with this they may have typical movement patterns (e.g. Rett syndrome).
- Children with a known neurological disorder such as cerebral palsy are more likely to have paroxysmal movement disorders and also seizures.

It is important to correctly identify paroxysmal disorders to be able to give appropriate advice and, if needed, treatment. In order to be able to diagnose these conditions you need to be aware of the key symptoms.

Disorders characteristically starting in infancy

Non-epileptic disorders

NEONATAL JITTERS

These are fine tremulous movements of the jaw or limbs in term-born infants, which can be prolonged. They are triggered by light or sudden noise but are not associated with eye deviation or cardiovascular signs. They are associated with hypoxic encephalopathy and drug withdrawal. This is a benign disorder and usually resolves by 7 months.

HYPOXIC–ISCHAEMIC ENCEPHALOPATHY

Hypoxic–ischaemic encephalopathy affects infants who suffer birth asphyxia and have altered consciousness level within hours of birth. In addition, in affected infants tremor is triggered by stimuli such as sound and also multifocal segmental myoclonus; they may also have epileptic seizures, which may be subtle and difficult to diagnose.

BENIGN NEONATAL SLEEP MYOCLONUS

In infants affected by benign neonatal sleep myoclonus, myoclonic jerks in the limbs develop within a few days of birth. They occur only during sleep and stop immediately on wakening. The prognosis is good.

HYPEREKPLEXIA

In this condition the infants have a pronounced and repetitive startle without habituation in response to touch or sound. This can be tested for by tapping the bridge of the nose of the infant, which leads to a startle response that does not habituate. It is present from birth and the infant is generally hypertonic; there may also be a family history. Development is usually normal but the condition can be severe and interfere with activity, in which case treatment with clonazepam can be helpful.

PAROXYSMAL EXTREME PAIN DISORDER

This is an autosomal dominant disorder with onset in infancy and presents with episodes of extreme pain that can be either ano-rectal (associated with defecation), ocular or jaw. These episodes of pain can last minutes or hours, during which the child is terrified and inconsolable. Usually the symptoms improve in early childhood. Carbamazepine may help some children.

Epileptic seizures

Seizures can be subtle and difficult to diagnose in infancy. They should be considered if an infant has movements that tend to have the same repeated pattern, particularly if there is an alteration in cardiorespiratory parameters.

Disorders starting in early childhood

Non-epileptic

REPETITIVE SLEEP STARTS

These are brief body jerks, often bilateral, that coincide with the onset of sleep. They are seen in 60% of the population.

BENIGN MYOCLONUS OF EARLY INFANCY

These occur in healthy children towards the end of the first year of life and remit by the age of 3 years. They are repetitive jerks of the neck or upper limbs, leading to flexion or rotation of the neck and extension with abduction of limbs. They occur in clusters when the child is awake, separated by 3 to 4 minutes. The prognosis is good.

SHUDDERING

Shuddering is brief shuddering movements of the head, shoulders and arms. During an episode the child's neck is flexed and the arms flexed and abducted. Episodes can last 5 to 15 seconds, and can be very common. They do not cause distress or alteration of consciousness. The prognosis is good.

STOOL WITHHOLDING

Stool withholding is seen in children who are constipated or soiling. The episodes are painful (abdomen or anus) and lead to a distinct posture with back arching. Children will respond well to treatment of the underlying constipation.

INFANTILE MASTURBATION/GRATIFICATION

Around 90% of males and 50% of females will masturbate at some point in their life. Female infants are more likely to masturbate than males. It often occurs when the child is sitting in a seat with straps across the groin. The females can be seen posturing with rocking motion and in association with this there is grunting and flushing. These episodes can last minutes to hours and can be repeated many times. There is no loss of consciousness.

TONIC REFLEX SEIZURE OF EARLY INFANCY

These episodes can occur in healthy infants in the second to third month of life. Affected infants present with a tonic contraction of all four limbs which may be accompanied by brief apnoea lasting 3–10 seconds. They are precipitated by an upright rhythmical movement (e.g. being held and carried downstairs).

ALTERNATING HEMIPLEGIA OF CHILDHOOD

This is a rare disorder which starts before the age of 18 months. It presents with repeated attacks of alternating hemiplegia which occur approximately weekly. The hemiplegia is resolved by sleep but symptoms recur 10 to 20 minutes after wakening during an episode.

OCULOGYRIC CRISES IN INFANTS

These are episodes of conjugate eye deviation. They can be due to inborn error of dopamine metabolism, in which case infants have increased limb tone and myopathic facies. Affected children respond well to levodopa treatment. The episodes can also be precipitated by drugs, classically neuroleptics and metoclopramide.

Epileptic

INFANTILE SPASMS

Infantile spasms are episodes of lightening flexion of the trunk with arms extended or flexed (salaam) that occur in runs. The spasms usually occur when ths child is falling to sleep or waking and can be associated with eye deviation. The child often cries at the end of the seizure. In most cases the child's development either regresses or is static.

Disorders not closely linked with age

Non-epileptic

BREATH-HOLDING SPELLS

Breath-holding spells occur in preschool children. They are often precipitated by minor trauma or anger, which leads to a prolonged cry and then silence as the child becomes cyanosed with the mouth open. This can be followed by loss of consciousness and anoxic seizure with opisthotonic posture and flexion of limbs lasting several seconds. These episodes are involuntary and not a marker of an overindulged child. They usually stop by the age of 5 years and they have a good outcome.

REFLEX ANOXIC SEIZURES

Reflex anoxic seizures occur in preschool children. There is usually an obvious trigger such as a sudden unpleasant event. Initially, the child looks shocked and may grunt but not cry; then the child becomes grey and stiff or opisthotonic, during which time there may be irregular limb jerks. This lasts seconds and then the child comes around or goes into post-ictal sleep (ECG would show asystole). These are involuntary episodes but they can make disciplining the child difficult. They usually stop by the age of 5 years.

VASOVAGAL SYNCOPE

In vasovagal syncope there is often a clear precipitant such as prolonged standing or an unpleasant event. The child will describe a blurring out of vision and distortion of sound. An observer will see the child change colour, become pale and 'crumple'. This may be followed by extensor spasms or jerks. The eyes usually open but are not deviated. The child recovers quickly but can be left with a feeling of fatigue.

> **Red flag**
>
> A cardiac cause of collapse is more likely if the collapse occurs with exercise, on entering water or on 'emotional exertion'.

CARDIAC SYNCOPE

In cardiac syncope the episode is similar to vasovagal episodes but occurs during exercise, emotional response or sleep. There can be a family history of sudden unexplained death. These children require a cardiology assessment including exercise electrocardiography.

DAY DREAMING

This is when a child focuses on their internal thoughts rather than on events in their environment. Episodes are more likely when the child is bored rather than occupied. The child appears vacant but episodes can be terminated by calling the child's name.

EPISODIC ATAXIA

This is an autosomal dominant channelopathy which causes disturbed cerebellar function. It presents with episodes of ataxia and dysarthria which can last seconds to minutes. These episodes can occur a number of times a day. They can be precipitated by illness, anxiety or sudden movement. At rest myokymia (rippling of muscle) can be present.

PAROXYSMAL DYSKINESIA

These are episodes of abnormal movements that can last seconds to hours depending on the subgroup. They can be precipitated by anxiety, movement and sleep. There is no loss of consciousness.

PAROXYSMAL TORTICOLLIS

These episodes usually occur in infancy. They present with an abrupt onset of head tilting to one side with associated vomiting, pallor and agitation which can last minutes to days. There are no associated eye signs.

PAROXYSMAL VERTIGO

Paroxysmal vertigo is recurrent episodes of sudden vertigo which last minutes and are associated with nausea. There is no impairment of consciousness. It is considered to be a variant of migraine.

NARCOLEPSY

Narcolepsy is a condition in which there is excessive daytime sleepiness, with poor night-time sleep. Onset is typically during teenage years. It can be associated with cataplexy, in which the child collapses when he or she laughs.

HYSTERICAL EPISODES OR PSEUDO-SEIZURE

These events often occur when many people are around. The child will groan or shout for the whole duration of the seizure and often there are movements on both sides of body without loss of consciousness. Recovery is rapid but the child is disorientated afterwards (unlike true seizure, when the child may be drowsy but is orientated).

STEREOTYPIES

These are involuntary movements that are repetitive and purposeless (such as hand flapping, body rocking or head banging) lasting for at least 4 weeks. The movements interfere with normal activity and may have the potential to cause bodily harm. They increase during times of stress, frustration, excitement and boredom.

TICS

Tics are rapid, repetitive, involuntary contractions of a group of muscles. They can either be

- motor tics such as facial twitching, grimacing, blinking or shoulder shrugging
- vocal tics such as coughing, grunting, clearing the throat or sniffing.

Some people with tics may be able to suppress (control) a tic for a short period of time, but it leads to a feeling of increasing tension until the tic is finally released. Tics tend to wax and wane. They are worse when the child is anxious, stressed or tired (Chapter 18, p. 221).

Epilepsy

Generalized seizures

Generalized seizures are conceptualized as originating at a point and then rapidly spreading to both cerebral hemispheres.

- **Tonic seizures** cause a period of sustained muscle contraction.
- **Atonic seizures** cause a loss of muscle tone. These are usually brief.
- **Clonic seizures** are regularly repeating muscle contractions, typically at a rate of two or three per second.
- **Absence seizures** involve an interruption to consciousness during which the person experiencing the seizure seems to become vacant and unresponsive for a short period of time (usually up to 30 seconds). The person may have simple motor movements such as lip smacking.
- **Myoclonic seizures** involve an extremely brief (<0.1s) muscle contraction and can result in jerky movements of muscles or muscle groups.
- **Tonic–clonic seizures** involve an initial contraction of the muscles (tonic phase) which may involve tongue biting, urinary incontinence and the absence of breathing. This is followed by rhythmic muscle contractions (clonic phase).

Focal seizure

Focal seizures are conceptualized as originating at a specific point, with the epileptic activity being limited to that area.

- **Frontal lobe seizures** cause repeated episodes of abnormal body posturing, or repeated movements such as pedalling or pelvic thrusting. These movements are often similar in each episode. In rare cases the child may laugh uncontrollably or cry during a seizure. The child may not be aware of this episode and it can be followed by a brief period of post-ictal confusion. Often these seizures arise during sleep.
- **Temporal lobe seizures** cause the child to have odd feelings, most commonly an episode when he or she flushes, sweats or has a churning feeling in his or her stomach. But there can also be other unusual feelings such as euphoria, fear, panic and déjà vu. The child may be aware of the seizure or lose consciousness during these episodes. There may be simple movements during the seizure such as lip smacking or repeated hand movements.
- **Occipital lobe seizures** usually start with visual hallucinations such as flickering or coloured balls of light or brief periods of loss of vision.
- **Parietal lobe seizures** are unusual; they cause the child to have strange physical feelings such as a tingling or warm feeling down one side of their body.

Clinical approach to paroxysmal episodes (see Fig. 10.1)

Key questions

- What is the nature of the episode?
  - Obtain child and eye-witness accounts.
  - What was the child doing prior to the episode?; was there any precipitant?
  - What happened first?
  - Which parts of the body were affected?
  - Was there loss of consciousness?
  - What was the duration of the seizure?
  - How did the episode end?
  - What was the child like afterwards, and how long did it take for the child to recover?
  - What is the frequency of the seizures?
- What is the child's current general health?
  - Include, if appropriate, the child's bowel habit.
- Are there any clues to an underlying cause?
  - History
    - Past history (e.g. cerebral palsy, see Table 10.1)
    - Medications
    - Family history
  - Examination
    - Growth parameters including head circumference
    - Any dysmorphic features and neurocutaneous markers
    - Neurological examination
    - Cardiovascular examination for structural abnormalities

Investigations

- Consider 12-lead electrocardiography or exercise electrocardiography if the episodes occur during exercise.
- Ask the family to video the episode.
- Consider
  - electroencephalography – standard and sleep;
  - videotelemetry;
  - pH studies.

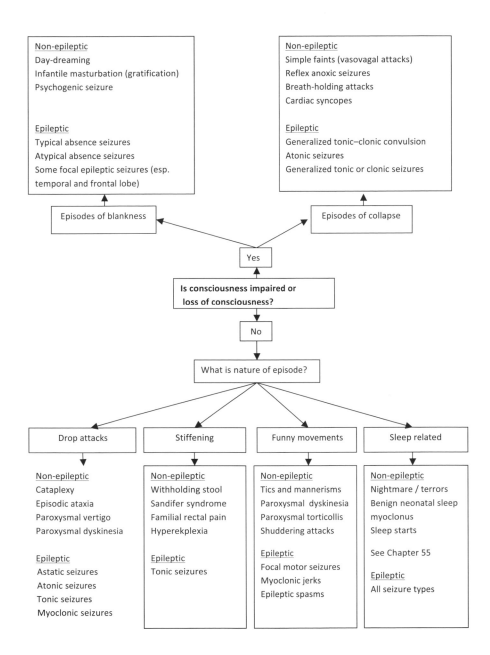

Figure 10.1 Flow chart for paroxysmal movement disorders.

Table 10.1 Cerebral palsy and non-epileptic paroxysmal episodes

Disorder	Clinical features
Dystonia	Abnormal movements precipitated by pain, sudden environmental stimuli
Muscle spasm	Precipitated by environmental stimuli such as noise or sudden movment and also pain
Sandifer syndrome	Episodes of opisthotonus or writhing related to eating
Myoclonus	Precipated by light, touch or sound
Gratification phenomena	Situational – boredom
Breath-holding	Provoked by pain
Reflex anoxic seizure	Triggered by startle or pain
Sleep starts	On settling to sleep
Obstructive sleep apnoea	History suggesting airway obstruction
Seizures	Both focal and generalized seizures more common (47% hemiplegia, 27% diplegia, 50% quadriplegia, 25% dyskinetic cerebral palsy)

Key messages

- If you are not sure of the diagnosis, the evidence suggests that it is probably not epilepsy – find out more information from seizure diaries and videos.
- An eye-witness account is key to making a diagnosis. If there is not an eye-witness in the clinic then ask if you can phone someone who has seen an episode.
- Characteristics of the seizures:
  - random occurrence;
  - precipitants rare with the exception of photosensitive epilepsy;
  - stereotyped – each event being similar to previous events.

11
Scoliosis

Gillian Robinson

Case vignette

Caroline is an 11-year-old female who has moved up to high school and is struggling. Her mother tells you that she is lazy and it is very difficult to get her out of bed in the morning. Caroline tells you that her chief difficulty is moving between classes and she has been pushed over on the stairs on a number of occasions. She is very reluctant to be examined and after removing a baggy jumper you see she has a thoracic scoliosis.

Learning points

- Teenage years are the classic time for idiopathic scoliosis to present; remember this is a diagnosis of exclusion.
- Cardiorespiratory difficulties can present with symptoms of overnight hypoventilation and this needs further assessment if present; it also makes an underlying cause more likely.

There are two roles for a paediatrician when seeing a child with a scoliosis. The first is to consider the underlying cause of the scoliosis and if there are any secondary consequences (Table 11.1). The second role is to refer the child on to an appropriate spinal surgeon. Spinal surgery is now organized into centres to ensure that expertise is maintained.

Table 11.1 Differential diagnosis of scoliosis

Group	Problem	Example
Apparent	Leg length discrepancy	
Idiopathic	Congenital Later onset	
Neurological	Cerebrum	Cerebral palsy Tumour
	Spinocerebellar	Friedreich ataxia Spinal cord tumour
	Anterior horn cell	Spinal muscular atrophy
	Peripheral neuropathies	Hereditary sensory motor neuropathy
Muscle	Dystrophy	Duchenne muscular dystrophy Myotonic dystrophy
	Myopathy	Mitochondrial myopathy Minicore myopathy
Bony or ligamentous	Congenital bony malformations	Spina bifida Hemivertebrae
	Marfan syndrome	
	Neurofibromatosis	

Key questions

History

- What are the present difficulties?
  - How long has the scoliosis been noted for and is it progressing?
  - Is the child in any pain?
  - Has there been any weakness, clumsiness or frequent falls?
  - Has there been any loss of sensation or unusual sensation?
  - Has the child experienced any bladder or bowel difficulties?
- Are there any secondary complications? (cardiorespiratory compromise)
  - Are there any symptoms of nocturnal hypoventilation such as
    - morning headache;
    - slowness to wake;
    - daytime somnolence?
- Is there any underlying diagnosis?
  - Was there any scoliosis, dimples, pits or hairy tufts noted at birth?
  - Examine the child's past medical history.
  - Look for any previous surgery, in particular thoracotomy or ventriculoperitoneal shunt.
  - Examine the developmental history, particularly motor development.
  - Is there any family history of neuromuscular disorders or tuberculosis?

Examination of the scoliosis

- Look
  - Is there dimpling or hair tufts?
  - What is the site and side of convexity of the curve?
  - Has the curve affected the scapulae and shoulder?
- Feel
  - Is there any spinal tenderness on percussion?
  - Examine the child while putting gentle upwards traction in the child's armpits to see if the scoliosis is correctable (i.e. positional rather than fixed).
- Move
  - Examine the child as he or she is sitting, standing and bending forward (ask the child to touch his or her toes and look at both the spine and for rib hump).
  - Is this real or apparent scoliosis? An apparent scoliosis is caused by leg shortening and this is easy to spot on clinical examination as the curve resolves when the child sits down.

Examination for underlying cause

- General examination
  - Look at the skin for signs of neurofibromatosis.
  - Are there any dysmorphic features which could indicate Marfan, Turner or Noonan syndrome?
  - Does the child have myopathic facies: an expressionless face with open mouth?
- Legs (including feet)
  - Are there any abnormalities such as champagne legs and pes cavus as in hereditary sensory motor neuropathy or Friedreich ataxia?
  - Is there any discrepancy in leg length?
  - Are there any scars, muscle wasting or contractures?
  - Feet: look for asymmetrical foot size or any deformity.
- Neurological examination
  - Power – include, if appropriate, the Gower manoeuvre
  - Coordination
  - Examination for anal tone
  - Sensation, including vibration sensation in lower limbs
  - Gait
- Cardiorespiratory examination

Investigations for the severity of the scoliosis

- Radiography: posteroanterior and lateral.
- Cardiorespiratory compromise.
  - Forced vital capacity.
  - Overnight saturation monitoring if a forced vital capacity of less than 40% is predicted.

Investigations into the underlying cause are guided by the examination and may include the following (see Table 11.2):

Table 11.2 Potential causes of scoliosis

Clinical clue	Diagnosis	Test
No other clinical signs	Idiopathic (80%)	By exclusion, largely on clinical and radiological examination
	Bony abnormality	Seen on radiography to assess curvature
Dysmorphic features	Neurofibromatosis	Diagnosis on clinical criteria
	Marfan syndrome	Diagnosis on clinical criteria
	Turner syndrome	Chromosomes
Upper motor neurone signs	Cerebral palsy Tumour	Brain MRI
Lower motor neurone signs	Spina bifida Spinal tumour	Image spine
	Spinal muscular atrophy	SMN deletion
	Hereditary sensory motor neuropathy	EMG ± genetic testing
Muscular weakness	Creatine kinase Neurology opinion	Muscular dystrophy
	Lactate	Mitochondrial myopathy
	DMPK	Myotonic dystrophy

MRI, magnetic resonance imaging; SMN, survival motor neurone; EMG, electromyography; DMPK, dystrophia myotonica protein kinase.

- head and spine MRI
- creatinine kinase test
- electromyography/nerve conduction studies
- Tensilon test.

Management

- Ensure that primary vaccinations are complete and vaccinate the child against pneumococcus and influenza.
- Refer the child to a spinal surgeon for curves of greater than 20 degrees, or for progressing curves.
- Refer the child to a paediatric neurologist if there are neuromuscular signs (opinion plus muscle biopsy/molecular genetics).
- The child should also be referred to cardiology if there are signs of cardiorespiratory compromise.
- Ensure that the school is aware of the physical limitations of the child by contacting either the school directly or the school medical service.

12
The clumsy child

Gillian Robinson

Case vignette

Philip is a 7-year-old who is an able reader, but who has poor written work. He was born at 26 weeks, but had an unremarkable neonatal course. He gets into trouble at school as he is always fidgeting. He is becoming increasingly reluctant to join in play-time games and refuses to go to any out-of-school activities.

Learning points

- Comorbidities are common in children with coordination difficulties and these need to be screened for: attention difficulties, autistic spectrum difficulties and dyslexia.
- Children with coordination difficulties may have low self-esteem. Working with children, particularly in groups of children, with similar difficulties can help.
- The child's coordination will improve with time and practice.
- Children who were born preterm have an increased risk of coordination and attention difficulties.

In this chapter we will consider the differential diagnosis of a child presenting with clumsiness (Table 12.1) and provide a framework for history taking, assessment (Fig. 12.1) and management (Fig 12.2) of any child with coordination difficulties.

Table 12.1 Differential diagnosis for a clumsy child

	Subgroup	Example
Neurological disorder	Upper motor neurone	Cerebral palsy Tumour Stroke Trauma Treated hydrocephalus
	Cerebellar	See causes of ataxia (Tables 9.4 and 9.5)
	Peripheral	Hereditary sensory motor neuropathy
Muscle disorder	Myopathy	Minicore myopathy Mitochondrial myopathy
	Dystrophy	Duchenne – early stages Becker
Connective tissue disorder		Ehlers–Danlos syndrome Hypermobility syndrome
Sensory impairment	Visual impairment Vestibular disorders	
General learning difficulty	Motor skills in line with overall learning	
Attention and planning		Born preterm Fetal alcohol syndrome Autistic spectrum disorder Attention-deficit–hyperactivity disorder
Developmental coordination disorder		

Key questions on clinical assessment

- Does the child have motor problems or is he or she a 'bull in a china shop', lacking planning and thought?
  - Does the child have problems with gross motor skills including running, jumping, climbing stairs, ball skills, riding a bike and swimming?
  - Does the child have problems with fine motor skills including handwriting, building and jigsaws?
  - Can the child carry out activities of daily living including
    - dressing – zips, buttons, laces;
    - using knife and fork;
    - organizing skills – packing bag for school?

- Is there any history suggesting a neuromuscular cause?
  - Are there any pre-, peri- or postnatal problems that may have led to a brain injury?
  - Is there a past medical history of neuromuscular problems?
  - Has there been any loss of skills?
  - Is there a family history of neurological disorder?
- What is the overall level of learning?
  - Discuss the child with his or her school or perform a developmental assessment for children who are of preschool age.
- Are there any concerns about vision?
- Is there any history suggesting comorbidities?
  - Are there behaviour problems with concentration, impulsivity or distractibility; can the child sit still?
  - Are there problems with social interaction: relationship with peers, repetitive interests? Again, a discussion with school will quickly highlight any difficulties.
- Are there any examination findings that suggest an underlying cause?
  - Are there any neuromuscular signs?
  - Is there any evidence of joint hypermobility?
- General
  - Head circumference (micro- or macrocephaly)
  - Dysmorphic or myopathic features
  - Involuntary movements
  - Nystagmus
- Neurological examination
  - Look for asymmetry
  - Tone (if altered consider cerebral palsy)
  - Power (myopathy)
  - Coordination
    - Dysdiadochokinesia, finger tapping (cerebellar)
    - Stand with feet together (test for cerebellar difficulties)
    - Feet together, eyes closed (dorsal column or peripheral neuropathy)
    - Balance – stand single leg
  - Sensation – light touch, pinprick and proprioception
  - Deep tendon reflexes
  - Gower sign
  - Fogs' test
- Range of joint movements – hypermobility tests such as Beighton criteria
- Did you notice any difficulties with social communication or attention during your assessment?

Age (y)	Paper and pencil	Standing	Ball skills (tennis ball)
4	Draw + Person – 3 parts	Stand on one foot for 3s	Throw ball with direction to person 1.5m away
5	Draw △ Write first name	Hop five times	Catch a ball with two hands Throw from 1.5m away (can use body to trap ball)
6	Draw ✳ Write first and last name	Stand on one foot for 10s	Catch a tennis ball thrown from 1.5m away (cannot use body to trap ball)
7	Draw ⊛ Draw a person – 8 parts	Skip forward for 6m	Bounce and catch ball with two hands
8	Draw ◇ Copy 'The quick brown fox jumps over the lazy dog'	Stand on one foot for 20s	Bounce and catch ball with one hand
9	Draw ⬠ Copy 'The quick brown fox jumps over the lazy dog' in 30s	Hop forward five times, stop and balance on foot for 5s	Throw tennis ball at wall from 1.5m and catch with two hands before it bounces
Note	Is head close to paper? Immature grasp? Failure to stabilize paper with non-dominant hand Inappropriate force Rotates body to paper	Looks at feet Exaggerated arm movements Lacks rhythm in hop Heavy or flat footed landing Holds body rigid	Throwing Can adjust body position Poor aim Poor judge of force required Catching Turns away or flinches Arms do not 'give' Positions self incorrectly

Figure 12.1 Assessment of the clumsy child.

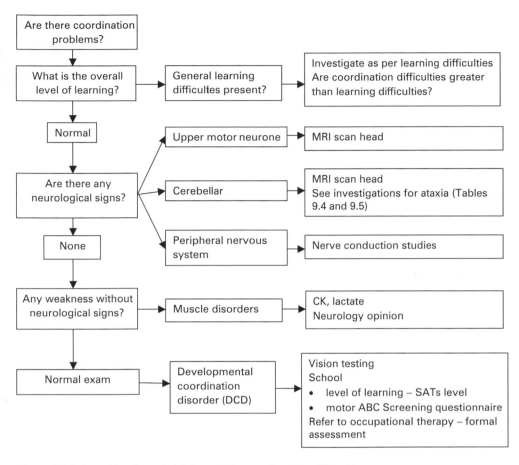

Figure 12.2 Investigation of children with coordination difficulties.

Key messages

- The medical examination needs to exclude neuromuscular disorders as a cause of the child's difficulties.
- If the difficulties are asymmetrical or there is progression then there is an underlying medical cause and the child should not be given a label of developmental coordination disorder.
- If the child has a global developmental delay then his or her motor skills will be in line with intellectual functioning.
- Look for comorbidities or you may not address the child's key difficulty.

Further reading

Aicardi J (2009) *Diseases of the Nervous System in Childhood*, 3rd Edition. London: Mac Keith Press.

Bax M, Gillberg C (2010) *Comorbidities in Developmental Disorders: Clinics in Developmental Medicine No 187*. London: Mac Keith Press.

Fernandez-Alvarez E, Aicardi J (2001) *Movement Disorders in Children*. London: Mac Keith Press.

Ferrie CD, Stephenson J. (2010) Special issue: non-epileptic paroxysmal disorders. *J Ped Neurol* 8: 1–125.

Gibbs J, Appleton A, Appleton. (2007) Dyspraxia or developmental coordination disorder? Unravelling the enigma. *Arch Dis Child* 92: 534–9. http://dx.doi.org/10.1136/adc.2005.088054

Gupta R, Appleton RE (2001) Cerebral palsy: not always what it seems. *Arch Dis Child* 85: 356–60. http://dx.doi.org/10.1136/adc.85.5.356

King M, Stephenson JP (2009) *A Handbook of Neurological Investigations in Children*. London: Mac Keith Press.

Lisi EC, Cohn RD (2011) Genetic evaluation of the paediatric patient with hypotonia: perspective from a hypotonia speciality clinic and review of the literature. *Dev Med Child Neurol* 53: 586–99. http://dx.doi.org/10.1111/j.1469-8749.2011.03918.x

Missiuna C, Gaines R, Soucie H (2006) Why every office needs a tennis ball: a new approach to assessing the clumsy child. *CMAJ* 175: 471–3. http://dx.doi.org/10.1503/cmaj.051202

Sanger T, Delgado MR, G Gaebler-Spira D, Hallett H, Mink JW (2003) Classification and definition of disorders causing hypertonia in childhood. *Pediatrics* 111: e89. http://dx.doi.org/10.1542/peds.111.1.e89

Section 5

Communication

13
Communication disorders

Anne M Kelly and Joanne Sandiford

Learning objectives

- To understand the current classification of communication disorders and its limitations.
- To know how to assess and manage communication disorders with the multidisciplinary team.
- To build an awareness of alternative and augmentative communication and the advancing role of computer-assisted technology.

The term 'speech, language and communication needs' is now often used to recognize the breadth of difficulties encompassed in this area. Language is the most complex and fragile of the developmental systems. Whatever the developmental difficulty, language is most often affected. It is inherently difficult to break down this complex, interactive process into its component parts, but we can attempt to do so in order to understand the possible difficulties (Fig. 13.1).

- 'Speech' refers to the actual ability to organize and articulate speech sounds.
- 'Language' needs to be broken down into receptive and expressive language. The receptive side of language is the ability to decode the words, grammatical structures and inherent meaning of the phrase in context. Expressive language refers to the thought process of having an idea to convey, organizing the words to do so, sequencing them into the correct syntactic order and employing the speech system to audibly produce those words.
- 'Communication' encompasses 'speech' and 'language' and also relates to the understanding of and ability to interact with people, as well as the understanding and use of non-verbal communication skills and metalinguistic features such as intonation, volume and rhythm.

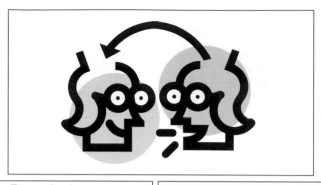

Receptive language	**Expressive language**
• decode the words	• wishing to convey an idea
• understand the grammar	• organizing words
• be aware of context	• sequencing them (syntax)
• interpret rate and rhythm	• articulating sound (speech)

Non-verbal communication
Eye contact
Facial expression
Gesture

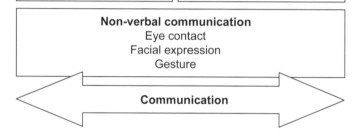

Communication

Figure 13.1 Essentials of communication.

Impaired language development

The incidence of communication problems in the school-age population is rated as high as 1 in 10 children.

It is difficult to apply a specific label to many children's language difficulties. There is a spectrum of competence ranging from, at one end, highly articulate children who talk early to, at the other end, those who have significant difficulties learning one or more aspects of language. Some may never learn to speak at all. There is a large number of children in the middle for whom it is not easy to decide the precise cause of their difficulties.

The causes fall into several broad categories:

- *Delayed language*, in which the child's language appears to be developing along normal lines but at a slower rate than expected or predicted from his or her intellectual ability. It implies that the child will 'close the gap'. Some delays may resolve with time but a more severe delay can represent a more persistent problem that might require intervention and could lead to lifelong difficulties. It is not always possible to predict the outcome at the initial presentation. Parents should not be told that 'delay' always means that their child will catch up.

- *Disordered language*, in which language acquisition is not following a normal pattern. This means that the various components of language – sounds, sentence construction and social communication – are misaligned with each other. On assessing children, their profile will be patchy, showing areas of strength and weakness. Outcomes are difficult to predict and can be more positive than for those with delay.
- *Disordered speech.*
- *Social communication disorders.*
- *Dysfluency.*

Communication disorders

There is no completely consistent classification of communication disorders as many children have difficulties that overlap several categories. If children who have an obvious cause (such as cleft palate, deafness, cerebral palsy or severe learning disability) for their communication problem are excluded, a proportion of children remain with problems that are thought to have a developmental origin. This implies that the biological and environmental processes for language development have faltered in some way.

Patterns of speech, language and communication impairments

- Specific language impairment (SLI)
  - Problems with language, and/or comprehension or expression, with no identifiable explanation.
- Impaired speech production
  - Impaired neuromuscular control of speech apparatus
  - Oropharyngeal structural causes
  - Stammering
  - Selective mutism
- Impaired language development and social interaction (pervasive developmental disorders)
  - Speech and language delay is the most common presentation of autistic spectrum disorder.
- Children who stop talking

Differential diagnosis of delayed language

- Learning difficulties
  - Delayed speech and language may be the most obvious marker of a general developmental delay. If this is the case, the severity of language delay should be in keeping with the degree of delay in other areas of development.
- Neurological disorders
  - Affecting overall development.
  - Specific damage to Broca's area, the area of the brain responsible for language development. This is more so for children with an acquired brain injury.
- Hearing impairment
  - Hearing impairment will lead to impaired speech development. All children with speech and language delay therefore require a hearing assessment.
- Environment
  - A lack of input may lead to delay, particularly in children who are linguistically vulnerable. Other signs of neglect may be present.

Clinical assessment of a child with a language difficulty

- Key questions
  - Is there any evidence for an underlying neurological disorder?
  - Does the child have solely a language problem or is this a marker of a more general learning disability?
  - Does the child have any dysmorphic features or malformation in other systems?
  - Is the difficulty specifically involving comprehension, expression or both?
  - Is there any evidence of rituals or routines?
- Assessment
  - Language
  - Early communication skills
    - Smiling
    - Babbling
    - Turn taking
    - Eye contact and facial expression
    - Use of pointing
  - Comprehension – see Chapter 4.
  - Expression and oral motor development – see Chapter 4.
- Feeding
- Development
  - How is the child's development in other areas?
  - Has there been any loss of skills?

- Past medical history
  - Genetic diagnoses
  - Other major malformations
  - Seizures
- Family history
  - Developmental or language delay
  - Learning difficulties – it may be helpful to ask if anyone in the family has attended special school
  - Hearing impairment
- Social history
  - Early life experiences, particularly neglect and maternal mental health difficulties
  - Language spoken at home
  - Involvement with play group and nursery session
- Examination
  - General
    - Growth parameters
    - Dysmorphic features
  - Head and neck
    - Tongue shows macroglossia such as in Down syndrome, Hurler syndrome and Beckwith syndrome
    - Malocclusion of jaw; micrognathia
  - Ear, nose and throat examination
    - Any cleft palate or submucous cleft?
    - Any adenotonsillar hypertrophy?
    - Are there any abnormalities of dentition?
  - Neurological examination
    - A full cranial nerve assessment including palatal movement
    - Reflexes including assessment of the jaw jerk
    - Coordination (dyspraxia) – ask the child to imitate licking, chewing movements, sucking, blowing, whistling, tongue protrusion and repetition of syllables

Language assessment

Chapter 4 has suggestions about how to approach this. You should certainly comment on

- use of eye contact, facial expression and gesture
- comprehension
- expression, including whether there are difficulties with articulation.

If you have concerns then a speech and language therapy assessment will be helpful.

Speech and language therapists assess:

- Concentration – some children with language difficulties have very poor concentration and flit from one activity to another.
- Non-verbal communication – use of eye contact, facial expression and gesture.
- Inner language – does the child understand that miniature toys and pictures represent real objects as evidenced through pretend play?
- Comprehension – can be assessed by asking the child to follow two-part instructions (e.g. 'Put the *spoon* in the *cup'* and progressing onto three and more objects, negatives, etc.).
- Expression – can the child name objects in picture books and tell a story from pictures?
- Articulation – some sounds are naturally acquired later than others.
- Syntactic difficulties – this relates to grammar and word order.
- Semantic difficulties – this refers to vocabulary and word meaning.
- Pragmatic difficulties – social use of language including taking turns and empathy.

Feeding assessment

Children with swallowing/feeding difficulties may require a feeding-trained speech and language therapist to carry out a clinical assessment (Table 13.1) of feeding and upper airway auscultation. They may feel that further assessment with *video-fluoroscopy* could be helpful, particularly if there is a history of coughing on feeding and recurrent chest infections.

Investigation of communication disorders

Most children with speech and language problems are managed outside the child development centre (CDC), in the community, where they may be seen and assessed by a speech and language therapist. A referral to a paediatrician is necessary only if the child has more severe or complex difficulties that are likely to be longer lasting or if there may be an underlying cause for the communication difficulty that requires investigation. Children with other difficulties co-occurring with communication problems are also likely to require input from the CDC.

Investigations

- *Every child with a significant speech and language delay should have a hearing test.*
- If a male is generally clumsy, is late to walk or has difficulty climbing stairs as well as speech and language delay, then Duchenne muscular dystrophy needs to be excluded. Serum *creatine phosphokinase* levels should be measured and, if raised, further investigation will be needed including genetic screening for survival motor neurone.
- An *electroencephalogram* (EEG) should be considered for any child with definite regression in speech and language, especially if preceded by a history of behavioural difficulties and/or seizures.

Table 13.1 Signs in children with neurological disorders and language difficulties

Category	Example	Clinical features
Upper motor neurone	Four-limb spastic cerebral palsy	Hypertonia and hyperreflexia affecting all four limbs Slow laborious speech May have significant learning difficulties, which may significantly contribute to speech and language delay
	Dystonic cerebral palsy	Dysarthric speech Marked dystonic movements Learning may not be as significantly affected
Lower motor neurone	Moebius syndrome	Congenital facial nerve palsy with bilateral external rectus muscle palsy
	Recurrent laryngeal nerve palsy	Hoarse voice, but often no other deficit
Muscular disorders	Myotonic dystrophy	Expressionless face

- In some children the delay in speech and language is a marker of a global developmental delay (see section on generalised developmental impairment/learning disability, Chapter 14).
- Other investigations are worth considering only if there are other neurological symptoms or signs or other factors such as epilepsy or a history of regression.

In the multidisciplinary team context, it is useful for children presenting with communication difficulties to be assessed by a speech and language therapist, clinical psychologist and occupational therapist. The speech and language therapist will offer a detailed assessment of communication and feeding skills; the clinical psychologist will assess cognitive levels, which is necessary if considering a diagnosis of SLI; and the occupational therapist will look at fine motor and functional hand movement skills and provide an assessment of their sensory processing that is often delayed alongside language skills.

Specific language impairments

Specific language impairments are thought of as *primary* language difficulties and are *specific* to language with no other major contributory factors. They are diagnosed by the exclusion of other potential causes.

- Language skills are two standard deviations below the mean for child's age (third centile).
- Language skills are one standard deviation below non-verbal IQ.
- There are no neurological, sensory or physical impairments that directly affect the use of spoken language.
- There is an absence of pervasive developmental disorder (PDD).

The exact prevalence of this group of disorders is not known, as there is disagreement about the definition of an SLI in relation to levels of cognitive ability. Between 3% and 8% of children perform below the third centile on formal tests of their language skills, depending on their age, the test used and the sample tested.

This does not imply that they require intervention or, conversely, that those children whose language scores are above this level have necessarily normal language development. SLI diagnosis implies a discrepancy between the child's language abilities and his or her non-verbal IQ performance, but this difference should not be greater than one standard deviation, as a larger difference would suggest that learning difficulties are more likely.

Children with an SLI usually have an atypical developmental profile and it can be difficult to predict their prognosis. Although their problems may resolve by school entry age, those with severe speech and language difficulties that persist beyond the age of 4 years are highly likely to have literacy difficulties. Some children require placement in a specialist language unit and some may require further support with literacy in high school. A very small proportion of children have such severe difficulties that they may never acquire socially useful speech, in which case an alternative means of communication such as signing will be required.

Subtypes of specific language impairments

Receptive language difficulties (comprehension difficulties)

Case vignette

Eddie was referred to the CDC team aged 2 years 6 months, with a history of late walking (23mo), delayed fine motor skills, limited attention and no spoken language. His parents thought he understood them. Assessment showed that Eddie did not comprehend any spoken language but was using environmental cues, for example when he saw his mother fetching her car key, he would fetch his shoes. His cognitive skills were at the low end of normal for his age. A standard battery of tests for developmental delay showed nothing causative. He went on to develop some understanding of single words and expressive babble but no single words by 3.5 years.

Learning points

- Eddie's assessment showed a distinct discrepancy between non-verbal and verbal skills, and therefore he fulfilled the criteria for specific language impairment. When talking about prognosis it is important to consider if there are delayed skills in other areas, as if so there is a high chance of future learning difficulties.
- Children with receptive language difficulties struggle to understand the spoken word, and cannot retain and process spoken language. These children may be socially 'tuned out' and unresponsive or may be desperately seeking clues from their environment to help them understand what is happening around them, i.e. trying to read gestures and facial expressions to cue them in. Detailed assessment is needed to identify the areas of difficulty, for example assessment that is specific to verbs or concepts such as prepositions.

Expressive language difficulties

> ## Case vignette
>
> Fay is 4 years and 6 months old and presented to speech therapy services aged 3 years with markedly delayed expressive language skills and milder delay in comprehension and some social interaction difficulties. She had communicated using some speech sounds, Makaton signs and a few words. There was no prior history of feeding difficulties or drooling. The rate of acquisition of speech sounds was very slow and inconsistent and there was evidence of her 'groping' for sounds. She had good non-verbal skills and her cognitive score did not suggest any associated learning difficulties.
>
> ## *Learning points*
>
> * Verbal dyspraxia is the most likely diagnosis provided there is confidence in Fay's cognitive abilities.
> * Neurological disorders are unlikely as there are no feeding difficulties.

Children with expressive language difficulties may or may not have comprehension difficulties. No cause is identified. A family history of delayed speech milestones may be elicited. Most children acquire functional speech before school entry age, but it can take longer for some to reach typical standards for their vocabulary, grammatical development and fluency of speech. It can be difficult to predict how long this will take and not all will necessarily reach that level.

More sophisticated methods of assessment have shown that some children who were previously thought to have a purely expressive delay may also have some subtle problems with comprehension.

The pattern in this group of children may be delayed or disordered relating to vocabulary or grammatical development. They often acquire a considerable noun vocabulary but have difficulties with verbs, and thus struggle to move on to phrase- and sentence-level speech. They often demonstrate the language they have been taught but do not absorb, acquire and assimilate new words and subsequently rehearse and use them as typically developing children would. They often develop compensatory strategies to help them to cope socially.

Phonological impairment

This refers to children whose speech sound system is delayed or disordered. Speech sounds may be pronounced incorrectly or not at all. There are critical periods for acquiring certain sounds. Typical errors made include /k/ replaced with /t/; deviations from these regular patterns are disordered processes. Breakdown at the phonological level means that the child thinks he or she is producing the correct sound as the auditory feedback loop is not working correctly, but he or she would be able to identify errors in others' speech. Phonological difficulties can have a significant effect on the development of the child's expressive language. Prolonged use of a bottle or dummy will affect speech sound development as well as dentition, i.e. (k, g) sounds made at the back of the mouth are used in preference to front sounds (t, d). The omission of certain sounds has a huge impact on what a child appears to say, reducing the intelligibility of his or her speech. Children with severe phonological impairment often retain a telegrammatic quality to their speech. For example, instead of saying 'Tomorrow I am going to go to John's for tea' the child might say 'Tomorrow John tea'.

Articulation impairment

This relates to specific sound production difficulties at the peripheral level because of misplacement of the articulators, for example extension of the tongue beyond the teeth when saying /s/ leads to production of /th/ – called a lisp. These difficulties are usually easily corrected with speech therapy, although monitoring and carryover into everyday speech may take some time.

Dyspraxia

Dyspraxia is defined as difficulty in carrying out the rapid, discrete and highly accurate patterned movements of the speech muscles required to produce fluent speech, in the absence of any obvious abnormality of neurological function. It is due to disruption in the motor programming that controls the organization and movements of the speech apparatus. It affects coordination of the tongue, lip and palatal movements. It can be subdivided into the following categories.

VERBAL DYSPRAXIA

Verbal dyspraxia affects only speech and not eating. The child appears to grope for speech sounds and is inconsistent in his or her production, i.e. he can produce sounds one day but not the next. The disruption to the motor programming means that sometimes speech sounds can be produced in isolation but not when combined with other sounds. Rhythm and sequencing are often also affected. The impact is particularly pronounced in polysyllabic words. Attempts are effortful, tiring and frustrating. Therapy is aimed at establishing, reinforcing and drilling motor pathways, but it is a long, hard slog.

ORAL DYSPRAXIA

Oral dyspraxia affects speech, eating and non-speech voluntary movements, for example the child can protrude his tongue to lick an ice cream, but not when specifically asked to do so. There is often a history of feeding difficulties in infancy. Assess whether the child is able to carry out a series of rapid repetitive movements such as blowing, sucking, whistling, chewing or protruding his or her tongue. Some will also have evidence of generalized dyspraxia affecting their general motor skills.

Causes of specific language impairments

Normal variation

There is evidence of biological programming of language acquisition that works even when the quality of stimulation is poor.

Chromosomal influences

Males are more commonly affected than females by SLIs, and therefore biological factors must play a huge part. Children with chromosomal anomalies including XYY, XXY and XXYY all have a higher than expected prevalence of language impairment. Individuals with fragile X syndrome have a variety of communication disorders ranging from social aversion or dyspraxia to autism with severe learning difficulties.

Genetic factors

There is a strong genetic influence on language development. A positive family history cannot, however, be assumed to be the sole cause of a child's difficulties.

Dysmorphic syndromes

These include Noonan syndrome, Williams syndrome and Angelman syndrome. The exact mechanism for the language difficulties in these syndromes is not known, but it seems likely that the language area of the brain is affected as a result of the underlying defect.

Impaired processing

Children with an SLI differ from typically developing children in the speed with which they process sounds when they listen to speech. This may be the physiological basis of language impairment.

Secretory otitis media (glue ear)

This may be a contributory factor but is not a major cause of SLIs, although it is a significant factor in early language delay.

Inadequate input

Children with an SLI may be exposed to a suboptimal communicative environment, but this may have occurred as the result of their difficulties rather than being the cause ('chicken and egg').

Severe neglect

Some children have language difficulties if their exposure to language is poor and some children are more vulnerable because of other factors such as an inherited predisposition to language problems. A move to a language-rich environment, such as a nursery setting, may result in a rapid improvement in speech. Children who have been exposed to chronic abuse or neglect may display some features seen in children with autism.

Bilingualism

Children cope well with hearing two languages and are able to distinguish between them from an early age. This is therefore not causal, but if major difficulties are identified it may be better to speak consistently in only one language.

Congenital auditory imperception (auditory agnosia)

The child's responses to sound are unpredictable from early childhood. The child cannot understand even simple everyday sounds such as his bath water being run. Audiological testing may suggest hearing loss but auditory brainstem response shows normal responses to pure tones. It can be difficult to distinguish this problem from severe learning disability or autism. Pure congenital auditory agnosia is a very rare condition and the prognosis for learning to speak is poor. Milder forms of the condition may resolve as the child gets older.

Overlap between categories

Children rarely have difficulty in a single specific area; many children present with comprehension and expressive language difficulties, perhaps with some phonological overlay.

Bloom and Lahey (1978) provide a useful model of form, content and use, which demonstrates the overlap between the various elements of communication and indicates how difficulties can arise in one or several areas (Fig. 13.2).

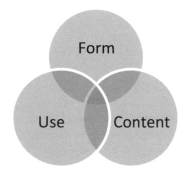

Form: grammar/syntax – includes word order and sentence length, as well as speech sound production
Content: vocabulary
Use: social use of language

Figure 13.2 Overlap of communication difficulties.

Predicting outcomes for children with an SLI

It is difficult to offer a prognosis for improvement because of the wide range of ages for language acquisition. Research shows that persistent language impairment at school entry is associated with literacy difficulties, and later academic underachievement. Some of this association may be explained by low intelligence, which often goes along with delayed language acquisition. If the child aged 4 is diagnosed as having an SLI, *the most important predictive factor is the non-verbal intelligence score.*

Impaired speech production

Case vignette

Adam, aged 2 years 8 months, presented at the CDC at 6 months with an evolving pattern of cerebral palsy. Involuntary writhing movements and fluctuating tone were both noted and athetoid cerebral palsy was diagnosed. Adam had little babble but occasional involuntary vowel or plosive (p, b) sounds produced with explosive uncontrolled quality. At about 2 years, Adam was taught to eye point at toys, food or DVDs when he wanted to make choices. Comprehension was developing well for his age.

Learning points

- Children with athetoid cerebral palsy can have spared cognitive and language skills.
- Eye pointing is the skill of looking at a carer's face, then at an object and then back to the carer to make sure he or she has understood the request.
- Developing eye pointing enables children to later choose between pictures to communicate, leading to communication aid use.

Speech production can be impaired due to specific physical impairments that impede the normal process of producing speech, structural causes and other psychological/emotional causes.

Neuromuscular causes: the dysarthrias

The Dysarthrias is the term used to denote speech impairments due to neurological damage, or to conditions that affect the muscles involved in speaking.

Children with extrapyramidal or pyramidal cerebral palsy often have a pseudobulbar palsy that causes dysarthria that, in the most severely affected cases, leads to absence of speech. Spasticity of speech muscles leads to disordered tongue movements and tongue thrusting. In dyskinetic (mixed spastic and dystonic) cerebral palsy, speech is often jerky, explosive and unclear.

Many children with severe cerebral palsy also have additional learning difficulties and hearing and vision impairment, which add to their communication difficulties. Children with athetoid cerebral palsy often have spared cognitive and language skills, and hence are often the most successful users of alternative and augmentative communication.

Other rare causes of dysarthria include *Moebius syndrome* (congenital facial nerve palsy and bilateral external rectus muscle palsy). This may present as paresis of the tongue, palate and larynx with severe dysarthria. There may be associated limb abnormalities such as talipes, pectoral muscle anomalies, mild pyramidal weakness, deafness and mild learning difficulties. It arises sporadically.

Red flags suggesting neurological disorder

- Severe problems with swallowing or chewing.
- Persistent dribbling beyond the age of teething.
- Facial immobility or other neurological deficits.

Structural causes of impaired speech production

Cleft lip and palate

This is a wide spectrum of defects ranging from minor notching of the lip or bifid uvula to complete unilateral or bilateral cleft lip, alveolus and palate. There are genetic and epidemiological differences between cleft lip with or without cleft palate and isolated cleft palate. Over 400 syndromes involving a cleft lip or palate have been described. The more common syndromes include velo-cardiofacial syndrome (22q11), Pierre Robin anomaly and Treacher Collins syndrome.

Cleft palate is far more likely to be associated with other anomalies than cleft lip. The most common additional findings are microcephaly, short stature, learning difficulties or other craniofacial abnormalities. Isolated cleft lip with or without cleft palate can be seen recurring within families and inheritance is probably multifactorial. Environmental factors including fetal exposure to alcohol and retinoic acid are also associated with cleft lip and palate.

The management of cleft lip and palate is now undertaken by a multidisciplinary team including a plastic surgeon, orthodontist, speech and language therapist, oral surgeon, dentist, ear, nose and throat (ENT) surgeon, psychologist and audiologist.

Velo-pharyngeal incompetence

This may result from neurological disorders or from an anatomical defect. The most common defect is a submucosal cleft, which is recognized by the triad of bifid uvula, notched or absent posterior nasal spine and translucent central area of the soft palate. The affected infant usually feeds slowly with nasal regurgitation and will later have hypernasal speech. Video-fluoroscopy and nasopharyngoscopy may help to establish the diagnosis. Velo-pharyngeal incompetence is a typical finding in the velo-cardiofacial syndrome, a multisystem disorder caused by a deletion on the short arm of chromosome 22 (22q11) that often includes cardiac abnormalities.

Nasal obstruction

Nasal obstruction is caused by chronic enlargement of the adenoids. This can give rise to defective articulation, particularly of the nasal sounds 'n', 'm' and 'ng'. Speech will be hyponasal. Review by an ENT surgeon is required, particularly if there is a history suggestive of sleep apnoea.

Macroglossia

Macroglossia occurs in syndromes such as Down, Beckwith and Hunter syndromes and hypothyroidism. The size of the tongue probably plays a very small role in the child's speech problems, but is linked to an open mouth posture and drooling. Parents may request surgery to reduce the size of the tongue to improve the appearance.

Tongue tie

Tongue tie is still widely believed to be a cause of late talking. This condition should be diagnosed only if the frenulum is so tight that the tongue cannot be protruded to the outer margin of the lower lip. If this is the case, then there is likely also to be a history of feeding difficulties but not necessarily speech difficulties later in life. If feeding is significantly affected, the tight frenulum may be released. The child should be referred to a maxillofacial surgeon for assessment.

Malocclusion of the jaws

This occurs when the lower jaw is underdeveloped so that the tongue is thrust out during speech, causing lisping. If the mandible protrudes then the lower incisors lie anterior to the upper incisors, causing a lack of clarity with several sounds. Malocclusion may occur as an isolated anomaly, sometimes as a familial abnormality or as part of a dysmorphic syndrome. Orthodontic or maxillofacial treatment may be required.

Dysphonia

Dysphonia refers to difficulty in voice production that often presents as a hoarse or weak voice. Any child with an unexplained and persistent voice disorder should be referred to ENT to undergo a laryngoscopy. This may reveal chronic inflammatory changes or, more rarely, nodules or papilloma. Recurrent laryngeal nerve palsy is a very rare cause of dysphonia in children.

Dysfluency

Dysfluency (stammering or stuttering in the USA) refers to in-coordination between respiratory and articulatory function, causing prolongation of word sounds, stopping or blocking of speech or repetition of one or more words or sounds. This is so common between the ages of 2 and 4 that it is regarded as 'normal developmental non-fluency'. About 3% of children stammer at some point during childhood but only 1% of school-age children stammer regularly. It is appropriate to reassure parents of an occasionally stammering 2- to 4-year-old. Advice about not correcting the child, but allowing the child sufficient time to speak, is appropriate. A child who stammers regularly benefits from seeing a speech and language therapist, but rarely requires a referral to a paediatrician. If the normal developmental non-fluency is overemphasized and the child becomes increasingly aware of it, a more significant stammer can develop. Stammering can be the result of emotional or functional disorders and it can cause troubling social anxiety; therefore, early intervention from a speech and language therapist is recommended.

Selective mutism

Selective mutism (previously elective mutism) is when a child will talk in selected social situations, such as at home, but not in others. More females than males are affected. It is usually a transient problem, with only 1 child in 1000 having a persistent problem. Most cases present soon after the child starts school. These children are often anxious, which may reflect

* parental depression and anxiety
* speech or language difficulties
* various types of abuse.

The child is usually heard speaking in situations outside school but, if not, it may be necessary to video him or her whilst playing or through a two-way mirror to confirm this. There are useful programmes to encourage children to communicate; initially this communication may need to be non-verbal. Educational psychologists have experience in these school-based programmes.

Social communication disorders

Case vignette

Laura, aged 5 years, was referred initially with suspected selective mutism as she did not speak outside her home. On assessment she had significant difficulties in her receptive and expressive language skills. Her mother complained that she showed rigidity in her behaviour and insisted on following certain routines. She had a preference for sameness and an obsessive interest in particular dolls. She attempted to engage her peers using phrases her teacher used, repeated verbatim, which sounded odd.

Learning points
Laura has pragmatic difficulties as well as comprehension and expressive language problems, but her difficulties did not meet the criteria for a diagnosis of autistic spectrum disorder, when assessed by the school-age autism assessment service. Diagnosing her with pragmatic difficulties enables her family and teachers to understand that her difficulties go further than a problem with language.

The pervasive developmental disorders (PDDs) are a group of disorders characterized by impairment of reciprocal social interaction, which is present in at least two social situations (hence the use of the word pervasive). Autism is the largest and most obvious subgroup of PDDs. PDD as a diagnosis is rarely used in the UK, but it is commonly used in the USA, particularly for those children whose symptoms do not satisfy all the criteria for a diagnosis of autism.

The triad of impairments (Wing 1981) that are the essential features of autism are

1   Impaired and abnormal social development that is not in keeping with the child's intellectual level.
2   Delayed and disordered language development that is, again, not in keeping with the child's intellectual level.
3   Repetitive behaviours – insistence on sameness, preference for routines, stereotyped play patterns, abnormal preoccupations and resistance to change.

In order to satisfy the criteria for a diagnosis of childhood autism, these features must be present before the age of 3 years. Multidisciplinary teams use the *International Classification of Diseases and Related Health Problems*, 10th revision (ICD-10), or the *Diagnostic and Statistical Manual of Mental Disorders*, fourth edition (DSM-IV), for diagnostic purposes.

In a proportion of children diagnosed with autism, intelligence is normal or near normal. However, many children who have a diagnosis of autism spectrum disorder have some learning difficulties.

Pragmatic language difficulties

In pragmatic language difficulties, higher-level language functions are involved. Affected children may develop language slightly later than average. There can be an early history of echolalia – immediate or delayed. They struggle to acquire the rules of social interaction and language use. Hence, taking turns in conversations and social participation is impaired. Their expressive language can sound quite sophisticated (although sometimes odd) but can be deceptive, as it is learned in chunks and is repetitive. They have difficulty integrating real-world knowledge and struggle to use language to negotiate, question and reason. They may show literal understanding and have difficulties following conversational rules such as initiating, terminating and interrupting conversations. Other features include poor listener awareness, topic maintenance and social timing. Non-verbal features such as eye contact, proximity and facial expression can also be problematic. They may therefore appear rude and insensitive.

This group was previously labelled as having semantic–pragmatic disorder by speech and language therapists in the UK. This term is no longer used and was never internationally recognized.

Children with pragmatic disorders merge into the spectrum of autistic disorders and Asperger syndrome and are considered a separate group from those with SLIs. Those affected may have other features including rigid thinking, difficulty with turn taking, poor empathy, preoccupation with routines and an obsession with certain topics or toys, and may indeed be better considered as part of the autism spectrum disorder continuum.

Differential diagnoses for delayed language and poor social skills development

* Primary language problem
* Autism
* Cognitive delay/global delay

- Severe neglect
- Hearing impairment
- Attachment difficulties

If a child presents with language delay, difficulties with socializing and behavioural difficulties such as overactivity, poor attention and oppositional behaviour, then other causes should be considered, such as a combination of developmental delay in speech and language and inconsistent parenting with inadequate boundary setting.

Children who stop talking

This is very rare and can be frightening for parents and carers. A full neurological work-up is required in the absence of an obvious explanation such as recent severe head injury, meningitis or acquired hearing loss.

Disintegrative process

The most common cause of regression in language and social skills occurs in association with the onset of autism spectrum disorders. Children may develop speech following a normal pattern up to the early/middle part of their second year, but then they appear to lose social interest, understanding and previously acquired words.

Acquired receptive aphasia (Landau–Kleffner syndrome)

In this condition, deterioration in language function is accompanied by the onset of seizures. The onset usually occurs between the ages of 3 and 9 years. The loss of receptive language may be preceded by behavioural difficulties. With the loss of language, behavioural difficulties continue to be a significant feature. Seizures may be generalized or focal. They are not necessarily frequent or severe. Some children recover completely whereas others continue to have major language difficulties.

Electrical slow waves in sleep

Children with electrical slow waves in sleep (ESWS) present at an average age of 8 years and they may have a history of seizures in the past. Accompanying the deterioration in their language is a fall in their IQ. A sleep electroencephalogram is the most relevant investigation in the diagnosis of this little understood and rare condition. This shows electrical status in sleep with continuous 2 to 2.5Hz spike–wave discharges. It is a difficult condition to treat and the prognosis is uncertain.

Neurological conditions

These include brain tumours, degenerative diseases, congenital infections, prolonged focal seizures, metabolic diseases (Wilson disease, glutaric aciduria, Sanfilippo disease), Rett syndrome and vascular lesions.

Psychosocial factors

This includes severe abuse and trauma due to separation or bereavement.

Management of speech and language difficulties

There is no medical treatment for communication disorders as such. Associated problems such as epilepsy may require treatment and hearing impairment will require appropriate management. However, this does not apply to most children with communication difficulties.

Parents should be encouraged not to focus on obtaining a diagnostic label and instead to concentrate on trying to help their child learn to communicate, guided by the advice from their speech and language therapist.

Those with the most severe communication difficulties may be referred to a genetics clinic, as parents may want advice on the possible recurrence risk. Generally severe communication disorders are sporadic and have a low risk of recurrence. The risks, however, with autism are higher, particularly if there are already two affected family members.

Advice to parents

- Talk to the child during daily routines and play.
- Minimize background noise – turn off the television so that the child can hear your voice.
- Face the child; call his or her name to gain attention; get down to his or her level if necessary.
- Show as well as say: use gestures and pointing to aid comprehension.
- Use simple language with short sentences and emphasize key words.
- Pitch you language a little higher than that of the child, for example at a two-word level if the child is using single words.
- Follow the child's attention and talk about what he or she is looking at, even if only for a brief period.
- Establish and follow the routine of a joint picture/story time. Talk about the pictures rather than just asking, 'What's that?'.

Speech and language therapy

Parents may mistakenly believe that their child requires intensive individual therapy sessions from a speech and language therapist in order to make progress. Early intervention is recommended as it is the most effective way to help the child, if all those in the child's environment are aware of how to support the child's communication development. Giving advice to parents or attending a language group can accelerate language development in a preschool child (Wake et al. 2011).

There are several well-established schemes devised to accelerate language development. Examples of such language schemes include the following:

- Hanen Early Language Parent Program
- I CAN Early Talk programme and
- Derbyshire Language Scheme.

Intervention may be offered individually by the speech and language therapist in a 'block' to a child, or he may be seen for a regular review with a programme of advice that is given to parents and childcare practitioners. Input may be offered for

- language – vocabulary and syntactic development, both receptive and expressive
- phonology
- articulation
- social communication and pragmatics
- early interaction (pre-language skills) or
- parent–child interaction.

Education and support

It is often suggested that time spent with other children in a day nursery may be beneficial in stimulating social interaction and language development. There is little objective evidence to support this, but much anecdotally reported and measured progress. Speech and language therapists may train nursery staff to carry out specific approaches with the child, but the skills of individual nursery staff differ and improvement may not always occur.

Some children require more specialist provision, which may include a language unit/ resourced provision attached to a mainstream school. Alternative methods of communication may be offered as another way of providing the child with a means of communicating and/or reducing frustration whilst language skills develop.

Signs of distress in children unable to communicate verbally

Children and young people who cannot communicate verbally may express their emotions, such as unhappiness, distress or pain, by other means. Parents and familiar carers usually recognize these vocal, social and motor behaviours and the potential significance of changes in them. You may be asked to assess such a child in order to exclude treatable causes, for example dental pain, constipation or gastro-oesophageal reflux. It is often more difficult to identify emotional health causes of distress such as sadness, anxiety or depression. Signs of distress may include

- louder than normal vocalizations, including screaming or screeching
- gestures more violent than usual, such as nodding, shaking of head
- change in posture, such as rigidity, extensor posturing, curling up
- aggressive behaviour such as biting, scratching, nipping, kicking
- self-injury such as banging fists on forehead, picking at hands
- social withdrawal, for example reduced eye contact and smiling, reduced engagement
- sadness, for example downcast facial expression, crying, excessive clinginess to familiar adults
- restlessness, changes in mood, apathy

- loss of appetite and
- changes in sleeping pattern.

Augmentative and alternative means of communication

It is vital to consider alternative means of communicating that can augment or replace the need for speech for these children. Without a means to communicate even their basic emotions, such children can remain distressed and difficult to care for. The term alternative and augmentative communication (AAC) is used to describe these systems. AAC includes simple methods such as eye pointing, body language, gesture and signing, extending to the use of pictures and symbols, a communication board, book or a sophisticated electronic aid.

Augmentative and alternative communication should be considered for any child with severely delayed language skills, although levels of communicative intent (the understanding of the need to communicate to another person) and cognitive skill levels must be considered. The use of such methods should not adversely affect efforts being made to speak. It can relieve frustration and improve quality of life as well as advancing language development. These alternatives cannot, however, work as quickly nor be as versatile as speech. This may disappoint parents, who may give up on using such methods because their child does not make the anticipated progress.

Methods

- The *Makaton* signing system, which is based on natural gesture rather than British sign language, may provide a means of communicating that can satisfy the child's basic needs, but it has a limited vocabulary (as it provides up to 450 concepts). It is not be suitable for children with a physical disability who lack the manual dexterity to perform the signs. Of note, key words are signed as well as spoken, so the system will not reduce the child's ability to acquire spoken language if he or she is able to do so.
- *Objects and picture boards.* These consist of a board to which a few pictures of objects are attached. The child is encouraged to point to these to indicate his or her needs or is shown an object to help him or her understand what is going to happen next, for example shown a nappy before having his or her nappy changed. Photographs or pictures can be used to make the system more transportable.
- *Picture Exchange Communication System (PECS).* Bondy and Frost (1994) developed this to enable children, particularly those with autism, to communicate their basic needs by passing a picture to their carer indicating the object/activity they desire. The child is given the object in exchange. Through this method the child learns that the pictures represent the object and he or she can obtain this only by interacting with his or her carer and giving him or her the appropriate card (Fig. 13.3).
- *Communication aid technology.* Computer-assisted communication has great potential for helping children with severe speech problems, but the system chosen must be suited to the child's physical abilities and his or her intellectual level. It may involve
  - using a joystick to operate the system
  - registering movements of any body part of which the child has reliable voluntary control
  - keyboards that can be adapted to meet the child's fine motor ability level.

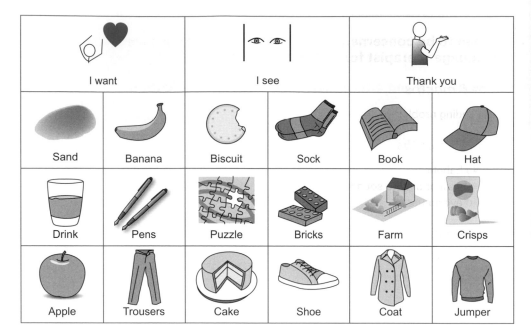

Figure 13.3 Examples of communication symbols from the Picture Exchange Communication System. Reproduced with kind permission of Pyramid Educational Consultants UK, Ltd.

Head switches and even eye gaze can be used to produce spoken words or words displayed on a screen. Applications for mobile phones, iPads or other tablets are now being developed and can be used as therapeutic as well as communication tools.

- Voice recognition technology is now available and can be used in the school or home not only to produce written work but also allowing opportunities for variable environmental influences (e.g. background noise). The limiting factors are the child's intellectual level and motivation.

Specialist speech and language therapists in AAC should assess the child. Parents, teachers and therapists should become familiar with the aid and be happy to use it. Otherwise, much money can be wasted and disappointment is inevitable. Other limitations are the poor reliability of the technology and the fact that sometimes the aids are not easily transportable. Aids are very expensive and rarely available on the NHS.

When to be concerned and consider referral to a speech and language therapist for further assessment

0 to 6 months

- Feeding problems

6 to 12 months

- No babble
- Not responding to sounds
- No eye contact

12 months

- Few sounds
- No exploratory play

18 months

- No words/gestures
- No communicative intent (understanding the need to communicate to others)
- Not using objects properly in play (hairbrush, telephone)
- No pretend play (feeding teddy)
- Not following simple commands ('put it in the bin')
- Fleeting attention

2 years

- Only a few single words, still jargoning (strings of unintelligible babble)
- Not understanding single words
- Dribbling and managing to eat only mashed foods (not chewing)
- Speech not intelligible to familiars
- Little pretend play
- Poor attention

2 years 6 months

- Not linking words ('Daddy shoe', 'Mummy gone')
- Limited vocabulary
- Immature play (still mouthing, exploring only)

3 to 4 years

- Only single words/learned phrases (whole chunks of repeated language)
- Unintelligible to less familiar adults
- Not understanding instructions of two or three words ('give Daddy the *apple*')

- Persistent hoarse voice
- Sounds – if mainly using 'k', 'g' and vowel sounds

4 to 5 years

- Not using four-word sentences
- Repetitive echoed language
- Word-finding difficulties
- Confused word order
- Unintelligible speech

5 years

- Difficulties in understanding, especially in groups
- Social difficulties – language goes off at a tangent, does not stay on topic, talk about special interests to exclusion of others, unable to take turns, no understanding of others' wants or needs

Key messages

- Our understanding of normal language development is still very limited; even more so when trying to establish why language delay or disorder occurs.
- Children with severe and complex communication difficulties require referral to the CDC for assessment and input. Speech and language therapist face-to-face input is not the only intervention.
- It is important to provide the child with an alternative means to communicate to lessen his or her frustration, reduce his or her isolation and facilitate his or her care.

References

Bloom L, Lahey M (1978) *Language Development and Language Disorders*. New York: John Wiley & Sons.

Bondy A, Frost L (1994) The Picture Exchange Communication System (PECS). *Focus Autistic Behav* 9: 1–19. Also available at: www.pecs.org

Wake M, Tobin S, Girolametto L et al. (2011) Outcomes of population based language promotion for slow to talk toddlers at ages 2 and 3 years: Let's Learn Language cluster randomized controlled trial. *BMJ* 18: 343. http://dx.doi.org/10.1136/bmj.d4741

Wing L (1981) Asperger's Syndrome: a clinical account. *Psychol Med* 11: 115–29. http://dx.doi.org/10.1017/S0033291700053332

Further reading

Cockerill H, Carrollfew L, editors (2007) *Communicating without Speech: Practical Augmentative and Alternative Communication Clinics for Children*. London: Mac Keith Press.

Great Ormond Street Hospital for Children NHS Trust (2012) *Speech and Language Development 0–2 Years. Information for Families*. London: Great Ormond Street Hospital for Children NHS Trust.

Law J, Garrett Z, Nye C (2010) Speech and language therapy interventions for children with primary speech and language delay or disorder. *Cochrane Database Syst Rev* 3: CD004110.

Sheridan MD (2008) *From Birth to Five Years: Children's Developmental Progress*, Third Edition. Revised and updated by Ajay Sharma and Helen Cockerill. New York: Routledge.

Williams P (no date) *Developmental Verbal Dyspraxia*. London: Nuffield Hearing Centre, Royal National Throat, Nose and Ear Hospital.

Support organization

Selective Mutism Information and Research Association (SMIRA): www.smira.org.uk

Websites

Afasic England: www.afasic.org.uk

Apraxia-KIDS: www.apraxia-kids.org

I CAN: www.ican.org.uk

Makaton: www.makaton.org

Picture Exchange Communication System (PECS): www.pecs.org.uk

Section 6

Learning difficulties and loss of skills

14
Disordered development and learning disability

Karen Horridge

Learning objectives

- To understand definitions of disordered development and learning disability.
- To understand epidemiology and aetiology of disordered development and learning disability.
- To know how to assess and manage a child with disordered development or established learning disability.
- To know how to assess and manage common secondary disabilities and comorbidities of learning disability.
- To understand the implications of disordered development and learning disability.

Introduction

Disordered development means development outside the broadly typical range for age. Disordered development is preferable terminology to 'developmental delay' as the latter implies that there will be developmental 'catch-up' to the broadly typical range at some point. This is not helpful for parents of children who in fact have a significant learning disability, as it sets unrealistic expectations from the outset that may become entrenched.

There are many different definitions that are related to learning disabilities. It is always important to check what is meant when these terms are used as parents and professionals from different agencies and different countries have different understandings of the same words. Many definitions have a statutory basis, but unfortunately have no consistency with each other. Some people with disabilities think that definitions of disability focus too much on a medical model, with social exclusion is seen as an inevitable result of their impairments or medical conditions. The social model of disability asserts that the poverty, disadvantage and social exclusion experienced by many people with disabilities is not inevitable, but rather stems from attitudinal and environmental barriers. Therefore, it is social barriers, not impairments or medical conditions, that cause disability. Parents' perspectives of their children's learning abilities vary enormously. For example, a child with mild learning disability may cause more anxiety in an academic family than in one with lower expectations of academic achievement.

The *International Statistical Classification of Diseases and Related Health Problems*, 10th revision (ICD-10), uses the term 'mental retardation', which is not widely used in the UK as some parents find it stigmatizing, although it is more regularly used in the USA and some other European countries. ICD-10 defines mental retardation as

> a condition of arrested or incomplete development of the mind, which is especially characterized by impairment of skills manifested during the developmental period, skills which contribute to the overall level of intelligence, i.e. cognitive, language, motor and social abilities. Retardation can occur with or without any other mental or physical condition.
>
> (WHO 2004)

ICD-11 is due to be published in 2015; watch this space. In this chapter learning disability will be used synonymously with mental retardation as defined in ICD-10. Around 1% to 2% of the UK's child population have a mild or moderate learning disability and 0.3% to 0.5% have a severe or profound learning disability. According to the literature, a medical diagnosis is found in up to 80% of children with a severe or profound learning disability (see Table 14.1 for a description of levels of learning disability). This is likely to increase further with the newer genetic investigation techniques, including microarray comparative genome hybridization.

Table 14.1 Overview of the different levels of learning disability

Level of learning disability	IQ	Equivalent mental age as adult	Functioning
Mild	50–69	9–12y	Sufficient speech for everyday purposes Full independence in self-care (eating, washing, dressing, bladder and bowel control), albeit at a slower rate of skill acquisition Many children struggle with academic work at school, especially with reading and writing Many adults will be able to work in roles that demand practical rather than academic abilities, e.g. unskilled or semi-skilled manual labour Many adults have good social relationships and contribute to society
Moderate	35–49	6–9y	Likely to lead to markedly disordered development in childhood Slow acquisition of language comprehension and use Most can learn to develop some degree of independence in self-care and acquire adequate communication and academic skills Adults will need varying degrees of support to live and work in the community
Severe	20–34	3–6y	Likely to result in a continuous need for support
Profound	<20	<3y	Severe limitation in self-care, continence, communication and mobility

Case vignette 1

Philip is a 7-year-old male with learning difficulties in special school. On paediatric assessment he is of significant short stature (4cm below the 0.4th centile) with dysmorphic features. In view of the clinical concerns, a skeletal survey for dysmorphology was arranged and revealed atlantoaxial instability. Subsequent magnetic resonance imaging of the cervical spine showed cervical cord compression. Philip was also referred for a genetics opinion. A diagnosis of Aarskog syndrome was suggested.

Action and outcome

Philip

Cervical spine fixation was undertaken, which was potentially life saving. This also led to a dramatic improvement in cognitive and language skills. Philip was reintegrated into a mainstream school setting.

His family

Philip had an older brother, Mark, who was also of short stature, had learning difficulties and attended a special support unit attached to a mainstream school. He had a diagnosis of 'epilepsy'. This was revisited: his 'seizures' consisted of him shaking his hands because they 'tingled'. Spinal radiography and magnetic resonance imaging were undertaken, which showed cervical cord compression more severe than that exhibited by his brother. Mark also underwent cervical spine fixation. He was undiagnosed with regards to his 'epilepsy' and was successfully weaned off anticonvulsants. The quality of life for both boys was dramatically improved. The family was fully informed about their condition.

Learning points

- Use diagnostic handles, for example short stature, physical disproportion and dysmorphic features, to guide investigations.
- In a child with dysmorphic features, look for abnormalities in other systems.
- Children and young people with learning disabilities, including those in special schools, should be offered up-to-date assessment and investigation with paediatricians competent in neurodisability.
- Short stature associated with learning disability should always be fully investigated, including linking with colleagues in endocrinology and clinical genetics.
- Diagnosis matters!

Population screening and case identification

All those working with children in the early years need to have a working knowledge of the broadly typical range of child development in order to recognize when development may be disordered. The Healthy Child Programme, launched in 2011 in the UK, empowers parents as well as professionals to learn about the broadly typical range of child development, and includes assessments with health workers, usually health visitors and general practitioners, at key intervals. An excellent e-learning resource for the Healthy Child Programme can be found on the website of the Royal College of Paediatrics and Child Health at www.rcpch.ac.uk/hcp.

Parents and professionals working in universal services need to be aware of 'red flags' of disordered development and be familiar with the referral pathways locally for further expert assessment.

Red flags of significantly disordered development

Any child who has

- lost developmental skills at any age
- difficulties with vision, fixing or following (simultaneous referral to paediatric ophthalmology) leading to parental or professional concern
- significant hearing loss at any age (simultaneous referral for expert audiological/ear, nose and throat assessment)
- suspected clinical diagnosis of cerebral palsy
- complex disabilities
- a head circumference that is above the 99.6th centile or below the 0.4th centile or which has crossed two centile lines upwards or downwards on the appropriate chart, or is significantly disproportionate to the parental head circumference.

Or any child who is not able to

- hold an object placed in his or her hand by 5 months of age (corrected for gestation)
- reach for objects by 6 months of age (corrected for gestation)
- sit unsupported by 12 months
- walk by 18 months (males) or 2 years (females) (check creatine kinase urgently)
- 'walk' other than on tiptoes
- speak by 18 months, especially if he or she does not attempt to communicate by any other means such as gesture (simultaneous referral for urgent hearing test)
- point at objects to share interest with others by 2 years
- run by the age of 2 years 6 months.

Goals for the paediatric assessment for a child with disordered development or learning disability

Assess the child's development to confirm or refute whether development is in fact disordered or within the broadly typical range for age. If there are significant difficulties, the advice below should be followed.

Assessment

- Emphasize the child's positive attributes and strengths as well as clearly describing areas of difficulty.
- Identify potential aetiological factors from history and examination, in order to
  - help plan investigations
  - explain to parents why their child is as he or she is and
  - reduce parental (usually maternal) self-blame.

Identify and manage secondary disabilities, particularly vision and hearing, as well as associated medical conditions, e.g. epilepsy, gastro-oesophageal reflux, drooling, constipation, spasticity, pain, postural deformities, dental problems, behavioural and sleep difficulties, growth and endocrine disorders.

Management plan

- Offer an appropriate package of multidisciplinary, interagency support, preferably with an identified keyworker or care coordinator. This should include early referral to education and social care, in order that interagency care plans can be in place, preferably by the time the child starts nursery or school.
- Hearing and vision screening if indicated.
- Medical investigations.
- Empower parents to remain in charge of their lives, which otherwise risk being over-run by an army of professionals, and ensure that family privacy is protected and respected.
- Signpost to further information in a range of formats tailored to the family's needs and circumstances. The early support materials are useful. It is also helpful to include guidance to accessing information on the Internet, such as the helpful leaflet from Contact a Family, which can be downloaded from http://www.cafamily.org.uk/pdfs/about_diagnosis_part9.pdf

---

Prior to the assessment

- Be able to access all relevant case notes, reports and previous assessments, including a common assessment framework where this has been completed.
- Have an appropriate, accessible environment in which to assess the child, including standardized equipment and support to accurately weigh, measure and assess nutritional status with a range of growth charts available, and appropriate toys.
- Be able to access facilities for investigations, including biochemical, haematological, neurometabolic, immunological and radiological.
- Have a knowledge of local therapy and support networks, e.g. physiotherapy, speech and language therapy (feeding, swallowing, dysphagia, communication, social communication), occupational therapy, dietetics and specialist teachers.
- Have a knowledge of experts with whom to discuss, or to whom to refer for further assessment and investigation, including experts in neurodisability, audiology, ophthalmology, neurology, neurophysiology, clinical genetics, metabolic paediatrics, endocrinology and child psychiatry.

A structured approach to paediatric assessment of the child with disordered development

As in other areas of paediatric neurodisability, this is composed of the following:

- detailed history
- assessment for behavioural syndromes or phenotypes
- systemic examination
- developmental assessment
- differential diagnosis or formulation, including identification of secondary disabilities and
- targeted tests.

Case vignette 2

Grace was admitted to hospital at 3 months with incessant crying and an astute junior doctor noted poor visual behaviour. She was discharged by a consultant upon the diagnosis and treatment of a urinary tract infection. She re-presented at 6 months with infantile spasms when a paediatric neurodisability assessment also elicited a history of jumps and jerks since birth and marked brachycephaly with associated marked central hypotonia – she 'slipped through the hands'. She had nystagmus (rapid involuntary movement of the eyes) in a neutral eye position and her best reported developmental skill was that she 'smiled when the sun shone brightly on her face'. She could suck and swallow and was thriving but had no independent movements. Investigations included an electroencephalogram that showed hypsarrhythmia and magnetic resonance imaging of the head showed lissencephaly. Genetic testing confirmed *LIS1* gene deletion.

Action, outcome and implications for family

An understanding of Grace's difficulties informed an appropriate choice of anticonvulsants and management plan. The greatest difficulty for the family was their housing and they were successfully rehoused. Grace had a 'death with dignity': she died in her sleep whilst at a seaside caravan with family (where they went so the sun could shine brightly on her face).

The clear diagnosis avoided the need for a coroner's inquest and facilitated appropriate genetic counselling for the family.

Learning points

- Always take a holistic approach in all settings and do not jump to conclusions that all presenting symptoms are the result of one pathology.
- Look for 'handles', in this case infantile spasms, marked hypotonia with associated brachycephaly, nystagmus and delayed developmental milestones.
- A structured approach can sometimes limit the number of appropriate tests to be ordered to be able to reach a precise diagnosis.
- The more precise the diagnosis, the more accurate the management plan and the better the family can be prepared for the journey ahead, including the death of their child where this is inevitable.

History

History is the cornerstone of all paediatric assessment for the child with disordered development, and is likely to give the highest yield in terms of clues or diagnostic 'handles' to inform diagnostic formulation.

It is important to understand the child's current difficulties:

- Always listen to and heed parents' concerns, as they often know intuitively when all is not as it should be, even if they sometimes struggle to openly acknowledge this.
- Establish at the outset who has which concerns, as parents' and referring professionals' concerns may differ.
- Use structured history sheets to underpin history taking, as these can ensure a consistent, holistic approach. If they are sent to parents for completion ahead of the appointment, they give parents time to reflect on why they are attending and allow details such as family history to be checked. They can facilitate time management during the consultation, as areas with no concerns can be dealt with quickly, leaving more time to focus and probe further where there are difficulties. Confirm parental reports of neonatal or past history from contemporaneous case notes or discharge summaries wherever possible.
- Be alert for potential diagnostic pointers or 'handles' throughout the consultation.

Potential pitfalls

- Be guided but not distracted by first impressions. The child who has to be carried kicking and screaming from the waiting room to the consulting room, runs up and down repetitively, hand flaps and twiddles and shows no interest in the people or toys in the consultation room may well be on the autism spectrum, but there may be other diagnoses to consider instead of, or in addition to, this.
- Consider that there may be more than one diagnosis, e.g. visual impairment and autism.
- Do not be led astray by red herrings. A story of birth asphyxia may not be the full explanation; there could be an underlying genetic or metabolic disorder.

Past medical history

- Pregnancy and early history.
- Early feeding and weaning.
- Past medical history.
- Specific questions about aspects of general health can reveal secondary disabilities that require management, such as
  - chest infections, breathing, wheezing, chest noises during feeding
  - chewing and swallowing, vomiting, acid brash (smelly burps), bowel function and
  - seizures or any other paroxysmal episodes.

Family history

Three generations of family history, including specific enquiries, should be taken. Consider the following:

- Extra help at school or attending special school (more likely to yield a response than asking about family history of learning disabilities, which parents may not perceive themselves as having).
- Consanguinity.
- Physical difficulties, speech or language difficulties.
- Behavioural or mental health difficulties, autism spectrum disorder, etc.

Development and play

- Ask open questions about how the child plays, which can be very revealing and guide further probing enquiries.
- Establish a timeline of developmental milestone acquisition and profile of current functioning across a range of domains including
  - posture and movements
  - hand function and personal care
  - vision
  - hearing
  - communication:
    - speech
    - language
    - social communication and relationships
  - feeding, including chewing and swallowing
  - behaviour
  - sleep
  - learning, including specific enquiry about any loss of previously acquired developmental skills.

Social situation

- Enquiring about current sources of support, from both family and friends and other professionals already involved, helps build a picture of resources available, in order to precisely identify and plan for any identified unmet needs.
- Sensitive enquiry about housing, along the lines of 'we can sometimes help if there are any issues', and a supporting letter to housing providers when issues are identified, can result in an improved environment for the child and family, which in turn can improve the wellbeing of the whole family.

Physical examination

General presentation

- Overall impressions are important; be aware of any unusual or dysmorphic features, variations in hair or skin pigment or texture and any potential skeletal anomalies.
- Notice whether there are any striking behaviours.
- Consider clinical photographs, which may allow more careful consideration of, for example, possible dysmorphisms after the clinic or facilitate other expert opinions. Always obtain consent, including for teaching if need be.
- Home photographs of parents as children or of the index child when he or she was younger, or a home video of the child at home and playing, can reveal vital information not evident during the consultation.

Growth

- Height, weight and head circumference should be measured and plotted on appropriate growth charts, remembering that some conditions have specific growth charts, e.g. Down syndrome, Turner syndrome, achondroplasia.
- A head circumference that is below the 0.4th centile or above the 99.6th centile may require further evaluation – consider magnetic resonance imaging of the head and if in doubt discuss with a paediatric neurologist, neurodisability specialist or neuroradiologist.
- Pubertal status should also be checked for and recorded and trends over time should be monitored, as overgrowth, short stature, faltering growth or early or delayed puberty may be key diagnostic 'handles' and have implications for treatment.

Neurological examination

Look for neurological signs and remember to examine the eyes.

General physical examination

Genetic and metabolic disorders can be associated with abnormalities in other systems.

Behaviour

Note the child's behaviour as certain patterns of cognitive functioning, personality and behaviour can be associated with specific disorders. This is referred to as the behavioural phenotype (Table 14.2).

Table 14.2 Behavioural phenotypes

Condition	Behavioural phenotype
Down syndrome	Relative strength with visual processing, receptive language and non-verbal social functioning Relative weakness in gross motor and expressive language skills
Williams syndrome	Remarkable conversational verbal abilities ('cocktail party chatter') Excessive empathy
Prader–Willi syndrome	Temper tantrums Obsessive–compulsive features, autistic features Stubborn and argumentative Skin picking and spot picking Lying and blame shifting Sleep disorder Insatiable appetite with food seeking/hoarding
Angelman syndrome	Excitable personality with inappropriately 'happy' affect, bouts of frequent laughter unrelated to context Sociable and inquisitive Hyperactivity Stereotypies, e.g. hand flapping or twirling Absent or limited expressive language Mouthing objects Difficulties falling or staying asleep Attraction to water or shiny objects
Cri du chat syndrome (5p– syndrome)	High-pitched, infantile, cat-like cry Feeding problems, poor suck, regurgitation Frequent respiratory and ear infections Pronounced inattention and hyperactivity Self-stimulatory and repetitive behaviours
Rett syndrome and MECP2 mutations, deletions and duplications	Stereotypic hand movements, e.g. wringing or flapping often in the midline Social withdrawal during phase of regression, later alert and interested in the world, but little or no speech – autistic-like features Spontaneous outbursts of laughing or crying, including in sleep Reduced response to pain Disturbed sleep–wake cycle Teeth grinding

Differential diagnosis or formulation

Time and pattern recognition are important clinical tools. Diagnosis is rarely an event, more often requiring time and careful thought, consultation with books, the Internet and other experts. It is important to explain this process to children and families, so that they know what to expect in terms of timescales and remain engaged.

If there is no clear diagnosis or insufficient evidence to make a clear diagnosis, it is much better to be honest with families about this, rather than jump to what may later turn out to be the wrong diagnosis that will then be much harder to unpick. Sharing uncertainty is an important part of neurodisability clinical practice and, although difficult for parents, they much prefer an honest approach; this is more likely to lead to a relationship of trust between the clinician and the family in the long run.

Tools to assist differential diagnosis or formulation

- List all the key pointers, 'red flags' or 'diagnostic handles' from the clinical assessment and available case notes, previous assessments and reports.

 Pause and reflect

- Consult books, the Internet and published literature.

 Pause and reflect

- Discuss with expert colleagues or refer on for further expert opinions.

 Pause and reflect

- Check for supporting evidence of any existing diagnoses.

 Pause and reflect

- Formulate a differential diagnosis, which may need to be 'no unifying diagnosis at this time'.

Investigations

Gathering further information, particularly from the child's school or nursery, can help to clarify the level of learning ability. Where uncertainty remains or there are concerns about loss of skills, a more detailed or accurate assessment of cognition is required. This can be requested from clinical or educational psychology colleagues, who can access a broader range of assessment tools. The medical component of the assessment is to consider whether there is an underlying medical cause. Be careful when interpreting the assessments of others to ensure that these were done at a time when the child was well, settled and able to demonstrate his or her 'usual' level of performance.

Top tips for investigating children with early developmental impairment or learning disabilities

- Do not draw up a list of investigations until you have considered whether there are any features suggesting a specific diagnosis.
- For any unusual tests, it is best to check with the laboratory in advance in case special arrangements are required, for example if transport on ice is required the sample must arrive in the laboratory on the next working day, or to confirm which tube to put the specimen in.
- If in doubt about which investigations to do, network with expert colleagues, as this may save the child from unnecessary, expensive and/or painful tests.
- Do check that whoever is reporting the results from the MR imaging is confident and competent in the assessment of the developing brain. If in doubt, ask for an expert neuroradiological opinion.
- Remember to clearly indicate that the skeletal survey is to look for evidence of skeletal dysmorphology, otherwise the report will probably read 'no fracture seen'.
- Accurate diagnosis of the epilepsies in the context of learning disabilities and complex disabilities can be complex, as can management. Work with colleagues in neurodisability or paediatric neurology.
- If investigations do not reveal a diagnosis, clinical reassessment after an interval can be helpful, when the child may have 'grown into' a more recognizable pattern, or when technology may have advanced and new tests have become available.

Secondary disabilities and comorbidities associated with disordered development and learning disability

Regardless of the specific diagnosis, it is important to think about secondary disabilities and comorbidities (Table 14.3). It is essential to maintain a broad vision throughout consultations and consider the following:

- underlying diagnosis
- any secondary difficulties

- any sensory difficulties
- any self-injurious behaviour
- any comorbidities
- the family's strengths and difficulties.

Table 14.3 Secondary disabilities and comorbidities

Secondary disability	Associated medical conditions	Comorbidities	Associated behavioural issues
Visual impairment	Pain	Social	Sleep
Hearing impairment	Epilepsy	communication	Anxiety
Communication	Feeding difficulties	difficulties	Obsessive–
impairment	Gastro-oesophageal	Attention difficulties	compulsive disorders
Continence	reflux	Hyperactivity	Challenging
	Drooling	Coordination	behaviours
	Aspiration/chest	difficulties	Psychosis
	infections	Organization and	
	Constipation	planning difficulties	
	Spasticity		

Secondary disabilities are covered in detail in other chapters.

Once you have understood all the needs of the individual child or young person you can then write a comprehensive care plan that addresses all of the issues. This should help towards achieving the best possible quality of life for the child or young person and family.

Handy hints: the child with learning disabilities and acute illness

PRESENTATION

- Those with disordered development and learning disabilities can have the same range of illnesses as other children and young people, but presentation may be different and it may be harder to elicit clinical signs. For example, children on the autism spectrum and with some specific syndromic diagnoses can have exceptionally high pain thresholds that can mask the usual expected clinical findings (e.g. fractures, acute abdomen, etc.); those with neuromuscular disorders can quickly slip into respiratory failure without evidence of increased work of breathing – check P_{CO_2} early.
- Those with metabolic disorders can decompensate with intercurrent illness and require condition-specific treatment.
- Aspiration can be silent, with no outward vomiting in the child or young person with complex disabilities who may have significant gastro-oesophageal reflux.
- Constipation can be severe and cause significant pain. Remember to check for it.
- Other possible causes of pain include the hips and teeth, postural deformities, bony fractures, foreign bodies.

- Those with difficult epilepsy are likely to have had emergency treatment at home. Check what has been given in all settings, especially how many doses of benzodiazepines, to avoid accumulation and secondary respiratory depression.
- Always keep an open mind to potential safeguarding issues.

EMERGENCY HEALTH CARE PLANS

- Does the child have an emergency healthcare plan or personal resuscitation plan? This may contain information about diagnoses, treatment, specific secondary disabilities to look out for, what has been discussed about levels of intervention, resuscitation, intensive care and so on.
- If there is no such plan, the child must be assessed and managed as per advanced paediatric life support guidelines. Also ask the child's lead clinician to prepare one to make communication easier for the next visit, especially clarifying what has been discussed and agreed about appropriate levels of intervention.

ONGOING CARE

- If the child has no obvious lead clinician and no evidence of thorough aetiological work-up, discuss with/refer to paediatric neurodisability, neurology, metabolic paediatrics, clinical genetics, and so on as appropriate.

Self-injurious behaviour is covered in Chapter 19.

Learning disabilities: links with other services

It is essential to manage children and young people with disordered development and learning disabilities within a multidisciplinary and multiagency framework from the outset. Families can be overwhelmed and confused by the number and range of professionals involved, so coordination of care, preferably by a keyworker, can be extremely helpful.

Linking early with colleagues in education, including educational psychology and in social care, including the social work and occupational therapy teams, is essential if clear, multiagency care plans are to be in place. These help families to make informed choices about educational placement and social care support. These coordinated packages are needed to ensure that each child has the best possible chance of reaching his or her full potential.

The paediatrician has an important advocacy role for the child and family, ensuring that appropriate support is in place from all agencies and the family is aware of the support available from the voluntary sector. A telephone call or letter from the paediatrician chasing up on equipment or other resources can make a big difference.

Sometimes team meetings involving key professionals along with the family can help to address the complex needs of the child. Such meetings are expensive in terms of professional and family time and can be intimidating for some families. Careful thought should be given to whether there are equally effective ways to achieve the desired outcomes.

Implications for the future

The outlook for children and young people with a learning disability is determined by the

* specific diagnosis;
* degree of learning disability;
* sensory impairments;
* resilience of the individual;
* environment and family support.

Honesty and openness with families from the outset is essential, about both what is known and what is *not* known. Some parents spend many years and precious family time and resources in pursuit of unachievable goals and lose track of the 'big picture' for the whole child and their family. Whilst always striving for optimizing and maximizing functioning in all domains, striving towards goals that are completely beyond reach will mean the child is repeatedly set up to fail. It is important always to celebrate each child's achievements and positive attributes, no matter how small, and to encourage a positive approach, emphasizing enjoyment of life and getting an appropriate balance between this and academic achievement.

Transitions

All transitions require careful thought and planning: into first nursery, from nursery to school, primary school to secondary, secondary to tertiary education. Transition to adult services is especially important and depends very much on the range of adult services available in the young person's locality to link up to. Care must be taken throughout childhood to keep the general practitioner (GP) in the loop and to ensure that the family makes appropriate use of primary care along the way; otherwise, there is a risk that the paediatrician will inadvertently disempower the GP by taking over all aspects of care in childhood, then expect the GP to pick up the baton when the young person leaves statutory education and graduates from paediatric care.

Careful, person-centred transition planning should ensure that care plans in adulthood continue to be relevant and comprehensive, towards ensuring the best possible quality of ongoing life.

Paediatricians should not fall into the trap of 'hanging on' to patients beyond 19 years, as we are not competent in the recognition and management of health issues that may present in adult life. If we believe that we are indispensable to families, then we may have inadvertently encouraged dependencies that are not sustainable or appropriate. We must empower families to use appropriately the broad range of agencies and professionals available to them, very importantly including their GP. For many young people, it is the GP who will carry the main responsibility for coordinating their health care throughout their life.

Key messages

- Diagnosis is important.
- Identify 'clinical handles' that can help to tailor investigations.
- If a diagnosis cannot be made, remember to review this regularly, as the child or young person may 'grow into' a recognizable pattern.
- Never be afraid to seek further expert clinical opinions, for example paediatric neurology or neurodisability, clinical genetics, metabolic paediatrics, learning disability and child psychiatry.
- Remember to think about secondary disabilities and comorbidities in order to be able to meet all the needs of the child.
- Beware of neurodegenerative disorders that can be missed if not specifically considered.

References

Oliver C, Richards C (2010) Self-injurious behaviour in people with intellectual disability. *Curr Opin Psychiatry* 23: 412–16. http://dx.doi.org/10.1097/YCO.0b013e32833cfb80

Oliver C, Murphy G, Hall S, Arron K, Leggett J (2003) Phenomonology of self restraint. *Am J Mental Retard* 108: 71–81. http://dx.doi.org/10.1352/0895-8017(2003)108<0071:POSR>2.0.CO;2

World Health Organization (2004) *International Statistical Classification of Diseases and Related Health Problems 10th Revision (ICD-10)*. Geneva: World Health Organization.

Further reading

Horridge KA (2011) Assessment and investigation of the child with disordered development. *Arch Dis Child Educ Pract Ed* 96: 9–20. http://dx.doi.org/10.1136/adc.2009.182436

King MD, Stephenson JBP (2009) *A Handbook of Neurological Investigations in Childhood*. London: Mac Keith Press.

McClintock K, Hall S, Oliver CJ (2003) Risk markers associated with challenging behaviours in people with intellectual disabilities: a meta-analytic study. *Intellect Disabil Res* 47: 405–16. http://dx.doi.org/10.1046/j.1365-2788.2003.00517.x

Website

Healthy child programme: www.rcpch.ac.uk/hcp

15
Educational underattainment or the child failing at school

Gillian Robinson

Learning objectives

- To understand factors affecting school attainment (Fig. 15.1).
- To have an approach to children who are failing to achieve at school (Fig. 15.2).
- To have knowledge and management strategies for children with specific learning difficulties.

Case vignette

John is an 8-year-old boy who had no initial difficulties in school, but lately he has had difficulties with reading. His mother is being contacted on a weekly basis about his behaviour. She is finding this very difficult to manage as she has recently split up from her husband and is struggling to manage both financially and emotionally. John has had chest difficulties, and has now been diagnosed with asthma.

Learning points

- If children are struggling with learning, and if this in not acknowledged or support is not given, then behaviour often deteriorates.
- Physical ill health affects learning, particularly if significant periods of school are missed.
- Children, like adults, struggle with concentration during traumatic periods in their lives.
- If it is only reading and writing then dyslexia should be considered.

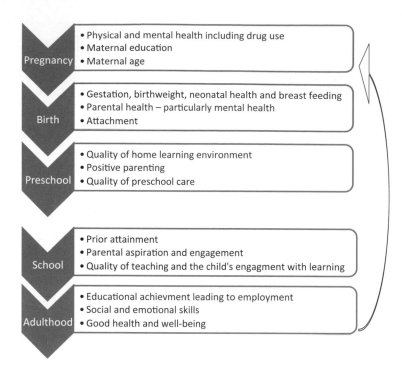

Pregnancy
- Physical and mental health including drug use
- Maternal education
- Maternal age

Birth
- Gestation, birthweight, neonatal health and breast feeding
- Parental health – particularly mental health
- Attachment

Preschool
- Quality of home learning environment
- Positive parenting
- Quality of preschool care

School
- Prior attainment
- Parental aspiration and engagement
- Quality of teaching and the child's engagment with learning

Adulthood
- Educational achievment leading to employment
- Social and emotional skills
- Good health and well-being

Figure 15.1 Factors affecting school attainment.

Educational underattainment describes a group of children who are falling behind in their learning compared with their peer group, or who are making poor or slow educational progress.

Poverty affects children's school achievement, and there is clear evidence that by school age children from poorer backgrounds do worse cognitively and behaviourally than those from more affluent homes. Schools do not effectively close that gap; children who arrive in the bottom range of ability tend to stay there. In fact, the brightest 5-year-olds from poorer homes are overtaken by the progress of their less gifted but richer peers by the time they are 10 years old (Perry and Becky 2010).

Handy hints: factors that help the home learning environment

- Reading to children
- Taking children to the library
- Helping children learn the alphabet
- Teaching children numbers or counting
- Teaching children songs, poems or nursery rhymes
- Painting or drawing

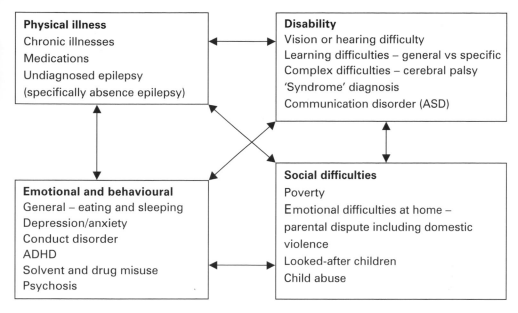

Figure 15.2 Reasons why a child might be failing at school. ASD, autism spectrum disorder; ADHD, attention-deficit–hyperactivity disorder.

Effect of failure at school (Fig. 15.3)

As we all know, once you are behind in your work, it is always difficult to catch up. This is more so if you have a specific difficulty affecting your learning. This can often lead to a vicious cycle. Also, often children would rather be seen to be silly or awkward than to let their classmates know they are struggling with their learning.

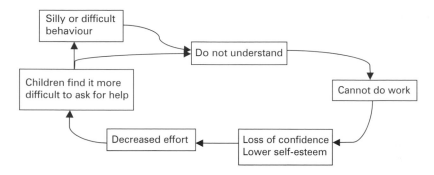

Figure 15.3 The consequences of failing to understand.

Assessment

Aims of assessment

- Does the child have difficulties in all areas of learning or specific areas?
- Is the learning difficulty new or ongoing?
- Is the child's school attendance good? If it is poor, why is this the case?
- Are there any difficulties with vision or hearing?
- Are there difficulties with behaviour?
- Are there safeguarding concerns?
- Examination should exclude neurological, genetic and general paediatric cause.

History

Learning

- What are the present difficulties and strengths?
- Has there been any loss of skills?
- What is the current attainment and how was this assessed?
- What support for learning is currently available?
- How is the relationship between the teacher and the child and between the school and family?
- What is the child's school attendance record?
- Has there been any bullying by either children or adults?
- What is the child's coordination like?

Behaviour

- What is the child's attention to tasks and impulsivity?
- How is the child's behaviour at school and home, including his or her relationship with peers and repeated behaviours?
- What are the child's eating and sleeping patterns?
- Have there been any episodes of unusual behaviour, such as epilepsy (especially absence epilepsy)?

Current health

- General health and medications.
- Concerns about hearing or vision.
- Concerns about use of street drugs.

Past history

- Pregnancy history, including alcohol and drug usage, and history of births, especially any preterm births.
- General health – including a history of epilepsy.

Developmental history

- How is the child's progress at nursery and school, including current abilities?
- Enquire about self-help skills and activities of daily living.

Family history

- Is there a history of learning or educational difficulties?

Social history

- Who does the child live with, and have there been any recent changes?
- Are there any safeguarding concerns? Talk to the child separately.

Examination

- General demeanour
  - mood
  - attention, impulsivity
  - social interaction including eye contact and facial expression.
- Relationship with parent.
- Dysmorphic features (including fetal alcohol syndrome).
- Skin – look for signs of neurocutaneous disorder (neurofibromatosis, tuberous sclerosis, bruises).
- Growth, particularly head circumference, height, weight.
- Neurological assessment.
- Coordination (see Chapter 12 on the clumsy child).
- Consider assessing attention, if appropriate, with Conners' questionnaires.

Simple functional assessments

Reading age

A simple test takes around 3 minutes. Various tests are available, such as the Burt reading test (www.syntheticphonics.com/burtreadingtestpage.htm).

Memory – forward and reverse digit span

This is a test of short-term memory and is commonly impaired in dyslexia. A sequence of random numbers are read at 1-second intervals – starting with around three numbers and then increasing. The normal digit span in 8- to 10-year-olds is 5 ± 1 and this increases to 6 ± 1 by adulthood. Reverse digit span is usually one less than forward span.

Drawing – Goodenough draw a person test

Ask the child to draw a person. At 3 years old a child is able to draw a circle, which scores three points. Each additional body part drawn gains a point. Children progress by adding on four body parts each year, i.e. the formula $3+(n/4)$ gives an approximate developmental age.

Writing

The child writes a sentence and then copies a sentence.

Coordination

See Chapter 12 on the clumsy child.

Investigations

- Low threshold for vision and hearing tests.
- Consider speech and language therapy assessment; if the child does not understand the instruction, he or she is likely to struggle. Speech and language therapists will also think about social communication.
- Discussion with school
  - teacher's assessment of difficulties
    - learning
    - child's behaviour with teachers, peers and family
  - child's ability on national curricular assessments
  - request to see any educational psychology assessments.
- Consider standardized questionnaires for attention (Conners' questionnaires) or mood.

Understanding school progress – England and Wales

National curriculum levels

The UK national curriculum has descriptions of different standards of work. These are then used to grade children's school progress. These descriptions are not age specific, and therefore, in theory, any child can be at any level.

For example, at maths level 2, pupils

- count sets of objects reliably, and use mental recall of addition and subtraction facts of 10
- begin to understand the place value of each digit in a number and use this to order numbers up to 100
- use the knowledge that subtraction is the inverse of addition
- use mental calculation strategies to solve number problems involving money and measures
- recognize sequences of numbers, including odd and even numbers.

Children functioning under 5 years

Children who are working towards the first level, which can be written as 'W', use a pivot scale, which is organized from P1 (lowest) to P8 (highest). Within each 'P' level there are further subdivisions, from a (highest) to e (lowest). So, for example, a P4a score is higher than a P4e. P4a is almost a P5e. Children with marked learning difficulties may be on the pivot scales throughout their school career.

Children aged 5 years and over

There are national standard assessments that are completed in year 2 (6–7y) and year 6 (10–11y). In addition, there is non-statutory testing available for each school year, which the majority of schools will complete. The normal rate of progress is two subgrades a year (Fig. 15.4).

Age	0-6m	6-12m	12-18m P2	18-24m P3	24-30m P4	30-36m P5	P6	P7-8	1c	1b	1a	2c	2b	2a	3c	3b	3a	4c	4b	4a	5c	5b	5a	6c	6b	6a	GCSE
0-6m																											
6-12m																											
12-18m																											
18-24m																											
24-30m																											
30-36m																											
nursery																											
reception																											
Year 1																											
Year 2																											
Year 3																											
Year 4																											
Year 5																											
Year 6																											
					Move to High School																						
Year 7																											
Year 8																											
Year 9																											
Year 10																											
Year 11																											

	Above national expectations
	Achieving national expectation
	Below national level of expectation – school action
	Further below expected level – for assessment by education psychology and external agencies
	Individual support needed – consider statement of special educational need

Figure 15.4 Levels of attainment and additional support.

Management

- Optimize medical treatment. Look to see if all the appointments are needed.
- Address any specific diagnoses raised and explain these to the parent including impact on learning. In particular, emphasize that if the child has a specific learning difficulty, the child is not 'stupid' or lazy, but that he or she has a particular problem with... It is helpful to say that he or she is also good at...
- Suitable educational support.
- Address areas of conflict at either home or school.
- Help families to understand the process for supporting children with additional needs in school (see Chapter 47 on special educational needs).
- Think about family resources and about how they can help their child.

Suitable educational support

In most classes the teacher will already be differentiating the work, probably to three groups, so it is important for children to be in the correct group so that they can understand, but are suitably stretched by, the activity.

Children who are struggling within the lowest group may be taken out for specific booster classes with a small group of other children. These happen for around 20 minutes three times a week. Most commonly, these are run by a learning support assistant under direction from a member of teaching staff. These children should be known to the school's special needs coordinator (SENCO), who can also be called the inclusion manager, and should have an individual education plan (IEP) written with specific targets that should be reviewed each term.

Children who are still struggling should then have additional assessment via educational psychology. If the child is functioning around 2 years behind their peers it is difficult for them to be included in the classroom setting without additional support. This should be sought through the procedures involved in special educational need.

Specific learning difficulties

These are a group of disorders exhibited by children who have normal overall intelligence but have difficulties in specific areas.

Dyslexia:	difficulties with reading
Dysgraphia:	difficulties with writing
Dyscalculia:	difficulties with numbers
Developmental coordination difficulties:	difficulties with coordination

As a group of disorders they have common themes and are defined in similar ways.

- General learning is normal.
- Difficulties in one area of learning that is around 2 years behind that of peers or, in children with other learning difficulties, where one area is significantly more delayed than others.

- This has always been the case.
- These difficulties are affecting the child.
- Difficulties are not due to an underlying medical disorder.
- The child has been in school regularly.

Key message

- For all of these conditions an understanding that the child has a particular difficulty with learning the skill rather than being obstructive or obtuse is key to making progress and maintaining the child's self-esteem.

It is well recognized that these difficulties do coexist, and part of assessing the child is to consider other comorbid diagnoses. All of these skills are based in the prefrontal cortex; it is therefore likely that the neurological deficit is in that area.

Clearly, multiple comorbidities merge into children with general learning difficulties (Fig. 15.5).

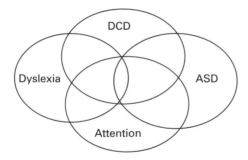

Figure 15.5 The effect of comorbidities on learning. DCD, developmental coordination disorder; ASD, autistic spectrum disorder.

Dyslexia-specific difficulties with reading and spelling

Dyslexia is the most common specific learning difficulty and its core feature is a marked reading difficulty. It is estimated to affect 5% to 10% of the population, and is more common in males. Dyslexia should be recognized as a spectrum disorder, with symptoms ranging from mild to very severe. People with dyslexia have difficulties with the following.

Phonological awareness

People with dyslexia struggle to understand the relationship between speech sounds and letters or letter groups (phonological coding deficits). The processing of language in the course of reading or writing is constantly compromised by the struggle to decode or encode words. This is particularly true when children meet new or made-up words.

Word attack skills

This is the understanding of how to break down words into smaller known groups of letters, e.g. sun/bath/ing.

Verbal memory

This is the ability to remember a sequence of verbal information for a short period of time, such as red, blue, green.

In the past it has been suggested that there is a visual component to dyslexia. There is little evidence to support this, but some people do feel that coloured glasses or overlay sheets help them.

Underlying cause

Dyslexia frequently is familial, occurring more often in sons (35–40% risk of occurrence) than in daughters (17 18% risk). Susceptibility loci have been identified on eight different chromosomes and, recently, four candidate genes have been identified. Clearly, there is significant heterogeneity. The available evidence suggests that dyslexia could be due to the abnormal migration and maturation of neurones during early development. Functional neuroimaging techniques have shown minor structural abnormalities in the temporal–parietal region and also the cerebellum, which would fit with these findings (Shastry 2007).

Presentation

Primary school children

- will have slow and halting reading
- have difficulty with comprehension
- put letters and figures the wrong way round
- have difficulty remembering days of the week, the alphabet, times tables
- leave letters out of words or put them in the wrong order.

Secondary school children

- still read inaccurately
- still have difficulties with spelling
- need to have instructions and telephone numbers repeated
- get 'tied up' using long words, for example 'preliminary', 'philosophical'
- confuse places, times and dates
- have difficulty with planning and writing essays.

Diagnosis

If the child has a marked discrepancy between written language skills and general learning (verbal skills, maths, science and coordination) then dyslexia is a likely diagnosis. Formal diagnosis requires appropriate testing by either a psychologist or appropriately trained teacher. This can be arranged by schools, but often they struggle for psychology and learning support time, and therefore, sadly, children with specific learning difficulties may not be prioritized. Families can arrange for a private assessment by an educational psychologist. Information from these reports can then be used to support the child's education.

> **Key message**
>
> The medical role in this process is to:
>
> 1   exclude underlying neurological disorder
> 2   consider comorbidities, including developmental coordination disorder or attention problems.

Management

Explanation

Provide an explanation of the problem.

A quiet environment for reading and writing

Suggest a quiet or non-distracting environment for reading and writing.

Structured teaching

Structured teaching approaches will help the majority of children with dyslexia to learn to read. These include

- Phonics alphabet, including the concept of long and short vowels, e.g. 'a' as in apple and 'a' as in ape. To help with this process use pictures and movements (such as the Jolly Phonics programme), making large letters in play dough and sand paper.
- Sound out words and break down words into syllables, such as in *Toe by Toe* (Cowling and Cowling 1993), which the family can use with their child.

Reading

The parent and child should spend time reading together. Normally the parent assists only with the words the child finds difficult. Also, paired reading, during which the parent and child read at the same time, can be helpful. Encourage the child to read anything he or she likes, including comics! This needs to be at a level at which he or she can read comfortably.

It is also important to assist with comprehension skills because, as the child struggles to decode individual words, an overall understanding can be lost.

Help with organization

Planners – if needed, the teacher should write down the homework.
Lists – making use of technology, for example a laptop.

Dysgraphia (Table 15.1): specific difficulties with writing

The child displays poor writing skills despite paying attention to the task. This includes spelling errors, letter reversals, unfinished words or omitted words and random or poor punctuation.

Table 15.1 A summary of the causes of writing difficulties

	Dyslexia	*Motor*	*Poor visuospatial skills*
Spontaneously written	Illegible	Illegible	Poor
Oral spelling	Poor	Normal	Normal
Copy written text	Normal	Poor	Poor
Drawing	Normal	Poor	Severe difficulty
Finger tapping speed	Normal	Decreased	Abnormal

Management

Writing

- Explanation.
- Good seating – feet should be on the ground and the desk should be at an appropriate height.
- Good positioning of paper – a slope might help (try using an A4 folder).
- Pen grips may help.
- Allow more time.
- Use technology – keyboard/dictate ideas/voice recognition software.
- Writing practice.
  - Mazes, dot to dots.
  - Handwriting practice – this is boring, but with continued practice handwriting will improve (the Handwriting Rescue Kit, which can be bought online, is a useful resource).

- Completing work – use POWER
  - P – plan your paper
  - O – organize your thoughts and ideas
  - W – write your draft
  - E – edit your work
  - R – revise your work and produce a final draft.

Spelling difficulties

Encourage students to write and correct key spellings only.

- Encourage the use of spellchecker – either electronic or aurally coded dictionary, such as the ACE spelling dictionary (Moseley 1995).
- Break down spelling lists into manageable chunks – three spellings a time, get the child to look, look away and spell out loud, and then write down the words in order to learn them.
- Use computer-based spelling games (e.g. Word Shark).

Dyscalculia (Table 15.2): specific difficulties with numbers

Dyscalculia is a common problem that affects 5% to 6% of the population and affects males and females equally. Difficulties with numbers can persist in more than half of those affected. There is a familial component, with more than half of children affected having a sibling with a similar problem.

Table 15.2 Normal mathematics skills

Age	Skill
3–4y	Count by rote Count four items with meaning Understand size concepts such as bigger and smaller
5y	Count up to 15 items with meaning Understanding the concepts of more or less, and larger and smaller Understand the relationship between written number and quantity Simple addition up to 10
8y	Recognize symbols Simple addition and subtraction Place numbers in the correct sequence Understand three-digit numbers Count in twos, tens and fives Managing money
11y	Three-digit number addition and subtraction Multiplication and division Understand about money

Diagnosis

The use of school testing can be helpful in suggesting the diagnosis – if there is a 2-year gap between the general and the expected level of achievement, dyscalculia is highly likely. There is a battery of standardized maths tests administered by educational psychology experts that will confirm the diagnosis.

Management

- Explain that this is a specific difficulty rather than a behaviour problem.
- Allow more time.
- Numeracy skills should be developed from the child's current level of understanding; ensure understanding of number and concepts.
- Use technology such as calculators once basic concepts have been mastered.
- There are many information technology maths resources to help, e.g. Mathletics.

Developmental coordination disorder

Developmental coordination disorder (DCD) has had a number of earlier names including dyspraxia and, before that, clumsy child. It is a common condition, with 6% of the childhood population affected and 1% severely affected. It is more common in males, with a male–female ratio of 3:1. Problems with coordination are seen more commonly in children who were born preterm or with intrauterine growth retardation.

Minor motor difficulties may not seem to be an important diagnosis, but the self-perception of failure when young children struggle with motor tasks can impact on their self-esteem and ability to engage in learning. Early assessment and understanding that poor skills are not deliberate, together with practical strategies to tackle the difficulties, will help in limiting the impact of DCD (Table 15.3).

The underlying pathophysiology is not clear but it can be demonstrated that children have the following problems:

- poor motor planning (e.g. how to jump)
- struggle with the amount of force and timing (e.g. poor ball skills)
- dependent on visual information rather than joint position sense (e.g. stair climbing)
- poor balance
- slower reaction time.

Table 15.3 Presentation of developmental coordination disorder

Preschool	Primary school	Secondary school	Adult (50% have ongoing difficulties with coordination)
Difficulty with dressing and toileting	Poor jumping	Poor hand writing	Handwriting difficulties
Poor drawing skills	Dressing problems	Academic failure	Independence difficulties
Poor ball skills	Messy eating	Poor organization	Organization difficulties
Difficulty using cutlery	Late in learning to ride a bicycle	Socially isolated – less participation in team games	Driving difficulties
Difficulty with jigsaws	Avoids active play	Low self-esteem	Less fit – increase in obesity
Difficulty using scissors	Low self-esteem	Bullying	Social isolation
	Bullying		Anxiety and depression
			Substance misuse

Assessment

Medical

The medical assessment has been discussed in the assessment of the clumsy child.
   The medical role is to

* identify any undiagnosed neurological difficulty
* have an understanding of the child's overall level of learning (this information can be obtained from school)
* assess the level of difficulty in coordination on clinical examination (see clumsy child) and also using appropriate screening questionnaires, such as the Movement ABC checklist. This can be quickly completed by the child's class teacher and gives a risk level of DCD. Refer to therapy colleagues only those children with significant difficulty.

Therapy assessment – occupational therapist or physiotherapist

Therapy assessments use standardized tools and can take between 20 minutes and 2 hours to administer depending on the test. These include the Movement ABC checklist and the Bruininks–Oseretsky Test of Motor Proficiency.

Therapeutic interventions

As with all skills, more practice leads to improved performance. Children with coordination difficulties progress more slowly than other children, but they can benefit from the skills being practised and taught. Not only is the skill learned, but also there is a boost to self-esteem and then children are more likely to participate with their peers.

There are different approaches:

- *Adaptations*: Are there any adaptations that will make life easier, such as avoiding the use of shoelaces by using Velcro fastenings (see dressing), using adapted scissors and pen grips.
- *Task-orientated therapy* looks at a specific skill that the child and family wish to improve and aims to improve this specific task through practice. It is helpful to break down the task into stages in order to aid learning the skill, giving appropriate feedback to the child so he or she can understand how to progress, such as dressing skills, ball skills, bike-riding skills and organization skills. Completing this in a group is helpful as children discover there are other people like them.
- *Process-orientated therapy* concentrates on developing sensory modalities involved in motor performance, such as the sensory integration approach, or kinaesthetic (movement perception) training. The evidence base for these approaches is similar to general stimulation programmes and they do not offer specific benefits.

Key messages for all learning difficulties

- Be positive – tell children about what they are good at.
- Praise children for making the first step in completing a task rather than at the end of the whole task.
- Tell children you know it is harder for them.
- Frequent short practices are better than infrequent long ones.
- Encourage children in areas where they can succeed – self-esteem is very important.

References

Cowling K, Cowling H (1993) *Toe by Toe: A Highly Structured Multi-sensory Reading Manual for Teachers and Parents*. Shipley: Keda Cowling.

Moseley D (1995) *Aurally coded dictionary – ACE spelling dictionary*. Wisbech, UK: LDA.

Perry B, Becky F (2010) The social class gap for educational underachievement: a review of the literature. Royal Society for the Encouragement of Arts, Manufactures and Commerce. Available at: www.thersa.org/__data/assets/pdf_file/0019/367003/RSA-Social-Justice-paper.pdf (accessed 4 November 2012).

Shastry B (2007) Developmental dyslexia: an update. *J Hum Genetics* 52: 104–9. http://dx.doi.org/10.1007/s10038-006-0088-z

Further reading

Demonet JF, Taylor MJ, Chaix Y (2004) Developmental dyslexia. *Lancet* 363: 9419. http://dx.doi.
org/10.1016/S0140-6736(04)16106-0.

Goodenough FL (1926) *Measurement of Intelligence by Drawings*. Chicago, IL: Harcourt.

Hadders-Algra M (2010) *The Neurological Examination of the Child with Minor Neurological Dysfunction*,
3rd edition. London: Mac Keith Press.

Missiuna C, Gaines R, Soucie H (2006) Why every office needs a tennis ball: a new approach to assessing
the clumsy child. *Can Med Assoc J* 175: 471–3. http://dx.doi.org/10.1503/cmaj.051202

Parry TS (2005) Assessment of developmental learning and behavioural problems in children and young
people. *Med J Aust* 183: 43–8. www.mja.com.au/public/issues/183_01_040705/par10304_fm.html

Sugden DA (2006) Developmental coordination disorder as a specific learning difficulty. Leeds Consensus
Statement. Economic and Social Research Council. Available at: www.dcd-uk.org (accessed 4 November
2012).

Websites

British Dyslexia Association: www.bdadyslexia.org.uk

Burt Reading Test: www.spontingrac.com/html_files/burt_test.html

Dyslexia Action: www.dyslexiaaction.org.uk

Jolly Phonics (phonic alphabet): www.jollylearning.co.uk/2007_UKGuide.pdf

Mathletics (Internet-based maths skills): www.mathletics.co.uk/

The Dyspraxia Foundation: www.dyspraxiafoundation.org.uk

The Handwriting Interest Group: www.handwritinginterestgroup.org.uk

16
Loss of previously acquired skills

Arnab Seal

Learning objectives

- To learn the various clinical presentations of neurodegeneration (regression).
- To know when to suspect a neurodegenerative disorder.
- To know how to investigate and when/where to refer for further evaluation.

Regression or loss of previously acquired skills is an uncommon but serious clinical problem. Concerns raised by parents/family or any professional regarding regression in any child must always be taken seriously and carefully evaluated. Clinicians should be mindful of the trap of an 'established diagnosis', most commonly cerebral palsy. Regressive neurological disorders can follow different trajectories (Fig. 16.1).

Regression may follow a period of normal development or may occur against the background of an existing developmental disorder. Those disorders that show a slow rate of loss of skills, such as some leukodystrophies, can be misdiagnosed as a non-progressive disorder. On the other hand, non-progressive, static conditions such as cerebral palsy can also present with functional loss from long-term disuse and mimic degeneration. The approach to any child presenting with a loss of skills requires an open mind, careful clinical evaluation and selected investigations.

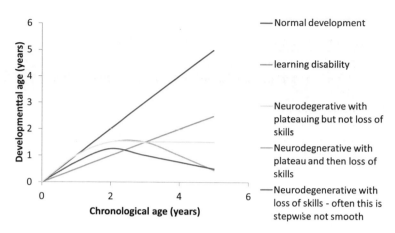

Figure 16.1 Developmental trajectories.

Case vignette

Anna, aged 2 years 6 months, presents to clinic with slow acquisition of walking. At 20 months she is not walking but is sitting. She is tearful and miserable in clinic and her mother says she has been like this since an admission for a respiratory tract infection some weeks before. She is observed to be crawling reciprocally. At review, after 3 months, she appears stiffer and is unable to demonstrate any crawling. Detailed investigation reveals a white matter disorder, subsequently diagnosed as vanishing white matter disease.

Learning points

- Is this a late presentation of significant delay – was it missed or was it not present at a younger age?
- Post-illness deterioration may be a characteristic of a metabolic illness.

Loss of skills or regression can result from degenerative disorders or from non-degenerative conditions (Table 16.1). A word of warning: a number of the presentations mentioned in Table 16.1, such as intractable seizures, deafness, visual loss, psychosis and autism, can themselves be clinical manifestations of a static or progressive condition. The loss of skills in these children may well be explained by the clinical finding itself, e.g. intractable seizures, but does not necessarily rule out the possibility of an underlying progressive condition. For instance, a child with difficult-to-control seizures and epileptic encephalopathy may lose skills as a result of the encephalopathy itself, but the seizures and encephalopathy may have been caused by a progressive neurological condition such as Alper disease.

Table 16.1 Loss of skills from non-neurometabolic conditions

Central nervous system disorder	Brain/central nervous system tumours
	Chronic central nervous system infection, e.g. human immunodeficiency virus
	Raised intracranial pressure
	Uncontrolled seizures (epileptic encephalopathy)
	Specific epilepsy syndromes, e.g. Landau–Kleffner syndrome, West syndrome
Poisons and toxins	Heavy metals and other neurotoxins, e.g. lead poisoning
	Substance misuse, e.g. drugs, alcohol
	Prescribed medication, e.g. sedatives, antiepileptics
Mental health disorders	Child abuse/bullying/severe psychological trauma/bereavement
	School failure/refusal (see Chapter 15)
	Severe psychiatric disorders, e.g. chronic disintegrative disorder
	Autism spectrum disorder
Other medical disorders	Chronic/progressive hearing or visual loss
	Endocrine dysfunction, e.g. hypothyroidism
	Chronic sleep deprivation (commonly from using the Internet, playing video games or watching television too late)
	Encephalopathy from any cause, e.g. chronic kidney or liver disease
	Non-progressive disorder with progressive skill loss from disuse, e.g. cerebral palsy

Most children presenting with deteriorating school performance and no other abnormal clinical signs or symptoms do not have a neurodegenerative condition. Commonly there are other reasons for educational failure such as specific learning disorders, bullying, chronic sleep deprivation, hearing loss, drug/alcohol misuse, etc. Taking a good history, including an exploration of psychosocial circumstances, coupled with information obtained from teachers, can usually point towards the correct diagnosis. Identifying and tackling some of the underlying causes, such as hearing loss or sleep deprivation, can be very rewarding.

In addition, there is a group of children with 'pseudo' degeneration who appear to be, or you are told, falling or tripping more. This group may already be known to you as having some motor difficulty, such as developmental coordination disorder, and at school entry start falling more. After examination and observation, this is often because the child is now trying to 'keep up' and attempt more complicated motor skills or those that are in the way of their more motor-sophisticated peers.

Red flags for children presenting with loss of skills

- Rate of progression or stability of an illness can give diagnostic clues.
- Multiple neurological involvement makes neurodegenerative illness likely.
- Multisystem involvement makes a neurometabolic condition likely.
- Fluctuation of symptoms make neurometabolic and seizure disorders likely.
- Asymmetry of symptoms and signs can be common (contrary to common belief).
- Family history of similar condition and/or consanguinity increases likelihood of neurometabolic/genetic disorder.

Clinical approach (Table 16.2)

Table 16.2 The age at onset can give useful clinical clues to the underlying cause

Age	Presentation
First week	Non-ketotic hyperglycinaemia Hyperammonaemia Type 1 gangliosidosis Type 1 glycogen storage disorder Biotinidase deficiency Peroxisomal disorders (adrenoleukodystrophy, Refsum, Zellweger)
1mo	Galactosaemia Pompe disease (type II glycogen storage disorder) Maple syrup urine disease Infantile neuronal ceroid lipofuscinosis Menke syndrome
2–6mo	Gaucher disease Tay–Sach disease Krabbe disease Niemann–Pick disease Phenylketonuria (particularly if not born in the UK) Canavan disease Alexander disease
6–12mo	Lesch–Nyhan syndrome Pelizaeus–Merzbacher disease Homocysteinuria
6mo–2y	Autistic regression Rett syndrome Adrenoleukodystrophy GM1 gangliosidosis type II Hurler syndrome Metachromatic leukodystrophy Mitochondrial disorders (Leigh disease) Niemann–Pick type C

Age	Presentation
2–6y	Infantile-form neuronal ceroid lipofuscinosis Hunter syndrome GM2 type III gangliosidosis Subacute sclerosing panencephalitits HIV Wilson disease
4–8y	Juvenile form of neuronal ceroid lipofuscinosis Sanfillipo syndrome
8y and over	Adrenoleukodystrophy Huntington chorea Lafora body disease Niemann–Pick disease Juvenile metachromatic leukodystrophy Gaucher disease type III (juvenile) Hallervorden–Spatz syndrome

HIV, human immunodeficiency virus.

Key questions for clinical assessment

Is there any loss of skills?

- In one or a number of areas?
- What is the age and nature at onset?
- What is the nature of the progression? Slow and relentless, fluctuating, stepwise?
- Are there any clear precipitants?

Are there any other neurological symptoms?

- Seizures?
- Symptoms suggesting raised intracranial pressure?

Are there other health issues?

- General health
- Are there previous neurological diagnoses – who made the diagnosis and on what evidence?

Is the child taking any drugs?

- Prescribed (especially antiepileptics) or non-prescribed?

Are there any concerns about hearing or vision?

- Has there been any changes in behaviour, including sleep?

Has anyone in the family had similar problems?

- Take a history going back three generations, asking specifically about consanguinity and human immunodeficiency virus.

Social history

- Family structure and changes.
- Housing (carbon monoxide and lead poisoning).
- Schooling, including attendance and bullying.

Examination

General

- Growth, including head circumference.
- Body proportions and any skeletal abnormalities.
- Skin – neurocutaneous markers, pigmentation, disorders, xanthomas.
- Dysmorphic features, including coarse facies

Neurological (Tables 16.3 and 16.4)

- Eyes – cornea, iris, lens, fundus, visual acuity and eye movements.
- Ask child to gently rest hands on yours (any abnormal movement can be made more obvious).
- Observe hands at rest and with active movements.
- Formal central nervous system examination.

Systems examination

- Particularly hepatosplenomegaly, cardiac signs and symptoms.

Table 16.3 Important neurological symptoms/signs in a child with loss of skills

Symptom/sign	Clinical correlation and example
Seizures	Age at onset, e.g. onset in infancy in Krabbe disease Type(s) of seizures, e.g. spasms in SSPE Seizure control; difficult to control, e.g. ring chromosome 20
Spasticity	See movement disorders (Chapters 9 and 10)
Ataxia	Progressive ataxia – see movement disorders (Chapters 9 and 10)
Extrapyramidal signs	Chorea, e.g. Lesch–Nyhan syndrome Dystonia, e.g. Wilson disease – see movement disorders (Chapters 9 and 10)

Symptom/sign	Clinical correlation and example
Cognitive decline/ language decline	Usually present in all but may be a late sign Insidious language decline can be Landau–Kleffner syndrome
Psychosis/ behavioural disturbance	Attention difficulty, e.g. Sanfillipo syndrome (MPS type 3) Self-injury, e.g. Lesch–Nyhan syndrome Hand wringing, e.g. Rett syndrome
Head size	Macrocephaly, e.g. MPS Microcephaly, e.g. mitochondrial disorder
Sensory loss	Visual loss, e.g. X-linked adrenoleukodystrophy Hearing loss
Family history	Consanguinity and family history of similar illness or loss

The examples cited are not the only condition in which the clinical sign/symptom can be found. SSPE, subacute sclerosing panencephalitis; MPS, mucopolysaccharidosis.

Table 16.4 Useful non-neurological signs/symptoms in a child with loss of skills

Symptom/sign	Clinical correlation and example
Eye signs	Corneal haze, e.g. mucopolysaccharidosis Cataracts, e.g. Lowe syndrome Retinitis pigmentosa, e.g. Refsum disease Optic atrophy, e.g. leukodystrophies Cherry red spot, e.g. gangliosidosis Kayser–Fleischer ring, e.g. Wilson disease Conjunctival telangiectasia, e.g. ataxia telangiectasia
Skin or hair changes	Kinky/steel-wool hair, e.g. Menke disease Angiokeratoma, e.g. Fabry disease Xanthomas, e.g. cerebrotendinous xanthomatosis Ichthyosis, e.g. Refsum disease Fair skin, blonde hair, e.g. phenylketonuria Pigmentation, e.g. X-linked adrenoleukodystrophy Seborrhoeic dermatitis/alopecia, e.g. biotinidase deficiency
Skeletal changes	Dysostosis multiplex, e.g. mucopolysaccharidosis Joint swelling, e.g. Farber disease Rachitic changes, e.g. Lowe syndrome Scurvy-like changes, e.g. Menke disease
Visceral	Hepatosplenomegaly, e.g. mucopolysaccharidosis, peroxisomal disorders Vomiting, e.g. urea cycle disorders Diarrhoea, e.g. cerebrotendinous xanthomatosis
Facial dysmorphism	Coarse facies, e.g. mucopolysaccharidosis Typical facies, e.g. Zellweger syndrome

The examples cited are not the only condition in which the clinical sign/symptom can be found.

In children who present with loss of skills and associated other clinical signs and symptoms, further evaluation for a neurometabolic, degenerative and/or genetic cause should be undertaken (Fig. 16.2).

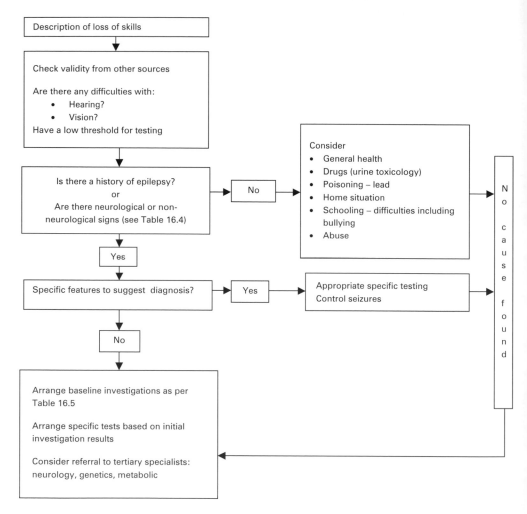

Figure 16.2 Flow chart for investigating the underlying cause in children who have lost skills.

Table 16.5 Investigations to consider in any child who is losing skills

Blood	Full blood count
	Urea and electrolytes, liver function test, creatinine, bone profile
	Thyroid function
	Uric acid
	Plasma amino acids
	Plasma lactate
	Blood sugar
	Blood gas
	Serum ammonia
	Where clinically indicated lead levels, copper/caeruloplasmin, acylcarnitines, very long-chain fatty acids
	Bile salts, biotinidase, white cell enzymes, cholesterol, vitamin E, phytanic acid
Urine	Urine amino acids and organic acids
	Urine mucopolysaccharides and oligosaccharides
	Urine creatinine
	Urine uric acid
	Urine toxicology (if substance misuse or poisoning suspected)
Imaging	MRI of brain ± spine
	Skeletal survey
Ophthalmology	Fundus examination
	Slit lamp examination
Electrophysiology	EEG if seizures
	VEP, ERG if visual loss (specialist teams)
	EMG if peripheral neuropathy is suspected
CSF (second line)	Preferably specialist paediatric neurology/metabolic team decision
	Glucose, protein, lactate, folate, amino acids, neurotransmitters, virology
Genetic tests (second line)	Karyotype/CGH array
	DNA tests including mitochondrial DNA
	Specific test for any condition suspected
Biopsy (second line)	Skin, muscle, liver, brain, according to situation

Second-line tests and tests done only when a specific condition is suspected and after discussion with paediatric neurology and other specialist teams as necessary. MRI, magnetic resonance imaging; EEG, electroencephalography; VEP, visual evoked potential; ERG, electroretinography; EMG, electromyography; CSF, cerebrospinal fluid.

The number and complexity of possible conditions is ever expanding and it is advisable to refer the child to a specialist paediatric neurology, paediatric metabolic and/or genetic service as deemed appropriate. An initial battery of tests that may be considered is provided in Table 16.5, but this must be individualized based on the clinical presentation. Treatment is dependent on the underlying cause. A number of conditions are treatable and should be specifically tested for. Enzyme replacement therapy, substrate/end product replacement and bone marrow transplant have been effective in some enzyme deficiencies. Gene therapy and stem cell research hold promises for the future. Symptomatic management, therapy, family support and counselling for carers, siblings and other family members are important for both treatable and untreatable conditions.

Key messages

- Loss of skills or regression is extremely worrying and needs urgent assessment and investigation.
- Most children presenting with deteriorating school performance and no other abnormal clinical signs or symptoms do not have a neurodegenerative condition.
- Clinical features may evolve over time. Initial clinical signs may be isolated signs for a long time, especially with spasticity. Loss of skills in a child previously diagnosed with cerebral palsy or any static neurological illness warrants diagnostic review and further investigation.
- Progressive spasticity without a history of perinatal or postnatal brain injury (such as preterm birth, hypoxia, trauma or infection) requires investigation. Consider a trial of levodopa and CSF studies for neurotransmitters and folate.
- Search for evolving neurological and non-neurological signs, which may give clues.
- Consider repeat neuroimaging if there is progressive loss of skills or new neurological signs, especially if the previous scan was under 2 years age (prior to completion of myelination).
- Referral to specialist paediatric neurology/paediatric metabolic/genetic service is recommended when neurometabolic condition is suspected.

Further reading

Dale RC, Vincent A, editors (2010) *Inflammatory and Autoimmune Disorders of the Nervous System in Children*. London: Mac Keith Press.

King M, Stephenson JBP (2009) *A Handbook of Neurological Investigations*. London: Mac Keith Press.

Section 7

Behaviour disorders

17
Behaviour and understanding and coping with disability

Martina Waring and Arnab Seal

Learning objectives

- To understand the effect of chronic illness and disability on behaviour.
- To be able to describe the clinical presentation and functional impact of the common behavioural disabilities.
- To be able to discuss the management of common behavioural disabilities in isolation or in the context of an associated developmental disability.

Understanding normal behaviour patterns

Behavioural difficulties can have a significant negative impact on a child's functioning. Behavioural disturbance is often referred to as 'challenging behaviour' to reflect the challenge it poses to carers and does not imply that the child is deliberately challenging authority. Certain patterns of behaviour are recognized as an identifiable biological condition, such as attention-deficit–hyperactivity disorder, whereas other behavioural patterns are known to be associated with a diagnosed disorder, for example 'cocktail party' behaviour in Williams syndrome. The latter are referred to as 'behavioural phenotypes', which, when recognized, can help in diagnosis, targeted assessment and intervention (see Section 6). In other instances, injury to the developing brain, e.g. by exposure to drugs, alcohol and toxins, can result in a higher risk of behavioural difficulty in later life. Risks of behavioural dysfunction may also increase with pre-existing conditions such as epilepsy, communication disorders and sensory impairments.

Being affected by a disability can have a significant impact on a child's mental health and behaviour. There is usually a complex interaction between biological, environmental and psychosocial factors. Children with a disabling condition often have a low self-esteem from negative social attitudes at school or home. Depression, anxiety, aggression, self-injury, mental health conditions and high parental stress levels are much more common in children with learning difficulties or communication difficulties and those experiencing pain.

Parental attitudes can be influenced by negative cultural and community experiences. In cultures where disability is not accepted as part of mainstream community life, the child and family can experience social isolation and exclusion. This can sometimes lead to distress for the child and family and difficult family relationships as a consequence. On the other hand, adopting a model of care that is overprotective and which focuses on disability rather than ability can lead to dependence and further disablement of the child.

Early recognition and effective management of behavioural disorders is important for these children and their families. When the disorders go unrecognized or untreated, children can fail to function in educational and social settings, become unmanageable at home and often display self-injurious behaviour. A multidisciplinary approach involving the family, paediatric team, child mental health team, the educational setting and social support is required for effective intervention.

Understanding and coping with disability

Chronic illness affects around one in six children but only 1% to 2% of children experience significant behavioural difficulties. The idea that most children with a chronic disability will experience psychological morbidity is outdated. Most children adapt to their circumstance and often do not experience any behavioural difficulty. The way in which children react to their illness depends on several factors, including the child's personality, the specific illness and their family. Family structure, attitudes, resilience and coping mechanisms play an important role in the child's adaptation to disability. One major factor is the child's developmental stage and his or her understandings of what causes illness. It is important to provide the child with the appropriate level of information and the right kind of support at the right time. This helps boost resilience and coping ability. Health practitioners will do well to remember that the medical condition itself and the medical establishment are not high on the list of priorities in the lives of most children with disabilities. It is usually regarded as one more of the regular mundane things that one has to comply with to get on with life. It is a bit like homework: an inconvenience that needs to be complied with as otherwise there will be consequences to face!

Infants and toddlers have very little understanding of their illness. They experience pain, restriction of motion and separation from their parents as challenges to developing trust and security. Reassurance, consistency of care and comfort from caregivers provides a sense of security and control. Preschool children may understand what it means to get sick, but they may not understand the cause-and-effect nature of illness. Any impairment can challenge the child's developing independence. The child may try to counter lack of control over their world by challenging limits set by parents. Parents can help by being firm with things that the child does not have a choice over and offering choices where possible. For example, never ask 'Do you want to take your medicine now?' unless there really is a choice – almost all children will say 'NO!'. However, 'Do you want the medicine from a red or blue spoon?' may be feasible.

Early school-aged children can describe reasons for illness, but these reasons may not be entirely logical. Children of this age often have 'magical thinking'. They may believe that they caused illness by thinking bad thoughts or by not eating their vegetables. Children also begin to sense that they are different from their peers. Parents can help by allowing children to help in the management of their illness (with close adult supervision). They should reassure their child that the illness is not their fault. Older school-aged children are more capable of understanding their illness and its treatment, but they should not be expected to react as adults do. They may feel left out when they miss school or activities with their peers. Parents may feel the need to protect their children by restricting them from activities with other children. This is a natural reaction, but it can interfere with the child's independence and sense of mastery. Parents should encourage their child to participate in school or other activities as far as practicable and to the extent allowed by medical advice.

Adolescents begin to develop their own identity separate from their family. Self-image becomes extremely important during the teenage years. That can be a problem when the teen-ager's appearance is altered by illness or medication. Often children feel they themselves are not disabled but perceive others to be. Teenagers are also beginning to develop a real independence from their families. Parents who have been very involved in their teenager's care for many years may find it difficult to let go of their role as primary caregiver. This can be particularly challeng-ing for any teenager. Many teenagers will go through times of denial of their illness when they may neglect to take medications or follow advice. In addition, the adolescent's body is rapidly changing, which may change the symptoms of the illness or the doses of medications needed. It is important to help the teenager to gain control of his or her condition and the environment. It is worth remembering that teenagers will be teenagers irrespective of their disability, and the important issues to them are independence, college planning, sexuality and so on.

Having a chronic disability may make the child feel depressed if excluded, anxious when not in control or angry with the world in general. Promoting resilience in the child and within the family can help reduce the chances of such problems appearing. Developing resilience involves behaviours, thoughts and actions that can be learned by children over time.

Tips for developing resilience in a child

- Teach the child how to make connections and friends. Community and social networks improve resilience.
- Encourage the child to help others.
- Maintain a daily routine and structure in the child's life.
- Teach the child how to take a break from anxieties and worries.
- Teach the child how to take care of him/herself (self-care). Provide a good role model at home and at school.
- Teach the child to set reasonable goals and then to move towards them one step at a time.
- Nurture a positive self-view. Teach the child to develop the ability to laugh at him/herself.
- Keep things in perspective and maintain a hopeful outlook.
- Encourage opportunities for self-discovery, e.g. coping in tough circumstances.
- Change can be scary. Help the child accept that change is part of living.

General behaviour management principles

All children and adults have certain needs that must be met in order for them to thrive and develop successfully into adulthood, as shown in Maslow's hierarchy of needs in Fig. 18.1.

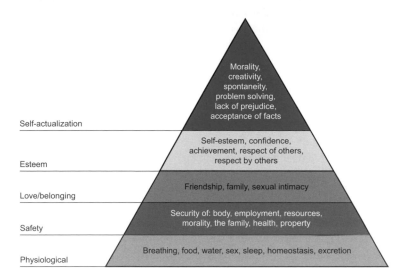

Figure 18.1 Maslow's hierarchy of needs.

For children there are additional things that are required to maximize their development in all areas, including encouragement, opportunities for play and awareness of boundaries, in the context of warm, loving relationships with key adults.

The pressures of modern life lead many parents to struggle to meet these needs, and their children can exhibit behaviour difficulties as a result. There is a wide range of parenting courses and materials now available to support parents in managing their child's behaviour more effectively, and while some have a particular focus they tend to share an emphasis on 'positive parenting approaches'. The quality of the parent–child relationship appears to be key to achieving positive behaviour change, so interventions that focus on improving parental attunement and the ability to engage and play with their child are also effective.

Key positive techniques

- Praise
- Using rewards as a motivator
- Promoting parent–child interactions through play and effective communication
- Effective limit setting
- Parental modelling of emotional regulation skills
- Appropriate parental expectations depending on the child's developmental stage

Websites

The Incredible Years: www.incredibleyears.com
Mellow Parenting: www.mellowparenting.org
Parenting.co.uk: www.parenting.co.uk

18
Behaviour in children with disabilities

Martina Waring and Arnab Seal

Learning objectives

- To know how to carry out an initial assessment of any type of challenging behaviour.
- To be able to identify the main risk factors which can lead to challenging behaviours.
- To identify some basic interventions that parents and carers may be able to implement to reduce challenging behaviours.

Caring for children with disabilities

To be able to thrive, children with disabilities have the same requirements as children without disabilities; however, they often have additional requirements from their parents and carers.

- *Predictability* – having a learning disability makes understanding the world very hard, and many children experience high levels of anxiety about what is happening to them, and what will happen next. Predictable routines provide a structure that will support children and reassure them about what is happening, thereby increasing their sense of control over themselves and their world.
- *Clear communication* – children with learning disabilities often have difficulties understanding and expressing complex information. Many children understand things better if the spoken word is supported with visual prompts, such as objects, photographs or pictures. Advice from a speech and language therapist can be invaluable in promoting 'total communication' using all modes of communication and interaction.
- *High levels of consistency* are effective in reducing behaviour difficulties in all children, but because children with learning disabilities can become easily confused and unsettled by mixed messages or too much change, it is particularly important for them. This can be especially important when children spend time in several different settings with many different carers.

- *More support* in maintaining friendships, staying healthy and getting their needs met timeously and appropriately. Having friends and accessing appropriate activities promotes development and protects children from mental health difficulties. Negotiating complex professional systems can be a time-consuming and daunting task, but many parents and carers succeed in becoming formidable advocates for their children.

Behavioural difficulties

Children with learning disabilities are at least four times more likely to experience behavioural difficulties or 'challenging behaviour' than their non-disabled peers; the more severe their level of disability, the higher the risk.

Definition

Challenging behaviour is any behaviour that places the individual or others at significant risk of harm or leads to the individual being excluded from normal community activities.

There is no definitive list of what types of behaviour are challenging, as it is often the context in which they occur which makes them problematic. The children who are most at risk of developing severe challenging behaviours are those with a dual diagnosis of learning disability and autism. Self-injurious behaviours are especially difficult for carers to cope with and are most often seen in children with profound disabilities and/or genetic conditions such as Lesch–Nyhan, Cornelia de Lange, Smith–Magenis, fragile X and Angelman syndromes.

Behaviours which are often seen as challenging

Aggressive behaviours – hitting, biting, scratching, kicking or head butting others. These are difficult to change as they can cause fear in others, making them reluctant to implement management strategies. When other children get hurt it can be very emotive for carers and lead to negative attributions about the child, and the risk of punitive approaches such as exclusion from school.

Self-injurious behaviours – hitting, biting, scratching oneself, head banging, eye poking or skin picking. These behaviours can evoke extreme responses in carers and are therefore powerful and effective in achieving the child's desired outcomes. Minimizing injury is paramount, making the implementation of strategies such as ignoring or withdrawal of attention very difficult to achieve.

Elimination behaviours – urinating, soiling, spitting, vomiting and smearing. Behaviours that involve bodily fluids also evoke powerful responses in others. They can be linked to a child's sensory needs, physical health problems or abuse.

Sexualized behaviours – stripping, masturbating, touching other people inappropriately. Again, these behaviours can evoke powerful responses in others, making them very effective in gaining adult intervention. They can be linked to sensory needs or abuse, but need to be viewed in a developmental context.

Repetitive behaviours – screaming, rocking, hand flapping, spinning. Often linked to sensory needs, commonly associated with autism, and can be a risk factor for later development of self-injurious behaviours. These behaviours can be a child's way of coping with situations or environments that feel overwhelming.

Understanding challenging behaviour

The first question you should ask yourself when faced with a child who is displaying problematic behaviours is 'What is the child getting out of behaving in this way?'.

Understanding the function of any given behaviour is crucial to deciding what form of intervention is needed. The aim of the behaviour tends to fall into one of the following categories:

- to secure interaction with a preferred adult
- to obtain something tangible and highly valued, e.g. food
- to avoid doing something undesirable, e.g. difficult school tasks or
- to gain sensory experiences that are wanted or needed.

If a particular behaviour results in a desired outcome for a child, that behaviour quickly becomes reinforced and is much more likely to occur again. This is known as operant conditioning, and this type of learned behaviour can occur irrespective of the extent of a child's intellectual impairments.

Case vignette

Carla is an 8-year-old female with cerebral palsy and a severe learning disability. She is reliant on the care of adults for all of her day-to-day needs. She has no speech but enjoys social interaction. One day she has a headache and she begins to make noises to try to get someone to come to her and make her feel better. This is unsuccessful so she begins rocking in her wheelchair, but still no one comes. She then begins to hit herself on the head with her fist and immediately her support worker rushes to her. Her worker cuddles her, talks to her, sings to her and makes her feel better. The next time Carla feels unwell she does not waste time calling or rocking; she instantly starts to hit herself and she quickly has her needs met.

Learning point

This type of situation creates a powerful cycle of reinforcement which can be very resistant to change.

The second question to ask is 'What is this child's developmental level?'.

If a child aged 2 years screams, kicks and throws him- or herself on the floor, it can be seen as developmentally appropriate. If a child aged 14 years behaves in the same way it would be seen as 'abnormal'; however, a 14-year-old child who has a severe learning disability may function in many ways at the level of a 2-year-old, and so his or her behaviour needs to be understood as being in line with the developmental stage that he or she is at.

The third question to ask is 'How does this child communicate how he or she is feeling?'.

Difficulties with expressive language and managing social interactions are widespread in children with learning disabilities and they mean that often the children do not have the necessary understanding or skills to tell others how they are feeling in words. Instead, they may show how they are feeling through their behaviour, leaving the adults around them to work out what the behaviour means.

Assessing challenging behaviour

Difficult behaviours can take many forms as listed earlier, but whatever a particular behaviour looks like, the method of assessment remains the same.

Step 1 – Record the behaviour

In order to fully understand the function of any behaviour it is essential to gather as much relevant information about it as possible. This includes when it happens, where it happens, who it happens with, what happens just before it happens (the triggers) and what happens afterwards (the reinforcers). A simple ABC chart is very useful and most parents will be able to complete one if they are given clear directions about what type of information is needed (see Appendix VI).

Step 2 – Use the recordings to identify patterns of behaviour

Often the process of recording allows parents/carers to see the patterns in a child's behaviour for themselves, for example it always happens when their sibling is around and taking the parent's attention away, or it tends to happen most on a Friday when the child is more tired. Sometimes a parent is so involved in the situation that someone who is more removed from the child may be needed to complete the recording sheets, e.g. a teacher, support worker or grandparent.

Step 3 – Consider other explanations

If no obvious patterns emerge then it is possible that the child's behaviour is linked not to environmental triggers but to internal triggers such as pain or distress (see Chapter 53). Constipation and tooth decay are common causes of behavioural disturbance in children with severe learning disabilities, and should always be excluded as part of a behavioural assessment. Post-traumatic stress disorder (PTSD) also needs to be considered in children who become extremely distressed for no apparent reason, especially in view of the higher number of negative life events to which young people with disabilities are exposed. Anxiety and low mood could also be contributing factors; young people with learning disabilities are at a heightened risk of both because of their experience of the world as hard to understand and control and the high levels of social isolation that they often experience.

Intervening with challenging behaviour

Once you have an understanding of why a child is behaving in a certain way, you are in a position to intervene to change it if appropriate. In cases where a child is communicating that there is something wrong with their care or their environment then the focus should be on improving their environment. If a child hits out because he or she does not understand what is being asked of him or her, then the intervention should aim to promote understanding of the child's comprehension skills via training or involvement of a speech and language therapist. If children bite themselves when they feel stressed or worried, then they may need to be taught ways of relaxing or other ways of telling people how they feel. Involvement of other key professionals may be required in order to look at what interventions are available and how best to implement these changes in a way that parents and carers can manage.

Case vignette

Max is a 9-year-old boy with a visual impairment and a moderate learning disability. Every time his teacher asks him to go to the hall he begins screaming and climbs under the tables in the classroom. When staff try to remove him he kicks and hits them. In the end he is left behind while his classmates go to the hall for singing practice.

Over time the school staff realize that Max is scared of being in the hall because it is too loud and busy, and because Max cannot see what is happening he feels unsafe. In order to address this situation the staff start taking Max into the hall at quiet times so that he can get used to it. They gradually reintroduce the other children into the hall while allowing Max to stand at the side with a familiar adult who can reassure him. Over time Max feels more confident in the hall and is able to join in with singing along with his classmates, and he no longer needs to sit under the tables.

Learning point

If you understand why a child behaves in the way he or she does, then the intervention should be aimed at finding a more desirable way for the child to meet that particular need, thus removing the need for the undesirable behaviour in the future.

Self-injurious behaviour

> ### Risk factors for self-injurious behaviour
>
> - Severe intellectual impairment
> - Severely limited communication skills
> - Additional sensory impairments
> - Physical health problems, for example pain and/or discomfort

Although self-injurious behaviours can be some of the most distressing for parents and carers to cope with, the process of assessment is the same as any other type of behaviour. Having said this, particular attention should be paid to excluding physical pain as a contributing factor, and the child's sensory needs also need special consideration. Sensory overload can be experienced as a form of pain, and for this reason a full assessment of a child's sensory profile may be needed. Self-injurious behaviours are often the most resistant to change. This is because of the biofeedback loop (Fig. 20.1) that quickly becomes established in any self-injurious behaviour and which gives the child the powerful experience of being able to make himself feel better.

If interventions are to be effective in reducing self-injury they need to happen quickly; the longer the cycle is established, the lower the chances of success.

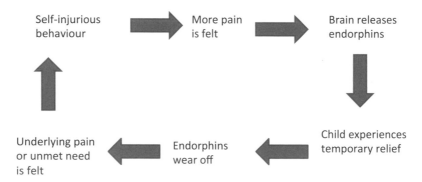

Figure 20.1 The feedback loop in self-injurious behaviour.

Case vignette

Daniel is a 10-year-old male with a moderate leaning disability and a physical disability that severely restricts his ability to move around his environment unaided. Daniel used to bite his hands and scream at sudden changes when he was a toddler, and recently this behaviour has re-emerged. He is biting through his skin and is exposing his hands to repeated infections, which is causing a high level of concern at home and school.

The recording charts show that the behaviours are more likely when he is tired, when there are unexpected changes to his routine and when he is exposed to loud, busy places. Once these triggers are identified the interventions focus on improving his sleep routines and introducing a symbol system so that he can express his worries more appropriately and the adults around him can communicate what is happening in advance. He is also given more choices about whether he goes to busy places and when he can leave, and, over time, the frequency of the behaviours reduces.

Learning points

- Look out for children at heightened risk of developing self-injurious behaviours.
- Encourage active involvement of services as soon as self-injury develops.
- Always investigate physical health problems and pain.

Useful resources

The Challenging Behaviour Foundation (www.thecbf.org.uk or www.challengingbehaviour.org.uk) has a large number of easy-to-download resources including information sheets/packs for parents and professionals.

The Contact a Family (www.cafamily.org.uk/pdfs/behaviour.pdf) parent information booklet on behaviour management in children with disabilities is comprehensive and provides a range of behaviour management ideas for families.

Further reading

Gillberg C, O'Brien G (eds.) (2000) *Developmental Disability and Behaviour*. London: Mac Keith Press.

Howlin P (ed.) (2000) *Behavioural Approaches to Problems in Childhood*. London: Mac Keith Press.

Websites

Contact a Family: www.cafamily.org.uk

Mencap: www.mencap.org.uk

19
Common behavioural disorders

Arnab Seal

Attachment disorders

Attachment can be disordered as a result of difficulties in the child, the parent or the environment (Table 19.1).

Parent

If parents cannot understand their infant's feelings because of their own difficulties in noticing or regulating their own feelings, they will be less able to meet the infant's needs in a empathetic and predictable way. This is particularly true if parental care is

- inconsistent or indifferent
- hostile or rejecting
- rigid or intrusive
- unpredictable or uncertain.

Child

If the child is not able to respond in a normal manner to the parent because of either illness or developmental difficulty, this will impact on the care that the parent will be able to offer.

Table 19.1 Risk factors for disordered attachment

Parent	Child	Environment
Mental health difficulties	Illness	War
Learning difficulties	Sensory impairment – vision	Displacement
Drugs and alcohol use	Significant developmental	Domestic violence
Poor early parenting	delay	

Assessing attachment

Whilst it can be helpful to describe observed child–parent interactions in the clinic, and these can be very helpful when considering emotional abuse, you should *not* label children as having an attachment disorder. By definition, attachment behaviour can be observed only when the child attachment system is 'activated' by a mild stress when the child's search for safety and security can be seen.

Useful observations regarding attachment

- Does the child seek comfort from the mother/carer when distressed?
- How does the mother/carer respond?
- Does her response comfort the child?
- Is the balance between secure base versus exploration instinct age appropriate?
- How does the child relate to you?

In order for the observations to be meaningful this should be completed in a standardized manner by appropriately trained staff (usually a psychologist who has been on a dedicated course lasting several days; see Table 19.2).

It is only after such an assessment that a formal label should be attached to a child. It is, however, important for paediatricians to be aware of different patterns of behaviour seen in attachment disorder so that appropriate assessment and help can be sought.

Table 19.2 Formal assessments of attachment

Developmental period	Method of assessment	Length of assessment (minutes)	Requirements (all require observation room and video equipment)
Infancy	Observation: stranger situation	21	Extra person (stranger)
Preschool and primary school	Observation: stranger situation	21	Extra person (stranger)
	Story stem: Manchester child attachment story test	30	Dolls' house and figures
Adolescence	Interview: child attachment interview	45	None

Described attachment disorders

INSECURE ATTACHMENT

If the attachment process does not progress normally the child may become

- emotionally self-reliant (suppress his or her feelings, avoid intimacy and withdraw socially)
- angry, demanding and attention seeking
- confused and distressed
- fearful and anxious and finding it hard to concentrate. In later life this can become hyperactive and impulsive behaviour, often with sleep problems.

This can present itself as a number of different patterns, as seen in Table 19.3.

Table 19.3 Recognised patterns of attachment disorders

Avoidant–unwilling parent (seen in 22% of parent–child relationships)

Parent	Distressed
	Rejecting or unwilling
Child	Passive, avoids his or her parents
	Little preference of parent over stranger
	Temper outbursts
	Little display of emotional distress
Teenager/adult	Problems with intimacy – dismisses importance of relationships
	Avoids stress
	Wants to be accepted as he or she thinks others want them to be

Ambivalent–resistant attachment (unable to parent) (seen in 8% of parent–child relationships)

Parent	Erratic
	Unpredictable
	Unreliable
	Find parenting difficult as they feel they are failing this relationship
	Insensitive parent who looks to meet own needs
Child	Demanding and clingy behaviour – exaggerated distress
	Angry or preoccupied with carer
	Struggles to learn about and make sense of emotions
	Poor levels of concentration
	Seeks attention
Teenager/adult	Unpopular with peers and lacks self-confidence
	Often angry, dissatisfied and disruptive
	Does not accept responsibility in relationships
	Dependent on others and fearful of relationship breakdowns

Disorganized – carer can be both a source of fear and potential safety (seen in 15% of parent–child relationships)

Parent	Abuses the child and exposes him or her to angry, violent behaviour
	Not available to comfort the distress felt by the child
	Behaves negatively towards his or her child
	Feels disappointed by his or her child and uses harsh discipline
Child	Feelings of distress remain high and unregulated
	Can perceive him- or herself as powerful and bad
	Feels out of control
Teenager/adult	Angry and finds it difficult to empathize
	Self is seen as unloved and bad
	Others seem unavailable, threatened, frightened or frightening
	Volatile or violent close relationships
	Socially isolated
	Higher risk of psychiatric problems and criminal behaviour

What helps?

PSYCHOLOGICAL ASSESSMENT OF THE CHILD

If there are severe problems or if the child is involved in child protection proceedings.

UNDERSTANDING THE CHILD AND HELPING CARERS UNDERSTAND THEIR CHILD

Advise the parent or carer of the following.

- The child is doing the best that he or she can.
- The child wants to improve.
- Acknowledging that change is stressful for these children and therefore they try to control their environment.
- The child's attacks and resistance to you reflect his or her fear of your motives.
- The child may have poor affect, regulation/control of behaviour, fragmented thinking, sense of shame and an inability to trust.

BUILD UP A RELATIONSHIP OF TRUST BETWEEN THE CHILD AND HIS OR HER CARERS

- Accepting the child for who he or she is.
- Increasing the child's emotional awareness by *listening* and tuning in to the child's emotions and reflecting back in a non-critical way what you are seeing and hearing
  - 'I guess you're feeling…'
  - 'I wonder if you're feeling…'
  - 'I think you're showing me you're feeling…'
- Labelling emotions has been shown to have been helpful for young people, enabling them to recover more quickly from upsetting incidents.
- The aim is to help them develop a vocabulary with which they can express their emotions – not to tell them what they should be feeling.
- Try to use 'thinking' rather than 'fighting' words:
  - Not saying 'You're not going to stay in this group and act like that' but saying 'You're welcome to stay with us if you give up on that behaviour.'
  - Not saying 'You're not going to talk to me that way' but saying 'I'll be happy to discuss this with you as soon as the arguing stops.'

Useful resources

Bessel van der Kolk: www.traumacenter.org

Bruce Perry: www.childtrauma.org

Attention difficulties (see also Chapter 28)

There are many causes of attention difficulties (Fig. 19.1) other than attention-deficit–hyperactivity disorder (ADHD), and when assessing children this broad differential needs to be borne in mind. In particular, if the difficulties are largely with school and around learning, having an appropriate individual education plan and support in place is essential. During the assessment you should also bear in mind that comorbidity is common in this group and consider if the child could have a developmental coordination disorder or be on the autistic spectrum.

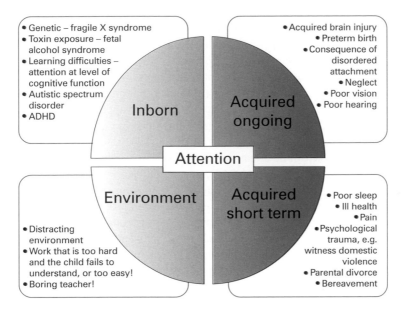

Figure 19.1 Causes of difficulties with attention. ADHD, attention-deficit–hyperactivity disorder.

Tics and Tourette syndrome

Tics are sudden, rapid, involuntary, repetitive, non-rhythmic movements or vocalizations. They are a form of paroxysmal motor/movement disorder. Simple motor tics affect one muscle group (e.g. eye blinking, facial twitch, shoulder shrug). Complex motor tics affect groups of muscles, usually resulting in facial or body contortions. Tics are non-purposeful or can be semi-purposeful (e.g. jumping, smelling, gestures), but actually serve no useful function. Vocalizations or phonic tics include simple grunting, barking, throat clearing or complex vocalizations including phrases. The type, frequency and severity of a tic disorder can wax and wane over time. Video recording of the episodes can be useful in correctly differentiating them from any other paroxysmal motor disorder.

Tics are fairly common and have an estimated prevalence of 6% to 12%. The highest prevalence is in the 9 to 11 years age group and they are three times more common in males. They are more common in children with ADHD and special needs.

Most tic disorders are idiopathic. They can be a primary inherited disorder or present as a secondary phenomenon associated with infection, head trauma, surgery, drugs and toxins. The exact cause of tics is unclear; abnormality of neurotransmitter function, in particular dopamine, is hypothesized.

Tic disorders can be transient (duration < 1y) or chronic (duration > 1y). The tics can be of only one type or there may be multiple motor tics with or without vocalizations. The transient variety is usually mild and does not necessarily come to medical attention.

A type of primary chronic tic disorder is Tourette syndrome, which is characterized by onset before 21 years age, multiple motor tics and at least one vocal tic. All secondary causative factors such as drugs, infection and brain injury need to be ruled out. Onset is usually around the age of 6 or 7 years, with subsequent motor and vocal tics. Coprolalia, a tic of obscene words, is commonly portrayed in the media as being a major sign of Tourette syndrome, but actually it is present in less than 10% of affected people. Tourette syndrome is often associated with behavioural difficulties, in particular obsessive–compulsive disorder (OCD; 20–60%). Behaviours such as biting, hitting and self-injurious behaviour (SIB) can occur and may be more disabling than the tics. ADHD is a common comorbidity (50%) and usually appears before the onset of tics. The comorbidities of OCD, SIB and ADHD significantly increase the functional impairment in Tourette syndrome.

Tic disorders and OCD can be a feature of paediatric autoimmune neuropsychiatric disorders associated with streptococcus (PANDAS), which is a disorder thought to be caused by an immune-mediated cross-reactivity between group A beta-haemolytic *Streptococcus* and neuronal antigens. Response to immune-modulatory therapy has been promising.

Most tic disorders are transient and will disappear spontaneously. It is important not to bring attention to them, for example by asking the child to stop or by name calling/mocking. The child, parents and school need to be counselled regarding the nature of the condition and reassured. Anxiety and excitement sometimes can aggravate symptoms. Behavioural therapies aimed at managing aggravating factors and boosting self-confidence may be helpful. Identification of comorbidities of ADHD, OCD and any other behavioural disorder is important as these are likely to cause more functional impairment and may indicate a more chronic course. The severity of tics does not predict chronicity or likelihood of comorbidities.

In situations where there is an adverse effect on a child's life in school, home or his peer group, drug treatment can be considered. For mild tics, clonidine, baclofen or clonazepam can be effective. More severe tics can be treated with pimozide, haloperidol or newer and atypical antipsychotics such as risperidone. The use of these medications should preferably be by experienced clinicians.

Obsessive–compulsive disorder

Obsessive–compulsive disorder (OCD) is an anxiety disorder characterized by obsessions or compulsions or both. Obsessions are recurrent, intrusive thoughts, images or impulses that cause anxiety. Compulsions are repetitive behaviours (e.g. repeatedly checking if the door is locked) or mental acts (e.g. counting, praying) that are done to neutralize an obsession or performed as part of following some rigid rules. It is not unusual for anyone to experience brief spells of repetitive thoughts, urges or impulses, but these can be dispelled easily and do not cause anxiety or discomfort. In some children these thoughts become entrenched and the child becomes stuck in repetitive cycles of doing something over and over again, for example repeated hand washing. When these kinds of behaviours become a persistent problem and interfere with the child's life for more than an hour a day, it is termed as OCD. In younger children sometimes compulsions are present without obsessions (e.g. the need to perform an elaborate ritual as part of a rigid routine such as a mealtime routine). The child is usually unaware that the obsessions are unreasonable and that the consequences of ignoring them are not harmful. Cognitive–behavioural therapy (CBT) can be successful in creating this awareness and result in symptomatic improvement. It is the treatment of first choice. Drug treatment (usually with selective serotonin reuptake inhibitors such as fluoxetine) is reserved for significant and persistent symptoms and is usually not curative. OCD is a well-recognized comorbidity in developmental disabilities, especially autism spectrum disorder, Tourette syndrome and ADHD. In its more severe form it can cause significant problems with a child's normal functioning and participation.

Oppositional defiant disorder and conduct disorder

Oppositional defiant disorder (ODD) is characterized by disobedient, negative, hostile and defiant behaviour towards parents, teachers and authority figures, which is beyond what is expected for a child's developmental age. The behaviours should be present for at least 6 months and are usually seen in multiple settings. The diagnosis is usually made in pre-adolescents and, if persistent, can often progress to a conduct disorder in adolescence. Oppositional behaviours are common in toddlers and teenagers but in children with ODD and conduct disorder it is of a pathological degree resulting in impaired functioning in school, home and social settings. The behavioural characteristics of children with ODD and those with conduct disorders are outlined in Table 19.4.

Conduct disorder is usually diagnosed in adolescents and young people who display a pattern of behaviour in which other people's rights are violated, norms are ignored and rules are broken deliberately. The behaviour pattern must have lasted at least 12 months. Both ODD and conduct disorder are more common in males and can be a frequent comorbidity (30–50%) of ADHD.

Table 19.4 Behavioural characteristics of oppositional defiant disorder and conduct disorder

Oppositional defiant disorder	Conduct disorder
Temper tantrums (frequent, severe)	Aggression towards people and animals
Cannot take 'no' for an answer	Destruction of property, including arson or
Argumentative	vandalism
Breaks rules, non-compliant	Deceitful
Deliberately annoys people	Theft, stealing
Blames others for own mistakes	Violation of rules
Easily annoyed	Antisocial and criminal behaviour; truancy
Mean and hateful when upset	
Angry and resentful	
Spiteful and vindictive	

Both ODD and conduct disorder are multifactorial in origin. There are biological, psychological, environmental and social factors which contribute. Assessment should include a careful look for comorbidities including ADHD, learning disabilities, mood disorders and anxiety disorders. Behavioural therapy is the treatment of choice in ODD and conduct disorder. Parent training programmes can help parents learn behavioural management techniques. Individual psychotherapy can help the child develop better anger management skills, family therapy can improve family functioning and social skills training may increase flexibility and improve frustration tolerance. Identification and treatment of comorbidities such as ADHD is important. Drug treatment of

ODD and conduct disorder with stimulants can be beneficial but should be considered only in conjunction with behavioural therapy.

Advice for parents of a child with oppositional defiant disorder or conduct disorder

- Set consistent limits/boundaries and behavioural expectations
- Use sanctions judiciously. Be fair and consistent with boundaries and sanctions
- Apply the same rules in all settings, e.g. at home, school, grandparents' house
- Build on positives. Praise good behaviour. Reinforce using a reward programme (e.g. stickers)
- Walk away or take time out when conflict with the child is likely to exacerbate
- Pick your battles carefully. Let minor issues go by. Prioritize the major desired behaviours
- Remain calm and in control as much as possible
- Maintain other interests to avoid burnout. Manage your own stress healthily

---

Anxiety disorders

Anxiety disorders are characterized by an exaggerated fear, worry or dread that impairs the child's ability to function normally and that is disproportionate to the circumstance. Anxiety is a normal experience of most children and it is a normal aspect of development. Separation anxiety in toddlers, fear of monsters or bugs in childhood, shyness in some children and fear of not conforming to peers in teenagers are examples of anxiety experienced during normal growing up. Pathological anxiety is anxiety that is so exaggerated that it impairs function and causes severe distress.

Anxiety disorders include generalized anxiety disorder, social phobia, specific phobias, separation anxiety disorder, panic disorder, post-traumatic stress disorder (PTSD) and OCD (see page 228). Anxiety disorders often have a genetic predisposition but are heavily influenced by psychosocial experience. Anxiety in parents is often picked up by children, who in turn find it difficult to stay calm and composed. This can be a particularly common problem in children with disabilities, whose parents can be anxious regarding their child's condition and may be overprotective.

Diagnosis of generalized anxiety disorder requires persistent excessive anxiety and worry about a variety of things, in various settings, which is hard to control and has been ongoing for more than 6 months. There should be problems with the child's ability to function at home and/ or at school because of the anxiety and it should not be related to any other illness or social/ environmental factors.

Symptoms that accompany the worry include the following:

- feeling tense, restless or keyed up;
- easy fatigue;
- concentration problems;
- irritability;

- muscle tension and cramps;
- poor appetite;
- sleep disturbance.

Panic disorders are more common in adolescents and females. In panic disorders there are recurrent panic attacks brought on by triggers or by the worry of having more panic attacks. Typical panic attack symptoms can include the following:

- palpitations
- feeling short of breath, resulting in hyperventilation
- sweating, trembling or shaking
- chest pain or discomfort
- choking sensation
- nausea and abdominal discomfort
- feeling dizzy and lightheaded. Feeling unreal or detached
- fear of losing control, going mad or dying
- numbness and tingling
- hot flushes or chills.

The urge to avoid triggers may lead to other comorbid phobias, for example avoiding small, closed places (claustrophobia) or avoiding going out of the home (agoraphobia). There is often a history of anxiety disorders and/or panic attacks in other family members.

A *phobia* is an irrational fear resulting in anxiety and extreme avoidance behaviours. An important phobia in children is social phobia, which includes school phobia or school refusal. In a child affected by social phobia there is an extreme and persistent fear of one or more social or performance settings where the child is exposed to strangers. It should not be confused with normal shyness, which causes minimal or no functional impairment and which usually improves with familiarity. The child has normal relationships with family members and close friends, but is afraid of other peers and adults. When exposed to social situations the child may cry, have a tantrum, refuse to engage or completely freeze. In some situations the reaction is so marked and persistent that it can be mistaken as a major communication disorder. The clue is in the history (or a video) of the child displaying normal communication in familiar settings. Social phobia is generalized if it is present in multiple settings, if it causes impairment in social functioning and lasts more than 6 months. In extreme situations a child may refuse to go to school or refuse to go to the cafeteria, use the toilet, etc. A variant of social phobia is selective mutism, in which a child refuses to speak to unfamiliar people or children. Phobias can be comorbid in children on the autism spectrum and in females with fragile X syndrome.

Post-traumatic stress disorder is an anxiety disorder that occurs after exposure to a traumatic physical or psychological experience. The symptoms are of the child re-experiencing the trauma, feeling intense fear with numbness and displaying aroused, agitated behaviour. There may be disturbed behaviour, nightmares, flashbacks and avoidance of all things (people, places, objects, thoughts, feelings) associated with the trauma. Increased arousal results in sleep disturbance, irritability, hypervigilance and an exaggerated startle response. In children with developmental disabilities PTSD may be caused by physical, sexual or severe emotional abuse. It is more common in children with learning disabilities because of their limited coping abilities.

Mood disorders

Mood disorders in children include major depression and bipolar disorders. The symptoms of major depression include the following:

- depressed mood (compared with the child's normal behaviour)
- decreased interest or pleasure in most activities
- change in appetite
- change in sleep (insomnia or hypersomnia)
- psychomotor agitation or retardation
- fatigue and loss of energy
- feeling of worthlessness or guilt
- indecisiveness
- recurrent thoughts of death or dying.

Symptoms should not be secondary to bereavement, must be present for more than 2 weeks and be associated with impairment of daily function.

Bipolar disorder swings between depression and mania or both may occur together (mixed bipolar disorder). Manic symptoms include the following:

- delusions of grandeur
- decreased sleep requirement
- very talkative and forced/pressured speech
- flight of ideas
- distractibility
- psychomotor agitation
- increased dangerous pleasure-seeking behaviour.

Symptoms must be present for more than a week. Hypomania is associated with less severe symptoms or of lesser duration and causing little or no impairment.

Other psychiatric and behaviour disorders in children

Psychotic disorders are uncommon in childhood. Schizophrenia is a primary psychotic disorder and can occur from the age of around 12 years. Clinical indicators of psychoses include

- delusion (fixed irrational false belief), e.g. paranoia (persecution), grandeur ('I am the king')
- hallucination (sensory perception without stimulus), e.g. hearing voices, seeing imaginary people
- confused and disturbed thoughts and behaviour, e.g. confusing film/television/dreams with real life, flight of ideas, bizarre speech and behaviour, 'word salad' – jumbled incoherent speech, catatonia
- lack of insight and self-awareness.

Important differential diagnoses to consider are

- drug and alcohol misuse/drug withdrawal/poisoning
- encephalitis/encephalopathy from any cause
- epilepsy
- brain tumours or raised intracranial pressure from any cause
- child abuse
- other psychiatric disorders such as mood disorders, anxiety disorders, depression and ASD.

Symptoms of psychosis should ring alarm bells. Accurate diagnosis (remembering the differential diagnosis) and early treatment of the cause is essential. The treatment of primary childhood psychosis includes psychotherapy and antipsychotics under the supervision of a child psychiatrist.

Eating disorders in developmental disabilities

Three types of eating disorders are common in children with developmental disabilities: binge eating, fussy/restricted diet and rumination.

Binge eating is characterized by an insatiable appetite, eating large amounts rapidly and aggression when food is refused. There are no associated attempts at vomiting/purging or any distortion of body image. Resulting risks include obesity and choking, both of which can be life-threatening. The behaviour can be associated with Prader–Willi syndrome and as a side effect of medication (valproate, risperidone). Treatment involves dietary restriction (low calories, small portion size, no snacking, supervised mealtimes) and a regular exercise regime.

Children with ASD can sometimes have very *restricted eating* patterns. This can take the form of having only one or two types of foodstuff, e.g. potato crisps, or particular brands, e.g. one particular brand of crisps, or specific colours/smells/textures or arrangement of food. Most of these children consume adequate amounts and grow well but may suffer from mineral and vitamin deficiencies due to the restricted dietary pattern. Evaluation by a dietitian and appropriate supplementation (sometimes by hiding it in food or drink) should be considered.

Rumination is a process by which stomach contents are repeatedly regurgitated into the mouth and chewed for comfort. It is a learned habit and a form of self-stimulatory behaviour. It is common in children with moderate to severe learning disabilities and some children with ASD. It tends to occur more with boredom, anxiety or for pleasure. It can result in bad teeth, mouth odour and great parental concern. Treatment is difficult and is by distraction and good dental care. The usefulness of antireflux medication, antacids and laxatives is debatable.

Chronic fatigue syndrome

Very occasionally you may be asked to consider chronic fatigue syndrome (CFS) as a cause of severe and persistent tiredness in a child, or more likely an adolescent, with a disability.

CFS refers to severe and continued tiredness that is not relieved by rest, cannot be directly attributed to any medical cause and has been present for 6 months or more. Its cause is unknown but it is recognized that it can develop after viral infections, such as that due to Epstein–Barr virus, but no specific virus has ever been identified as the cause. It is thought that age, genetics, previous illness, stress and environment may play a role in its causation.

Apart from persisting chronic tiredness, the child may complain of cognitive difficulties, forgetfulness, attention problems, irritability and headaches, as well as a mild fever, sore throat, lymphadenopathy, myalgia, arthralgia and weakness not due to the child's underlying condition. He may become socially withdrawn.

Clinically, it would be wise to consider and rule out other causes of extreme tiredness such as the following:

1 Iron deficiency anaemia and other deficiencies, e.g. folate and B12, particularly if diet is poor.
2 Vitamin and mineral deficiencies, e.g. if diet is restricted or parentally fed.
3 Rickets – causes 'stones, bones and groans' – general lethargy, particularly in dark-skinned children and those who do not play outside often. Adolescents may complain of non-specific tiredness.
4 Hypothyroidism.
5 Mental health disorders, particularly depression and anxiety.
6 Other autoimmune disorders.
7 Infections and rarer causes such as tumours.

Management is supportive. There is no diagnostic test for CFS. History, clinical examination and appropriate tests should identify any treatable disorders. Therapy includes advising on graded rehabilitation, cognitive–behavioural therapy, if appropriate, sleep management and healthy diet. Medications to manage fever, pain, anxiety and depression, and sleep problems may be used if indicated and supervised by paediatricians and child and adolescent mental health services. Management may be jointly delivered by these teams.

Section 8

Sensory impairment

20
Hearing impairment and deafness

Arnab Seal, Gillian Robinson and
Anne M Kelly

Learning objectives

- To understand the normal physiology of hearing.
- To understand the epidemiology and aetiology of hearing impairment.
- To know when to arrange a hearing assessment.
- To know how hearing impairment is assessed and managed in childhood.
- To understand the implications of childhood hearing impairment.

Introduction

'Hearing impairment' or 'hearing loss' are synonymous terms in this context and are used to imply less than perfect hearing. The degree of hearing loss can be mild to profound.

There are two main causes of hearing loss:

- *Conductive hearing loss*, in which the lesion is in the external or middle ear, i.e. the external ear canal, tympanic membrane or middle ear cavity. It is most commonly caused by secretory otitis media (SOM, also known as glue ear or otitis media with effusion [OME]), which causes temporary and often fluctuating loss.
- *Sensorineural hearing loss* (SNHL), in which the lesion is in the inner ear, auditory nerve or auditory pathway in the brain. SNHL is likely to be congenital in origin and permanent. In SNHL, sound is both diminished and distorted, whereas in conductive loss sound is diminished only.

Each type can be unilateral or bilateral, and can cause adverse affects on the child's communication, cognitive and psychosocial functioning. Deafness that occurs before speech is acquired is described as prelingual deafness, as is the case in about half the cases of childhood SNHL.

The degree of hearing disability is not merely dependent on the hearing thresholds. Children need to be able to process sounds, and this is an ability that is dependent on higher cortical function. Therefore, two children with identical pure tone audiograms (PTAs) may show significant variation in their ability to discriminate the complex sounds of speech, which will consequently affect their response and function.

Permanent hearing impairment for a long period has been shown to have a significant detrimental effect on children's communication skills and ability to socialize with others. This may lead to educational underachievement and, in the longer term, to poor employment prospects and mental health problems. Identification and rehabilitation of the child with suitable aids before the age of 6 months has been shown to reduce the fall in the average verbal IQ score from 25 points to 6 points. Hence, the importance of the National Universal Neonatal Hearing Screening Programme, which was rolled out to all areas of the UK in 2004 with the aim of identifying and offering suitable habilitation to infants less than 6 months old (Davis et al. 1997).

Epidemiology

Hearing impairment (Table 20.1) is the most prevalent sensory deficit in the human population.

Table 20.1 Levels of hearing (described by the quietest sounds heard at 0.5, 1, 2 and 4Hz frequencies)

Level	Volume or threshold heard in the better ear (dB)
Normal	≤20
Mild hearing loss	21–40
Moderate	41–70
Severe	71–90
Profound	>91

The Newborn Hearing Screen detects SNHL in about 1 in every 1000 live births, but 50% to 90% *more* children are diagnosed by the age of 9 years, giving a total estimated prevalence of 1.65 to 2.05 per 1000.

Most cases of SNHL are congenital and should be detected soon after birth. Some children present later for the following reasons:

• Approximately 10% to 20% of all cases of SNHL are acquired postnatally and therefore will be missed by the Newborn Hearing Screen.
• Some cases of autosomal dominant genetic deafness cause late-onset or progressive deafness that only becomes apparent with age.

Conductive hearing loss is, by contrast, much more common, affecting 4% of all schoolchildren. It is found most commonly in preschool children and can persist into adolescence. It can be particularly troublesome in some syndromes, particularly Down syndrome and craniofacial anomalies. Most conductive loss is usually temporary and often fluctuant, but occasionally can be significant and persistent enough to require surgery and/or hearing aids.

SNHL and conductive loss may coexist, resulting in mixed hearing loss. Amongst children with SNHL, 33% have persisting OME requiring grommets and a further third have intermittent OME.

Case vignette

Aiya is a 5-year-old female born in Eritrea who presents to the orthopaedic team with a limp. The orthopaedic team refers her to a neurodisability paediatrician, who diagnoses a hemiplegia. Aiya was born preterm. Her parents are also concerned about her communication and development. Basic tests and magnetic resonance imaging (MRI) of the head are requested. The MRI reveals encephalomalacia and hearing tests reveal severe SNHL. An initial diagnosis was made of SNHL resulting possibly from preterm birth and neonatal insults. Further investigations, which look at other possible causes of SNHL, find a connexin deletion.

Learning points

- Never automatically attribute hearing loss to preterm delivery.
- Apply the hearing loss guideline for investigation of any hearing loss as often multiple causes can coexist. The correct diagnosis has significant management implications for the child and family.

Normal hearing

Sound has the following two components:

- Pitch, or the musical note of the sound, measured in hertz.
- Volume, measured in decibels.

Fig. 20.1 shows everyday sounds, their pitches and volume. Note the range of pitch and normal volume range for speech sounds.

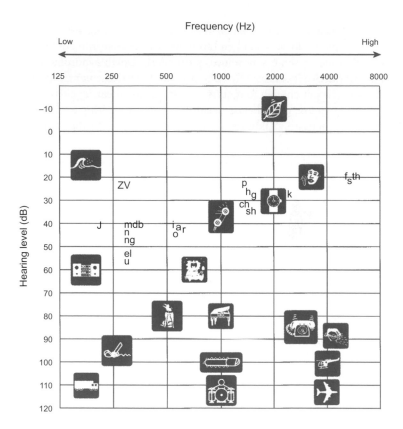

Figure 20.1 Normal range of hearing.

Normal anatomy and physiology

Fig. 20.2 shows the normal anatomy of the inner ear. Sound enters the ear canal, causing the tympanic membrane to vibrate. These vibrations are magnified through the ossicles, resulting in a pressure wave in the cochlea. The hair cells are organized along the cochlea so that different pressure waves stimulate cells at different points, resulting in the perception of pitch. The pressure wave causes a deflection in the sensitive hair cell bundle, causing the calcium channels to open, which leads to the depolarization of the VIII nerve and subsequently the sending of a signal to the cochlear nucleus.

The sound message passes rapidly through brainstem nuclei, including some crossover of sound signals, before ending in the temporal cortex, where the meaning of the sound is decoded by comparing with previous sound experiences.

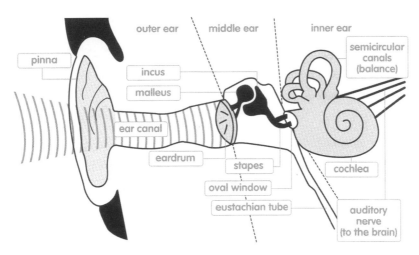

Figure 20.2 Normal anatomy of the inner ear.

Table 20.2 Normal hearing milestones

Age	Development
20wk gestation	The cochlea is formed and the fetus demonstrates a startle response to sound and is able to recognize its mother's voice
4–7mo after birth	The infant is able to start to localize, responding to sounds of 15dB. Myelination of the auditory nerve is complete
7–9mo	The infant is able to localize sounds at the level of the ear
9–13mo	The infant is able to localize sounds at all levels

High-risk groups for hearing impairment

The following factors are associated with a high risk of hearing impairment:

- family history of hearing loss
- craniofacial syndromes
- developmental delay
- visual impairment
- bacterial meningitis or measles encephalitis
- head injury with base of skull fracture or auditory symptoms
- prolonged course of ototoxic drugs (including oncology drugs)
- extreme preterm birth
- severe neonatal jaundice
- history of congenital infection
- history of hypoxic–ischaemic encephalopathy.

Key messages

Sixty per cent of children with sensorineural hearing loss will be identified by screening. They include the following:

* graduates from the neonatal unit
* children with a family history
* children with craniofacial abnormality.

Parental or professional concern at any age should always be taken very seriously. It is useful to know the normal hearing milestones in order to recognise hearing impairment at an early stage (see Table 20.2). Warning signs of hearing impairment are detailed in Table 20.3.

Table 20.3 Warning signs of hearing impairment

Infant	Preschool child	School-aged child
Lack of startle to loud sounds	Limited or poor speech	Limited or poor speech
Delayed vocalization	Fails to respond to conversational speech	Inattentive
'Quiet or good infant'	Behavioural problems	Difficulties in learning
	Poor attention	Increases the television's volume
	Recurrent ear infections	Fails to respond to conversational speech
		Deteriorating school performance
		Recurrent ear infection
		Behavioural problems

Which children need a hearing assessment?

The following children require a hearing assessment:

* those with warning signs
* those who have missed the Newborn Hearing Screening
* those in a high-risk group (see above)
* those for whom there is parental or professional concern regarding hearing.

Tests of hearing

There are several methods of testing a child's hearing. The method chosen depends in part on the child's age, development or health status. There are some tests based on utilizing normal physiology of hearing (physiological tests) and others based on hearing behaviours (behavioural tests).

Physiological tests

Otoacoustic emission (OAE) test

The otoacoustic emission test is commonly used as the neonatal screening test. It works on the principle that a healthy cochlea will produce a faint response when stimulated with sound.

A small earpiece (containing a speaker and microphone) is placed in a settled or sleeping child's ear. A clicking sound is played and, if the cochlea is working properly, the earpiece will pick up the cochlear response. A computer averages these recordings. A normal recording is associated with normal outer hair cell function and this typically reflects normal hearing.

ADVANTAGES

* Simple and quick to perform, but its performance is affected by ambient noise or an unsettled infant.

DISADVANTAGES

* Relatively high false-positive rate in the first 24 hours of life due to amniotic fluid in the ear canal. If this happens the test is usually repeated. If the infant fails again, an auditory brainstem response (ABR) and full assessment is arranged (around 15% of infants).
* It is not a test of hearing, but a test of cochlear function.
* Misses auditory neuropathy (also known as auditory dys-synchrony), which is a condition in which sound enters the inner ear normally but the transmission of signals from the cochlea to the brain is impaired.

The auditory brainstem response (ABR) test

The ABR test works by recording brain activity in response to sounds. An infant may be sleeping naturally or may have to be sedated for this test. Older cooperative children may be tested in a silent environment while they are visually occupied. Tiny earphones are placed in the infant's ear canals. Usually, click-type sounds are introduced through the earphones and electrodes measure the auditory pathway's response to the sounds. A computer averages these responses and displays waveforms. There are five waveforms in a trace, representing different areas of the auditory pathway. There are characteristic latencies and amplitude of waveforms for normal hearing.

ADVANTAGES

* Screens entire hearing pathway from ear to brainstem.
* Low false-positive rate.

DISADVANTAGES

* Affected by movement, so the child needs to be asleep or still.
* Complex computerized equipment required, but this is portable.
* Certain neurological disorders will lead to an abnormal result.

Auditory steady state response test

An infant is typically sleeping or sedated for the auditory steady state response (ASSR) test. This is a new test that currently must be done in conjunction with the ABR to assess hearing. Sound is transmitted through the ear canals, and a computer picks up the brain's response to the sound and automatically establishes the hearing level.

Behavioural tests

Behavioural tests involve careful observation of a child's behavioural response to sounds such as warble tones or frequency-specific or narrow-band noise. Sometimes other calibrated signals are used to obtain information about hearing at different frequencies.

Visual response audiometry

Visual response audiometry (VRA) is suitable for children aged from 6 months to about 2 years 6 months. The child is conditioned with a loud sound accompanied by a visual reward, e.g. a squealing monkey. When conditioning is achieved, the child turns to progressively frequency-specific quieter sounds until thresholds are determined.

ADVANTAGES

• Screens the hearing pathway in the speech frequencies.
• Can check different frequencies.
• No sedation required.

DISADVANTAGES

• The child needs to have good head control and be cooperative.
• Does not give specific information about each ear without using earphones or inserts.
• Can be time-consuming.
• Requires appropriate soundproofed room and equipment.

Performance testing

Before children accept earphones, warble tones can be played through a speaker, which can establish thresholds in the better ear.

Pure tone audiometry

From about the age of 3, children are actively involved in testing by using a technique known as conditioning. Younger children are shown how to move a toy (for example, putting a peg into a board) each time they hear a sound.

Older children are asked to respond to sounds by saying yes or pressing a button. The sounds come through headphones, earphones placed inside the child's ear, or sometimes through a speaker (when the test is known as soundfield audiometry).

ADVANTAGES

- Criterion standard.
- Full range of frequencies.

DISADVANTAGES

- Requires cooperation and equipment.

Bone conduction

All of the tests above are described as testing using air conduction. These are sounds that pass through the ear canal and middle ear before reaching the cochlea. Abnormalities in air conduction can be cause by either middle ear disease (e.g. SOM) or nerve deafness. Sound can also be transmitted directly to the cochlea via the skull bones. ABR, VRA and PTA can also be tested using bone conduction. A small vibrating device is placed behind the child's ear and this passes sound directly to the inner ear through the bones in the head, i.e. using bone conduction. This gives an abnormal result if there is a sensorineural component but is normal for pure conductive hearing loss as it bypasses the air conduction pathway.

Audiograms

Hearing test results are depicted as audiograms. On the x-axis is plotted pitch, in hertz, and on the y-axis is volume, in decibels. Normal hearing is in the range of –10 to 15dB. By convention, air conduction thresholds for the right ear (i.e. the softest sounds the right ear can hear at each frequency) are marked as an 'O' and those for the left ear as an 'X' on the audiogram. Masked bone conduction thresholds are marked on the audiogram as] (right ear) or [(left ear). Masking means that a constant noise is presented to the non-test ear to enable testing of the subject ear. The purpose of masking is to prevent the non-test ear from detecting the signal. Figs 20.3 and 20.4 show examples of audiograms for different types of hearing loss.

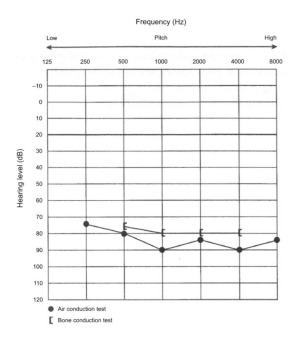

Figure 20.3 Example of a severe sensorineural hearing loss.

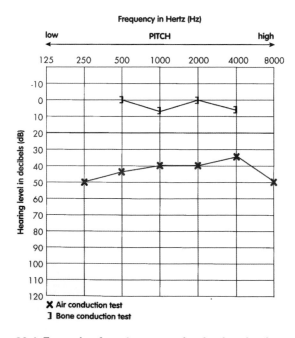

Figure 20.4 Example of moderate conductive hearing loss.

Speech discrimination tests

Speech discrimination tests check the child's ability to discriminate words at different 'listening levels'. The tester asks the child to identify toys or pictures, or to copy words spoken by the tester or from a recording. From this the tester can assess the quietest level at which the child can correctly identify the words used, by using a sound level meter.

Tympanometry

Tympanometry is not a test of hearing; it is used to check middle ear function. A small earpiece is held gently in the ear canal. A pump causes the pressure of the air in the ear canal to change. The normal eardrum compliance changes with a change in pressure. The earpiece measures this by checking the sound reflected by the eardrum. If the eardrum is not moving freely, there is likely to be some problem with the middle ear or tympanic membrane, e.g. acute or secretory otitis media (Figs 20.5 and 20.6).

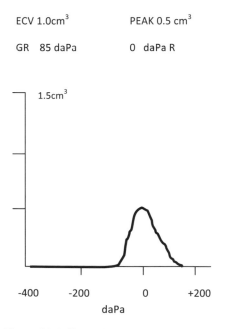

Figure 20.5 Normal tympanogram.

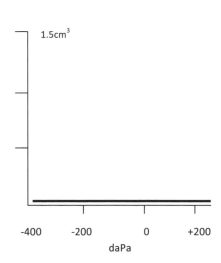

Figure 20.6 Tympanogram showing middle ear disease.

Sensorineural hearing loss

Aetiology

The aetiology of childhood sensorineural hearing loss (SNHL) has changed in the new millennium (Fig. 20.7). Fewer cases are now attributed to childhood infections such as mumps, measles, meningitis or congenital rubella. The prevalence of these infections has been successfully reduced by vaccination programmes. The relative importance of genetic causes has now grown, with approximately 50% of cases now being attributed to single gene mutations. The proportion of infants admitted to newborn units who are later found to have SNHL has also steadily risen.

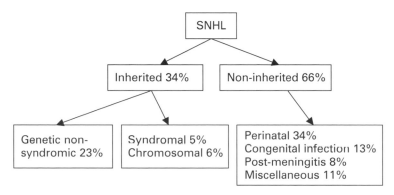

Figure 20.7 Causes of sensorineural hearing loss (SNHL).

The clinical characteristics of syndromal deafness are outlined in Table 20.4. The most common genetic cause of SNHL is non-syndromic or isolated deafness, with no other recognizable features. Fifty different chromosomal loci are associated with this form of deafness. To date, 41 autosomal dominant and 32 autosomal recessive genes have been identified as associated with deafness. Different gene defects can cause the same clinical picture. Conversely, the phenotype may vary within one genotype, and therefore prognosis is not always possible.

The molecular basis for the deafness has been identified in certain cases. In deafness due to the Connexin family of genes, the faulty gene codes for abnormal gap junctions involved in recycling K^+ in cochlear hair cells. These genes are thought to be responsible for up to 70% of cases of deafness in European populations and are situated at a single locus on chromosome 13q. In Usher syndrome there are 10 possible genes involved, all of which code for myosin.

There may be a clear environmental determinant such as congenital cytomegalovirus (CMV) infection, but in other cases genes and the environment interact, causing deafness. Carriers of the mitochondrial mutation of *A1555G* in 12srRNA are predisposed to deafness caused by aminoglycosides. The use of this group of antibiotics should be avoided if there is a family history of aminoglycoside-induced deafness.

Table 20.4 Clinical features associated with syndromal deafness

Sign	Associated syndrome
Abnormal external ear	Treacher Collins syndrome
	Goldenhar syndrome
Eye – retinal pigmentation	Usher syndrome
	Alström syndrome
	Refsum syndrome
Skeletal abnormalities	Klippel–Feil syndrome
Skin, hair (white forelock) and nail pigmentary abnormalities	Waardenburg syndrome
Renal disease – haematuria	Alport syndrome
Endocrine – goitre	Pendred syndrome
Prolonged QT syndrome	Jervell and Lange-Nielsen syndrome
Sinus in neck; preauricular pit	Branchio-oto-renal syndrome

Aetiological investigations

Why and when is early investigation of causative factors indicated?

- For couples contemplating further children to enable early genetic counselling on the risk of recurrence.
- To treat some conditions, including
  - long QT interval to avoid risk of syncope and sudden death
  - post-meningitis, to fast track to cochlear implant if indicated
  - congenital cytomegalovirus (CMV) infection.
- To manage progressive loss, for example
  - attempt to arrest progression in congenital CMV with treatment
  - avoid trauma such as contact sports in wide vestibular aqueduct (WVA) syndrome
  - familial cases to obtain advice on likely progression.

Case vignette

Newborn female infant Rosie did not show clear responses during the Newborn Hearing Screen. Further testing confirms severe high-frequency sensorineural deafness. Rosie is seen by the community paediatrician, who notices she has heterochromia of the iris. Her mother has a white patch of hair. Further genetic appointments confirm Waardenburg syndrome.

Learning points

- All children with SNHL should see a paediatrician. Community paediatricians are particularly well placed to see this group.
- All children with deafness should have a detailed physical examination.
- Deafness can be the presenting complaint of a genetic diagnosis that can have individual and family implications. Forewarned is forearmed!

Assessment and investigation

1. History and examination

HISTORY

- Obtain a detailed history of pregnancy and neonatal and postnatal periods (obtain maternal and neonatal notes).
- Check specifically for ototoxic drugs, infection, preterm birth, hypoxia.
- General health- ear disease, meningitis, head trauma, immunization status.
- Family history – obtain three-generation pedigree. Any early deaths? (Jervell and Lange–Neilsen syndrome with long QT and hearing loss).
- Developmental milestones.

EXAMINATION (SEE TABLE 20.4 ABOVE FOR SYNDROMIC ASSOCIATIONS)

- General systems
- Look for dysmorphic features especially involving ears, eyes and face
- Neck
- Skin, nails, hair – pigmentary anomalies
- Eye examination and fundoscopy
- Developmental assessment

Case vignette

Tom was born at 36 weeks' gestation. He was known before birth to have a congenital cardiac malformation – this was confirmed as tetralogy of Fallot after birth. Physical examination showed Tom to have a coloboma of the left iris and preauricular tags. Subsequent hearing tests revealed SNHL and a diagnosis of CHARGE association was made. Tom was fitted with hearing aids and early referrals to the Teacher of the Deaf and the cochlear implant team were made.

Learning points

- If you see one congenital anomaly, look for others.
- Ear anomalies can be associated with hearing impairment

2. Specific investigations

RADIOLOGY

Neuroimaging is usually indicated in bilateral severe or profound loss.
Early imaging is recommended for

- post-meningitis hearing loss
- cochlear ossification
- cochlear implant assessment
- progressive hearing loss
- renal anomaly associated
- establishing the recurrence risk for parents/professionals.

MRI of internal auditory meatus, inner ears and brain shows cerebral structures, VII and VIII nerves and membranous labyrinth. Computed tomography shows bony structures including middle ear ossicles and mastoid air cells.

GENETIC TESTS

Connexin 26 and 30 gene mutations.

- Some geneticists prefer to see the family first – agree and follow local protocol.
- Perform karyotype analysis if dysmorphic features or developmental delay/disability are present.

INFECTION SCREEN

- Congenital CMV infection affects 0.5% of all births in UK; 4% of affected infants will be deaf, which increases to 8% by 5 years. Check the urine for CMV and the blood for CMV and immunoglobulin M (IgM) at birth. Guthrie cards collected in the newborn period may be available to test the child if he or she presents beyond the newborn period.
- Rubella-specific IgM.
- Toxoplasma-specific IgM.

OPHTHALMOLOGY SCREEN

Deaf children are more likely to have eye conditions. Eye examination may establish diagnosis in Usher syndrome, CHARGE, congenital rubella, Alström syndrome and congenital CMV infections.

ECG

Long QT interval and severe/profound deafness in Jervell and Lange-Nielsen syndrome. Cardiac syncope and sudden death may occur. Incidence is 1 in 160 000.

OTHER INVESTIGATIONS TO CONSIDER

- Full blood count: congenital infections.
- Biochemistry: Alström and Alport syndromes.
- Urine dipstick/microscopy for haematuria: Alport syndrome.
- Urine metabolic screen: if developmental delay is present.

Case vignette

Sophie is a 6-year-old girl with communication and social difficulties who has a routine hearing test. SNHL is found, though earlier tests were normal. Further neurological investigation and imaging reveals findings associated with previous encephalitis. A diagnosis of SNHL – both acquired and progressive – is made. Cochlear implant referral is made and 2 years after the implant Sophie is in mainstream school and is happier and interacting with peers.

Learning points

- Hearing loss can be acquired.
- There may be multiple diagnoses.
- A cochlear implant should be considered for any child with significant SNHL who meets the referral criteria.

Management and rehabilitation

The best outcome for SNHL is dependent on early detection and early intervention to make optimum use of residual hearing. The early years offer an enhanced opportunity for better functional outcome because there is increased brain plasticity at this age. Children who lose their hearing ability after having learnt to talk usually retain speech. Addressing educational, social, communication and family issues in conjunction with amplification of residual hearing enhances outcome.

Measures to prevent hearing loss is an important public health issue. These include immunization against mumps, measles, rubella and meningitis, effective management of neonatal jaundice, reducing environmental noise pollution and educating young people regarding the long-term risk of hearing loss from exposure to high-volume noise from electronic devices, e.g. personal music systems.

Hearing aids

Hearing aids are used to make the best use of residual hearing. The goal of habilitation is to make speech and other environmental sounds comfortably audible while avoiding high sound intensity levels that may pose a risk to residual hearing. Hearing aids are fitted when educationally significant hearing loss cannot be corrected by medical or surgical means. Surgery is usually tried first when there is significant conductive loss or mixed hearing loss.

Timing of fitting aids

INFANTS UNDER 6 MONTHS OLD

Hearing aids are fitted in infants by using estimates of the hearing sensitivities derived from neonatal ABR in response to a combination of frequency-specific and broadband stimuli. These results are 'fine tuned' as soon as the infant is able to participate in behavioural testing, which is usually after 6 months of age.

OLDER CHILD

Hearing aid amplification and habilitation can begin almost immediately after the hearing loss has been confirmed. Hearing aid fitting is a challenge in infants and young children because of:

* the size of the pinna and ear canal
* the limited ability of children to communicate information on sound quality and loudness tolerance
* the fact that small ears are more likely to produce acoustic feedback (whistling) and the resonant frequency is higher than in adult ears.

Fortunately, the electro-acoustic characteristics of the hearing aid can be preset by computer and do not require the child's cooperation.

Hearing aid types

- Behind the ear (BTE) is the usual style of choice. The aid sits behind the pinna with amplified sound routed to the ear canal via a custom-fit ear mould. It can be adapted for use on the telephone and direct audio input. Most BTEs are now digital aids.
- In the ear (ITE) is less suited to small ears.
- Bone-anchored aids are suited for children with atresia of external canal or chronic OME.
- Body style in which the child wears a 'box' connected to ear moulds with a cord. These are now much less common with improvements in BTE aids.

Steps in fitting a hearing aid

- Ear mould impression taken using quick-setting silicone. Soft and flexible material used for moulds in children to improve tolerability.
- Measurements taken to correct for shape and length of ear canal.
- Selection of hearing aid characteristics (frequency and loudness).
- Assess aided performance using probe microphone measures.
- Assess the ability to discriminate and understand speech as soon as developmentally able (usually 3 years).
- Use information from a teacher of the deaf and parents to inform review.

Follow-up

Children younger than 2 years old with aids are monitored frequently as they are unable to communicate complaints and because their rapid growth necessitates frequent ear mould changes.

Management of unilateral hearing loss

Children with unilateral hearing loss are still at risk of academic failure and social difficulties. Strategies to improve hearing in the classroom include a classroom amplification radio aid in the affected ear or a unilateral hearing aid. For severe loss, particularly in the adolescent age group, amplification to the poorer ear may not help. The signal from a radio aid may be rerouted to the normal hearing ear (see section on Educational implications of hearing impairment, page 258).

Cochlear implants

Children who have profound hearing loss in the better ear may require a cochlear implant. There are clear referral criteria for this. Cochlear implants (Fig. 20.8) provide a sensation of hearing to children who have severe to profound permanent deafness and cannot hear the full range of speech sounds with hearing aids. A cochlear implant is different from a conventional hearing aid because it directly stimulates the auditory nerve using electrical signals, rather than simply amplifying sounds. It is an electronic prosthetic device that is implanted in the cochlea to stimulate the auditory nerve.

Cochlear implants were originally used in older children with acquired deafness (e.g. following meningitis). Results of a follow-up revealed that speech perception and production continued to improve even up to 4 years after the implant. There is a measurable improvement in the simple auditory behaviours, e.g. responding to name and alerting to environmental sounds, soon after the implant is in place and the electrodes are 'switched on'. Implants are now considered for younger children who are prelingually deaf. They must learn to extract important information from the pattern of stimulation presented to the brain by the implant, a process that can take considerable time and effort from the child, his family and the staff involved.

Assessment for implant can be a lengthy process and will be initiated only if the child is failing to achieve benefit from conventional hearing aids. To be considered, the child must have some intact afferent cochlear neurones that can be stimulated. Some parents may decide not to proceed despite advice from their audiologist.

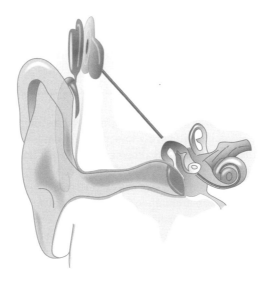

Figure 20.8 Cochlear implant.

Conductive hearing loss

Causes of conductive hearing loss

- Otitis media with effusion (OME), secretory otitis media (SOM), glue ear.
- Acute suppurative otitis media with or without perforation of tympanic membrane.
- Chronic suppurative otitis media (CSOM).
- Cholesteatoma.
- Congenital external auditory meatus abnormalities.
- Wax causes hearing loss only when it completely occludes the meatus. Middle ear disease is often found with impacted wax. It is essential to remove the wax before retesting the child's hearing.
- Otosclerosis.

Case vignette

Four-year-old Rhys has been referred to the local speech and language therapist because of concerns about his communication, articulation and attention levels. He is reported to have severe behavioural problems with major tantrums. Assessment shows delayed language skills and inattention. His parents report multiple episodes of ear infections, one of which led to a perforation. Hearing assessment showed bilateral moderate hearing loss with glue ears and stiff eardrums. He was referred to the ENT doctor with a view to myringotomy. Rhys's behaviour settled once his communication started to improve.

Learning points

• Conductive hearing loss is very common in young children and can present with language, attention and behavioural problems.

A normal newborn hearing test will pick up only congenital hearing loss, which accounts for less than half of the total of significant hearing losses in children.

Conductive deafness due to congenital malformations, such as congenital anomalies of the ossicles, is very rare and may occur in isolation. There may be some conductive hearing loss associated with ear malformations that occur in certain syndromes such as Treacher Collins syndrome. Otosclerosis is rarely seen in childhood. By contrast, acquired conductive loss is much more frequently encountered. Common causes are listed in the box 'Causes of conductive hearing loss'. Most acute otitis media cases are self-limiting and do not need any specific intervention apart from symptomatic relief. Hearing loss, if present, is usually temporary and often fluctuant. In chronic or SOM, it can be significant and persistent enough to require surgery and/or aiding.

Otitis media with effusion (also known as 'glue ear' or secretory otitis media)

OME occurs when there is a middle ear effusion behind an intact ear drum. The consistency of the effusion may vary from watery to a very thick, almost rubbery consistency. Suggested causes of the effusion include upper respiratory tract infection, allergy, inadequate treatment of an acute otitis media and Eustachian tube dysfunction. It is particularly troublesome in children with Down syndrome, cleft palate, Turner syndrome, primary ciliary dyskinesia and craniostenosis syndromes.

HISTORY

• Hearing loss, usually in the mild to moderate range.
• Delayed language development.
• Poor attention and poor listening skills.
• Behavioural problems.
• Underperformance at school.
• Poor balance and clumsiness.

DIAGNOSIS

- Hearing tests to assess hearing thresholds across the frequencies.
- Otoscopy showing
    - a pink infected or yellowish dull ear drum.
    - bubbles of fluid in the middle ear.
    - indrawing of the ear drum, which can be difficult to recognize.
- Tympanogram to measure impedance.

MANAGEMENT

Refer to National Institute for Health and Clinical Excellence guidance CG 60 (www.guidance. nice.org.uk/cg60/NICEGuidance/pdf/English).

- The majority of cases of OME will resolve spontaneously and antibiotics are not routinely indicated.
- There is no evidence to support the use of prolonged courses of antibiotics, antihistamines, steroids or decongestants in SOM.
- For most children, SOM is often little more than a transient problem.
- For children with persistent bilateral OME documented over a period of 3 months with hearing loss, surgery should be considered. Surgical treatment involves insertion of ventilation tubes. In addition, adenoidectomy can be performed if there are signs of persistent or frequent upper respiratory tract symptoms. Surgery is effective in the short term but it is not free of complications. There may be continuing discharge and infections and some ears scar. This can have a slight but negative effect on hearing thresholds in the longer term.
- Hearing aids may be needed for those with significant hearing loss who fail to respond to surgical treatment. Bone-anchored hearing aids may be helpful in chronic cases.

Developmental and behavioural impact of hearing loss

Early childhood hearing loss has been shown to have a significant effect on a child's language acquisition and cognitive, social and emotional development. Bilateral hearing loss, even of a mild degree, often affects development and adversely influences the child's educational and social progress.

Any type of hearing impairment interferes with detection and recognition of speech. SNHL can both filter and distort sound whilst conductive hearing loss is likely to cause fluctuating hearing levels. Either will adversely affect the acquisition of auditory skills, which is a prerequisite for receptive language and speech recognition.

Infants with hearing loss usually present with a reduced awareness of sound and delayed vocalization. Parents are often the first to notice that something is amiss. It is advisable to take their concerns seriously and arrange appropriate hearing tests.

The perception of sound is essential for the normal development of the hearing cortex in early life. This influences the development of appropriate connections for the acquisition of language, comprehension and attention skills. Disruption of the process affects the child's ability to learn and use an auditory–oral language system. The detection and management of hearing impairment in early life can reduce difficulties with language development. Studies following the introduction of the Newborn Hearing Screen, together with early remedial management, have demonstrated improved language acquisition and improved social and educational outcomes.

Educational implications of hearing impairment

Severe or profound hearing impairment is only the tip of the iceberg. Educationally significant hearing loss is common and under-recognized. The vast majority of children with all forms of mild to moderate loss experience speech and language delay and educational difficulties. Lack of awareness of warning signs and the subtlety of signs leads to under-recognition of the problem.
   Try this for yourself.

Lip reading exercise

In partial hearing loss the child can often hear only low-frequency sounds (vowel sounds), and misses out on the high-frequency sounds (e.g. 's' and 'f').
   Try deciphering the following instruction from a teacher:
   '…en ou av iid co..r..in tur o sh.'
   Did you get it right?
   'When you have finished colouring turn over your sheet.'

Strategies to help the preschool child

- Maximize hearing.
- 'Together time' with parent.
- Reading picture books together.
- Visual cause and effect toys.
- Use of gestures.
- Encourage peer group play.
- Encourage imaginative play.

Strategies to help the school-aged child (see also 'Handy hints')

Maximize hearing

- Hearing aids.
- Radio aids – the teacher can use a microphone to enhance his or her voice in the child's hearing aid and minimize background sound.
- Personal sound field systems that use speaker phones to enhance the teacher's voice.

Classroom organization

- Sitting at the front of the class.
- Position seating so that the better ear is directed towards the teacher or the child faces the teacher.
- Ask everyone to get the child's attention before speaking.
- Reduce ambient noise. Soft furnishings absorb noise so maximize the use of, for example, carpets, blinds, double-glazed windows and material on walls such as pin boards.

Alternative methods of communication

- *Sign language* is a visual method of communication involving signing and finger spelling. Signing uses gestures, facial expressions and body language. Finger spelling uses hand movements and agreed symbols. There are several sign languages of varying complexity. *Makaton* is the most commonly used basic sign language. This uses pictographic and uncomplicated signs alongside speech to communicate straightforward messages. *British sign language* is used for older children and has greater depth and complexity. Each language has its own dialects with local and regional variation. Learning to sign is easier for all children than learning to speak. It enables them to understand the concept of 'words', which they can use to communicate. Using sign language as an adjunct to spoken language has been shown to improve the child's communication. It does not delay spoken language.
- *Lip reading* can also be a useful adjunct, especially for older children. Only 50% of the English language is visible on the lips, making lip reading difficult. Learning this skill requires good vision, concentration and interest; therefore, it is difficult to teach to children with significant learning difficulties or multiple sensory impairments.
- *Induction loop systems* use electromagnetic waves to transmit sound to any receiver within the field of the loop. The sound is amplified and background noise is reduced. The loop system has three main components: a small microphone and transmitter, a receiver and an inductive neck loop. The microphone and transmitter pick up sound from a particular source and transmit it as electromagnetic signals to the receiver, which converts it back to amplified sound via the neck loop to the hearing-impaired listener (both receiver and neck loop are worn by the user and the user's hearing aid must be switched to the 'T' setting). A *radio aid* is a personalized induction loop system that works in conjunction with a hearing aid in order to amplify sound for the user. *Infrared systems* are similar but use infrared light instead of magnetic fields to transmit sound. Public places, such as theatres, cinemas, post offices and stations, often have access to loop systems. Personalized loop systems can also be set up relatively easily at home or in a car.

Other assistive aids

- Telephone amplification systems.
- Alerting systems, e.g. flashing lights on telephones, doors, alarm clocks and smoke detectors.
- Vibrating pillow attached to alarm clock; vibrating wrist watch.
- Text telephones.
- Subtitles and signing on television programmes, plays and films.

- The Internet has been a huge boon to deaf children's ability to communicate with their peers.
- Dogs for the hearing impaired.

Interpreting services for the hearing impaired

Deaf interpreting services should be used for any consultation for a child and/or parent with deafness and are important in engaging the child and obtaining his or her views. Children and young people with hearing impairment learn to communicate in different ways, which partly depends on the level of deafness. These include the use of hearing aids, signing, lip reading, written information or a combination of all approaches called total communication. It is important to check which method of communication the child would prefer for the consultation. Specialist interpreters using spoken language and sign language, and Braille can be used for deaf–blind children.

Family and social impact of hearing impairment

A significant proportion of children with hearing impairment diagnosed at birth have a family history of hearing impairment. Three-generational family trees and genetic studies are essential for counselling.

The diagnosis of deafness and hearing impairment has a profound impact on the family. Early on it may lead to attachment difficulties while at an older age there may be family disruption. The hearing-impaired child may also have other developmental difficulties, particularly with speech and language. A proportion of children will be born into hearing-impaired families, who may have issues about how the hearing world relates to them all. Thoughtful disclosure of diagnosis, with ongoing counselling, family support and advice about appropriate stimulation, is necessary to ensure progress for the child and family.

There are a large number of support groups, and the deaf community has a cohesive network with its own set of cultural values. Providing access to other families and information, much of which can now be accessed through the Internet, is helpful to families.

Children with hearing impairment are more likely to have social, emotional and behavioural difficulties. This is due to, in part, both communication difficulties and comorbid conditions. Deaf children are vulnerable and are more likely to be abused and bullied. Professional awareness of these issues and their early detection are essential to ensuring a good outcome. Children with permanent deafness can nevertheless achieve excellent social understanding and educational success with appropriate support.

Handy hints

Tips for optimizing communication with a child with hearing impairment

- Get the child's attention by using his or her name or physical contact.
- Sit opposite the child or have the child's best ear towards you.
- Decrease background noise. Carpeted and curtained rooms are better.
- Face the child and make sure all your face is uncovered and that there is adequate light. Do not have your back to a window as this creates shadows and makes it difficult to see facial expressions or lip read.
- Bring your head to the same level as the child.
- Be 1 to 2m away from the child to have space for signing and lip reading.
- Talk clearly with a normal speech rhythm; do not shout.
- Do not eat, smoke or block the view of your face. Beards and moustaches can make lip reading difficult; sunglasses and spectacles can interfere with eye contact.
- Use facial expression. Use body language and gesture when appropriate.
- Repeat the sentence if the child did not understand; as a last measure, write it down.
- If a word or sign is not easily understood, use a more common word.
- Inform the child when there is a new topic of conversation.
- When in a group, speak one at a time. It is helpful if the speaker raises his or her hand before talking so that the child knows who is speaking.
- Pause and check understanding – both yours and the child's.
- Be patient, friendly and take time to communicate.

Key messages

- Have a low threshold for arranging a hearing test, particularly if there are known risk factors.
- Mixed hearing impairments are common. The middle ear component needs to be managed well to optimize hearing.
- Always consider that there may be other abnormalities.

Reference

Davis A, Bamford J, Wilson I et al. (1997) A critical review of neonatal hearing screening in the detection of congenital hearing impairment. *Health Technol Assess* 1: 1–177.

Further reading

British Cochlear Implant Group (1998) Implant Centre Speech and Language Therapists Guidelines for Good Practice: Working with Paediatric Clients with Cochlear Implants. Available at: www.bcig.org.uk/downloads/pdfs/Paed%201CSLT%20Guidelines%202010.pdf (assessed 9 January 2013).

MacArdle B, Bitner-Glindzicz M (2010) Investigation of child with permanent hearing impairment. *Arch Dis Child Educ Pract Ed* 95: 14–23. http://dx.doi.org/10.1136/adc.2008.150987

Websites

British Cochlear Implant Group guidelines: www.bcig.org.uk

National Deaf Children's Society: www.ndcs.org.uk

NICE guideline on surgical management of OME: http://guidance.nice.org.uk/CG60

Royal National Institute for the Deaf: www.rnid.org.uk

Sense: www.sense.org.uk

21
Visual impairment

Alison Salt

Learning objectives

- To understand the definition of vision impairment.
- To understand the common causes of severe visual impairment in childhood.
- To be able to select appropriate methods of assessment of visual behaviour and acuity for different age groups.
- To know how to manage the child with reduced vision.
- To understand the assessment of strabismus.
- To be able to advise parents and teachers about the impact of visual impairment on development and education.
- To understand the principles of management of the 'deaf–blind' child.

Classification of visual impairment

Definitions of visual impairment are still generally described according to best corrected visual acuity. The World Health Organization's definition of visual impairment is described using the standard Snellen notation (Table 21.1), which gives the distance from which a standard letter can be seen by the person being tested over the distance from which this letter or line of letters can be seen by a person with no vision deficit.

Table 21.1 The World Health Organization's definition of visual impairment

Definition	Visual acuity
Normal vision	6/18 or better (slight visual impairment <6/9)
Visual impairment	
Low vision	6/18 to 6/30
Severe visual impairment	Worse than 6/30 to 6/60
Blind	3/60 to no light perception *or* fields <10° around central fixation

Visual impairment or strabismus is usually first noticed by parents. Therefore, listening to parents' concerns and observing the child's behaviour is often the most important first step in identification.

Risk factors for visual impairment

1 *Preterm infants* – infants born before 32 weeks' gestation (or weighing <1500g) should have been screened for retinopathy of prematurity. They are at higher risk of developing refractive errors and strabismus. They are also at higher risk of postretinal visual impairment as a result of damage to the optic radiations in periventricular leukomalacia.
2 *Neurological damage* – children who have suffered potential brain-damaging events and have other disabilities.
3 Congenital infections.
4 Family history of visual impairment.

Incidence

The cumulative incidence of severe visual impairment by 16 years of age was 5.9 (5.3–6.5) per 10 000 live births and, of these, 77% had additional non-ophthalmic disorders in the UK national study by Rahi et al. (2003). The common causes of severe visual impairment in childhood in the UK are outlined in Table 21.2.

Table 21.2 Causes of severe visual impairment in the UK by anatomical site

Area affected	%	Example	%
Whole globe and anterior segment	7	Micro-ophthalmia/anophthalmia	5
		Glaucoma (primary and secondary)	3
		Cornea (sclerocornea and corneal opacities)	2
		Lens (cataract or aphakia)	5

		Uvea
		  Aniridia
		  Uveitis
			3

Retina	29	Retinopathy of prematurity	3

		Retinal and macular dystrophies
		  Leber amaurosis
		  Ocular-cutaneous albinism
			10
			4

Optic nerve	28	Hypoplasia	12
		Atrophy	13
Cerebral/visual pathways	48	Hypoxic–ischaemic encephalopathy	12
Other	2		

Note: some children have multiple problems. Source: Rahi et al. (2003).

Normal visual development

Visual behaviour changes rapidly over the first year of life (Table 21.3) and relates to both cognitive development and maturation of the functions of the eye and cortex.

Table 21.3 Normal visual development

	Visual behaviour	
Age	Near	Distance
Neonate	Turns to diffuse light	
4wk	Fixes on mother's face	
6wk	Fixes and follows a face	Watches adult at <1m
3mo	Follows a small object (6cm) horizontal and vertical	
	Watches hands	
4mo	Able to converge	Watches adult at 1.5m
5mo	2.5cm brick	
6mo	1cm object, e.g. a sweet or raisin	Watches adult at 3m
12mo		2.5cm ball at 6m

Cognitive skills that develop alongside vision enable a more formal approach to visual assessment include the following:

- Naming objects: from 18 months
- Naming pictures: from 21 months
- Matching pictures: from 30 months
- Matching symbols/letters: from 33 months
- Naming letters: from 48 months.

Impact of severe visual impairment on development

Severe visual impairment constrains *all* areas of development and has a wide-ranging and cumulative impact that is related to the level of vision.

Visual impairment has an impact on

- visual development
- body awareness and posture
- movement skills
- fine movement coordination
- concept development, e.g. object permanence
- hearing and listening skills including sound localization
- language acquisition
- self-help
- socialization

Norms for the development of 'blind' and 'partially sighted' children were produced by Reynell and Zinkin in the early 1970s (Reynell and Zinkin 1979). Table 21.4 provides a comparison of developmental milestones between typically developing children and those with severe visual impairment. A good summary of the impact of visual impairment on development is set out in Sonksen and Dale (2002).

Table 21.4 Developmental milestones in visually impaired children

Milestone	Typically developing child (mean age, mo)	Child with severe visual impairment (mean age, mo)
Reaches for and touches object	5	11
Transfers objects from one hand to the other	5	16
Searches for removed object	6	20
Sits alone without support (5s)	7	16
Feeds self bite-size piece of food	7	20
Babbles	8	14
Moves 1m by crawling	9	20
Points to one body part	17	23
Follows direction for daily routine	20	37

Source: Dale and Sonksen (2002).

Recent research found that approximately 30% of children with profound visual impairment (awareness of light or light-reflecting objects only) are at risk of stasis or regression in cognitive development during the second year of life (Cass et al. 1994, Dale and Sonksen 2002). In this group disordered social communication was most prominent. There is likely to be a number of inter-related factors that lead to this vulnerability, including underlying associated structural brain anomalies and genetic factors. In addition, there are the challenges of development in the second year of life including the development of attention control, shared attention and social interaction. This highlights the need for intensive support and monitoring of development in these developmentally vulnerable children. The presence of even limited vision appears protective; therefore, visual promotion as early as possible is critical (Sonksen et al. 1991).

Assessing visual function

Vision is a complex multifaceted sense and the following are aspects to assess:

- Visual behaviour or the way a child uses his or her vision – response to people and objects.
- Visual detection (knowing that something is seen but not what it is).
- Visual acuity (or discrimination of two points, i.e. identification).
- Visual fields
- Vision for contrasts
- Vision for colour

Screening

The current best practice recommendations are

- At birth and at 6 weeks all children should be examined for the red reflex to exclude cataract and retinoblastoma.
- Parental concern. Parents will quickly note if their infant is not looking at their face in the first weeks of life. Any concerns should always be taken seriously and urgent action should be taken.

There is a lack of evidence for screening for visual impairments (Snowdon and Stewart-Brown 1997).

Assessing vision

Visual behaviour and abilities change with age, and therefore assessment must be tailored to the developmental level (Table 21.5).

Table 21.5 Visual assessment for children under the age of 3 years

	Method	Example of appropriate test
Near detection *at 30cm*[a]	Smallest object seen	Near detection scale – see below
Distance detection *starts at 3m then 2m, 1m, 0.5m and <0.5m*	Smallest object seen at a distance	Describe size and distance, e.g. a face or an object of defined size
Near acuity	Preferential looking (unable to letter/symbol match)	Keeler Acuity Cards Cardiff Cards
Visual assessment over 3y		
Near acuity	Letter match or name	Sonksen logMAR near acuity card
	Read words	MacClure Reading Test for Children
Distance[b] acuity at 3m	Letter match or name letters	Sonksen logMAR test
	Name letters	Any adult acuity test
Everyday visual function. State distance identified. Start at 3m then 2m, 1m, 0.5m and <0.5m	Vision for real objects	Simple everyday objects are best, e.g. shoe, brush, spoon, sock, toothbrush
	Vision for pictures	

[a]Also useful in older children with vision so low that formal acuity tests are not possible. [b]Preschool children perform best at 3 or 4m.

Functional assessments of vision

It is possible to assess visual behaviour to help to understand how a child is using his or her vision in everyday activities; this gives a good basis for advice to parents about what visual material will be seen by a child and at what distance they should be presented. The following tests measure visual detection and identification of objects and pictures.

Near detection

Near detection can be easily observed in the clinic with a few basic tools in children aged 8 to 9 months. The objects should be placed in front of the child, but the hand is swept slowly across the table and the object dropped in passing so that the child does not locate the object by following the examiner's hand.

The near detection scale has been designed to give a standard for assessment of the smallest sized object on which a child shows clear visual fixation (detection vision) and at what distance the object is seen. This is particularly helpful in the assessment of a young child with a significant visual impairment and allows monitoring of visual changes with time.

Near detection scale

- Penlight torch in a dark room
- Penlight torch glowing source (lights on)
- Mirror reflecting light
- Object in space (state furthest distance seen)
  - light-reflecting object (10cm tinsel ball)
  - non-light-reflecting yellow ball dangling (6cm)
- Fixation at (30cm) yellow or white objects on contrasting green background
  - ball (6cm)
  - cube (2.5cm)
  - Smartie (1cm)
  - saccharine (5mm)
  - Hermaseta (3mm)
  - 100 and 1000 (1mm)

Source: Sonksen et al. (1991).

Assessment of visual acuity

Acuity is the ability to discriminate two points (the retina's ability to resolve a particular subtended angle).

Forced choice preferential looking is used in young children. It is based on a child's inherent interest in patterned as opposed to homogeneous targets. Looking towards the target is interpreted as seeing the target. In the older child the task can be to point at the target. This test can be used from birth until other methods can be used. This is a near test and should be done at standard distance. Two commonly used tests are the Keeler Acuity Cards (striped black and white targets) and Cardiff Cards (pictograms), which are used for near vision.

It is important not to overinterpret the results as equivalent to results achieved with adult standard letter-based acuity tests, as the behavioural tasks are very different. It can, however, be helpful in defining a general visual level and to monitor changes in vision, for example monitoring a child after cataract removal.

Table 21.6 and the graph summarizes how visual acuity changes with age.

Table 21.6 Visual acuity changes with age (by forced choice preferential looking)

	Distance					
Vision	1m	2m	3m	4m	6m	12m
Central	6/180		<6/60	6/60 to 6/36	6/36 to 6/24	6/24 to 6/18
Peripheral		6/180		6/60		6/60

Also refer to norms for vision testing in older children (Salt et al. (2007) and Sonksen et al. (2008)).

The *Kay Picture Test* assesses vision by asking the child to match pictograms at a distance with those the child has on a card. This can be done as either a single pictogram or pictograms in a line (Crowded Kay pictures). This can be done by children aged over 2 years.

The *Snellen standard* was the original criterion standard. The Snellen standard specifies particular letter proportions and distances between letters (see figure below).

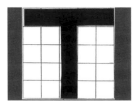

A visual acuity of 6/48 means that the 48th line of letters is seen (well enough to be read) by a fully sighted adult at 48 metres but is seen by the testee at only 6 metres. 6/6 (20/20 if measured in feet) is normal vision for an adult, although some people may be able to read one line lower and they would have 6/5 acuity.

The *logMAR standard* (Bailey and Lovie 1976) is now increasingly accepted as the standard. LogMAR refers to the log of the minimal angle of resolution. The advantages of the logMAR scale are a regular progression of both letter sizes and spacing from one level to the next (each step equal to 0.1 log unit) and an equal number of letters at each level. In addition, the method of scoring takes account of each letter correctly identified by the testee, which results in increased sensitivity and repeatability. (Each letter contributes 0.025 if there are four letters on a line.) The equivalent to 6/6 in this scale is 0.0 and to 6/60 is 1.0.

The *Sonksen logMAR test* is designed for use at 3 metres and has norms available that allow interpretation of results according to the child's age. A near card is also available as part of this test. It can be used from as early as 2.5 years. From this age more than 80% of individuals can get a result with both eyes open (Salt et al. 1995, 2007). To achieve this it is important that distractions are minimized, the child is seated at a small table and the examiner first trains the child at the table to match letters against a training card.

The *MacClure Reading Test* can be used in children who are literate to assess the print size which is appropriate for them. It is important to assess the font size of print that is read at a comfortable reading distance (about 30cm).

Refractive errors

It is essential to ensure that children with refractive errors are identified, especially children with disabilities, who may have a higher incidence of errors. In younger children refractive errors are assessed by cycloplegic retinoscopy, whereas in older children, as in the adult population, it can be completed by subjective refraction.

Myopia – also referred to as short sight. In this error the image is focused anterior to the retina.

Hypermetropia – also known as long sight. In this error the image is focused behind the retina and may be caused by the eye being shorter, the cornea flatter or the lens weaker than usual.

Astigmatism – optical asymmetry in the anterior segment of the eye leading to uneven focus on the retina, which may be due to pupillary position, corneal astigmatism or lenticular astigmatism.

Strabismus

Strabismus is a common childhood disorder (manifested in around 5% of children) for which there are a range of underlying diagnoses (Table 21.7). When assessing for strabismus simple observation may be misleading. Variations in shape and form of the palpebral apertures and ocular and orbital factors may either mask or simulate strabismus.

The symmetry of corneal reflections should be assessed in the straight ahead position, both fixing on a near target (about 50cm) and looking into the distance and in all directions of gaze.

They are described by their clinical presentation (Table 21.8).

Table 21.7 Aetiology of strabismus

	Aetiology
Abnormal anatomy	Anomaly of eye, e.g. optic nerve hypoplasia
	Abnormality of binocular vision, e.g. albinism
	Abnormality of the orbits, e.g. craniofacial dysostosis
Genetics	Close relative with strabismus (25%)
Refractive error	High hypermetropia (long sighted)
	High myopia (short sighted)
	Anisometropia (unequal refraction in each eye)
Neurological dysfunction	Cerebral palsy: 20–40% have a convergent strabismus (esotropia)
	Hydrocephalus
	Perinatal asphyxia
Preterm birth	Increased incidence of refractive error, retinal abnormalities (retinopathy) and neurological disorders
Developmental anomalies of extra-ocular structures	Congenital fibrosis of the extraocular muscles

Table 21.8 Clinical presentation of strabismus

Type of strabismus	Presentation
Esotropia	Convergent
Exotropia	Divergent
Concomitant strabismus	The angle of deviation is constant, irrespective of the direction of gaze, and the range of movement of each eye is full
Incomitant strabismus (Note: probably less than 1% of all incidences of strabismus)	There is a limitation of eye movement and the angle of deviation changes with direction of gaze

However, it is more practical to consider whether they are

- *Paralytic* – due to involvement of the cranial nerves. In this case the appearance of the strabismus will vary with the direction of gaze (incomitant strabismus).
- *Non-paralytic* when it relates to a problem with the visual axis and the angle of deviation is relatively constant (concomitant strabismus).

Paralytic strabismus

The clinical features of the strabismus will vary with the cranial nerve affected (Table 21.9).

Table 21.9 Strabismus and cranial nerves

	Cranial nerve		
	III	*IV*	*VI*
Pupil and limitation of movement	Pupil dilatation Decreased adduction Decreased elevation	Limited depression in adduction	Eye abduction
Head posture	No specific posture	Chin depression in order to have binocular vision and towards the affected side	Head tilt to affected side
Ptosis	Present	Absent	Absent
Apparent strabismus	Eye looks 'down and out' – esotropia	Only apparent on downwards gaze	Exotropia

CONGENITAL ABNORMALITY

All of the cranial nerves can be congenitally affected, but this is most common for the VI cranial nerve. When it occurs in isolation this is known as Duane syndrome. The VI cranial nerve can also be affected along with the VII cranial nerve in Moebius syndrome.

ACQUIRED

Trauma is the most common cause (42.5%). If trauma is minor, then consider other causes. Cranial nerve palsies, in isolation or in combination, can also occur after bacterial meningitis, when there is often recovery. Cranial nerve palsy can also be the presenting feature of a tumour, most commonly a brainstem glioma, craniopharyngioma or leptomeningeal sarcoma. It can also be a consequence of enlargement of the third ventricle with other brain tumours.

VI NERVE PALSY

1   You need to be aware of an acute presentation of VI nerve palsy as this can be a sign of raised intracranial pressure.
2   Transient unilateral VI nerve palsy in newborn infants is benign and more likely with forceps delivery. If there are no other neurological or other abnormalities, then no further investigation is required.
3   Benign recurrent VI nerve palsy occurs after a viral illness and is isolated and painless. All investigations including MRI are normal. Recovery usually occurs in 8 to 12 weeks, but the condition can be recurrent.

Non-paralytic strabismus

The features are most clearly demonstrated using a cover test (Fig. 21.1), in which a cover is placed in front of the strabismic and non-strabismic eye.

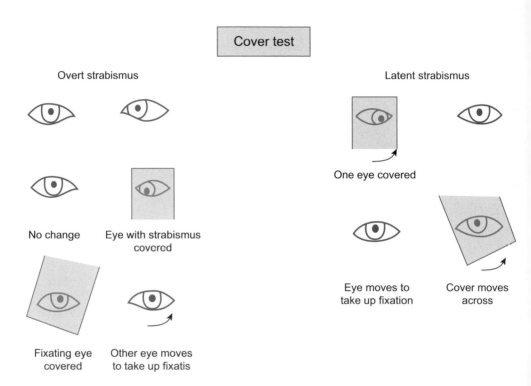

Figure 21.1 Cover test.

MANAGEMENT: PREVENTION OF AMBLYOPIA

Management of strabismus is important as misalignment of the eyes in adults leads to double vision (diplopia). In a child the vision of one eye may be suppressed to avoid this diplopia and the visual pathways then fail to develop normally. This leads to amblyopia or loss of vision in what was otherwise a normal eye.

Orthoptic and ophthalmological management may include

1 Correcting any refractive error (particularly if asymmetrical, as this may correct the strabismus).
2 Patching the non-strabismic eye.
3 Surgery.

Paediatric role in assessing and managing a child with decreased vision

> ### Case vignette
>
> A male infant born at term after a normal delivery is noted by his mother not to be looking at her face and she starts to worry at 3 weeks. She seeks help from the GP and is reassured. By 6 weeks there is no change and she presents to the accident and emergency department of a specialist eye hospital. Assessment includes examination of the eyes, which shows small (hypoplastic) optic nerves. Visual evoked potentials confirm reduced size and latency of signals. The child is assessed by an endocrinologist and a MRI of the head is arranged. A small pituitary gland, absent septum pellucidum and small optic nerves are found. Detailed assessment of pituitary function finds a low level of thyroid hormone. A referral was made to the local preschool service for children with visual impairment (qualified teacher for visual impairment).
>
> ### *Learning points*
>
> - Always listen to parents' concerns about their infant's visual behaviour. An infant not looking at his or her mother's face should always be investigated further.
> - Children with bilateral optic nerve hypoplasia are at risk of additional midline anomalies of the brain and should always undergo MRI and assessment of pituitary function.
> - Early support for the parent and child to promote development is essential.

Clinical approach to visual assessment

What is the degree of visual impairment?

- Do you think he or she sees normally? Why or why not?
- Does he or she look at your face?
- Does he or she watch as you walk away?
- What sort of things can he or she see?
- Does he or she recognize your face (not voice) and, if so, at what distance?
- Does he or she look at toys/pictures?
- Does he or she hold objects close to his or her eyes?
- Does he or she feel for objects?

What could be the underlying cause? Consider the following risk factors:

- Pregnancy, particularly features suggesting infection
- Perinatal and neonatal history
- Other disabilities
- Other malformations
- Family history of eye problems

How is the child progressing with the rest of his or her development?

Are there clues to the underlying cause in the general examination?

- Growth parameters – particularly head circumference.
- Dysmorphic features (including skin and hair colour, e.g. in albinism).

Are there any abnormalities in the child's eyes or eye movements?

Are there any abnormalities of appearance?

- Eyelids (e.g. ptosis)
- Size of eyes (e.g. micro-ophthalmia)
- Cornea
- Iris – coloboma and aniridia
- Pupil symmetry and reactions to light

Is there any strabismus?

- Corneal reflections and cover test

Are the eye movements normal?

- Nystagmus
- Are the movements conjugate (consider features of paralytic strabismus)?
- Smooth pursuit and fast (saccadic) eye movements

Are the visual fields normal?

Test by direct confrontation to assess peripheral visual fields: the examiner and child face each other with both eyes open. The child is instructed to look at the examiner's nose. The child's eye contact is engaged and then he or she is asked to point at whichever of the examiner's fingers are moving as they are held at the periphery of the examiner's own visual field.

Is the fundus normal?

- Retina (central and peripheral)
- Optic disc
- Macula

What is the child's visual acuity and functional vision (see above)?

Assess the child's development

Investigations to consider

Visual field testing – formal visual fields can be tested from around 7 to 8 years by Goldmann visual field examination.

Electrophysiological tests

ERG (electroretinography) is a test to assess retinal function. This measures the change in voltage across the eye in response to a sudden change in light level. Responses to a flash or a pattern at retinal level are measured from an electrode on a contact lens or under the eye.

VER, (visual evoked responses or potentials) are the change in bioelectrical activity sent from the retina along the optic nerve to the occipital cortex in response to a change in visual stimulation and are recorded from scalp electrodes positioned over the occipital cortex. Visual stimulus can be a flash or chequerboard or a striped pattern.

Ophthalmic management

Involve an ophthalmologist and orthoptist if they are not already involved. If there is a refractive error, ensure that this is corrected and the child has access to suitable glasses.

Consider if there is a need to perform any *investigations* into the underlying cause of the visual difficulty.

Check hearing

Support the family

Parents play a major role in promoting the development of their infants. However, when their child is diagnosed as visually impaired they need support not only to come to terms with the shock and sadness associated with the knowledge of their child's visual impairment but also to understand how to help their child learn about their world.

The early months are critical in the development of drive to learn. If the child's natural interest and responsiveness is not stimulated early, then it becomes increasingly difficult to promote them. Therefore, it is essential that parents receive early support and education about how to help their child. In the UK each education authority has an advisory service for visually impaired children, and in most areas a specialist peripatetic teacher will visit the family at home to provide practical advice and support.

A new national early intervention programme (part of the Department for Education in England) is available to all children born with a visual impairment. The documents that support this programme (*The Developmental Journal for Young Children with Visual Impairment*) are available to all parents and can be ordered through the Early Support website (www.ncb.org.uk/early-support/resources/development-journals/).

Education

When children start school, if this is mainstream, it is essential to continue to involve teachers for the visually impaired to support the class teacher.

Top tips

- Have and wear clean glasses with a good correction. It is often useful to have a spare pair as they are frequently broken.
- Consider lighting conditions. Avoid conditions that are too dim or too bright (e.g. for those with albinism or cone dystrophy).
- Ensure good contrast (avoid print overlying pictures).

Ensure that classroom teachers are receiving advice from a specialist teacher for children with visual impairment.

Classwork

- Sit the child at the front of the class (if the child has a minor impairment, ensure that he or she has been assessed and advice about the size of the letter that can be seen with ease is given).
- If assessment of vision suggests that seeing sufficient detail at a distance is not possible, then all written material must be presented at a distance of less than 50cm (i.e. at their desk) or visual aids, such as a CCTV linked to a screen at close range, should be provided.
- Print must be appropriately enlarged to a font size easily read at approximately 30cm.
- A sloping desk helps with near work without adversely affecting the child's posture and the lighting of the text.
- Tasks with high visual demand should be confined (if possible) to the early part of the school day because of additional demands they impose and the fact that they are tiring.
- Alternative means for producing written work will also be necessary, e.g. access to a laptop or audiotape.
- Consider low-vision aids.

Low-vision aids

Low-vision aids and magnifiers are usually useful only for accessing small amount of text and are rarely useful for longer spells of reading.

- CCTVs
  - useful where small amounts of text are too difficult to enlarge or for maps or pictures or distance access
- Computer software
  - to enlarge print and large letters on screen and keyboards
- Small magnifiers (from age 3 years)
  - useful to look at the small detail in pictures or to look at other small things such as insects
- Binoculars or a monocular (usually from age 5 years)
  - to help children to see detail in the distance, for example on outings (younger children can practise with toy binoculars)

Mobility

Enabling children to be confident about their movements can be helped by

- marking steps with a contrasting line on their edge;
- contrasting lines along corridors or around doorways.

Social understanding

It is important to remember that children with a visual impairment require additional verbal cues as they may not see facial expression and body language at a distance. This is particularly true for unstructured times as children need support to identify their friends in the playground and also to understand non-verbal social cues.

Underlying diagnosis

Visual disorders may be considered in the groups shown in Table 21.10.

Table 21.10 Diagnosis of visual disorders

Apparent eye anomaly	Abnormality behind the lens	Apparently normal eye but abnormal vision
Cataract	Retinoblastoma	Refractive error
Micro-ophthalmos	Retinitis pigmentosa	Optic atrophy
Cryptophthalmos	Retinal haemorrhage – shaking injury	Cortical blindness
Buphthalmos	Retinopathy of prematurity leading to retrolental fibroplasia	Delayed visual
Albinism	Congenital infection	maturation
Aniridia	Coloboma	
Oculomotor apraxia	Optic atrophy	

Apparent eye anomaly

Cataracts

Cataracts (lens opacities) range in size from tiny opacities to total obstruction of vision. The pupil is described by the parent as hazy or milky, but this appearance may be easily visible only in certain lighting conditions. Early and reliable detection is best accomplished by looking at the red reflex of the pupil through an ophthalmoscope.

Urgent referral to an ophthalmologist is recommended whenever cataract is suspected in infancy. After surgery, the aphakia (absence of lens) leaves the child severely hypermetropic, and spectacles, contact lenses or intraocular lenses correct this.

In about one-third of cases, cataracts are inherited as isolated defects, and the inheritance may be dominant, recessive or sex linked. Some of the other possible causes are shown in Table 21.11. Examination of other family members may be helpful.

Table 21.11 Causes of cataracts

Group		Specific condition
Congenital infection		Rubella
		Toxoplasmosis
		Varicella
Genetic	Isolated	Autosomal dominant or recessive
		Sex-linked recessive
	Chromosomal	Down syndrome
		Trisomy 13
	Systemic syndromes	Lowe syndrome
		Nance–Horan syndrome
		Hallerman–Streiff syndrome
		COFS syndrome
		Cockayne syndrome
Metabolic disorders		Galactosaemia
		Peroxisomal disorders
		Mitochondrial disorder
		Hypocalcaemia
Other ocular abnormalities		Micro-ophthalmos
		Anirida

COFS, cerebro-oculo-facio-skeletal.

Nystagmus

Nystagmus can be broadly divided into three categories.

1   nystagmus secondary to visual defect;
2   nystagmus secondary to intracranial lesions and drug toxicity;
3   congenital benign idiopathic nystagmus.

The first two are most common. The last can sometimes be diagnosed only by exclusion, but positive identification is possible by eye movement recording.

Congenital benign idiopathic nystagmus is thought to be due to a fault in smooth pursuit and fixation systems and can be sex linked, autosomal recessive or autosomal dominant.

Vision may be impaired but often is surprisingly good. Near vision is often better than distance vision. The individual does *not* have any sensation of apparent movement (oscillopsia).

Abnormality behind the lens

Retinopathy of prematurity (ROP) is seen in infants who weigh less than 1500g and are less than 31 weeks' gestation at birth. These children are routinely screened according to a nationally agreed protocol. Treatments for 'threshold' disease can include cryotherapy and laser treatment. All children who progress to stage 3 should be followed up as they are at risk of developing refractive error, visual and ocular motor problems. Consequences of ROP include retinal detachment, microcornea, micro-ophthalmos, secondary glaucoma, corneal opacity and cataract.

Retinoblastoma. This may present with strabismus or retrolental mass. About 25% of cases are familial with dominant inheritance, and these may be bilateral. Deletion of chromosome 13 has been described in association with retinoblastoma. Radiotherapy may be successful but enucleation may be needed.

Norrie's disease. This is characterized by vitreo-retinal dysplasia (retinal folds, retinal detachment, vitreous haemorrhage and retrolental masses) in the eyes, causing severe visual impairment in the early months of life. Cataracts, corneal degeneration and atrophy of the iris also develop. A significant number of affected individuals have learning difficulties and some develop deafness in later years. It is a sex-linked recessive disorder, so it is mostly males who are affected. However, some females have been affected, which suggests that heterozygotes may manifest symptoms.

Retinal dystrophies

The inherited retinal dystrophies are a genetically heterogeneous group of disorders, many of which become symptomatic in childhood. They may be isolated in an otherwise healthy child or be associated with systemic abnormalities.

Retinal disorders can be divided into two categories: stationary retinal dystrophies and progressive retinal dystrophies, either isolated or those associated with systemic disorders (Table 21.12).

Table 21.12 Retinal dystrophies

Stationary retinal dystrophies	
Stationary night blindness	Congenital
	With characteristic appearance of the retina are Oguchi disease and fundus albipunctatus
Stationary cone dystrophy	Rod monochromatism (achromotopsia)
	Blue cone monochromatism
Progressive retinal dystrophies	
Rod–cone dystrophies	Leber amaurosis (infantile rod–cone dystrophy)
	Progressive rod–cone dystrophies (retinitis pigmentosa)
Cone dystrophies	
Cone–rod dystrophies	

Progressive rod–cone dystrophy – retinitis pigmentosa is a degenerative disorder affecting the rods first and the cones in later stages. Pigment is deposited in clusters which resemble a bone corpuscle. It is unusual for this disorder to present before adolescence. The first complaint is usually poor vision in dim illumination; the child may have difficulty in going down stairs in the evening. There is increasing constriction of the visual fields, with preservation of a central tunnel of vision (the visual field is really cone shaped and increases in diameter with increasing distance from the eye). There are several types; it can be inherited in a dominant, recessive or sex linked manner (Table 21.13). Occasionally retinitis pigmentosa is associated with a variety of other abnormalities.

Table 21.13 Genetic inheritance of rod–cone dystrophy

Autosomal dominant	*Autosomal recessive syndromes*	*Metabolic*
Olivopontocerebellar atrophy	Laurence–Moon–Biedl	Abetalipoproteinaemia
Alagille syndrome	Bardet–Beidl	Mucopolysaccharidosis
Myotonic dystrophy	Usher	Peroxisomal disorders
	Cockayne	Mitochondrial disorders
	Joubert	Carbohydrate-deficient
	Jeune	glycoprotein syndrome
	Hallavorden–Spatz	Neuronal ceroid lipofuscinoses
	Osteopetrosis	Idiopathic infantile hypercalcaemia
	Alström syndrome	
	Cohen syndrome	

Leber's congenital amaurosis is an important cause of retinal dystrophy. It is an autosomal recessive group of disorders, with at least 10 different genotypes. They present with visual impairment from birth with normal-looking eyes and nystagmus. The diagnosis depends on eletroretinography findings, which are absent or poorly recordable. Several genes have been identified, which has given rise to different causes of the retinal degeneration. The manifestation can be quite variable and many different causal genes have been identified.

Cerebral visual impairment

In the developed countries, visual impairment is most commonly due to abnormality of the cerebral cortex or visual pathways. The reasons include the increasing survival of children following preterm birth or life-threatening illnesses, e.g. encephalitis or trauma of various causes, coupled with improved treatments for primary visual disorders, e.g. cataract and glaucoma. Children with cerebral palsy are likely to have associated visual problems. This is discussed in Chapter 25 on cerebral palsy.

As a developmental paediatrician it is important to draw attention to vision assessment in the child with a neurological disability and assessment. The methods described above should always be part of routine examination of such children. Clinical clues may be observed in the child's fixation, his or her capacity to follow an object with a smooth eye gaze, head posture and tilt when looking, coupled with your knowledge of the neuroimaging results.

In this group of children visual acuity may be severely impaired, or in a proportion within normal limits or only mildly impaired, but visual function may be a significant problem. Higher order visual dysfunction may be seen, in which perceptual or cognitive deficits lead to difficulties with more complex visual tasks.

The cortical visual pathways are divided into dorsal and ventral streams. Dysfunction in either pathway leads to well-described specific characteristics, although presentation in an individual child will vary. Dorsal stream difficulties lead to potentially impaired ability to interpret complex visual scenes such as finding a toy in a box or an item on a patterned background, reading crowded text and impaired visually guided movement, for example seeing floor boundaries or steps and impaired ability to perform more than one visual task at a time. Ventral stream dysfunction leads to impaired recognition and orientation for people, shapes or locations.

In order to appropriately help the child, these visual difficulties must first be identified. Assessment of these complex difficulties of visual function will require involvement of a paediatric ophthalmologist and paediatrician specializing in neurodisability, working closely with a psychologist (ideally a neuropsychologist), in order to provide a full understanding of visual and higher visuocognitive function. The specialist teacher for children with visual impairment will also provide helpful observations of the child's function and will be an important partner in implementing recommendations for the school and home.

Managing the deaf–blind child

A significant minority of children with hearing or visual impairment have impairment of the other sense. These children are sometimes known as 'deaf–blind' but rarely have total hearing and visual loss.

The term 'deaf–blind' normally refers to people with severe loss in both senses, but the issues that arise are relevant to children with some impairment in both senses. This is particularly the case for children with other impairments such as learning difficulties.

Causes of dual sensory impairment

- Congenital rubella (less common now as a result of immunization)
- Other congenital infections
- Usher syndrome
- CHARGE syndrome
- Meningitis/encephalitis
- Trauma including non-accidental injury
- Severe neonatal encephalopathy
- Extreme preterm birth

Many of these conditions will also cause physical and learning disabilities. Children who have profound and multiple disabilities must always be assessed carefully for hearing and vision impairments because management of these may significantly improve the child's abilities.

Usher syndrome

Usher syndrome is an important cause of isolated hearing and visual impairment. The major symptoms of Usher syndrome are hearing loss and retinitis pigmentosa. Many people with Usher syndrome also have severe balance problems. There are three clinical types of Usher syndrome, of which types 1 and 2 are the most common. The three clinical types together account for approximately 90% to 95% of all children with Usher syndrome. Those with Usher syndrome type 1 are born with profound hearing loss and may have problems with their balance. Typically their vision starts to change in the first and second decades of life, with tunnel vision and night blindness often being the first symptoms. Children with Usher syndrome type 2 are born with partial hearing, and often use hearing aids. Their vision often starts to deteriorate during the teenage years but their balance is unaffected. Young people with Usher syndrome type 3 may have normal hearing from birth, but develop retinitis pigmentosa in adolescence or later, when hearing loss also occurs.

Management

Most children with multisensory impairment have some function in one or both senses and use of this residual function must be maximized.

Children with severe hearing and visual loss will need to rely on touch for communication. As infants they cannot anticipate touching and handling and may cry in response, which may make parents reluctant to handle them. Early advice on touching and handling will help to overcome this.

Helping children with dual sensory impairment to communicate is key. A flexible approach using multisensory modalities is needed. This is often referred to as *total communication*. This could include

- use of facial expression, gesture and body language
- speech
- written words
- finger spelling or other sign language
- objects of reference
- models
- symbols or line drawings
- Braille or Moon.

Sense is an organization for people with dual sensory impairment. Their website (www.sense.org.uk) contains additional useful information.

Registration as sight impaired and benefits

To register as severely sight impaired/blind (SSI) or sight impaired/partially sighted (SI) in the UK, a child must be seen by a consultant ophthalmologist. The specialist will conduct an eye test and complete a Certificate of Vision Impairment (CVI). In Scotland, this is a BP1 form if the vision fulfils the criteria for registration. The CVI includes the results from the eye test, as well as information about a person's circumstances and preferred format for correspondence.

When registered as SSI the local social care department is informed and should make further assessments of need. Children or adults who are registered as SSI or SI are often eligible for allowances aimed at supporting them practically, for example a reduction in television licence fees.

Key messages

- Always listen to parents' concerns about their child's vision and refer for urgent assessment.
- Ensure that the child and family are supported by a teacher for children with visual impairment from as soon as possible after visual impairment is suspected.
- Ensure that parents receive immediate emotional and practical support to help them to know how best to interact with their child and support their child's development.
- Severe visual impairment affects all areas of development, but in particular social interaction and communication.
- Children with a neurological disability should always have their visual function assessed thoroughly.
- Work with orthoptists to ensure that a child with a strabismus has appropriate treatment to prevent amblyopia.

References

Bailey IL, Lovie JE (1976) New design principles for visual acuity letter charts. *Am J Opt Physiol* 53: 740–5. http://dx.doi.org/10.1097/00006324-197611000-00006

Cass HD, Sonksen PM, McConachie (1994) Developmental setback in severe visual impairment. *Arch Dis Child* 70: 192–6. http://dx.doi.org/10.1136/adc.70.3.192

Dale N, Sonksen P (2002) Developmental outcome, including setback, in young children with severe visual impairment. *Dev Med Child Neurol* 44: 613–22. http://dx.doi.org/10.1111/j.1469-8749.2002.tb00846.x

Rahi JS, Cable N, British Childhood Visual Impairment Study Group (2003) Severe visual impairment and blindness in children in the UK. *Lancet* 362: 1359–65. http://dx.doi.org/10.1016/S0140-6736(03)14631-4

Reynell J, Zinkin P (1979) The Reynell-Zinkin Scales. Developmental Scales for Young Visually Handicapped Children: Part 1 Mental Development. Windsor, UK: NFER-Nelson Publishing Co.

Salt AT, Sonksen PM, Wade A, Jayatunga R (1995) The maturation of visual acuity and compliance with Sonksen–Silver acuity system in young child. *Dev Med Child Neurol* 37: 505–14. http://dx.doi.org/10.1111/j.1469-8749.1995.tb12038.x

Salt AT, Wade AM, Proffitt R et al. (2007) The Sonksen logMAR test of visual acuity. Testability and reliability. *J AAPOS* 12: 589–96. http://dx.doi.org/10.1016/j.jaapos.2007.04.018

Snowden S, Stewart-Brown S (1997) Preschool vision screening: a review. *Health Technol Assess* 1, 8.

Sonksen PM, Dale N (2002) Visual impairment in infancy: impact on neurodevelopmental and neuro-biological processes. *Dev Med Child Neurol* 44: 782–91. http://dx.doi.org/10.1111/j.1469-8749.2002.tb00287.x

Sonksen PM, Petrie A, Drew KJ (1991) Promotion of visual development of severely visually impaired babies: evaluation of a developmentally based programme. *Dev Med Child Neurol* 33: 320–35. http://dx.doi.org/10.1111/j.1469-8749.1991.tb14883.x

Sonksen PM, Wade AM, Proffitt R, Heavens S, Salt AT (2008) The Sonksen logMAR test of visual acuity II: age norms from 2 years 9 months to 8 years. *J AAPOS* 12: 18–22.

Further reading

Ferrell K (2008) Project PRISM. A National Collaborative Study on the Early Development of Children with Visual Impairments. Available at: www.nationaldb.org/documents/products/2008cec/dbprism.ppt (accessed 4 November 2012).

Sonksen PM, Wade AM, Proffitt R et al. (2008) The Sonksen logMAR test of visual acuity. Age norms from 2 years 9 months to 8 years. *J AAPOS* 12: 18–22. http://dx.doi.org/10.1016/j.jaapos.2007.04.019

Websites

Early Support: www.ncb.org.uk/early-support/resources/development-journals/

Health Technology Assessment programme: www.hta.nhsweb.nhs.uk/htapubs.htm

RNIB: www.rnib.org.uk

Section 9

High-risk groups

22

Extremely preterm infants and neonatal encephalopathy

Arnab Seal

Learning objectives

- To recognize risk factors for negative developmental outcomes for the unborn child in pregnancy.
- To understand the risks associated with preterm birth.
- To understand the potential developmental outcomes after preterm birth.

Background

Some infants are at a higher risk of developing a disability. The risk factors can be inherent or a consequence of maternal factors, environmental influences or social conditions. Recognition of the 'high-risk child' allows prevention (see Chapter 3 on screening), early identification, early treatment and better planned care.

The most important factor influencing risk is the underlying cause of the disorder. For example, when considering cerebral malformations, a child with agenesis of the corpus callosum has a lower risk of developmental disability than the child with holoprosencephaly. Even within the same diagnostic label there can be a wide range of clinical severity. In some conditions the severity of the clinical presentation correlates with the severity of the lesion, e.g. the neurological deficit resulting from a myelomeningocele depends on its size and location. In other conditions, however, there may be little correlation between severity of the condition and subsequent clinical outcome, e.g. the developmental outcome of severe pneumococcal meningitis can be very variable. Exposure to risk factors at critical periods of development can cause significantly more damage than at other periods, e.g. rubella infection in the first trimester has a much worse outcome than later in pregnancy. Another important but little understood variable is each child's inherent genetic resilience.

Table 22.1 provides examples of underlying risk factors and the associated adverse outcomes. Some risk factors are dealt with in other sections of this book, as indicated. This chapter covers the developmental outcome risks associated specifically with preterm birth, neonatal encephalopathy, in utero infections and exposure to drugs and toxins.

Table 22.1 'High-risk' factors in the newborn period for future developmental disability

Risk domain	Aetiology	
Child	Congenital brain/spinal cord lesions (see Chapter 25 on CP and Chapter 31 on spina bifida)	Brain malformations, e.g. lissencephaly Brain injury, e.g. antenatal stroke Spinal cord malformations, e.g. spina bifida
	Inherited/genetic conditions (see Section 11 on genetics)	Syndromic, e.g. Down syndrome Non-syndromic inherited disorders, e.g. familial microcephaly
	Metabolic disorders	Inherited, e.g. PKU, MCAD Acquired, e.g. severe electrolyte disturbance with encephalopathy, severe hypoglycaemia
	Neonatal encephalopathy	With known cause, e.g. HIE, metabolic Idiopathic with or without seizures
	SGA/VLBW/LBW	Nutritional causes Placental dysfunction Maternal causes, e.g. illness/drugs Child causes, e.g. genetic, infection
	Preterm birth	Extreme preterm birth (23–27wk) Preterm (28–37wk)
	Multiple pregnancy (IVF/spontaneous multiple)	Risks of preterm birth, IUGR, developmental disabilities
Maternal	Illness/infections/inflammation/drugs	Maternal chronic illness, e.g. IDDM, PKU, SLE, thyroid disorders
		Acute illness during pregnancy, e.g. viral illness, UTI
		Pre-eclampsia/eclampsia
		Chorioamnionitis
	Substance abuse during pregnancy	Alcohol (FAS), cocaine, stimulants
	Medication taken during pregnancy	Anticonvulsant drugs, thalidomide
	Nutrition	Caloric deprivation, iron deficiency, mineral and vitamin deficiency
Environmental factors	Toxin exposure	Lead, mercury, arsenic
	Traumatic delivery	Acquired birth injury, e.g. brachial plexus, spinal
Socioeconomic	Teenage pregnancy	Higher risk of adverse pregnancy outcomes
	Social deprivation, impoverished parental situation	Developmental impairments

PKU, phenylketonuria; MCAD, medium-chain acyl-CoA dehydrogenase deficiency; HIE, hypoxic–ischaemic encephalopathy; SGA, small for gestational age; VLBW, very low birthweight; LBW, low birthweight; IVF, in vitro fertilization; IUGR, intrauterine growth restriction; IDDM, insulin-dependent diabetes mellitus; SLE, systemic lupus erythematosus; UTI, urinary tract infection; FAS, fetal alcohol syndrome.

High-risk outcomes of preterm birth

Preterm births (births before 37 weeks' gestational age) account for 5% to 7% of all births in industrialized nations. The figure is considerably higher (10–12%) in resource-poor nations. Preterm birth is a major cause of neonatal mortality and morbidity and has long-term adverse consequences for health and development. The survival of preterm infants has improved in developed countries over the past few decades but there has not been a corresponding fall in the number of children who have poorer neurodevelopmental outcomes.

For most preterm infants born after 36 weeks' gestation, the survival and outcomes are similar to those seen in infants born at term. There is emerging evidence that between 32 and 36 weeks' gestation there is a higher risk of some developmental problems, especially related to learning and attention. Children who are born between 22 and 32 weeks' gestation have higher rates of cerebral palsy, sensory deficits, learning disabilities and respiratory illnesses than children born at term. The most substantial impairments affect the 0.2% of infants who are born before 28 weeks' gestation or whose birthweight is <1000g (extremely low birthweight [ELBW]). The morbidity associated with preterm birth often extends to later life, resulting in enormous physical, psychological and economic costs.

Case vignette

Andrew was born at 26 weeks' gestation by Caesarean section because of maternal pre-eclampsia. His mother, Sara, received two doses of high-dose beclomethasone in the 3 days prior to delivery. Andrew was born in a good condition, weighed 750g at birth, was electively ventilated and transferred to the neonatal intensive care unit (NICU). His neonatal course was complicated by infant respiratory distress syndrome (IRDS), grade 2 intraventricular haemorrhage (IVH) on the right side and grade 3 IVH on the left, two episodes of sepsis and retinopathy of prematurity (ROP) requiring laser treatment. He developed chronic lung disease of the newborn infant and was on supplemental oxygen until 6 months of age. By 1 year of age it was apparent that Andrew was developing signs of bilateral cerebral palsy. At 5 years of age Andrew is now in a mainstream primary school with additional support for his learning needs (mild learning disability) and physical needs from a moderate diplegia. His vision is corrected with spectacles and his hearing is normal. He participates in all class activities and is a popular boy in school.

Cerebral palsy

Most children with cerebral palsy are not born preterm. However, preterm infants, especially those born before 32 weeks' gestation, are at higher risk. The risk increases with decreasing gestation. Additional risk factors include feto-maternal infection, sepsis and severe illness in the newborn period. Large intraventricular haemorrhage (IVH), periventricular haemorrhage and infarcts, periventricular leukomalacia (PVL) and posthaemorrhagic hydrocephalus (PHH) are associated strongly with a high risk of cerebral palsy and other neurodevelopmental problems. A prolonged course of high-dose corticosteroids in the newborn period has also been associated with an increased risk of cerebral palsy. Preterm infants are also at higher risk of coordination and attention difficulties and problems with sensory integration.

Visual impairment

Most visual impairment in preterm infants is secondary to retinopathy of prematurity (ROP) and/or cortical visual impairment (CVI) from damage to visual tracts and visual cortex. ROP affects infants <32 weeks' gestation and the incidence and severity are inversely related to gestational age. The risk is directly related to the concentration and duration of oxygen exposure. Careful monitoring of supplemental oxygen use can help prevent ROP. Appropriate screening of at-risk infants can ensure early detection and treatment of progressive disease (cryotherapy or laser photocoagulation). Progressive untreated ROP can lead to blindness, visual field defects and refractive errors. Extreme preterm infants without ROP are also at higher risk of refractive errors and strabismus.

Hearing impairment

Infants born at less than 28 weeks' gestation are at higher risk of sensorineural hearing loss. About 3% of this group is affected. Sepsis, hypoxia, severe neonatal illness, certain drugs (aminoglycosides), severe jaundice and extreme preterm birth can be important contributory risk factors. Newborn Hearing Screening programmes allow early detection and provision of hearing aids to minimize the impact on speech and language development.

Learning difficulties

Learning difficulties can manifest as part of more complex needs, e.g. cerebral palsy, or as an isolated problem. Nearly 50% of infants born at less than 28 weeks' gestation need some additional educational support. The IQ of ELBW infants is, on average, 10 points lower than the IQ of those born at term. There is also a higher incidence of specific learning difficulties (SLDs), e.g. problems with maths, reading and writing. However, other determinants of preterm birth such as socioeconomic deprivation also have a significant influence.

Behaviour, social and psychological development

Extremely low-birthweight and extreme preterm infants are at high risk of attention, social and thought processing problems. Attention problems along with minor cognitive and sensory difficulties can lead to educational failure that can manifest in the early/middle school years. This can be quite subtle or difficult to identify at first but can have a significant effect on the child's learning ability and social functioning.

Early social milestones are often delayed in preterm infants. Many of them need prolonged hospitalization, which can affect bonding and attachment. Infants who are very unwell in the first few months of life can miss out on stimulation and social cues. They may develop difficulties with sensory integration because of exposure to a multitude of adverse sensory stimuli in the NICU and special care baby unit. When the child goes home from hospital, parents can be understandably quite anxious about their child's health, which can result in overprotectiveness. This can have a detrimental influence on the child's behaviour and social development in the long term.

Outcomes of extreme preterm birth

Extreme preterm birth is defined as being born between 23 and 26 weeks' gestation. The mortality and morbidity in this group is considerably higher than among those born at higher gestations. The EPICure study (Johnson et al. 2007) in the UK has followed a group of infants born extremely preterm at 25 weeks' gestation or earlier in 1995 and assessed them at 2 years 6 months, 6 years 6 months and 11 years of age. A total of 4004 such infants were recorded, 811 of whom were admitted to intensive care after resuscitation. The assessment at 2 years 6 months included 302 surviving infants available for follow-up. Subsequently, 241 of the surviving children were assessed at early school age at an average age of 6 years and 4 months, and 219 were assessed at 11 years of age.

Table 22.2 Key findings from the EPICure study

- 39% overall survival below 25 weeks' gestation
- Male sex was a risk factor for poor outcome
- Some impairment of motor skills, visuospatial and sensorimotor function at 6 years
- Poor postnatal growth in the early years of life, especially if chronic lung disease had been treated with prolonged courses of postnatal steroids
- Poor respiratory health over the first 6 years of life
- Cognitive impairment at 11 years including some language and phonetic difficulties
- 22% had severe disability (12% had disabling cerebral palsy), 24% had moderate disability, 34% had mild disability and 20% had intact survival at 6 years
- Non-ambulant cerebral palsy was a rare outcome at 6 and 11 years

At 11 years of age the extremely preterm children had significantly lower scores than their classmates for cognitive ability, reading and mathematics. Twenty-nine (13%) of the children attended specialist educational provision. In mainstream schools, 105 (57%) children had special educational needs (SENs) and 103 (55%) required SEN resource provision. Thus, the follow-up at 11 years of age shows that the survivors of extreme preterm birth remain at high risk for learning impairments and poor academic attainment in middle childhood. A significant proportion of survivors require full-time specialist education, and over half of those attending mainstream schools require additional health or educational resources in order to access the national curriculum. The prevalence and impact of SEN are likely to increase as these children approach the transition to secondary school.

Neonatal encephalopathy

Neonatal encephalopathy is an important clinical diagnosis made on the basis of a constellation of findings, including a combination of abnormal consciousness, depressed tone and reflexes, poor feeding, difficulty with initiating and/or maintaining respirations and often seizures occurring in the term/near-term (>34wk gestation) neonate. Neonatal encephalopathy occurs in approximately 3.5 to 6 in every 1000 live births. It is important to recognize that neonatal encephalopathy can be caused by a number of different conditions; intrapartum asphyxia causing hypoxic–ischaemic encephalopathy (HIE) is only one of many implicated conditions.

Often these infants present as 'flat' or 'depressed' at birth, but sometimes the initial signs of encephalopathy may be delayed by up to 48 hours. There are three stages of encephalopathy (Table 22.3). Infants with moderate or severe encephalopathy are most likely to have increased mortality and increased risk of poorer long-term outcomes. Infants with mild neonatal encephalopathy usually have normal developmental outcomes.

Table 22.3 Stages of neonatal encephalopathy

Stage 1	Duration <24h with hyperalertness Uninhibited Moro and stretch reflexes Sympathetic effects Normal electroencephalogram
Stage 2	Significantly depressed consciousness Hypotonia Decreased spontaneous movements with or without seizures
Stage 3	Stupor Flaccidity Seizures Suppressed brainstem and autonomic functions The EEG may be isopotential or have infrequent periodic discharges

Causes of neonatal encephalopathy

Neonatal encephalopathy accounts for less than one-quarter of cerebral palsy in term or near-term infants. Only a minority of infants with neonatal encephalopathy as neonates have definite antecedent intrapartum asphyxia. What accounts for the remainder? There are a number of risk factors for neonatal encephalopathy (Table 22.4) and some of these risk factors are also known to be risk factors for cerebral palsy. Nearly two-thirds of infants with neonatal encephalopathy have only antepartum risk factors and a number of infants with intrapartum asphyxia also have associated antepartum risk factors.

Table 22.4 Risk factors for developing neonatal encephalopathy

Maternal factors	Fetal factors
Maternal fever in labour	Intrauterine growth restriction
Thyroid disorders	Intrapartum hypoxia
Family history of neurological disorders and/	Fetal infection and/or chorioamnionitis
or seizures	Metabolic disorders causing, for example,
Coagulation disorders, e.g. factor V Leiden,	hypoglycaemia, hyperammonaemia,
antithrombin III, protein C	hyperglycinaemia
Maternal drugs and toxins	Neurological disorders, e.g. degenerative
Hypertension	disorders, muscle diseases, lower motor
High maternal age	neurone disorders, antenatal stroke
Infertility	Coagulation disorders in the fetus
Socioeconomic deprivation	Genetic/inherited/chromosomal disorders
Placental anomalies	Genetic susceptibility

Hypoxic–ischaemic encephalopathy (HIE) is neonatal encephalopathy with intrapartum hypoxia in the absence of any other identified cause. HIE is associated with less than one-third of the total number of neonates with neonatal encephalopathy in developed countries. Most children with HIE do not go on to develop cerebral palsy. For HIE to result in cerebral palsy, it would need to be severe enough to have caused neonatal encephalopathy in the newborn period. Usually there would be associated stage 3 or prolonged stage 2 encephalopathy. Term infants who develop long-term neurological sequelae from intrapartum asphyxia may not have low Apgar scores but will always demonstrate encephalopathy within the first 48 hours. The historical markers used to define perinatal asphyxia, such as meconium-stained liquor and low Apgar score, are not specific to the disease process leading to the neurological damage and should not be used as such. The 'essential criteria' to define an acute intrapartum event sufficient to cause cerebral palsy are provided in Table 22.5.

Table 22.5 Essential criteria for an acute intrapartum event sufficient to cause cerebral palsy (must meet all four)

- Evidence of a metabolic acidosis in fetal umbilical cord arterial blood obtained at delivery (pH <7 and base deficit ≥12mmol/L)
- Early onset of severe or moderate neonatal encephalopathy in infants born at ≥34wk gestation
- Cerebral palsy of the total body, spastic quadriplegia or dyskinetic type
- Exclusion of other identifiable aetiologies, such as trauma, coagulation disorders, infectious conditions or genetic disorders

Apart from HIE there are a number of other important causes of neonatal encephalopathy. Specifically, it is important to exclude metabolic disease, electrolyte disturbance, infection (maternal, placental, fetal), drug exposure, genetic conditions, nervous system malformation and neonatal stroke as possible causes of the encephalopathy. The adverse effects of inflammatory mediators from infection and/or inflammation on the fetal brain are being increasingly recognized, as is the role of procoagulants and autoimmune disorders such as maternal thyroid disease. The identification of other risk factors (Table 22.4) may point towards an underlying cause, e.g. a family history of neurometabolic illness. The requirement to investigate and exclude these possibilities will depend on the presentation, history and clinical features of the individual case.

Genetic susceptibility seems to play a significant role in neonatal encephalopathy and its subsequent outcomes. It is unclear why some infants but not others develop neonatal encephalopathy in response to an insult and why some have poorer outcomes from the same degree of neonatal encephalopathy. Understanding this susceptibility and resilience factors can help with future preventative strategies.

Investigations for neonatal encephalopathy

The immediate assessment in the delivery room of a seriously depressed neonate, especially after an uncomplicated delivery, should include the following procedures to try and gather as much information as possible regarding possible aetiology:

- examination of the placenta, membranes and umbilical cord.
- samples of umbilical artery blood for pH and base deficit.
- culture between the membranes, after splitting the amnion from the chorion.
- close review of the maternal and family history.
- newborn blood cultures and C-reactive protein.
- evaluation for maternal and fetal thrombophilia.

In the absence of any obvious reason for the encephalopathy, investigations should be undertaken to look for infections (including central nervous system infections), drugs and toxins (including those used in labour), metabolic conditions, neurological disorders, coagulation problems and electrolyte disturbance. Neuroimaging techniques such as ultrasonography, CT and MRI can reveal specific findings over a period of time, which may be helpful in determining the timing and severity of the injury. However, they can serve to approximate only a window in time for the injury rather than determine the precise moment the injury occurred. Functional MRI is the most useful for predicting long-term outcomes, but it is not widely available.

Treatment of neonatal encephalopathy

Treatment depends on identifying the underlying cause and addressing it wherever possible. Treatment is generally supportive. Infants with moderate or severe neonatal encephalopathy should preferably be monitored and cared for in a tertiary care unit. Therapeutic cooling has been shown to reduce mortality and reduce the severity of disability in survivors of moderate and severe HIE. It also improves intact neurological survival. Use of magnesium in acute neonatal encephalopathy has also been reported to be beneficial.

Long-term outcomes of neonatal encephalopathy

Around half of infants with severe neonatal encephalopathy develop severe disability including neuromotor impairment (cerebral palsy) with a high risk of cognitive impairment, poor memory, attention problems and visual impairment. Those with severe neonatal encephalopathy who do not develop cerebral palsy are still at a high risk of cognitive and educational difficulties. The type of cerebral palsy associated with neonatal encephalopathy is predominantly spastic quadriplegia, with some children showing a dyskinetic pattern. Other types of cerebral palsy, including spastic diplegia, hemiplegia and ataxic cerebral palsy, are not associated with neonatal encephalopathy.

Infants with moderate neonatal encephalopathy are at much lower risk of significant neuromotor impairment than those with severe neonatal encephalopathy, and early follow-up data may show little difference from normal. However, a significant percentage of infants with moderate neonatal encephalopathy also show a small decrease in mean IQ compared with their peers, with associated increased SEN and lower educational achievement.

Mild neonatal encephalopathy usually has a good prognosis. However, this is influenced by the underlying cause and the genetic susceptibility of the individual infant.

Key messages

- Neonatal encephalopathy is a clinical syndrome.
- Neonatal encephalopathy can be caused by various conditions affecting the mother and fetus/neonate.
- HIE is responsible for less than one-third of neonatal encephalopathy cases in the developed world.
- Not all infants with HIE will develop cerebral palsy.
- Infants with stage 2 and stage 3 neonatal encephalopathy are at higher risk of adverse neurodevelopmental outcomes.
- Appropriate investigations should be performed to look for underlying causes.
- Treatment is mostly supportive. Therapeutic cooling reduces mortality and morbidity.
- Severe neonatal encephalopathy is associated with a high risk of long-term disability.
- Developmental follow-up of these high risk infants is advisable.

References

Johnson S, Fawke J, Hennessy E et al. (2009) Neuro-developmental disability through 11 years of age in children born before 26 weeks of gestation. *Pediatrics* 124: e249–57. http://dx.doi.org/10.1542/peds.2008-3743

Further reading

Baker PN, Sibley C (2007) *The Placenta and Neurodisability*. London: Mac Keith Press.

Gilles FH, Nelson MD Jr (2012) *The Developing Human Brain: Growth and Adversities*. London: Mac Keith Press.

Johnson S, Fawke J, Hennessy E et al. (2009) Neuro-developmental disability through 11 years of age in children born before 26 weeks of gestation. *Pediatrics* 124: e249–57. http://dx.doi.org/10.1542/peds.2008-3743

Johnson S, Wolke D, Hennessy E, Smith R, Trikic R, Marlow N (2009) Academic attainment and special educational needs in extremely preterm children at 11 years of age: the EPICure study. *Arch Dis Child Fet Neo Ed* 94: F283–9. http://dx.doi.org/10.1136/adc.2008.152793

Marlow N, Hennessy EM, Bracewell MA, Wolke D (2007) Motor and executive function at 6 years of age after extremely preterm birth. *Pediatrics* 120: 793–804. http://dx.doi.org/10.1542/peds.2007-0440

Preece P, Riley EP, editors (2011) *Alcohol, Drugs and Medications in Pregnancy: The Outcome for the Child*. London: Mac Keith Press.

23
Congenital infections and toxins

Anne M Kelly

Learning objectives

- To know common causes of congenital infections.
- To know how to investigate for these infections.
- To understand the risks and potential outcomes of congenital infections.
- To know common toxins and their effects on the unborn child.

Congenital cytomegalovirus infection

Congenital cytomegalovirus (CMV) infection occurs in 0.06 of every 1000 live births in the UK and is an important cause of deafness and disability in children. It is the *most common congenital infection worldwide*. Half of women of childbearing age in the UK show evidence of infection with CMV, but this rate varies with ethnicity, parity and social class. CMV infection can occur as a result of reactivation of a latent infection (as it is a DNA virus like herpesviruses) or as a result of a primary maternal infection in pregnancy. About 10% to 15% of congenitally infected infants are symptomatic at birth.

Clinical features

Most of these symptomatic infants experience serious long-term complications including cerebral palsy, cognitive impairment, sensorineural deafness, epilepsy, microcephaly and intracranial calcifications. Most asymptomatic infants develop normally but a minority may develop problems later in life, the most common of which is sensorineural deafness. Antenatal CMV infection can present with hydrops, polyhydramnios, microcephaly and pulmonary hypoplasia. In the newborn period, however, CMV infection has a non-specific clinical presentation with many signs similar to those found in other causes of congenital infection. They include hepatomegaly, splenomegaly, petechiae, thrombocytopenia, chorioretinitis, seizures, microcephaly and intracranial calcification.

One should be aware that a form of Aicardi–Goutières disease may present in a similar manner. This is a genetically inherited disease that can present in a similar way to congenital infections and causes severe learning disability and seizures. Brain imaging findings can be similar. Refer to a specialist paediatric neurology text for further information (e.g. Aicardi 2009).

Diagnosis

Serology to diagnose infection can be problematic as CMV-specific immunoglobulin M (IgM) can persist for up to 5 months after an acute episode. Detection of IgG antibodies does not identify those more likely to give birth to an affected child. Stored neonatal blood spots, however, are now being used to provide DNA for polymerase chain reaction (PCR) and this may help to confirm a suspected diagnosis.

Treatment

There is some evidence that intravenous ganciclovir may improve outcomes as regards hearing loss but its use is reserved for those infants with central nervous system (CNS) involvement because of its toxicity.

Toxoplasmosis

Toxoplasmosis is caused by infection with the protozoan parasite *Toxoplasma gondii*. Acute infections in pregnant women can be transmitted to the fetus and may cause severe illness, preterm delivery and even death.

Transmission to humans

- Ingestion of raw or inadequately cooked infected meat, especially pork, lamb and game.
- Ingestion of oocysts, an environmentally resistant form of the organism that cats pass in their faeces, with exposure to humans occurring via exposure to cat litter or garden soil (e.g. whilst gardening or from eating unwashed fruit or vegetables).
- A newly infected pregnant woman passing the infection to her unborn fetus.

Women infected with toxoplasma during pregnancy can transmit the infection to their fetuses transplacentally. Toxoplasmosis infection is generally weak in the mother and she may not be aware of it. Infection of the fetus, however, can cause severe problems and the earlier it occurs in pregnancy, the greater the likelihood of more severe problems later.

Incidence

In the UK, toxoplasmosis occurs in 1 to 2 per 1000 live births, but in other countries this rises to 3 to 6 per 1000 live births. A screening programme is in operation in France.

Clinical presentation

Clinical presentation in the neonatal period may include hepatosplenomegaly, diarrhoea or vomiting, eye damage from retinitis, feeding problems, hearing loss, intrauterine growth retardation and petechiae.

The classic triad of signs suggestive of congenital toxoplasmosis consists of chorioretinitis, intracranial calcifications and hydrocephalus.

Intracranial calcifications are scattered or occur in a cluster around the choroid plexus. Similar appearances are found in other congenital infections such as CMV and rubella. Most infants infected in utero will have no obvious signs, but up to 80% may develop some of the following problems over time:

- sensorineural hearing loss
- learning disabilities
- seizures
- neurological problems
- visual impairment; blindness, strabismus, chorioretinitis.

Diagnosis

Antenatal suspicion of toxoplasma infection is raised if there is ultrasonographic evidence of intracranial calicifications, ventricular dilatation, hepatic enlargement and increased placental thickness.

Prenatal testing can be carried out by

- PCR for toxoplasma DNA in amniotic fluid most commonly and, less frequently, in fetal blood.
- Antibody titres – toxoplasma IgG and IgM from maternal blood (needs careful interpretation as IgM can persist for years after delivery).

Postnatal testing can be done via

- PCR for toxoplasma DNA or antibody studies (specific IgG and IgM) on cord blood, urine and cerebrospinal fluid
- CT/MR imaging of the head
- neurological and standard eye examination.

Treatment

Treatment of pregnant women is with the antibiotics spiramycin or sulfadiazine alone or a combination of pyrimethamine and sulfadiazine to reduce the risk of transmission to the fetus, depending on the gestational age and whether the fetus is known to be infected.

Treatment of infants is with pyrimethamine, sulfadiazine and folic acid for 1 year. Steroids are also given if vision is threatened or if the protein level in the spinal fluid is high.

Congenital rubella syndrome

This is now rare as a result of high levels of community immunity in the UK population. Cases of congenital rubella occurred before the introduction of the whole-population childhood immunization programme with the measles, mumps and rubella (MMR) vaccine in 1988. However, there are some cases that do occur each year, particularly in women who come to the UK from countries with no immunization programme.

Rubella is known to be a teratogenic virus and, as with other intrauterine infections, the most severe effects occur when the infection occurs in the first trimester (Fig. 23.1). Contracting rubella either just before conception or during the first trimester of pregnancy could give rise to the following additional problems:

- microcephaly
- delayed motor, intellectual and language development
- failure to thrive
- learning disability.

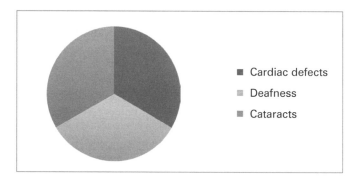

■ Cardiac defects

▨ Deafness

■ Cataracts

Figure 23.1 Typical triad of features in rubella.

Late effects of congenital infection that may appear years later include insulin-dependent diabetes mellitus (IDDM) and hypothyroidism.

The viral infection itself in the mother is often subclinical or difficult to diagnose clinically because of its non-specific signs. In the newborn infant, however, the following findings are seen: hepatosplenomegaly, jaundice due to hepatitis, bone lesions, thrombocytopenia, anaemia, myocardial damage and CNS damage. Damage to the eyes can be particularly common, with signs of cataracts, micro-ophthalmia, glaucoma retinopathy or cloudy cornea.

Contracting rubella in the later stages of pregnancy does not tend to lead to these major structural abnormalities, but sensorineural hearing loss is the usual clinical outcome for the child.

Treatment

There is no effective treatment. Most affected infants are severely damaged. Vaccination of all women of childbearing age is the effective prevention strategy.

Congenital herpes simplex infection

Clinical presentation

Herpes simplex virus (HSV) is the most common cause of sporadic encephalitis. Most HSV infections occur as a result of contact during the birth process. HSV infection presents in the newborn period either with an encephalitis-type picture with convulsions and fever or as an encephalopathy with neurological signs. Ulcers on the hard palate or intra-oral ulcers in a neonate should raise suspicion. Neuroimaging and EEG reveals abnormalities, especially in younger children. Most of those infected experience long-term neurological sequelae such as

- developmental delay
- motor abnormalities (e.g. hemiparesis, quadriparesis)
- visual problems
- epilepsy.

Those infected with the virus under the age of 1 year are at greatest risk of long-term sequelae. A small number of infants are affected by in utero infection rather than infection acquired at the time of birth. The infants with in utero infection have the classic triad of skin lesions, hydranencephaly and chorioretinitis. Significant brain damage is common.

Diagnosis

Diagnosis can be made using PCR for herpes simplex virus DNA or seroconversion to IgG or IgM within 2 weeks of the onset of infection. Among untreated cases, irrespective of the mode of transmission, the mortality rate is about 70%. Antiviral treatment with intravenous acyclovir should be started promptly as soon as the diagnosis is suspected.

Human immunodeficiency virus infection

Infection is via vertical transmission from mother to infant in more than 95% of cases. Human immunodeficiency virus (HIV) can also be acquired through unprotected sexual activity and from unscreened blood products.

Diagnosis

Maternally acquired HIV antibodies (IgG) persist for up to 15 to 18 months after birth. PCR for HIV DNA should be checked after 18 months. This is not done in resource-poor countries routinely.

All women attending antenatal clinics in the UK undergo HIV testing. If a woman is found to be positive then antiretroviral therapy is offered during the pregnancy and at the time of delivery.

Mother to child transmission (MTCT) occurs in 15% to 20% of cases in the UK and Europe without interventions. This rises to 30% in Africa, probably because of the longer duration of breastfeeding. The risk of transmission can be reduced by offering perinatal antiretroviral therapy (ART), elective Caesarean section and avoidance of breastfeeding.

Clinical presentation

One-fifth of children infected perinatally develop rapidly progressive disease presenting with *Pneumocystis* pneumonia aged 3 months. The remaining four-fifths present later with other signs including lymphadenopathy, persistent parotid enlargement, hepatosplenomegaly, shingles, extensive molluscum, recurrent or difficult to clear oral thrush, reduced platelets, recurrent infections and failure to thrive. Both groups require treatment with highly active antiretroviral therapy (HAART). The infections which should raise concerns regarding the possibility of HIV infection (AIDS-defining conditions) in infancy include *Pneumocystis* pneumonia, CMV infection, toxoplasmosis and tuberculosis.

Developmentally, the mean rate of development of infected infants is significantly slower than that of non-infected infants born to seropositive mothers but there is no gross cognitive deficit in preschool children infected with HIV compared with matched comparison children.

Treatment

Maternal infection can be treated using HAART during pregnancy.

Zidovidine was the first available antiretroviral drug. There are now 17 other similar drugs. The drugs do not eradicate the virus and children require lifelong therapy. Most children remain well as long as they comply with their medication.

Lymphocytic choriomeningitis virus infection

Lymphocytic choriomeningitis virus (LCMV) infection can be a cause of fetal infection that leads to serious developmental sequelae. LCMV is acquired by inhalation of the virus, or through contact with chronically infected mice or hamsters. Adult infection is biphasic with an initial flu-like illness followed by a variety of neurological complications, e.g. transverse myelitis, deafness, Guillain–Barré syndrome.

Intrauterine infection with LCMV, especially in the first trimester, causes chorioretinitis (in approximately 90%), retinal scarring, optic atrophy, microcephaly and periventricular calcifications. Clinical presentation is with severe visual impairment and physical and intellectual impairment.

Diagnosis

Diagnosis is by an enzyme-linked immunosorbent assay (ELISA).

Intrauterine inflammation and developmental disabilities

In addition to causing damage as a result of direct infection of the brain, there is emerging evidence that non-specific antenatal infections and inflammation at critical periods of brain formation can cause brain damage. White matter damage resulting in periventricular leuko-malacia (PVL) has been linked to maternal antenatal inflammation resulting in cerebral palsy. Although the exact mechanisms are unclear, the damage is thought to be caused by inflammatory mediators such as cytokines. In addition to maternal infection and/or inflammation, clinical and/or histological evidence of chorioamnionitis is associated with an increased risk of cerebral palsy. Examining the placenta in infants who are preterm or of low birthweight, develop neonatal encephalopathy or have other high-risk factors is being increasingly recognized as an important part of the diagnostic process (see Chapter 22 on high-risk infants).

Toxicity due to drugs and/or alcohol in pregnancy

This section will include

- substance misuse and the effects on the fetus
- fetal alcohol spectrum disorder (FASD)
- fetal anticonvulsant syndrome (FACS).

Substance misuse (e.g. heroin misuse in pregnancy)

Heroin can be smoked on its own or with tobacco, swallowed, dissolved, injected or snorted. It crosses the blood–brain barrier and binds to opiate receptors. It is twice as powerful as morphine and is used mainly for its pain relief properties but it also causes euphoria, cough suppression, reduced consciousness, constipation and itching.

Heroin use is associated with an erratic lifestyle, with some women using prostitution or crime to fund their drug habit. Many women conceal their drug use from medical professionals. Heroin is not considered to be teratogenic but it readily crosses the placenta and is associated with spontaneous abortion, intrauterine growth restriction (IUGR), preterm delivery and antepartum haemorrhage.

Neonatal abstinence syndrome

Infants may show signs of narcotic withdrawal with *fever, irritability, sneezing, sweating, stiffness, diarrhoea, increased appetite accompanied by weight loss, and seizures*. Admission to a neonatal unit for monitoring and treatment is required. Withdrawal symptoms may begin 12 hours after delivery but can be delayed until the second week of life or sometimes even later.

Treatment

Antenatal treatment with methadone may result in stabilization of substance misuse, decreased injecting and increased uptake of health services by heroin-using pregnant women. However, methadone is associated with longer withdrawal, lower birthweights and smaller head circumference in the newborn infant.

Clinical presentation

In the long term, affected infants grow poorly in the neonatal period and during the first 3 years. Head growth can be slower but catch-up head growth may also occur. Earlier studies demonstrated no evidence of long-term neurodevelopmental problems but now there is evidence to show that maternal opiate use adversely affects the fetal brain as it causes neurochemical changes that subsequently give rise to behavioural deficits. Affected infants have:

- Lower cognitive scores at 18 months than typically developing infants. This difference persists at 3 years of age with reduced motor performance scores and social maturity.
- Visual defects such as strabismus, nystagmus, refractive errors and delayed visual maturation. Nystagmus is particularly common in those treated for neonatal abstinence syndrome (NAS).

Confounding factors such as polydrug use, ongoing social deprivation and child abuse make it difficult to separate out the effects of each of these factors.

Other drugs such as cocaine and benzodiazepines are misused and can affect the developing fetus. Maternal cocaine use does not lead to withdrawal in the newborn period but it can affect the developing brain through its ability to constrict blood vessels.

Alcohol

Alcohol is now recognized as the most common non-genetic cause of learning difficulty and the leading preventable cause of congenital birth defects in the USA.

Fetal alcohol spectrum disorder (FASD) is the umbrella term for the set of disorders caused by exposure of the fetal brain to the teratogenic effects of alcohol. The spectrum includes the following subgroups (see also Fig. 23.2):

- fetal alcohol syndrome (FAS), confirmed exposure
- FAS, exposure not confirmed
- partial FAS – not all features present but some facial and CNS defects are present
- alcohol-related birth defects (ARBDs) – structural abnormalities (e.g. cardiac, ocular) or behavioural features are pronounced
- alcohol-related neurodevelopmental disorder (ARND) – prominent neurocognitive features.

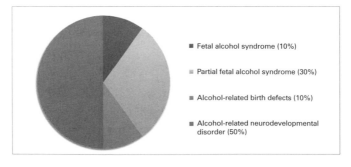

Figure 23.2 Fetal alcohol-related subtypes.

Prevalence

- FAS: 1 to 4.8 per 1000 live births.
- FASD: worldwide prevalence of 0.97 per 1000 live births.
- There are higher rates of FASD in lower socioeconomic groups and amongst certain ethnic groups.

Alcohol is a known teratogen. The first and third trimesters in pregnancy are thought to be the most vulnerable periods when drinking is thought to cause the greatest harm. Alcohol affects the growth and development of the cerebellum, hippocampus and prefrontal cortex areas of the brain. Higher alcohol intakes are linked to a higher risk of fetal alcohol syndrome. Lower rates of drinking are more likely to be linked to a diagnosis of partial FAS, ARND or ARBD.

The threshold for damage is not defined because of the varying susceptibility of women genetically and nutritionally, but there may be synergistic reactions with other drugs being taken. Binge drinking is thought to be more harmful than chronic drinking, but even low levels of drinking are now thought to be harmful.

The Royal College of Obstetricians' advice to pregnant women was altered in 2007 to advise that alcohol should be avoided during pregnancy. Twenty per cent of women acknowledge that they drink during pregnancy and 1% continue to drink heavily.

Consumption of alcohol during pregnancy is often concealed because of social stigma. Some women of childbearing age may binge drink unaware that they are pregnant, particularly during the first trimester of an unplanned pregnancy. The UK has the highest rates of teenage and unplanned pregnancies in Europe.

Drinking levels

Low to moderate	Fewer than one drink a day (1.5 units)
Heavy drinking	More than six units per day for women or more than eight units per day for men

Diagnosis of FASD

DIAGNOSTIC CRITERIA FOR FETAL ALCOHOL SYNDROME (INSTITUTE OF MEDICINE, USA)

- Maternal alcohol history.
- Facial anomalies (Fig. 23.3).
- Growth retardation: pre- and postnatal growth restriction.
- Showing one example of CNS abnormalities, such as small brain size; structural abnormalities (e.g. small cerebellum, agenesis of corpus callosum); neurological signs (e.g. poor gait, poor hand–eye skills).

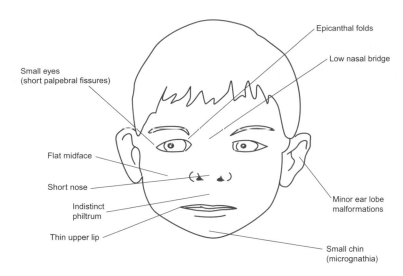

Figure 23.3 Fetal alcohol syndrome facial features.

CANADIAN GUIDELINES FOR THE DIAGNOSIS OF FETAL ALCOHOL SYNDROME

All criteria must be satisfied for FAS to be diagnosed.

- CNS: one structural or three domains of significant impairment.
- Growth: less than the 10th centile for height and weight.
- All three facial features: palpebral fissure length <10th centile on available chart; lips 4 or 5 (visual scoring system, fullest=1, thinnest=5); philtrum 4 or 5 (visual scoring system: deepest=1, smoothest=5).

Behaviour

Adverse behavioural aspects have been recognized in children exposed to low and moderate as well as risky levels of alcohol. These include

- *Preschool child* – decreased reaction time, inattention and hyperactivity.
- *School-aged child* – learning problems such as visual spatial problems, concrete thinking, attentional difficulties, impulsivity, memory problems, difficulties making and keeping friendships and mental health problems such as mood disorders.
- *Adult* – attentional problems, executive functioning difficulties (i.e. problem-solving, planning and mental organization), antisocial behaviour, high rates of drug and alcohol and nicotine dependence.

Management

Management is aimed at reducing the effects of the impairments (e.g. cardiac, ocular or neurodevelopmental/behavioural difficulties) affecting the child. Most will require additional educational support, particularly if the cause of their needs is diagnosed. Families, too, will require additional social support, recognizing the burden imposed on them by caring for an affected child. These will be long-term needs and many affected adults will struggle to find employment, maintain relationships, avoid alcohol/drug dependency and manage their mental health needs.

Fetal anticonvulsant syndrome

Between 6% and 9% of children exposed to antiepileptic drugs in utero are born with congenital malformations. Further proportions have learning difficulties or behaviour problems. As epilepsy affects about 5 out of every 1000 mothers, a large number of children are potentially affected. Particular drugs are associated with certain patterns of abnormalities, including

- neural tube defects with sodium valproate and carbamazepine
- fingernail hypoplasia with carbamazepine and phenytoin
- congenital heart disease with all three drugs.

Each syndrome is associated with its own characteristic facial appearance.

Table 23.1 Assessment for fetal anticonvulsant syndrome

Clinical problem area	Typical features
Neonatal withdrawal	Jittery, seizures, apnoea, hypoglycaemia, feeding problems
Facial appearance	Epicanthic folds, infra-orbital groove, convergent strabismus, broad or flat nasal bridge, anteverted nares, broad or flat nasal tip, shallow philtrum, thin upper lip, broad or tall forehead, low-set ears
Congenital malformations	Cardiac, genital, neural tube defect, cleft palate, talipes, other limb anomalies, congenital dislocation of hip, hernia, craniosynostosis, upper airway malformation
Childhood medical problems	Myopia, strabismus, otitis media with effusion, joint laxity
Neurodevelopment	Communication difficulties with speech and language delay, gross motor delay sometimes and/or fine motor delay
Behaviour	Attention-deficit–hyperactivity disorder, autism, Asperger syndrome, behaviour problems associated with attention deficit or communication

In 2009 draft diagnostic criteria were proposed for the diagnosis of fetal anticonvulsant syndrome (Table 23.1), as there is no reliable diagnostic test as yet. Clinical signs in different body systems are assessed and a scoring system has been developed based on major and minor features. The following six clinical areas should be considered when a potentially affected child is seen:

- History of neonatal withdrawal syndrome.
- Observations of the facial appearance.
- Occurrence of particular medical problems.
- A pattern of developmental delay, especially in speech and language.
- Pattern of behaviour ranging from poor social skills to autism at the extreme end.
- Other causes of congenital abnormalities, medical, learning or behavioural problems should be excluded first.

Diagnosis requires four positives, i.e. one positive finding in each category.

Diagnostic criteria

- History of exposure to an antiepileptic drug in utero.
- Characteristic facial appearance.
- The presence of at least one of the following:
  - neonatal withdrawal
  - compatible malformation
  - compatible childhood medical problem
  - compatible developmental delay
  - compatible behavioural problem.
- Normal relevant investigations for an alternative cause, e.g. karyotype; fragile X mutation studies and catch-22 deletion.

The risk of developing fetal anticonvulsant syndrome, including poor cognitive outcome, may be greater for sodium valproate than for other anticonvulsants, particularly when it is used at a moderate (>1g/day) or high dose during pregnancy. The child's IQ is negatively correlated with in utero exposure to anticonvulsant drugs, and polytherapy exposure during the last trimester may be the most harmful. Monotherapy carries less risk to the fetus than polytherapy. The anticonvulsant drug of choice for a particular woman should be used at the lowest effective dose for maintaining seizure control during pregnancy.

References

Aicardi J (2009) *Disease of the Nervous System*, 3rd edition. London: Mac Keith Press.

Further reading

Dean JCS, Moore SJ, Turnpenny PD (2000) Developing diagnostic criteria for the fetal anticonvulsant syndromes. *Seizure* 9: 233–4. http://dx.doi.org/10.1053/seiz.2000.0392

Dudgeon JA (1967) Maternal rubella and its effect on the foetus. *Arch Dis Child* 42: 110. http://dx.doi.org/10.1136/adc.42.222.110

Elliott EJ, Payne JM, Morris A, Haan E, Bower CA (2008) Fetal alcohol syndrome: a prospective national surveillance study. *Arch Dis Child* 93: 732–7. http://dx.doi.org/10.1136/adc.2007.120220

Kini U, Adab N, Vinten J, Fryer A, Clayton-Smith J, on behalf of the Liverpool and Manchester Neurodevelopmental Study Group (2006) Dysmorphic features: an important clue to the diagnosis and severity of fetal anticonvulsant syndromes. *Arch Dis Child Fetal Neonatal Ed* 91: F90–5. http://dx.doi. org/10.1136/adc.2004.067421

Koren G, Nulman I, Chudley AE, Loocke C (2003) Fetal alcohol spectrum disorder. *Can Med Assoc J* 169: 1181–5.

Mactier H (2011) The management of heroin misuse in pregnancy: time for a rethink? *Arch Dis Child Fetal Neonatal Ed* 96: F457–60. http://dx.doi.org/10.1136/adc.2009.181057

Manning MA, Hoyme HE (2007) Fetal alcohol spectrum disorders: a practical clinical approach to diagnosis. *Neurosci Biobehav Rev* 31: 230–8.

Preece PM, Riley EP (2011) *Alcohol, Drugs and Medication in Pregnancy*. London: Mac Keith Press.

The Scottish Government (2006) Substance Misuse Research: Neonatal Abstinence Syndrome: A New Intervention: A Community Based, Structured Health Visitor Assessment. Available at: www.scotland. gov.uk/Publications/2006/09/04102243/8 (accessed 8 November 2012).

Sharland M, Gibb DM, Tudor-Williams G (2002) Advances in the prevention and treatment of paediatric HIV infection in the United Kingdom. *Arch Dis Child* 87: 178–80. http://dx.doi.org/10.1136/adc.87.3.178

Townsend CL, Peckham CS, Tookey PA (2011) Surveillance of congenital cytomegalovirus in the UK and Ireland. *Arch Dis Child Fetal Neonatal Ed* 96: F398–403. http://dx.doi.org/10.1136/adc.2010.199901

Ward KN, Ohrling A, Bryant NJ, Bowley JS, Ross EM, Verity CM (2011) Herpes simplex serious neurological disease in young children: incidence and long-term outcome. *Arch Dis Child* 97: 162–5. http://dx.doi. org/10.1136/adc.2010.204677

24
Abuse resulting in disability

David Cundall and Gillian Robinson

Learning objectives

- To understand the possible presentation of child abuse – physical, neglect, emotional or sexual abuse.
- To understand the potential outcomes of child abuse.
- To know the warning signs and differential diagnoses.

Background

Child abuse in any form can result in short- and long-term damage to children's physical and psychosocial development. It remains an important cause of a range of disabilities and should always be considered when thinking about causation.

Shaking injuries or inflicted traumatic brain injury or non-accidental head injury

Shaking injuries occur in approximately 1 in 10 000 children under the age of 1 year. Unexplained fractures or bruises in infants, retinal haemorrhages and subdural haemorrhages raise concern regarding possible associated shaking injury. Shaking injuries can cause profound neurological damage, with up to one-quarter of children dying at the time of presentation. Of those who survive, around two-thirds of children will have difficulties, of whom one-third will have severe difficulties and be totally dependent. More severe problems are related to a greater degree of injury at presentation.

Infants present in a variety of ways, some with a profoundly decreased consciousness level. Subsequent MRI findings, in particular degree of cerebral oedema and changes in the basal ganglia, predict outcome.

Problems include

- motor deficits (60%)
- visual deficits (25–50%)
- epilepsy (20%)
- speech and language abnormalities (60%)
- behavioural problems (50%)
- sleep problems (25%)
- cognitive abilities with a mean IQ of 70 (60–70%).

Be aware that methylmalonic acidaemia and glutaric aciduria can present with chronic subdural effusions and developmental difficulties and can be confused with shaking injuries.

Neglect

Neglect is defined as the persistent failure to meet a child's basic physical and/or psychological needs likely to result in the serious impairment of the child's health or development. The earlier the insult, the higher the likelihood of long-term damage.

There are many reasons why some parents are neglectful (Table 24.1), including

- alcohol and drug usage with episodes of intoxication
- parental learning difficulties
- parental mental illness
- parent not being parented adequately themselves as a child.

Table 24.1 Causes, presentations and effects of neglectful parenting

Form of abuse	Presentation	Consequence
Maternal substance misuse	Fetal alcohol spectrum disorder Effects of cocaine	Developmental and behavioural difficulties
Inadequate supervision	Attachment difficulties Avoidable injury	Emotional abuse Physical disability
Inadequate access to medical care	Acute Chronic	Delay in presentation of serious illness Ongoing untreated illness, e.g. deafness secondary to secretory otitis media
Failing to meet a child's emotional needs	Attachment disorders	Confused and angry child Attention problems Conduct disorder Adult mental health problems
Failing to support a child's development	Not playing or reading to child	Delayed development and/or attachment difficulties

Emotional abuse

The impact of emotional abuse on early life and brain development is extremely damaging. By the time of birth the essential structures of the brain are obviously present, but there continues to be massive growth and organization during the early years of life. The result of this process is the sequential learning of new skills. This progression is affected by both genetic and environmental factors. Neurones and neuronal connections change in an activity-dependent fashion. Therefore, the more certain areas of the brain are used, the greater the connectivity in that area – 'What fires together, wires together'. Early experiences enable an infant's brain to develop an internal representation of the external world. These connections provide the basis for memory and learning.

Adverse life experiences during this early period lead to raised cortisol levels, which can lead to adaptive fear-related brain activation. This leads children to be hypervigilant, watching for clues of threat, and to have increased muscle tone, anxiety and impulsivity. These behaviours are helpful at times of threat, but when constantly present they significantly impede development and can lead to children who are perpetually insecure. This maladaptive process can occur in children who have undergone significant and persistent emotional abuse, particularly from their primary caregiver. The long-term effects on the 'wiring' of the brain have been demonstrated on MRI, which shows the volume of the corpus callosum to be decreased.

The brain continues to have the ability to change its underlying pathways throughout childhood. If these children are identified early and cared for in a stable, predictable and nurturing environment, most of these changes can be ameliorated with time, although this may be many years. The very act of intervening, however, can contribute to the child's catalogue of fearful situations. The investigation, removal, placement, relocation, court proceedings and reunification may all contribute to the unknown, uncontrollable and, often, frightening experiences of the abused child. Having good systems, with few moves and carers who understand these children's emotional needs, can decrease this distress. These key elements are frequently missing in the poorly coordinated, overburdened and reactive systems mandated to help these children.

The effects of early deprivation on long-term psychosocial and physical outcomes have been studied in a longitudinal study of children adopted into the UK from Romania in the early 1990s (Rutter et al. 2009). The vast majority of the 165 adoptees studied experienced extreme early global deprivation up to 3 years and 6 months of age as a consequence of early placement in Romanian institutions. The findings from the assessments at 4, 6 and 11 years were striking in showing that there was a dramatic degree of cognitive and physical catch-up to norms in the institution-reared group, but that significant deficits remained in a substantial minority of individuals who had experienced institutionalization to beyond the age of 6 months. The follow-ups at 15 years of age, and into young adulthood, have revealed unusual, persisting, specific patterns of deficits that include difficulties with social attachment, attention and learning. Thus, in some individuals there seems to be irreversible consequences of severe deprivation starting early and lasting beyond 6 months of age.

Sexual abuse

Around three-quarters of children subject to child sexual abuse have mental health problems that persist into adulthood. Difficulties include post-traumatic stress disorder, major depressive episode, panic disorder, agoraphobia, substance abuse, borderline personality disorder, bulimia and suicidal ideation. These difficulties are seen more in families from lower socioeconomic backgrounds who use alcohol and drugs or have experienced domestic violence and in those for whom sexual abuse started at a younger age and involved multiple perpetrators.

> ## Key messages
>
> - Child abuse presents in various ways.
> - It is not confined to any one social class.
> - It has marked effects on the developing nervous system whether the abuse is physical or from neglectful or emotionally abusive parenting.
> - Be aware of a few rare neurometabolic conditions that can present in a way that mimics non-accidental head injury.

Reference

Rutter M, Beckett C, Castle J, Kreppner J, Stevens S, Sonuga-Burke E (2009) Policy and Practice Implications from the English and Romanian Adoptees (ERA) Study: Forty Five Key Questions. London: BAAF. Available at: www.nuffieldfoundation.org/english-and-romanian-adoptee-study (accessed 30 November 2012).

Further reading

Jayawant S, Parr J (2007) Outcome following subdural haemorrhages in infancy. *Arch Dis Child* 92: 343–7. http://dx.doi.org/10.1136/adc.2005.084988

Minns R, Brown K (2006) *Shaking and Other Non-accidental Injuries in Children*. London: Mac Keith Press.

Section 10

Specific conditions and disorders

25
Cerebral palsy

Jane Williams and Anne M Kelly

Key messages

- Many children in the early years of life have various motor patterns that may need review.
- Motor signs may resolve or alter with time. Do not rush into making a diagnosis.
- The major risk factors for developing cerebral palsy (CP) are antenatal: 'born too early, born too small'.
- The mainstay of assessment and treatment is paediatric physiotherapy. No child is too young to be referred for an opinion if you are concerned, or if there is a major risk factor.
- All children with CP should undergo neuroimaging of their brain, ideally brain magnetic resonance imaging (MRI) to gather evidence to support the clinical picture. In approximately 16% of children with CP findings on MRI are normal.
- There are several pharmacological and surgical interventions that offer new avenues of adjuvant treatment. The merits of such approaches should be discussed on an individual basis.

Background

In general 1 to 2 out of 1000 live born children are diagnosed with cerebral palsy (CP) by the age of 3 to 5 years. Approximately half of the affected children are born at term and the other half are born preterm. Among those children born before 32 weeks' gestation or with birthweights below 1500 grams, the prevalence of CP rises to 80 to 100 per 1000 live births. Postneonatal causes account for approximately 5% of children with CP.

Definition of cerebral palsy

Cerebral palsy describes a group of permanent disorders of movement and posture causing limitation of activities and which are attributable to a non-progressive disturbance that occurred in the development of the brain. The motor disturbances are often accompanied by disturbances of vision, sensation, perception, cognition, communication and behaviour, epilepsy and secondary musculoskeletal problems (Rosenbaum et al. 2007).

Risk factors

- Birth under 32 weeks' gestational age or birthweight below 1500 grams.
- Neonatal seizures, encephalopathy, hyperbilirubinaemia or hypoglycaemia.
- Suspected or proven abnormalities on early neuroimaging, usually neonatal brain ultrasonography but also brain MRI (periventricular leukomalacia, infarction, thalamic lesions).

Case vignette 1

Billy was born at 31 weeks' gestation and had no major neonatal problems apart from some minor initial feeding difficulties. At 10 months of age he was not sitting, but the clinician reassured his mother. At the age of 1 year his mother thought his legs were stiff.

On examination, Billy had a strabismus, bilateral hypertonia (stiffness) in his arms and legs with markedly increased adductor tone in his lower limbs, hyperreflexia and bilateral ankle clonus.

His brain MRI showed periventricular leukomalacia. The diagnosis was bilateral cerebral palsy.

Learning points:

- Failure to sit independently at 10 months was a concerning sign as this is the upper age limit for achieving this milestone.
- All children with an abnormality of tone and posture warrant neuroimaging.

Presentations

- A concerning neonatal history leading to the child's development being monitored.
- Reduced spontaneous motor behaviour, including sucking and feeding difficulties.
- An unsettled infant, often with feeding difficulties.
- Abnormal muscle tone (e.g. initial hypotonia), later hypertonia with increased extensor tone in the trunk and neck, scissoring, or fisting (thumb in palm).
- Early hand preference or limb neglect.
- Delayed motor milestones; however, this factor alone is not specific to CP.
- Bottom shuffling and delay in crawling and symmetrical walking.

Clinical signs

- Pathologically brisk deep tendon reflexes together with other upper motor neurone signs and increased tone.
- Persistent primitive reflexes and clonus.

In the first months of life it is rare to find any hypertonicity or stiffness in a child even if you suspect the infant has reason to develop motor difficulties and CP. This also applies to unilateral CP, even when there is a demonstrable cause such as a porencephalic cyst. An infant may not show any features at all until after 3 to 6 months, when it may be noted that the affected arm and hand is not being moved or used as much as the other side, and there is a tendency to hold the hand pronated and fisted with the thumb adducted across the palm.

Clinical approach

Case vignette 2

An 8-month-old infant, born at 26 weeks' gestation weighing 850 grams with known intra-ventricular haemorrhage and feeding difficulties, presented with persistent head lag and not yet rolling (motor delay). By 1 year of age it was clear the infant had bilateral increased tone and disordered posture with brisk bilateral deep tendon reflexes.

Learning points:

- This was a high-risk infant who should be reviewed regularly.
- Although the diagnosis may appear obvious neuroimaging is still required to provide information about aetiology.

Histories taking into account the above situation: key points

- A detailed history is required with attention to pre-, peri- and postnatal events.
- A developmental history is also necessary.
- Family history (there are genetic forms of CP) should be examined.
- Enquire about feeding and weight gain.
- Enquire about bowel movements (constipation is frequent in CP).
- Enquire about sensory behaviour: seeing and hearing.
- Enquire about sleep: quality and length and general behaviour (e.g. irritability, easy to settle).

Examination

- Measure and plot the weight, height and head circumference of the infant on the appropriate centile chart.
- While taking the history, observe the infant's spontaneous motor and visual behaviour.
- Watch while the child is undressed and see whether this is easy or difficult.
- Perform a complete system examination.
- Perform a neurological examination including
  - cranial nerves;
  - examination of tone (resistance to passive movement) and posture in supine, prone, pull to sit, supported sitting and standing;
  - observe and examine the quality of spontaneous movements;
  - elicit deep tendon reflexes;
  - motor reactions: look for persistence of primitive reflexes (e.g. asymmetrical tonic neck reflex) and emerging protective or saving reflexes (see Chapter 4).
- Examine the child's hips for stability and the spine for straightness.
- Perform a developmental examination: offer objects that are suitable for the developmental age and observe visual interest, reaching and grasping. Listen for vocalization.
- Use the information gained from these assessments to help decide the classification of cerebral palsy.

Classification of cerebral palsy

In order to standardize the way that the findings in CP are described, the Study of Cerebral Palsy in Europe (SCPE) has devised a classification strategy that is shown below (see also Figs 25.1 and 25.2):

- motor abnormalities
  - tone
  - spasticity, dystonia, ataxia
- anatomical and radiological findings
  - parts of body affected
  - scan findings

- associated impairments
- causation and timing.

Clinicians should try to follow the suggested schema to ensure that the necessary findings are recorded.

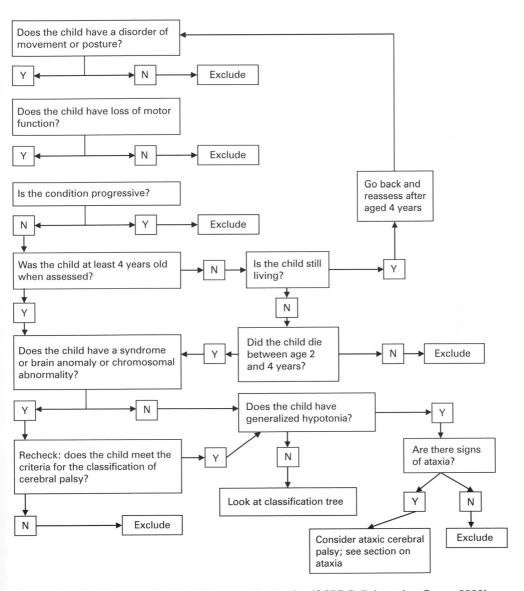

Figure 25.1 Decision tree for identifying cerebral palsy (SCPE Collaboration Group 2000).

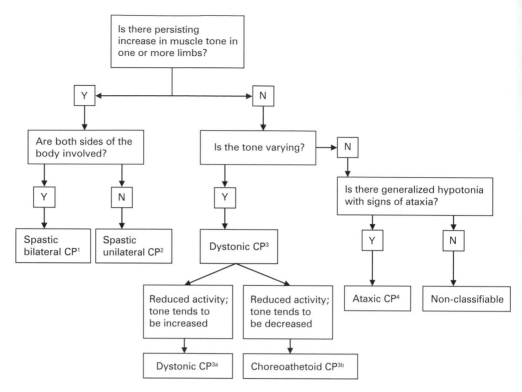

Figure 25.2 Decision tree for deciding subtypes of cerebral palsy (SCPE Collaboration Group 2000).

Abnormal muscle tone

The type of abnormality is almost entirely dependent on the site of the lesion. However, neuroimaging findings are not totally predictive of the type and severity of the motor disorder.

- *Spasticity* is defined as the velocity-dependent increase in the tonic stretch reflex causing hypertonia and brisk reflexes on clinical examination. There is coexistent weakness which is more difficult to treat than spasticity.
  - If limbs on both sides of the body are involved, this is referred to as bilateral spastic CP.
  - If the limbs on one side of the body only are affected, it is called unilateral spastic CP.
- *Dyskinetic CP* is characterized by abnormal posture with involuntary, uncontrolled recurring and occasionally stereotyped movements.

This can be either

- *Dystonic*, in which there is hypokinesia (reduced activity) with stiff movements and hypertonia due to sustained muscle contraction. It occurs secondary to basal ganglia damage.
- *Choreoathetosis*, in which there is increased 'stormy' muscle activity but reduced tone. This is also associated with basal ganglia damage.
- *Ataxic CP*, which leads to reduced tone but, more significantly, there is a loss of orderly muscle coordination that leads to movements that are performed with abnormal force, rhythm and accuracy. It is associated with cerebellar impairment. It is rare, and may be familial, but other neurometabolic disorders must be excluded.

After deciding that CP is the correct term, consider the type according to the abnormality of muscle tone (as above) and whether it is bilateral or unilateral. Then grade the functional severity using the Gross Motor Function Classification System (GMFCS), with GMFCS level I being the least severely affected and GMFCS level V being the most severe (see Table 25.1 and Fig. 25.3).

Table 25.1 GMFCS levels (before 2nd birthday)

Level I	Infants move in and out of sitting, floor sit with both hands free to manipulate objects Infants crawl on hands and knees, pull to stand and take steps cruising (holding on to furniture) Infants walk between 18m and 2y of age without the need for any assistive mobility device
Level II	Infants maintain floor sitting but may need to use their hands for support to maintain balance. Infants creep on their stomach or crawl on hands and knees Infants may pull to stand and take steps holding on to furniture
Level III	Infants maintain floor sitting when the low back is supported Infants roll and creep forward on their stomachs
Level IV	Infants have head control but trunk support is required for floor sitting Infants can roll to supine and may roll to prone
Level V	Physical impairments limit voluntary control of movement Infants are unable to maintain antigravity head and trunk postures in prone and sitting Infants require adult assistance to roll

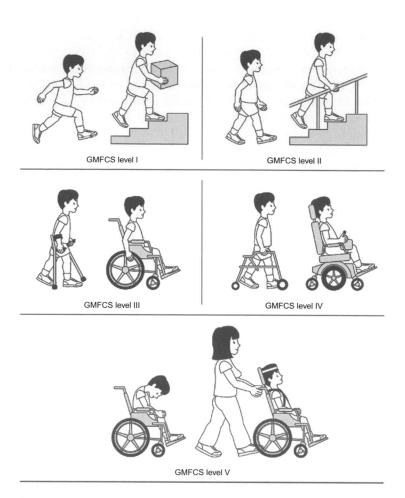

GMFCS level I

GMFCS level II

GMFCS level III

GMFCS level IV

GMFCS level V

Figure 25.3 The Gross Motor Function Classification System (GMFCS) for children aged 6 to 12 years. GMFCS level I: Children walk indoors and outdoors and climb stairs without limitation. Children perform gross motor skills including running and jumping, but speed, balance and coordination are impaired. GMFCS level II: Children walk indoors and outdoors and climb stairs holding onto a railing, but experience limitations walking on uneven surfaces and inclines and walking in crowds or confined spaces. Children have, at best, only a minimal ability to perform gross motor skills such as running and jumping. GMFCS level III: Children walk indoors or outdoors on a level surface with an assistive mobility device. Children may climb stairs holding onto a railing. Children may propel a wheelchair manually or are transported when travelling for long distances or outdoors on uneven terrain. GMFCS level IV: Children may continue to walk for short distances on a walker or rely more on wheeled mobility at home and school and in the community. Children may achieve self-mobility using a power wheelchair. GMFCS level V: Physical impairments restrict voluntary control of movement and the ability to maintain antigravity head and trunk postures. All areas of motor function are limited. Children have no means of independent mobility and are transported (see Palisano et al. 1997). Illustrations copyright Kerr Graham, Bill Reid and Adrienne Harvey, The Royal Children's Hospital, Melbourne.

You will be able to use the GMFCS to gain an impression of the severity of CP by the second year of life. Re-evaluate the score each time you see the child. There are different GMFCS descriptors for different age groups (see http://motorgrowth.canchild.ca/en/GMFCS/resources/GMFCS_English.pdf). You should discuss your estimated GMFCS level with the child's parents or carers and with your colleagues. The GMFCS score after the first year of life can be used to guide predictions for longer-term motor developmental outcomes for the child. Children will usually progress so that they operate at either the same level or one level above or below their early level.

In addition, there are other classification scales that can be helpful: in relation to the degree of communication difficulty there is the Communication Function Classification System (Table 25.2; see www.faculty.uca.edu/mjchidecker/CFCS/CFCS-hcr.html) and to classify the ability of a child or young person (4–16y) to use their hands to handle objects there is the Manual Ability Classification System (MACS; Table 25.3; see also www.MACS.nu), which can be particularly helpful for children with unilateral CP (hemiplegia).

Table 25.2 Communication Function Classification System for individuals with cerebral palsy

Level I	Effective Sender and Receiver with unfamiliar and familiar partners
Level II	Effective but slower-paced Sender and/or Receiver with unfamiliar and/or familiar partners
Level III	Effective Sender and Receiver with familiar partners
Level IV	Inconsistent Sender and/or Receiver with familiar partners
Level V	Seldom effective Sender and Receiver even with familiar partners

Table 25.3 Manual Ability Classification System for children with cerebral palsy

Level I	Handles objects easily and successfully
Level II	Handles most objects but with somewhat reduced quality and/or speed of achievement
Level III	Handles objects with difficulty; needs help to prepare and/or modify activities
Level IV	Handles a limited selection of easily managed objects in adapted situations
Level V	Does not handle objects and has severely limited ability to perform even simple actions

Neuroimaging

Approximately 16% of children with CP have normal findings on MRI. See Table 25.4 for MRI findings in CP.

Table 25.4 Magnetic resonance imaging findings in cerebral palsy[a]

Type of CP	MRI abnormality (%)	Finding
Bilateral spastic	90%	60% periventricular leukomalacia (90% if preterm) 15% cortical or subcortical/basal ganglia/thalamus lesions (4% if preterm) 10% malformations (1.5% if preterm) 3% unclassified
Unilateral spastic	90%	35% periventricular leukomalacia (85% if preterm) 30% infarction 20% malformations 5% unclassified
Dyskinetic	60–70%	50% basal ganglia/thalamus lesions 15% periventricular leukomalacia Rare: basal ganglia lesions ('kernicterus')
Ataxic	40–50%	Cerebellar hypoplasia (not correlated with clinical severity)

[a]MRI findings in different types of cerebral palsy (Krageloh-Mann and Horber 2007). MRI, magnetic resonance imaging.

If no aetiological contributory factors can be identified either in the antenatal, perinatal or postnatal history or from the brain MRI then one should always consider an alternative diagnosis and consider a paediatric neurology opinion. Alternative important diagnoses such as dopa-responsive dystonia, which is treatable, or hereditary spastic paraparesis are important to consider, especially if there is a positive family history.

Paediatric neuroradiologists vary in their recommendations as to when to perform brain MRI. Some centres with well-established neonatal imaging expertise perform an early MRI, but most paediatric neuroradiologists feel that a further scan (or first MRI) by 24 months will be more helpful, as sufficient myelination of white matter will have occurred by that point. It is more likely that changes seen on MRI at this age will be long-lasting and may provide an answer as to the aetiology of the child's difficulties.

Additional testing may be needed if the clinical picture appears to be like CP, but there are other features in the history such as

- late presentation given the degree of spasticity
- other organ system involvement (e.g. liver disease)
- a family history of CP or infant death
- progression of stiffness or loss of skills or
- episodes of deterioration/illness with associated loss of skills.

Always be vigilant for other non-obstetric causes of neonatal encephalopathy (e.g. spinal muscular atrophy type 1) and remember that there can be other causes even in children born preterm; do not always presume that the latter has led to the encephalopathy.

> **Key messages**
>
> - Brain MRI is abnormal in 80% to 85% of children with CP.
> - History, clinical examination and investigations usually identify aetiology.
> - Metabolic and genetic testing are rarely helpful but should be performed in children in whom there are any warning features such as progression or loss of skills or family history.

Unilateral cerebral palsy: congenital hemiplegia

Children with congenital hemiplegia usually present with an early hand preference on the non-affected side or fixed hand posture (fist) on the affected side. This finding should prompt a detailed examination, looking for asymmetrical posturing, increased tone and hyperreflexia. Often there is no history of prenatal or perinatal adversity. Neuroimaging is essential and commonly reveals a middle cerebral artery infarct, cortical dysplasia and focal periventricular tissue loss. In 20% of cases, the brain MRI may be normal.

The child with a hemiplegia will almost always learn to walk, but the school-age child and young person is at risk of experiencing added difficulties that include problems with attention, perception, behaviour and sensory issues. These difficulties may not be apparent until the child starts school. They should be discussed with the family, in a supportive and reassuring way, in order that support and management can be proactive rather than reactive. Epilepsy can occur in children with hemiplegia, in around 30% of cases, and families should be advised about the possibility that their child may develop seizures, particularly if brain MRI shows a definite unilateral lesion. The organization HemiHelp is a valuable resource with regards to information and advice for this group of children and families (see www.hemihelp.org.uk).

In order to classify the degree of severity of upper limb function, refer to the Manual Ability Classification Scales in Fig. 25.2.

Management of cerebral palsy: general principles

A multidisciplinary team of paediatrician and therapists work in partnership with parents to provide care for children with CP. They, ideally, should meet with parents at regular intervals to report progress and plan interventions collaboratively and proactively. Understanding parents', carers' and the child's concerns and priorities at that time is crucial to ensuring good-quality care. This approach is known as 'Team around the child'. Agreeing shared aims should optimize function, improve quality of life and encourage the child's participation in society.

There are two mainstays of treatment:

Management of the motor and movement disorder

- Physiotherapy and occupational therapy
  - Orthotics
  - Postural care

- Adjuvant therapy
  - Oral muscle relaxants
  - Intrathecal baclofen pump
  - Selective dorsal rhizotomy
  - Deep brain stimulation
  - Oral antidystonia drugs.

Management of the comorbidities, both medical and developmental

- Epilepsy, vision and hearing difficulties
- Communication
- Feeding and gastro-oesophageal reflux (GOR)
- Constipation
- Respiratory
- Bladder
- Dental
- Drooling
- Orthopaedic.

Motor disorder

Motor function and signs can change markedly in the first few years of life. Some children with milder CP will not be diagnosed until the age of 3 years or older. In one study of at-risk infants, 50% of those suspected to have CP at 12 months of age did not have it when reviewed at the age of 7 years, but there was an increased prevalence of other problems such as learning disability, behaviour difficulties and epilepsy in this group.

The management of the motor problems lies predominantly with physiotherapy and paediatric occupational therapy. In partnership with paediatric physiotherapy, paediatric occupational therapists have a major role in assessing and assisting the needs of a child with CP. The paediatric occupational therapist, in particular, will advise in relation to seating, feeding and positioning and will recommend practical solutions to difficulties with fine motor control (e.g. handwriting and activities of daily living). Often the therapists will work together and undertake joint assessments.

There are several different 'schools' of physiotherapy that advocate different methods (e.g. Bobath, and Peto/Conductive Education). None of these has been proved to be superior to the others.

The Bobath method:

- follows the neurodevelopmental sequence of physical development
- aims to inhibit abnormal movements
- uses handling, positioning and guiding movements to improve the quality of tone and movement
- recognizes the potential for enhanced function (i.e. neuroplasticity of the central nervous system).

Peto/Conductive Education

- was developed with the aim to help children walk
- must be started before 5 years of age
- requires good vision and understanding
- requires the child to be able enough to attend school and comprehend the conductor's instructions
- aims to integrate cognitive, emotional, social and sensorimotor development.

In the Peto/Conductive method, motion is performed in whatever way the child can, whereas the Bobath method emphasizes quality of movement. No single approach has been proved to be superior to the others. Most UK paediatric physiotherapists will use an individually tailored programme combining some elements of these approaches. Parents may choose to supplement this with alternative approaches or with more intensive programmes of standard physiotherapy. The focus of current treatment is on strengthening and stretching muscles, but looking at function and having a goal-orientated approach is essential.

Orthotics

Orthotics are splints made of rigid plastic or flexible Lycra or neoprene that are used to improve the child's posture in sitting, standing and lying and during activities such as walking and toileting. The most common are ankle–foot orthoses (AFO), which are used to keep ankle joints in positions that are otherwise not possible owing to spasticity or weakness. The orthoses are individually tailored to the child's foot and are made of rigid plastic with Velcro straps to secure them in place. Piedro boots provide ankle support and, with the help of AFO, aim to keep the foot in a neutral position. Some children may not tolerate wearing their AFO throughout the day. The evidence supports use of orthoses for over 4 hours to maintain joint movement, but there is not currently much evidence for other splinting and support.

Positioning and prevention of deformity: postural support

The therapist will assess the child to establish their level of physical ability. The objectives will be to understand the child's difficulties in order to prevent deformity, reduce the influence of primitive reflexes such as asymmetrical tonic neck reflex (ATNR), and improve independence. Motor ability has obvious effects on other areas of development including communication, feeding, fine motor skills and play. Understanding the child's difficulties helps to explain their fear and lack of willingness to alter their position. Some may feel insecure and frightened of falling unless handled and or supported correctly. The typically developing child can keep his/her body balanced without conscious effort, but this is not the case for many children with CP.

Children with CP do not move as well as typically developing children and they may adopt preferred postures. Excess activity in certain muscle groups exacerbates this. The preferred positions are often asymmetrical, as the result of primitive reflexes such as ATNR, and may not facilitate function (e.g. rolling is difficult or impossible because of the extended arm). This can be addressed with advice on positioning, supports and splints. If these poor postures are left unchallenged, they may progress to become fixed deformities, in which non-bony structures (e.g. tendons and muscles) become shortened or lengthened. This may progress to become structural, whereby bony changes occur.

The typical asymmetrical complex of deformities includes

- preferred head turning
- preferred hand use
- scoliosis
- windswept hips with the risk of the adducted hip dislocating (abductors of the other hip may become shortened, causing difficulty with positioning in lying, sitting and standing)
- ankle–foot deformities.

Correct positioning is fundamental to enable functional activity as well as making the child feel comfortable and enable ease of handling. It is also important to prevent deformity that will naturally occur if no intervention is offered. This can be encouraged by

- attention to postural care (see below)
- teaching parents to perform passive movements
- attempting to improve those abilities that are lacking.

Postural care is now the focus of therapy for the child with severe motor disability with the aim of protecting body shape, function and comfort long term. It involves providing gentle but adequate support to enable the individual to maintain a variety of comfortable symmetrical positions whilst they enjoy everyday activities. This support should be provided over 24 hours and will therefore include a sleep system. In the young child, a rolled-up towel or sheet may suffice to keep him in abduction or side lying. Older children require more specialized equipment, an example of which is shown in Fig. 25.4.

Adaptive seating may be required to enable feeding and also facilitate play. Gross and fine motor movements in the upper limbs will be improved if the child is sitting securely with a good posture. Examples of seating that may be suitable include

- corner seats
- moulded seats
- activity tables
- saddle seating for adductor spasm.

Standing support

Any child who is not standing well by 18 months independently should be stood regularly in a frame as weightbearing is necessary to encourage formation of the acetabulum and femoral head. The child should have his hips extended, slightly externally rotated and abducted. Feet should be flat and the foot in a neutral position. Asymmetry should be avoided.

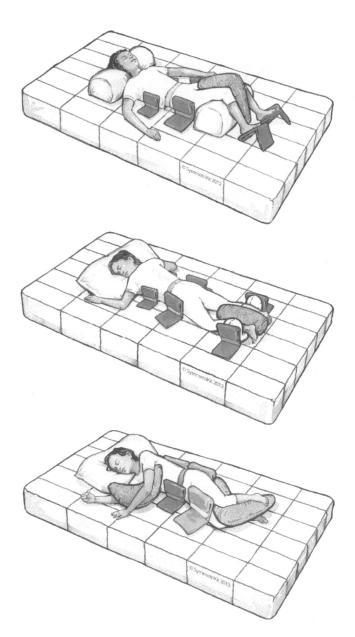

Figure 25.4 An example of specialized sleeping equipment for older children with cerebral palsy. Reproduced with kind permission of Andrew Wilson, The Helping Hand Company.

Role of adjuvant treatments

Medical interventions to treat the whole child or a particular part of the child (i.e. a limb) can be offered and may be fully or only partly reversible. Fig. 25.5 provides a summary of what is available and how each intervention fits into this model. These interventions are adjuncts to physiotherapy, which remains the mainstay of management despite the development of these newer interventions.

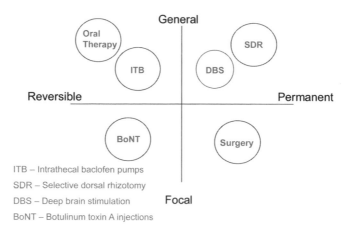

ITB – Intrathecal baclofen pumps
SDR – Selective dorsal rhizotomy
DBS – Deep brain stimulation
BoNT – Botulinum toxin A injections

Figure 25.5 Medical management of problems with tone (courtesy of Dr C Fairhurst).

Both medical and physical therapies attempt to address the secondary problems of a movement disorder that have arisen as a consequence of the primary brain impairment. There is, as yet, no effective treatment available to treat the initial insult to the developing brain, although research is ongoing. Infusions of stem cells have been tried in some countries, including Russia, without any effect on the underlying brain lesion.

Most interventions are targeted at

- spasticity;
- dystonia;
- secondary comorbidities.

ORAL MUSCLE RELAXANT DRUGS

Oral medicines are rarely necessary in the first 2 years of life but should be considered, particularly if there is painful spasticity or night spasms. Muscle relaxant drugs can be used but care should be taken to avoid excessive hypotonia in the case of baclofen and sedation due to diazepam. See NICE guidelines on spasticity in children and young people (NICE 2012).

BOTULINUM TOXIN TYPE A

Botulinum toxin type A is a neurotoxin which is taken up in the neuromuscular junction and end plates. It irreversibly blocks the motor end plate action potential. It is given by preferably guided injection into the target muscle, using either ultrasound or, less commonly, EMG. It will produce muscle relaxation that is apparent within a few days to a week and can last up to 3 to 4 months. The injections are helpful for local or focal problems as they can give relatively quick muscle relaxation allowing a 'window of opportunity' for increased muscle stretch therapy, often augmented by splinting (e.g. with orthoses or casting providing opportunities to work on improving function). There are concerns that overuse of this medication can precipitate weakness that is undesirable for maintaining posture and stability. Long-term use may precipitate the development of antibodies to the toxin, necessitating the need for larger doses in order to produce the same effect.

INTRATHECAL BACLOFEN

In the UK intrathecal baclofen is considered only for those children or young people with bilateral CP of GMFCS levels IV and V. An indwelling pump is surgically placed under the skin of the anterior abdominal wall and is connected to catheter tubing inserted into the cerebrospinal space at spinal level. The pump, which is refillable, is programmed to deliver a predetermined dose of the antispasmodic directly into the CSF. Children who are assessed as being potential candidates are offered a test dose as an inpatient and, if this produces a suitably positive response, the pump is implanted under general anaesthetic. It can be particularly helpful in those children with distressing stiffness (e.g. of hip flexors and adductors) causing difficulties in providing personal care. Doses need to be monitored in order to avoid truncal hypotonia. Only a few specialized paediatric centres are currently performing this type of treatment, but each region should have access to assessment for a suitable candidate.

SELECTIVE DORSAL RHIZOTOMY

Selective dorsal rhizotomy involves surgical resection of a proportion of the dorsal spinal nerve rootlets in order to reduce the stimulation of the spinal reflex arc. The percentage of rootlets resected varies between centres, as does the surgical approach. At present, it is thought to be a potential treatment for the ambulant, bilateral lower limb involvement, cognitively cooperative child. A definitive evidence base from long-term multicentre outcome studies is awaited. Assessment for suitability by the regional spasticity service is helpful. A 3-month period of intensive postoperative physiotherapy is essential for the surgery to be successful.

DEEP BRAIN STIMULATION

Deep brain stimulation involves implanting electrodes into the basal ganglia to deliver continuous electric signals to target nuclei. This treatment is proving to be helpful in children with certain rare movement disorders and it is sometimes considered in those with refractory dystonia associated with CP. The evidence for a consistent positive effect in this group of patients is not yet available. Cases need to be considered on an individual basis.

ORAL ANTIDYSTONIA DRUG TREATMENT

Dystonia often becomes more evident in children as they get older and there is often a mixture of spastic and dystonic CP in those with more severe CP as they move towards adolescence. There is some research evidence at this time for using medication to treat difficult dystonia; this is an area where new studies in the use of medication would be of value. Levodopa, trihexiphenidyl, clonidine and dantrolene may be considered but it is essential to seek advice from a paediatric neurologist before considering treatment within this group of drugs.

There is a condition called status dystonicus in which dystonic spasms become uncontrollable. This is a paediatric emergency and requires attention from your local paediatric neurology team.

Management of the comorbidities, both medical and developmental

Epilepsy, vision and hearing difficulties

Epilepsy, vision and hearing difficulties are all more common in CP. See Chapters 20, 21 and 26 for further information.

Communication

Many parents will ask you 'Will he walk?' when they are told their child has CP. Few, however, will ask 'Will he talk?' Communication is a major problem in CP and often neglected in early therapy as so much attention is given to postural control and motor development. Communication difficulties are seen in 80% of children with bilateral CP (GMFCS IV and V) and 40% of children with unilateral CP and diplegia (Bax 2006).

There are many reasons why communication is affected by CP:

- neurological damage to motor pathways
- neurological damage to communication centres and pathways
- disordered articulation
- associated sensorineural hearing impairment
- cognitive difficulties.

One can make some predictions that communication is more likely to be affected if neuroimaging reveals bilateral damage, particularly damage involving the basal ganglia. If MRI shows any lesion and involves the left hemisphere in particular, then language development may be more of a problem. In unilateral CP of congenital origin there can be reorganization of language centres to the other hemisphere, leading to less marked difficulties.

Improving the child's efforts to communicate should involve providing an environment in which communication is facilitated. Appropriate strategies taught to families and school by a speech and language therapist are important to aid this process, but the time spent directly with a therapist does not correlate directly with outcome. For specific techniques see Chapter 13 on communication. The Communication Function Classification System (see Table 25.2 can be used to classify the everyday functional performance.

Feeding, swallowing and chewing

One of the most common problems in the child with CP that is often recognized in retrospect is the difficulty the infant has in establishing how to suck, chew and swallow safely in order to gain weight. Feeding difficulties can be an ongoing problem in children with CP, particularly in those who function at GMFCS level II or higher. These difficulties can prolong feeding times (>3h/d) and be a cause of significant stress for families.

Key questions to ask

- **Is the feeding achieving adequate nutrition?**
  - This can be assessed from standard growth parameters. It is important to remember that children with CP have a different growth potential to typically developing children as they have limited muscle bulk that alters with their motor ability. There are some CP-specific charts which can be found at: http://www.lifeexpectancy.org/articles/GrowthCharts. shtml. Triceps skinfold thickness is a useful standard measure. These measurements should be considered in conjunction with a dietetic review.
- **Is the swallow safe?**
  - A specialist speech and language therapist should observe the child being fed. The specialist may suggest considering a videofluoroscopy if he or she is concerned about aspiration.
- **Is feeding efficient, comfortable and enjoyable?**
  - Prolonged and difficult feeding significantly impairs the quality of life of both the affected child and his family. These issues are considered in more depth in the section on nutrition. For children with CP a multidisciplinary approach is helpful to assess the whole process of feeding, from observation of the child's posture, seating, tools, food texture and consistency to the management of medical complications such as gastro-oesophageal reflux. Advice will be shared with carers on the best methods to be used during the feeding of their child and to make eating and the oral experience as pleasurable as possible.

Gastro-oesophageal reflux (GOR)

Many infants with an evolving abnormality of tone and posture present as distressed infants, with feeding difficulties that may be associated with slow weight gain. It is essential to consider GOR in this group, even if there is no vomiting. Impedance or pH studies (which enable evaluation of the amount of acid and non-acid reflux) are helpful but a trial of medication can be beneficial.

Sandifer syndrome describes children with GOR who present with unusual posture: hyperextension, often with twisting of the head to one side.

Constipation

This is a frequent complaint. It can also be the underlying cause of pain and distress without the symptoms of constipation being obvious. Children with CP are at risk from this for many reasons:

- a diet that may be low in fibre
- poor hydration due to poor drinking

- excessive drooling, which leads to additional fluid loss
- difficulties with posture and movement leading to difficulties with evacuation
- lack of physical movement, which reduces peristalsis.

Management is discussed further in Chapter 55.

Respiratory infections

Children and young people with more severe forms of CP are at risk of lower respiratory tract infections because of

- a poor cough
- aspiration due to abnormal swallow
- gastro-oesophageal reflux
- positioning problems
- scoliosis.

Anticipating this risk can be of help.

- Support carers with advice on safe feeding techniques.
- Investigate and institute appropriate treatment if there is gastro-oesophageal reflux. This could include a fundoplication.
- Ensure that the child is fully immunized, including annual influenza immunization.
- Early intervention by a paediatric respiratory physiotherapist can be markedly beneficial to the child and prevent hospitalization. Physiotherapists will also teach parents techniques to improve drainage.
- Early treatment with antibiotics and, in some children with more severe CP who are prone to recurrent infection, prophylactic alternate-day antibiotics can be very beneficial.

Case vignette 3

Ahmed is 9 years old and has bilateral CP of GMFCS level IV. He has a gastrostomy and is fed some foods orally by his mother. He enjoys school but has had a lot of absenteeism because of illness. He has had three admissions this winter for respiratory tract infections with tachypnoea and fever.

You discuss with his mother that Ahmed may benefit from prophylactic alternate-day antibiotics and she is taught by a paediatric physiotherapist to perform regular chest physiotherapy. You consider that he may be experiencing 'silent' aspiration. You decide that if there is no improvement after these measures then pH studies will be arranged. If these are abnormal a fundoplication may be required.

Ahmed improves with the initial interventions and there is a marked decrease in admission frequency.

Drooling

Drooling is more common in children with CP. This is not because of increased salivation but due to multiple factors including difficulties in the coordination of swallowing. For advice on the management of drooling see Chapter 51.

Dental care

Dental care needs consideration as medication, difficulty in cleaning teeth, antidrooling medications that lead to a decrease in saliva, and so on, can all make dental health more challenging (see Chapter 51).

Bladder function

Urinary tract infections can be more common in cerebral palsy because of:

- poor hydration
- constipation
- bladder emptying difficulty: this may be due to difficulties with posture and seating or autonomic dysfunction.

Urinary tract infections should be treated and managed as per current guidelines. Some individuals do then benefit from low-dose antibiotic prophylaxis. Again, you need to consider other underlying causes not associated with CP and consult nephrology or urology colleagues if necessary.

Orthopaedic problems

Skeletal health

Children with CP mature into teenagers and then into adults with CP. Early nutrition is essential for long-term bone health, and the group who are most at risk are those with early feeding problems, faltering growth, immobility, and those who are predominantly non-weightbearing and take medication (e.g. anticonvulsant drugs). All these factors will increase the chance of problems with bone mineralization. Osteopenia is a frequent radiographic observation in this group, but there are insufficient standardized data of bone density in young people to make, as yet, evidence-based recommendations as to how to treat this problem. Fractures are reported to occur spontaneously or with minimal force in those children who are severely affected with CP. However, one should also consider safeguarding issues and investigate carefully.

HOW TO PREVENT FRACTURES

1. Consider that there is a risk.
2. Ensure optimal nutrition throughout life.
3. Encourage weightbearing exercises (physiotherapy will be the lead here).

4　If a fracture happens with minimal force, consider bone density measurements (dual-energy X-ray absorptiometry).

5　Seek advice from a bone endocrine specialist if in doubt.

Hip and spine surveillance

All units and teams should have a policy for monitoring the hips of their patients with CP. There is now an overwhelming body of evidence highlighting the need for surveillance for hip and spine problems in children and young people with CP. These problems can be painful, particularly those relating to the hip. Hip subluxation/dislocation may impair quality of life and cause functional difficulties in sitting, standing and even lying in bed. It occurs because

- Hips that are normal at birth develop structural abnormalities as they are not subject to normal forces of weightbearing.
- The major deformity that occurs in spastic quadriplegia involves the hips taking on a windswept position due to strong ATNR. This leads to asymmetrical sitting, hip dislocation and secondary scoliosis.
- Hip subluxation/dislocation risk in children with CP increases with the severity of the impairment and the risks are greatest in children who do not walk independently.
- Hip subluxation/dislocation occurs in 60% of children with CP who are not walking at the age of 5 years. This can result in pain, increasing deformity, the inability to sit, functional restrictions and daily living problems and may lead to spinal deformity.
- Botulinum toxin A has a role in the management of spasticity in this group, but there is no evidence that it will absolutely prevent the need for hip surgery.

Australian recommendations in this area have been well evaluated and are based on reliable evidence. They are based on monitoring the migration percentage, which reflects acetabulum formation and the degree of subluxation (see Fig. 25.6). The guidelines in Fig. 25.7 suggest that baseline radiography in all children with CP should be carried out by the age of 2 years; the flow diagram shows how treatment should then proceed along the appropriate pathway. Studies indicate a significant decrease in hip dislocation after implementation of a surveillance plan.

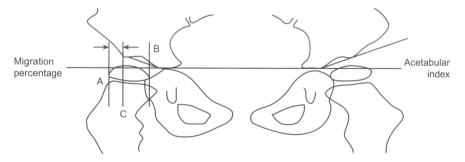

Figure 25.6 Measurement of hip migration percentage and acetabular index. Migration percentage=(Ac × 100)/AB. Acetabular index in measured in degrees (Scrutton and Baird 1997).

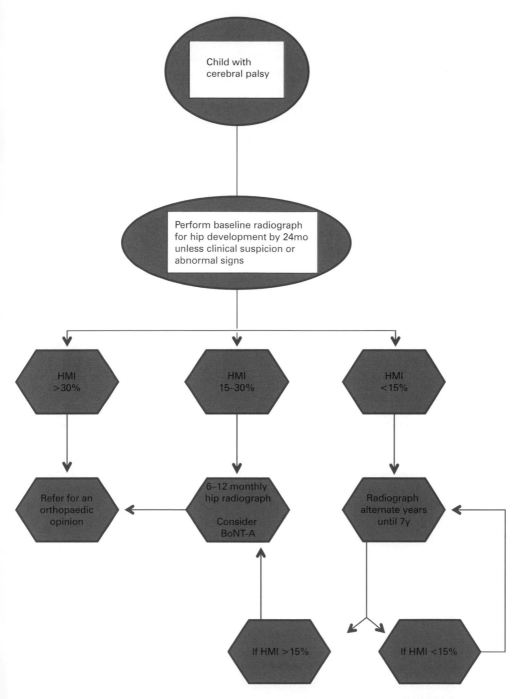

Figure 25.7 Hip surveillance pathway. HMI, hip migration index; BoNT-A, botulinum toxin type A.

Orthopaedic surgery

The orthopaedic surgeon should be experienced in the treatment of children with CP and work as part of a network with the paediatric physiotherapist, paediatrician and with or without a neurologist involved with the child.

Today, there is a much better understanding of the forces that affect posture, gait and function in CP and of the role that orthopaedic surgery plays in the overall management. Each child's difficulties should be considered in the context of their overall clinical picture; this includes consideration of communication, cognition, motivation and pain, as well as mobility. The family's involvement in managing their child's care should be considered too. A multidisciplinary team working with the child and parents should consider the nature of the problem and if surgery can help to move the child forwards, or prevent deterioration.

Common orthopaedic problems

- Dislocated hips.
- Contractures.
- Scoliosis.

Orthopaedic surgical procedures carried out in cerebral palsy

- Soft tissue releases around the hips/knees/ankles to lengthen shortened muscle tendon complexes in children usually over the age of 7 years. The aims of this surgery include the prevention of hip dislocation, improvement of gait and the maintenance of a neutral foot position.
- Occasionally, multilevel procedures are considered rather than successive procedures on ankles, knees and hips ('birthday party syndrome'). Gait analysis is carried out before and after to plan such interventions and assess the outcomes.
- Occasional procedures on feet to correct equinus or valgus deformity to improve walking, stability or orthotic wear.
- Procedures to correct severe anteversion of the femoral neck in children with windswept posture in bilateral CP with a derotation osteotomy.
- Procedures to reduce pain in children with established dislocated hip by reducing hip or performing proximal femoral excision, 'Castle' procedure, if femoral head is severely damaged
- Occasional interventions on the upper limbs to correct permanently adducted thumb to improve hygiene. Correction of persistent elbow flexion and finger flexion after puberty to ease dressing and improve cosmetic appearance.
- Rarely, prevention of progression in scoliosis.

The intended goals for each intervention should be clearly articulated and agreed beforehand with parents. Common goals include the following:

- Easing activities of daily living such as washing, dressing and maintaining hygiene in children with total body involvement.
- Facilitating transfers, use of standing frame and wearing of orthoses, and to maintain independence.
- Maintaining independent walking in children with spastic diplegia.

- Amelioration of pain due to hip dislocation, if this is thought to be a likely cause of a child's pain.

Orthopaedic intervention in the clinical categories of cerebral palsy

Unilateral CP (spastic hemiplegia)

Intervention is rarely needed, if ever, as usually children diagnosed with unilateral CP have good function, though there is emerging evidence that the hemiplegic person with more severe gait asymmetry does have a higher chance of developing hip problems.

Bilateral CP – lower limbs more severely affected (spastic diplegia)

Many children are referred for gait analysis as this provides a more objective assessment of which intervention is appropriate.

Four limbs affected (spastic quadriplegia)

Intervention will be required to

- prevent hip dislocation
- reduce pain in established dislocation and to facilitate care
- reduce the risk of progression in scoliosis. Spinal monitoring is a routine element of the examination. Any suggestion of a spinal curve, progressive kyphosis (hump) or lordosis needs radiological evaluation and referral to an orthopaedic/spinal colleague for monitoring. There is no evidence, however, that spinal corsets/jackets prevent deterioration.

After expert analysis non-surgical interventions may be recommended such as

- oral baclofen or other drugs to reduce spasticity and manage pain and spasms
- orthotics
- botulinum toxin followed by serial casting and intensive physiotherapy
- intrathecal baclofen.

Medical and surgical interventions are usually aimed at reducing spasticity or reducing the secondary postural effects of increased tone. The results will be better in children with spastic CP rather than in those with mixed spastic and dyskinetic CP who require other approaches including for example a trial of antidystonia drugs, and even, in some cases, consideration of deep brain stimulation in severe dystonia.

Care planning

For some children and young people the time may come when less aggressive treatments are considered to be more appropriate (e.g. after several pneumonias and persistent respiratory impairment). This can, and should, be discussed with the family if there is an anticipated risk of respiratory failure. Individual emergency healthcare plans planned with the young person, if possible, and family, can recommend how best to treat an individual child during an acute episode of ill health (see Chapter 52 and Appendix V).

Transition

There are always transitions that need consideration, such as when the child moves from nursery to school, moves school class, or moves from primary to secondary school; however, the largest transition occurs during the move from paediatric to adult care teams after 19 years of age.

Each young person's needs are different and your choice of team to pass on the leadership in care will vary according to those needs. If the young person with CP has seizures or significant cognitive needs then an adult neurology team would be relevant, or referral to the local adult learning disability team may be appropriate. If the young person is a wheelchair user then referral to an adult rehabilitation specialist with access to seating teams would be an appropriate team for referral. However, of increasing importance is the young person's general practitioner, who will be the key person in advocating and signposting the young person's health needs. Communication between the paediatrician and the general practitioner before transition is crucial.

Longevity

Life expectancy in CP is dependent on functional ability and skills for independent living. Several studies in the USA and UK have looked at this and the conclusions are the same (e.g. Hutton et al. 1994, Baird et al. 2011). For those with no severe disability, 20-year survival is thought to be over 95% and for those with severe functional disability survival is 50%. Life expectancy in adulthood can vary by 40 years or more dependent on functional dependency.

Quality of life

Studies in young people with CP reveal that professionals and carers underestimate quality of life compared with self-estimates by the young people themselves, who estimate their quality of life to be similar to their able-bodied peers. Hopefully further research will facilitate greater understanding and treatments to improve the experience of children and young people with CP.

Summary of objectives for follow-up consultation in a child with cerebral palsy

Presenting problems

- Assess the current concerns and problems.
- Review the achievements and ambitions for the child or young person and carers.

Motor problems

- Review the GMFCS motor development curves.
- Assess tone and spasticity: does the child need consideration for adjunctive treatment in addition to 'routine' therapy?
- Consider what are the individuals' and carer's goals for treatment or therapy; reflect on whether these goals have been achieved and consider whether to redefine the goals.
- Ensure that the local hip surveillance programme is 'on track' (Fig. 25.2) The method of choice to detect inadequate positioning of the head of femur is measuring Reimer's migration index: a standardized radiographic imaging of the pelvis in patients *around 24 months of age*. In general, a hip at risk in children with CP is defined as a migration index greater than or equal to 30% (Fig 25.6).
- Check the spinal position.
- Check the equipment needs and activities of daily living requiring occupational assessment and social care in the home.

Managing associated problems

- Check the child's growth, height and weight and consider nutritional needs.
- Does the child's vision or hearing need rechecking?
- Have the child's communication needs been considered adequately?
- Does the child have any pain or night spasms?

Education

- Have educational staff been informed and are they clear about medical needs?

Home and leisure

- Are leisure opportunities being considered?
- What respite support is being offered (e.g. short breaks)?
- Are the emotional health needs of the family, child or young adult being considered?

Finally

- Always pause to consider diagnostic accuracy: is CP the right diagnosis?
- Was neuroimaging done and, if not, why not?
- Are the history and imaging findings consistent with the clinical picture?
- Are there any new factors (e.g. family illnesses, genetic disease of relevance)?

References

Baird G, Allen E, Scrutton D et al. (2011) Mortality from 1 to 16–18 years in bilateral cerebral palsy. *Arch Dis Child* 96: 1077–81. http://dx.doi.org/10.1136/adc.2009.172841

Bax M (2006) Clinical and MRI correlates of cerebral palsy: the European study *JAMA* 296: 1603–8. http://dx.doi.org/10.1001/jama.296.13.1602

Graham HK (2005) Classifying cerebral palsy. *J Pediatr Orthop* 5: 127–8.

Hutton JL, Cooke T, Pharoah POD (1994) Life expectancy in children with cerebral palsy. *BMJ* 309: 431–5. http://dx.doi.org/10.1136/bmj.309.6952.431

NICE (2012) Spasticity in Children and Young People with Non-Progressive Brain Disorders: Management of Spasticity and Co-existing Motor Disorders and the Early Musculoskeletal Complications [CG145]. Available at: www.nice.org.uk/CG145 (accessed 7 January 2013).

Palisano R, Rosenbaum P, Walter S, Russell D, Wood E, Galuppi B (1997) Development and validation of a gross motor function classification system for children with cerebral palsy. *Dev Med Child Neurol* 39: 214–23. http://dx.doi.org/10.1111/j.1469-8749.1997.tb07414.x

Rosenbaum P, Paneth N, Leviton A et al. (2007) A report: the definition and classification of cerebral palsy April 2006. *Dev Med Child Neurol* 109: 8–14.

SCPE Collaboration Group (2000) Surveillance of cerebral palsy in Europe. A collaboration of cerebral palsy surveys and registers. *Dev Med Child Neurol*: 42: 816–24.

Scrutton D, Baird G (1997) Surveillance measures of the hips of children with bilateral cerebral palsy. *Arch Dis Child* 76: 381–4. http://dx.doi.org/10.1136/adc.76.4.381

Further reading

Barnes L, Fairhurst C (2011) *The Hemiplegia Handbook: For Parents and Professionals*. London: Mac Keith Press.

Bobath K (1992) *A Neurophysiological Basis for the Treatment of Cerebral Palsy*. London: Mac Keith Press.

Cans C (2007) Surveillance of cerebral palsy in Europe: a collaboration of cerebral palsy surveys and registers. *Dev Med Child Neurol* 42: 816–24. http://dx.doi.org/10.1111/j.1469-8749.2000.tb00695.x

Fairhurst C (2011) From cerebral palsy: the whys and hows? *Arch Dis Child Educ Pract Ed*, published online 4 November 2011. http://dx.doi.org/10.1136/archdischild-2011-300593

Dobson F, Boyd RN, Nattrass GR et al. (2002) Hip surveillance in children with cerebral palsy: impact on the surgical management of spastic hip disease. *J Bone Joint Surg* 84: 720–6. http://dx.doi.org/10.1302/0301–620X.84B5.12398

Dodd K, Imms C, Taylor NF (eds) (2010) *Physiotherapy and Occupational Therapy for People with Cerebral Palsy: A Problem-Based Approach to Assessment and Management*. London: Mac Keith Press.

Krageloh-Mann I, Horber V (2007) The role of magnetic resonance imaging in elucidating the pathogenesis of cerebral palsy: a systematic review. *Dev Med Child Neurol* 49: 144–51. http://dx.doi.org/10.1111/j.1469-8749.2007.00144.x

Leet AI, Mesfin A, Pichard C et al. (2006) Fractures in children with cerebral palsy. *J Paediatr Orthop* 26: 624–7. http://dx.doi.org/10.1097/01.bpo.0000235228.45539.c7

Pennington L, Goldbart J, Marshall J (2005) Direct Speech and language therapy in CP: findings from a systematic review. *Dev Med Child Neurol* 47: 57–63. http://dx.doi.org/10.1017/S0012162205000101

Rosenbaum P, Rosenbloom L (2012) *Cerebral Palsy: From Diagnosis to Adult Life*. London: Mac Keith Press.

Samson-Fang MD, Butler C, O'Donnell M (2002) Effects of gastrostomy feeding in children with cerebral palsy. An AACPDM evidence report. *Dev Med Child Neurol* 45: 415–26. http://dx.doi.org/10.1111/j.1469-8749.2003.tb00421.x

Wynter M, Hibson N, Kentish M, Love S, Thomason P, Kerr Graham H (2011) The consensus statement on hip surveillance for children with cerebral palsy: Australian standards of care. *J Paediatr Rehabil Med* 4: 183–95.

26
Epilepsy

Jane Williams

Learning objectives

- To know how to evaluate and manage a child with developmental problems presenting with a seizure.
- To understand the 'cause and effect' relationship between developmental problems and epilepsy.
- To understand the educational and social implications and comorbidities.

Background

If you are a paediatrician looking after children with disabilities, you will find that many children in this group will present with epilepsy or acquire epilepsy before or after their disability is recognized.

It is therefore essential that you have an understanding of this condition and a healthy respect for the difficulties of diagnosis and ensure that you are always familiar with current best practice. The current evidence-based recommendations can be found in NICE (National Institute for Health and Clinical Excellence) guidance (NICE 2012). It is also recommended that you work in a network of paediatricians with an interest in epilepsy led by your local paediatric neurology service. Discussing difficult cases and sharing management decisions and choices are all helpful, if not essential ingredients to facilitate you as a clinician to provide optimum and safe care for your patients.

The group of children with learning difficulties and epilepsy will be even more of a challenge in terms of diagnosis for a number of reasons:

- There may be a lack of a clear history from the individual.
- Many carers may be involved in the child's life leading to multiple potential historians, all with differing accounts of an attack.
- Other conditions can masquerade as an epileptic attack (e.g. autonomic disturbance in Rett syndrome or behavioural stereotypies of a person with autism).
- Several well-known common paediatric conditions such as self–gratification or day dreaming can be more common and hence can frequently be a presenting problem.

It is important to pause, reflect and consult with other colleagues, especially those in paediatric neurology, if there is uncertainty about the aetiology of episodic attacks. Visual recording of the onset and offset of attacks can be very helpful, but it is also important to consider the context of the child's other impairments, for example autism, oesophageal reflux, cerebral palsy, and so on, before making a decision. Details of these conditions can be found in current paediatric texts and paediatric neurology books, but this chapter aims at pointing you to definitions, aids for assisting accurate diagnosis, assessment and investigation principles, and the plans for treatment and training carers.

Epilepsy definition

Epilepsy is a chronic condition with spontaneous recurrent seizures. A seizure is caused by a sudden burst of excess electrical activity in the brain, causing a temporary disruption in the normal neuronal activity. Different areas of the brain have different functions, so there are different seizure types depending on the area of the brain in which the epileptic activity originates and how rapidly it spreads. Epilepsy affects people from all nations and of all races.

Some people can experience a seizure and not have epilepsy. For example, many young children have convulsions from fevers. These febrile convulsions are a type of recurrent seizure pattern which is not considered to be epilepsy. Other types of seizures not classified as epilepsy include those caused by electrolyte disturbance or by alcohol or drug withdrawal. Epilepsy by definition comprises recurrent electrical seizures and a single seizure usually does not mean that the person has epilepsy.

Classification

The International League Against Epilepsy (ILAE) has proposed several reclassifications of epilepsy and epilepsy syndromes over the years because of the rapidly changing understanding of the neural networks, genetics and other bases of diverse seizures and epilepsy (Berg et al. 2010). The progress in genetics, biochemical testing and structural and functional neuroimaging has caused the need for a more functional classification system which is flexible and can be more patient specific. Use of detailed seizure description (semiology) is important in classification and a uniform vocabulary is preferred (Fig. 26.1).

Any epilepsy can have an adverse effect on a child's overall development, in particular cognition, communication, behaviour and sleep. Earlier-onset epilepsy may potentially have a greater impact on a child's development than later-onset epilepsy. Age at epilepsy onset varies and often depends upon the underlying aetiology, especially in genetically determined epilepsies (Fig. 26.2). Seizures and cognitive function may vary over time, depending on the developmental

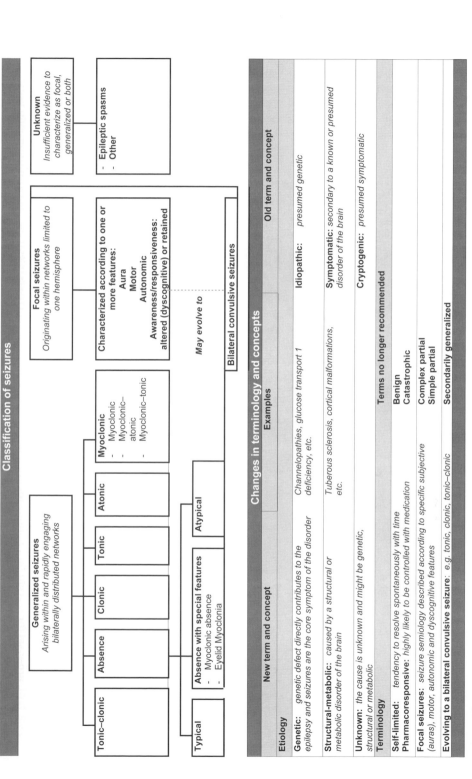

Figure 26.1 ILAE proposal for revised terminology for organization of seizures and epilepsies (classification of seizures) (Berg et al. 2010).

Electroclinical syndromes and other epilepsies group by specificity of diagnosis

Electroclinical syndromes

One example of how syndromes can be organized: arranged by typical age at onset

Neonatal period

- Benign neonatal seizures
- Benign familial neonatal epilepsy (BFNE)
- Ohtahara syndrome
- Early myoclonic encephalopathy (EME)

Infancy

- Febrile seizures, febrile seizures plus (FS+)
- Benign infantile epilepsy
- Benign familial infantile epilepsy (BFIE)
- West syndrome
- Dravet syndrome
- Myoclonic epilepsy in infancy (MEI)
- Myoclonic encephalopathy in non-progressive disorders
- Epilepsy of infancy with migrating focal seizures

Childhood

- Febrile seizures, febrile seizures plus (FS+)
- Early-onset childhood occipital epilepsy (Panayiotopoulos syndrome)
- Epilepsy with myoclonic atonic (previously astatic) seizures
- Childhood absence epilepsy (CAE)
- Benign epilepsy with centrotemporal spikes (BECTS)
- Autosomal dominant nocturnal frontal lobe epilepsy (ANFLE)
- Late-onset childhood occipital epilepsy (Gastaut type)
- Epilepsy with myoclonic absences
- Lennox–Gastaut syndrome (LCS)
- Epileptic encephalopathy with continuous spike-and-wave during sleep (CSWS)+
- Landau–Kleffner syndrome (LKS)

Adolescence–adult

- Juvenile absence epilepsy (JAE)
- Juvenile myoclonic epilepsy (JME)
- Epilepsy with generalized tonic–clonic seizures alone
- Autosomal dominant epilepsy with auditory features (ADEAF)
- Other familial temporal lobe epilepsies

Variable age at onset

- Familial focal epilepsy with variable foci (childhood to adult)
- Progressive myoclonus epilepsies (PME)
- Reflex epilepsies

Distinctive constellations/surgical syndromes

Distinctive constellations/surgical syndromes

- Mesial temporal lobe epilepsy with hippocampal sclerosis (MTLE with HS)
- Rasmussen syndrome
- Gelastic seizures with hypothalamic hamartoma
- Hemiconvulsion-hemiplegia-epilepsy

Non-syndromic epilepsies

Epilepsies to attribute to and organized by structural–metabolic causes

- Malformations of cortical development (hemimegalencephaly, heterotopias, etc.)
- Neurocutaneous syndromes (tuberous sclerosis complex, Sturge–Weber, etc.)
- Tumour, infection, trauma, angioma, antenatal and perinatal insults, stroke, etc.

Epilepsies of unknown cause

Figure 26.2 ILAE proposal for revised terminology for organization of seizures and epilepsies (electroclinical syndromes and other epilepsies group) (Berg et al. 2010).

stage of the child. Seizures may eventually stop in many children, but behavioural and cognitive problems may persist into adulthood.

Epilepsy syndromes are common in childhood. Correct identification of an epileptic syndrome will allow you to understand the cause, such as genetic aetiology or natural history (e.g. self-limiting), and help in deciding further investigations, treatment choices and management. It is important for paediatricians, especially neurodevelopmental paediatricians, to be acquainted with the common epilepsy syndromes of childhood as a number of them are associated with developmental problems and may initially present to your clinic with an evolving pattern. The common syndromes according to age at presentation are listed in Fig. 26.2. A detailed review of the epilepsy syndromes is outside the scope of this book.

Epileptic or epileptiform encephalopathies are characterized by slowing or regression of development that is attributed to ictal and/or interictal epileptic activity, often becoming more frequent in sleep. Deviation from a normal developmental trajectory in the presence of epileptiform electroencephalography (EEG) activity, including delay, plateauing or regression of cognitive abilities and/or behavioural regulation, should raise suspicion of a potential epileptic encephalopathy.

The epilepsy syndromes which are mainly associated with epileptic encephalopathies are:

- early myoclonic encephalopathy, early infantile epileptic encephalopathy (Ohtahara syndrome)
- West syndrome, severe myoclonic epilepsy in infancy (Dravet syndrome), migrating partial seizures in infancy, myoclonic status in non-progressive encephalopathies
- Lennox–Gastaut syndrome, Landau–Kleffner syndrome, and epilepsy with continuous spike-waves during slow-wave sleep.

However, it is useful to remember that uncontrolled frequent seizures of any aetiology may cause an encephalopathy. In any child with poorly controlled epilepsy presenting with symptoms of an encephalopathy it is also important to consider the possibility of a non-convulsive status epilepticus or drug adverse effect. An EEG can easily help differentiate a non-convulsive status.

Epilepsy and learning difficulties (Epilepsy Plus) coexist with a prevalence of 15% in those with mild learning disabilities and 30% in those with severe learning disability. Approximately 8% to 10% of children with Down syndrome have seizures. Epilepsy Plus patients have a reduced chance of seizure control and remission.

The majority of children who have epilepsy do not have learning difficulties, though learning disability is more likely to occur if the onset of epilepsy is in early childhood, and in those with late-onset epilepsy we may be under-recognizing additional learning needs.

However, the case remains that a significant proportion of children with learning difficulties do have epilepsy (Beghi et al. 2006). The term 'learning disability' is also misinterpreted on many occasions, but in the UK, at present, we use this term synonymously with the *Diagnostic and Statistical Manual of Mental Disorders*, 4th edition (DSM-IV) and *International Statistical Classification of Diseases and Related Health Problems*, 10th revision (ICD-10) definition. The ICD-10 uses the term 'mental retardation', which is not widely used in the UK as some parents find it stigmatizing, although it is more regularly used in the USA and some other European countries. However, DSM-5 is expected to replace the term 'mental retardation' with 'intellectual disability'. ICD-10 defines mental retardation as a condition of arrested or incomplete development of the mind, which is especially characterized by impairment of skills manifested during the developmental period, skills which contribute to the overall level of intelligence, i.e. cognitive, language, motor and social abilities. Retardation can occur with or without any other mental or physical condition.

Epilepsy itself, its treatment at times and the emotional impact of the illness can affect learning. However, it is more likely that the underlying central nervous system (CNS) cause of the epilepsy is the common factor that results in the learning difficulty. Sometimes, the CNS damage may have occurred many months or years before the epilepsy develops. Epilepsy is also associated with attention and behaviour difficulties, especially when there is poor seizure control. Studies have described that in autism, 20% to 30% of individuals have been found to have epilepsy by adulthood (Danielsson et al. 2005). There is a group of children with some rarer types of epilepsy such as Landau–Kleffner syndrome who initially have no cognitive problems, but who then develop aphasia, seizures and deterioration of learning, behaviour and communication abilities. Of course, this group needs urgent assessment from a regional paediatric neurology team.

Behaviour difficulties will be particularly common in the group of children with epilepsy: 10 438 children in the UK were surveyed and it was found that behavioural problems were three times more common in the epilepsy group than in those with other chronic illnesses (Meltzer et al. 2000). This will have an impact on our ability to investigate this group of children and may also have an impact on treatment compliance and treatment choice when discussing medication.

Anxiety and attentional problems are also frequently reported from detailed questioning of sufferers, but often poorly identified by clinicians, excluding potential therapeutic referral opportunities. All those with a learning disability and epilepsy deserve a personal care plan which the family and child should have taken an active part in writing.

Diagnosis

In epilepsy the diagnosis can be difficult, and particularly so if the child has learning difficulties.

A careful history is essential, including observational reports of the attacks and consideration of other features of the 'funny turns' (e.g. vasovagal, breath holding, self-gratification behaviour, stereotypies).

- A video of the seizure episode is extremely helpful. Note the onset of the seizure.
- Is there a precipitant?
- Is there any preceding feature such as aura?
- Does the seizure start on one side?
- Is consciousness maintained?
- Does the seizure terminate suddenly?
- What happens after the seizure stops?

Never feel unable to ask for another opinion as the difficulty of ensuring an accurate diagnosis in epilepsy is increasingly recognized.

A detailed examination is essential

Repeat the examination if this is a new problem, even if the child is well known to you. Pay particular attention to height, weight, head circumference, dysmorphism and cardiovascular and central nervous system examinations. This allows dose/weight to be accurately calculated if needed afterwards, to alert you to any underlying diagnosis that may require additional investigations such as short stature and epilepsy, micro- or macrocephaly and epilepsy. Ensure a normal cardiovascular examination and exclude a cardiac cause of seizure or collapse. Look for any focal neurological signs that may be new or old but may require new additional investigation, and similarly exclude any signs of a neurocutaneous disorder, for example neurofibromatosis type 1 or tuberous sclerosis. Using a Wood's lamp can be helpful in detecting the skin lesions. Note any obvious neurocutaneous markers in accompanying parents. Be aware that the cutaneous findings are not always present in infants and the café-au-lait spots and so on can, and do, develop over time.

The emergence of attacks may help you target investigations to look for an all-embracing underlying diagnosis (e.g. Angelman syndrome). Bear in mind that children with learning difficulties could also present with the other causes of non-epileptic seizures such as cardiac events or metabolic causes too. Children with epileptic seizures are at a much higher risk of experiencing non-epileptic seizures.

Investigations

EEG should not be used to make or exclude a diagnosis of epilepsy. EEG as clinically indicated (interictal, ictal, prolonged, ambulatory, sleep and sleep deprived) can be helpful in identifying an epilepsy syndrome. Photic stimulation and hyperventilation are routinely attempted but may be difficult in children with a learning disability. Videotelemetry (criterion standard) can be particularly helpful in selected patients when the diagnosis is unclear and is available in tertiary paediatric neurology centres.

Consider the need for other investigations (e.g. brain magnetic resonance imaging [MRI]) in order to look for lesions that may be causative of a learning disability with epilepsy (e.g. genetic syndromes such as tuberous sclerosis). In some disorders seizures tend to predate the learning difficulties, but not always. Of course, this group of young people may always have to have consideration for imaging under anaesthesia or sedation because of difficulties with cooperation.

MRI is the imaging of preference and is always indicated if seizures are

- diagnosed within the first 2 years of life
- are focal and
- do not respond to first line treatment.

Haematological, biochemical or genetic tests should be considered depending on clinical presentation.

Consider the need to look for an all-embracing underlying diagnosis that may link the learning needs and epilepsy. A paediatric neurologist/tertiary centre should be asked to see your patient if

- seizures begin in the first 2 years of life
- there is any loss of skill or regression or behavioural change
- there is no response to monotherapy within 2 years
- an epileptic syndrome is considered
- there is a hemispheric syndrome (e.g. Sturge–Weber syndrome), focal lesion on imaging, or Rasmussen's encephalitis or hypothalamic hamartoma
- there is diagnostic debate
- there is the opinion that the epilepsy may be amenable for an epilepsy surgical treatment.

Case vignette 1

Alex had early developmental impairment presenting at age 19 months with late sitting and walking, late speech, and difficulties with fine motor control compared with peers. Physical examination was unremarkable apart from hypotonia.

At age 20 months, Alex developed his first seizure associated with an intercurrent illness and followed within weeks by a cluster of tonic–clonic seizures and absences lasting less than 2 minutes, and not associated with any fever. New detailed investigations included chromosomal studies and revealed a small deletion on chromosome 15.

Some years later Alex continues to have infrequent seizures and takes two oral anticonvulsant treatments.

Learning point

The advent of epilepsy precipitated new targeted investigations that led to a diagnosis that was causing the learning difficulties and seizures.

Key points to aid the correct diagnosis of epilepsy

- Obtain a detailed history and eye witness account: the diagnosis is primarily based on history and rarely by investigations.
- A seizure diary with a detailed description of seizures, duration, date, time and preceding and post-seizure symptoms can be useful.
- Obtain a video of the episode if possible. Virtually everyone now has access to a video camera in their mobile phones, allowing easy recording.
- Always perform a detailed examination addressing the cardiac, neurological, development and mental state of the patient.
- Consider investigations such as electrocardiography (ECG, for convulsive seizures), EEG, and neuroimaging where appropriate.
- Classify the seizures. Consider the possibility of an epilepsy syndrome.
- If diagnosis is difficult and unclear, then consider further investigations and referral to a paediatric neurologist/ tertiary centre.
- First line drug choice is the same as those with no learning disability, but consider difficulties with self-advocacy.

Treatment

After consideration of the benefits and risks and in partnership with the individual (wherever possible), the family, and carer, medication may be introduced after more than one seizure. Refer to current treatment recommendations (NICE guidelines, and see Tables 26.1 and 26.2) for first-line drug medication according to seizure type, the child and their age, risk of side effects and tolerability of the side effects should they occur. Refer to up-to-date prescribing recommendations according to the most recent children's formulary.

Antiepileptic drugs (AEDs) are usually withdrawn over 6 to 8 weeks after a 2-year seizure-free period. Children with associated learning disabilities, complex needs (cryptogenic epilepsy) or an underlying CNS lesion (symptomatic epilepsy) are at higher risk of recurrence. When withdrawing AEDs additional consideration should be given to the risk of recurrence based on the epilepsy syndrome, personal circumstances (e.g. impending examinations) and personal wishes of the child and family.

Consider the need to prescribe a 'rescue medication' in a child with epilepsy who may be at risk from status epilepticus or who has had a prolonged seizure.

Currently, the first choice would be midazolam via the buccal route. Verbal, written and taught instructions regarding the situation and administration of such treatment need to be provided. All carers should be made aware of the risks of respiratory depression if and when the rescue medication is administered and when to call an ambulance. An example of a typical protocol would be 'buccal midazolam X milligrams (depending on age) to be administered for any convulsion continuing beyond 5 minutes, *or* four or more seizures within an hour. The dose can be repeated if necessary after 6 hours, but is not to exceed two doses in any 24-hour period'.

Other treatment modalities that may be considered, particularly in epilepsy that is difficult to control, are vagal nerve stimulation (VNS) and a ketogenic diet. These are usually available through tertiary paediatric neurology centres.

The emergence of epilepsy in a child with a learning disability may lead to new concerns from the school, respite centre, home-from-home carers and transport service. This diagnosis should not jeopardize any of these placements.

A personal care plan or emergency care plan (see Appendix XV) should be written to inform all carers and settings of what do to in the event of an epileptic attack; this should stay with the child wherever he or she is. Training from a suitably competent professional should be arranged in relation to sharing information as to what an epileptic seizure will look like for that child, and what to do in the event of a short attack or a prolonged attack. Consider the need to provide 'emergency' medication (e.g. buccal midazolam); this can help ameliorate anxiety in the family or carer, as witnessing a child having a prolonged seizure can be very frightening and, of course, it is the prolonged convulsion lasting over 30 minutes that, potentially, can lead to further CNS damage.

Table 26.1 Drug options by seizure type

Seizure type	First-line AEDs	Adjunctive AEDs	Other AEDs that may be considered on referral to tertiary care	AEDs to be avoided (may worsen seizures)
Generalized tonic–clonic	Carbamazepine Lamotrigine Oxcarbazepinea Sodium valproate	Clobazama Lamotrigine Levetiracetam Sodium valproate Topiramate		(If there are absence seizures or myoclonic seizures or if juvenile myoclonic epilepsy is suspected) Carbamazepine Gabapentin Oxcarbazepine Phenytoin Pregabalin Tiagabine Vigabatrin
Tonic or atonic	Sodium valproate	Lamotriginea	Rufinamidea Topiramatea	Carbamazepine Gabapentin Oxcarbazepine Pregabalin Tiagabine Vigabatrin
Absence	Ethosuximide Lamotriginea Sodium valproate	Ethosuximide Lamotriginea Sodium valproate	Clobazama Clonazepam Levetiracetama Topiramatea Zonisamidea	Carbamazepine Gabapentin Oxcarbazepine Phenytoin Pregabalin Tiagabine Vigabatrin
Myoclonic	Levetiracetama Sodium valproate Topiramatea	Levetiracetam Sodium valproate Topiramatea	Clobazama Clonazepam Piracetam Zonisamidea	Carbamazepine Gabapentin Oxcarbazepine Phenytoin Pregabalin Tiagabine Vigabatrin
Focal	Carbamazepine Lamotrigine Levetiracetam Oxcarbazepine Sodium valproate	Carbamazepine Clobazama Gabapentina Lamotrigine Levetiracetam Oxcarbazepine Sodium valproate Topiramate	Eslicarbazepine acetatea Lacosamide Phenobarbital Phenytoin Pregabalina Tiagabine Vigabatrin Zonisamidea	
Prolonged or repeated seizures and convulsive status epilepticus in the community	Buccal midazolam Rectal diazepamb Intravenous lorazepam			

Seizure type	First-line AEDs	Adjunctive AEDs	Other AEDs that may be considered on referral to tertiary care	AEDs to be avoided (may worsen seizures)
Convulsive status epilepticus in hospital	Intravenous lorazepam Intravenous diazepam Buccal midazolam	Intravenous phenobarbital Phenytoin		
Refractory convulsive status epilepticus	Intravenous midazolamb Propofolb (not in children) Thiopental sodiumb			

aAt the time of writing this drug did not have UK marketing authorization for this indication and/or population see specific details about this drug for this indication and population. Informed consent should be obtained and documented. bAt the time of writing this drug did not have UK marketing authorization for this indication and/or population see specific details about this drug for this indication and population. Informed consent should be obtained and documented in line with normal standards in emergency care. AED, antiepileptic drugs. Source: NICE (2012).

Table 26.2 Drug options by epilepsy syndrome

Epilepsy syndrome	First-line AEDs	Adjunctive AEDs	Other AEDs that may be considered on referral to tertiary care	AEDs to be avoided (may worsen seizures)
Childhood absence epilepsy or other absence syndromes	Ethosuximide Lamotriginea Sodium valproate	Ethosuximide Lamotriginea Sodium valproate	Clobazama Clonazepam Levetiracetama Topiramatea Zonisamidea	Carbamazepine Gabapentin Oxcarbazepine Phenytoin Pregabalin Tiagabine Vigabatrin
Juvenile absence epilepsy or other absence syndromes	Ethosuximide Lamotriginea Sodium valproate	Ethosuximide Lamotriginea Sodium valproate	Clobazama Clonazepam Levetiracetama Topiramatea Zonisamidea	Carbamazepine Gabapentin Oxcarbazepine Phenytoin Pregabalin Tiagabine Vigabatrin
Juvenile myoclonic epilepsy	Lamotriginea Levetiracetama Sodium valproate Topiramatea	Lamotriginea Levetiracetam Sodium valproate Topiramatea	Clobazama Clonazepam Zonisamidea	Carbamazepine Gabapentin Oxcarbazepine Phenytoin Pregabalin Tiagabine Vigabatrin

Table 26.2 (Continued)

Epilepsy syndrome	First-line AEDs	Adjunctive AEDs	Other AEDs that may be considered on referral to tertiary care	AEDs to be avoided (may worsen seizures)
Epilepsy with generalized tonic–clonic seizures only	Carbamazepine Lamotrigine Oxcarbazepine[a] Sodium valproate	Clobazam[a] Lamotrigine Levetiracetam Sodium valproate Topiramate		
Idiopathic generalized epilepsy	Lamotrigine[a] Sodium valproate Topiramate[a]	Lamotrigine[a] Levetiracetam[a] Sodium valproate Topiramate[a]	Clobazam[a] Clonazepam Zonisamide[a]	Carbamazepine Gabapentin Oxcarbazepine Phenytoin Pregabalin Tiagabine Vigabatrin
Infantile spasms not due to tuberous sclerosis	Discuss with, or refer to, a tertiary paediatric epilepsy specialist Steroid (prednisolone or tetracosactide[a]) or vigabatrin			
Infantile spasms due to tuberous sclerosis	Discuss with, or refer to, a tertiary paediatric epilepsy specialist Vigabatrin or steroid (prednisolone or tetracosactide[a])			
Benign epilepsy with centrotemporal spikes	Carbamazepine[a] Lamotrigine[a] Levetiracetam[a] Oxcarbazepine[a] Sodium valproate	Carbamazepine[a] Clobazam[a] Gabapentin[a] Lamotrigine[a] Levetiracetam[a] Oxcarbazepine[a] Sodium valproate Topiramate[a]	Eslicarbazepine acetate[a] Lacosamide[a] Phenobarbital Phenytoin Pregabalin[a] Tiagabine[a] Vigabatrin[a] Zonisamide[a]	
Late-onset childhood occipital epilepsy (Gastaut type)	Carbamazepine[a] Lamotrigine[a] Levetiracetam[a] Oxcarbazepine[a] Sodium valproate	Carbamazepine[a] Clobazam[a] Gabapentin[a] Lamotrigine[a] Levetiracetam[a] Oxcarbazepine[a] Sodium valproate Topiramate[a]	Eslicarbazepine acetate[a] Lacosamide[a] Phenobarbital Phenytoin Pregabalin[a] Tiagabine[a] Vigabatrin[a] Zonisamide[a]	

Epilepsy syndrome	First-line AEDs	Adjunctive AEDs	Other AEDs that may be considered on referral to tertiary care	AEDs to be avoided (may worsen seizures)
Dravet syndrome	Discuss with, or refer to, a tertiary paediatric epilepsy specialist Sodium valproate	Clobazama Stiripentol		Carbamazepine Gabapentin Lamotrigine Oxcarbazepine
Continuous spike and wave during slow sleep	Refer to a tertiary paediatric epilepsy specialist			
Lennox–Gastaut syndrome	Discuss with, or refer to, a tertiary paediatric epilepsy specialist Sodium valproate	Lamotrigine	Felbamatea Rufinamide Topiramate	Carbamazepine Gabapentin Oxcarbazepine Pregabalin Tiagabine Vigabatrin
Landau–Kleffner syndrome	Refer to a tertiary paediatric epilepsy specialist			
Myoclonic-astatic epilepsy	Refer to a tertiary paediatric epilepsy specialist			

aAt the time of writing this drug did not have UK marketing authorization for this indication and/or population (please see specific details about this drug for this indication and population). Informed consent should be obtained and documented. AED, antiepileptic drugs. Source: NICE (2012).

Case vignette 2

Amy was born at term with no difficulties. At 3 weeks of age she was found with arm and leg shaking and not responding to her mother. At the hospital it was found that Amy had had a cerebral haemorrhage secondary to a vascular malformation.

Amy grew up to have seizures, hemiplegia and learning problems. Her seizures required more than one anticonvulsant drug to control the attacks, but even then she had frequent daily attacks of different seizure types.

An epilepsy centre referral was made and after assessment she had epilepsy surgery. Her seizures stopped and after 2 years she no longer needs anticonvulsant drugs and has some words and phrases and improved cognition. Her hemiplegia remains but she no longer wears a helmet and she is happier.

Learning point

Epilepsy surgery outcomes are increasingly positive. Work with your local epilepsy network to consider suitable cases to refer. Referral should not be a last resort. Consider early assessment, particularly for focal lesions causing epilepsy.

Epilepsy and cerebral palsy

Overall, epilepsy occurs in 15% to 50% of children and adults with cerebral palsy (CP). Certainly, children with the more severe types of CP are more likely to suffer from more epilepsy, as are those with structural and focal abnormalities on brain imaging.

The same diagnostic dilemmas will exist in this group of children as recorded above. In addition, the same recommendations and guidelines for management exist.

The group of individuals with CP and epilepsy will generally be the more severely affected group within the CP spectrum. However, if epilepsy emerges in a child with CP, consider the need for further investigations as the onset of epilepsy may precipitate consideration that there is another underlying diagnosis.

Inclusion

The right to inclusion – advice for parents

If your child has epilepsy, he or she has the same right to use services and take part in activities as all other children and young people do. The law says that your child should not be discriminated against or treated less favourably by services because of his or her health needs or disabilities. Services have to take 'reasonable steps' to make sure that your child is included, and they do this through a process of 'risk management'. This means that services have to assess risk and then either eliminate it or minimize it by making 'reasonable adjustments' to the activities or by arranging additional support for your child. Risk assessments should not be used as an excuse for excluding your child but should be used to find a way of including your child safely wherever possible

(Council for Disabled Children 2010).

All children and young adults with epilepsy should have a safety risk assessment for

- bathing and showering
- preparing food
- using electrical equipment
- managing a prolonged seizure or serial seizures
- sudden unexplained death in epilepsy (SUDEP)
- suitability for independent living
- driving (where appropriate)
- choice of career.

Specific details for each of these can be found on the Epilepsy Action (the working name of the British Epilepsy Association) website at www.epilepsy.org.uk. Any clinician managing children with epilepsy should be fully aware of the current recommendations.

Planning for adolescence

Adolescence is the time when young people need more independence – this applies to those with learning disabilities and epilepsy too. Although the young person has the need for increased independence, the care needs may increase, leading to an increase in the number of carers and care environments.

In addition, there may be a need to reconsider the choice of anticonvulsant medication if the young person is female and of childbearing age, and in the case of profoundly disabled non-weightbearing young adults, who are at risk of osteoporosis. This may lead to reconsideration of the anticonvulsant drug of first choice based on current NICE guidelines; discuss with your local epilepsy specialists if necessary.

Rescue medication dosage may also need to be adjusted (an increase in dose) as the young person grows.

Quality of life

Various studies have drawn attention to the fact that quality of life (QoL) in young people with epilepsy varies with the severity of the illness and age. There is, in addition, evidence that a family's QoL will also be affected; however, children do appear to report their QoL assessments as being higher than their parents perceive. Compared with a chronic disease group of children with juvenile arthritis, young people with epilepsy have higher levels of depression, poorer educational achievement, lower percentages of long-term employment and marriage and higher rates of suicide (Camfield and Camfield 2007).

Sudden unexplained death in epilepsy (SUDEP)

Most of the time, people with epilepsy recover perfectly well after a seizure. A very small number of people die due to an injury that has happened because of a seizure. In some cases, there is no clear reason why a person with epilepsy has died. If a person with epilepsy dies unexpectedly, and no obvious cause of death can be found, it is called sudden unexplained death in epilepsy (SUDEP).
[…]
In the UK, about 620 000 people have epilepsy. It's estimated that SUDEP causes about 500 deaths each year. Some people with epilepsy have a higher risk of SUDEP than other people with epilepsy.
[…]
SUDEP has been shown to be connected with seizures, but the exact cause is not known. Research suggests that seizure activity in the brain may sometimes cause changes in the person's heartbeat or breathing. Very occasionally this may cause the person to stop breathing and not start again.
[…]
There is no way of predicting who will be affected by SUDEP. But the single most important risk factor is uncontrolled generalized tonic–clonic seizures.
[…]

Each person with epilepsy has their own level of risk of SUDEP. It can occur in people who have seizures very often or very infrequently. However, the risk is thought to be higher, the more seizures you have. The risk of SUDEP in people who are seizure-free is very, very low.

(Epilepsy Action 2011)

The risk of SUDEP seems to be significantly higher in children with complex needs. Here are some factors that may increase a person's risk.

- Not taking AEDs as prescribed (i.e. stopping or erratic compliance).
- Having generalized tonic–clonic seizures.
- Having seizures that are not controlled by AEDs.
- Having sudden and frequent changes to AEDs.
- Being a young adult (in particular male).
- Having sleep seizures.
- Having seizures when alone.
- Drinking large amounts of alcohol.

The most effective way to reduce the risk of SUDEP is to have as few seizures as possible

---

Advice for individuals with epilepsy in order to reduce the risk of SUDEP

- Always take AEDs as prescribed.
- Never stop taking AEDs, or make changes to them, without talking to a doctor first.
- Make sure that AEDs never run out and have instructions regarding what to do if medication is missed.
- If seizures continue, refer to an epilepsy specialist for a review of the epilepsy. This could lead to changes to the AEDs or other treatment options, which may include surgery or vagus nerve stimulation.
- Keep a diary of your seizures. This may help you see if there is a pattern to your seizures or anything that may trigger seizures.
- Avoid situations that may trigger seizures. Common triggers include forgetting to take AEDs, lack of sleep, stress, lack of food and too much alcohol.
- If seizures happen at night, consider using a bed alarm. Bed alarms can alert another person if there is a seizure. (Be aware that bed alarms are not always perfect. They may sometimes miss seizures or go off without a reason.) Information about bed alarms is available from the Disabled Living Foundation (www.dlf.org.uk).
- Tell other people that you have epilepsy and let them know how they could help. You may benefit from wearing identity jewellery or from carrying some form of epilepsy awareness card to alert other people that you have epilepsy.

Case vignette 3

Naheem was diagnosed with autism at 3 years of age. He attends a special school. At 11 years of age he was found on his bedroom floor shaking and he had been incontinent of urine; he failed to respond to his father's voice. An ambulance was called that took him to his local children's emergency unit, where on arrival he was his usual self. He was seen some days later by his paediatrician. No investigation was planned, but the family was told to be alert for another attack, to record any unusual event, to video an attack if possible and to be cautious in relation to bathing. The likely diagnosis was an epileptic seizure. A month later another attack happened whilst Naheem was playing on his PlayStation and 2 days later a staring attack was seen by his teacher. EEG was abnormal, MRI was normal, and a diagnosis of primary generalized epilepsy was made. Sodium valproate was prescribed and 2 years later Naheem is event free.

School and transport contacts and family members were taught what to do in the event of an attack and an emergency care plan was written and made available to carers and to the local emergency room and recorded in Naheem's hospital notes.

Learning point

Epilepsy can develop in people with autism and does not mean they have to change their life opportunities.

Reasons given for excluding children who have epilepsy

'It is too complicated' – Staff who provide services may be fearful about responding to seizures and giving emergency medication. Often this is because they assume that giving medication is more complicated than it actually is. They are unaware of the help and support that is available to ensure that children and young people with epilepsy can be included in services and activities.

'It can only be done by a nurse' – Many service providers wrongly assume that only a registered nurse or other health qualified person can be trained to give emergency medication.

'Something may go wrong' – Staff working in services are often fearful about something 'going wrong' and being personally responsible for the risk involved in caring for a child or young person with epilepsy.

'We cannot keep your child safe' – Service providers are worried that they will not be able to adapt the environment and activities to make them safe for children and young people who are likely to have seizures. They are unaware of the help and support that is available to ensure that children and young people with epilepsy can be included in services and activities. It is more about a 'can do' attitude than having technical skills.

'This service is not suitable for children with epilepsy' – This type of decision is made before the service really understands what is required and it assumes that all children and young people who have seizures are the same. It is a 'blanket rule' rather than one based on getting to know your child or making an individual assessment of your child's care and support needs.

(Council for Disabled Children 2011)

There is support available to prevent the response to the epilepsy becoming a problem such as

- the Disability Discrimination Act
- specific guidelines (see for example NICE guidelines)
- training and education.

Training is essential and is usually superbly carried out by the local specialist paediatric epilepsy nurse or a trained school nurse. This should be organized to be available for the carers and family, school, transport team and respite settings for the child or young person. A written care plan is therefore extremely helpful and supports the young person in all settings, and in turn supports staff to provide optimal and individual care as required.

Transition

Find out who in your area may be the adult neurologist who would be interested in seeing the young adult with epilepsy and learning difficulties. Some adult learning disability teams and the consultant in learning disability will be happy to look after the young adult on monotherapy and with no complex neurological needs, especially if there are learning and behavioural difficulties. However, in other cases, an adult neurology service is needed. A model in which there is an 'overlap' time between final discharge from the paediatric team and introduction to the adult team would be ideal.

This is a particularly vulnerable group of young people at a very vulnerable time when care and placement, both educational and social, may be changing.

Clarify who will be monitoring medication compliance. Is the young adult capable of self-administration or does a keyworker need to be appointed? This cannot be overstressed. Sometimes a specialist transition planning nurse can be needed or the paediatric epilepsy nurse can be involved. Ensure that there is someone who is appointed lead – too often everyone else feels everyone else is responsible. A multidisciplinary planning meeting would be of help (see Chapter 48).

Training

Training in epilepsy for professionals in the UK can be accessed through various organizations. The British Paediatric Neurology Association (www.bpna.org.uk) runs Paediatric Epilepsy Training (PET) courses, and the Royal College of Paediatrics and Child Health offers a module on epilepsy for trainees (www.rcpch.ac.uk).

Voluntary sector

A number of voluntary organizations provide a wealth of information for those affected, as well as for carers and professionals, relating to various aspects of epilepsy including education, safety, information for schools and teachers, impact on careers and impact on daily living activities (e.g. driving). Voluntary organizations also act as strong advocates for individuals and on a collective basis. The following are a few of the voluntary organizations working in this area:

- Epilepsy Action: www.epilepsy.org.uk
- National Centre for Young People with Epilepsy (NCYPE): www.ncype.org.uk
- National Society for Epilepsy (NSE): www.epilepsysociety.org.uk

---

Key messages

- Epilepsy is a complex disease.
- Epilepsy often affects the quality of life of young people and their families.
- We should look at a whole patient perspective in our treatment and management plans.
- It is essential that we look for and treat any comorbidities.
- We all need to work to eliminate 'stigma'.

References

Berg AT, Berkovic SF, Brodie MJ et al. (2010) ILAE revised terminology and concepts for organization of the epilepsies. *Epilepsia* 51: 676–85.

Beghi M, Cornaggia CM, Frigeni B, Beghi E (2006) Learning disorders in epilepsy. *Epilepsia* 47 (Suppl. 2): 14–18. http://dx.doi.org/10.1111/j.1528-1167.2006.00681.x

Camfield CS, Camfield PR (2007) Long-term social outcomes for children with epilepsy. *Epilepsia* 48 (Suppl. 9): 3–5. http://dx.doi.org/ 10.1111/j.1528-1167.2007.01390.x

Council for Disabled Children (2010) My Right's, Your Responsibility. Available at: http://www.ncb.org.uk/cdc/wider_projects/my_rights_your_responsibility.aspx (accessed 31 October 2012).

Danielsson G, Gillberg IC, Billstedt E, Gillberg C, Olsson I (2005) Epilepsy in young adults with autism: a prospective population based follow-up study of 120 individuals diagnosed in childhood. *Epilepsia* 46: 918–23. http://dx.doi.org/10.1111/j.1528-1167.2005.57504.x

Epilepsy Action (2011) Sudden unexplained death in epilepsy (SUDEP). Available at: www.epilepsy.org.uk/info/sudep-sudden-unexpected-death-in-epilepsy

Meltzer H, Gatward R, Goodman R, Ford T (2000) *The Mental Health of Children and Adolescents in Great Britain*. London: The Stationery Office.

NICE (2012) The Epilepsies: The Diagnosis and Management of the Epilepsies in Adults and Children in Primary and Secondary Care [CG 137]. Available at: http://www.nice.org.uk/_gs/link/?id=C1ED190B-19B9-E0B5-D4B6F98E316BE46E (accessed 31 October 2012).

Further reading

Aicardi J (2009) *Disease of the Nervous System*, 3rd edition. London: Mac Keith Press.

Appleton R, Gibbs J (2003) *Epilepsy in Childhood and Adolescence*, 3rd edition. London: Taylor & Francis.

Berg AT, Cross JH (2010) Towards a modern classification of epilepsies? *Lancet Neurol* 9: 459–61. http://dx.doi.org/10.1016/S1474-4422(10)70024-7.

Berg AT, Scheffer IE (2011) New concepts in classification of the epilepsies: entering the 21st century. *Epilepsia* 52: 1058–62. http://dx.doi.org/10.1111/j.1528–1167.2011.03101.x

Berg AT, Berkovic SF, Brodie MJ et al. (2010) Revised terminology and concepts for organization of seizures and epilepsies: report of the ILAE Commission on Classification and Terminology, 2005–2009. *Epilepsia* 51: 676–85. http://dx.doi.org/10.1111/j.1528-1167.2010.02522.x

Eeg-Olufsson KE (2007) *Paediatric Clinical Neurophysiology*. London: Mac Keith Press.

Russ SA, Larson K, Halfon N (2012) A national profile of childhood epilepsy and seizure disorder. *Pediatrics* 129: 256–64. http://dx.doi.org/10.1542/peds.2010–1371

Websites

Children's Epilepsy Workstream in Trent (CEWT): www.cewt.org.uk/

27

Autism spectrum disorders

Jeremy Parr

Definition and diagnostic classification

Autism spectrum disorders (ASDs) are developmental disorders characterized by

- qualitative impairments in communication and social interaction
- restricted, repetitive, and stereotyped patterns of behaviours and interests
- abnormal development that is usually present before the age of 3 years, although children's difficulties may only become obvious at a later age.

ASD is the term used to describe a heterogeneous group of disorders, which includes autism and Asperger syndrome. ASD is referred to as a 'spectrum' because the characteristics of the condition vary from one person to another, but all affected individuals have evidence of core impairments (see above).

Case vignette 1

A 2-year-old child's parents have concerns that their son is not yet speaking. He is less interested than his 18-month-old cousin in engaging with other children. He does engage with his parents but not as much as they expect. He does not look at them very frequently, and they have difficulty getting his attention. Unlike typically developing children, when he wants something, he pulls his parents to where it is and stands there; they have to guess what he wants. He is not concerned when either of his parents leaves the house or when one of them is unwell or upset. He is sometimes an affectionate child, but comes for hugs less often than expected. His parents have noticed that he tends to line toys up, or plays with certain parts of them, such as the wheels and doors. He plays in a much less interactive way than his cousin. When outside, he is very interested in the drainpipes, and drains in the garden; his parents struggle to keep him away from them, and he is very upset when he has to come back into the house. Twice or three times per day, he flaps his hands; at other times, he stares at the ceiling lights for 10 to 20 minutes at a time.

ASDs are referred to in psychiatric classification as pervasive developmental disorders (PDDs). The ASD subclasses of PDD are defined in both the *International Statistical Classification of Diseases and Related Health Problems*, 10th revision (ICD-10) and *Diagnostic and Statistical Manual of Mental Disorders*, fourth edition (DSM-IV) classification systems as shown in Table 27.1. Rett syndrome and childhood disintigrative disorder are both PDDs but they are not part of the autism spectrum. The different classification systems use slightly different terminology for ASDs; updates of both these systems are due in 2013, and terminology will change significantly (see below).

DSM-IV

- Autistic disorder
- Asperger syndrome
- Pervasive developmental disorder not otherwise specified (PDD-NOS)

ICD-10

- Childhood autism
- Atypical autism
- Asperger syndrome
- PDD

Table 27.1 Subclasses of autism spectrum disorder defined in DSM-IV and ICD-10 classification systems

- **Childhood autism** (core, classic, typical or Kanner autism): A PDD defined by the presence of abnormal and/or impaired development that is manifest before the age of 3 years, and by the characteristic type of abnormal functioning in the following three areas: reciprocal social interaction, social communication and restricted, repetitive behaviour and interests. Language delay is present.

- **Atypical autism**: Differs from autism in either the age at onset, absence of language delay, or because of failure to fulfil all three sets of diagnostic criteria.

- **Asperger syndrome**: No language delay. Good verbal skills. Average or above average IQ. Social difficulties pronounced compared with language ability and IQ. Classically, affected children present as a 'little professor'.

- **High-functioning autism**: As Asperger syndrome, but with language delay, and/or poorer verbal skills.

- **PDD-NOS/ASD**: A diagnosis for children who do not neatly fit into one of the other categories.

Looking towards DSM-5 and ICD-11

The lack of reliability between clinicians when assigning diagnoses, and a desire to see ASD as a single continuum, rather than a series of individual diagnoses under one umbrella term (PDDs), has led the classification systems to move to change diagnoses. There are a number of proposed changes, and discussion continues. Major changes will include the following:

- ASD will be considered to have two, rather than three, 'domains' (social communication and repetitive, restricted interest).
- The different ASD diagnoses listed above will be removed, and a single diagnosis of 'autism spectrum disorder' will be available to clinicians. There will be a separate scale on which to rate severity. Overall, this will reduce diagnostic complexity for clinicians, but it will not be popular with people who prefer individual diagnoses – particularly some individuals with Asperger syndrome. Clinicians anticipate that these changes will take many years to implement through diagnostic teams (see www.dsm5.org/and www.who.int/classifications/icd/revision/en/index.html).

Epidemiology

ASD was once considered an uncommon disorder, but in the last 15 years high-quality studies have demonstrated an increase in the detected prevalence. This is largely thought to be due to an increased recognition of autism and other ASDs; however, some parents and researchers continue to be concerned that there is a real rise in prevalence. Most data suggest that the rise in ASD diagnosis has been accompanied by a fall in the prevalence of other neurodevelopmental disorders. A study by Baird et al. (2006) showed that at least 1.2% of children in the UK have an

ASD, with around 0.4% having autism. A recent study from Korea (Kim et al. 2011) suggested that as many as 2% to 3% of children have an ASD; it is most likely that the prevalence falls between 1% and 2%. Males are affected more commonly than females (3–4:1). This makes ASD the most common neurodevelopmental disorder of childhood, after attention-deficit–hyperactivity disorder (ADHD).

History and aetiology

During the 1940s to 1960s, psychoanalysts thought autism occurred as a result of abnormally cold and distant parenting (the so-called 'refrigerator mother' hypothesis). This theory was refuted when the organic basis for autism was established during the late 1960s and early 1970s (through the association with learning disability and epilepsy, and the realization that autism was highly heritable).

Nowadays, we recognize that the ASD phenotype is seen in association with many other medical conditions, and also in children in whom 'cause' can be identified. This has led to the notion that there are multiple conditions of varying aetiologies that cause a similar behavioural phenotype – the 'autisms'.

Many medical conditions and other difficulties are associated with ASD; the full list of associated medical disorders is beyond the scope of this chapter. Some of the more common medical conditions associated with an increased prevalence of ASD are listed below:

1 fragile X syndrome
2 neurofibromatosis
3 tuberous sclerosis
4 down syndrome
5 cerebral palsy
6 preterm birth
7 epileptic encephalopathy (for example infantile spasms).

Genetics of autism

In the last decade, ASD genetic researchers have found no common causal genetic variants that are responsible for ASDs, although multiple rare genetic causes have been identified. Currently, the evidence is that there are unknown common genetic variants that exert a weak aetiological effect, and rare variants that have a large effect. Research evidence shows that there are gene–gene and gene–environment interactions that have yet to be discovered.

The genetic basis of ASDs is the presumed cause of

- the ASD-like behaviours sometimes seen in the relatives of those with ASDs (the broader autism phenotype)
- the 5% to 10% ASD recurrence rate in siblings of children with an ASD.

Genetic abnormalities in the regions 22q11, 15q11–13 and 16p11 are relatively common identified genetic causes, although together they cause only a few per cent of cases of ASD. In recent years, attention has turned to the role of some potentially pathogenic copy number variants (CNVs), each of which is likely to be responsible for a small number of cases (<1%) of ASD. CNVs (i.e. submicroscopic structural variations that result in a gain or loss of genomic material) alter genes and gene function (examples of potentially pathogenic ASD genes include neurexin [NRXN], neuroligin [NLGN] and SHANK). In combination, de novo and inherited CNVs may cause 15% to 20% of ASD cases. As the variants individually are very rare, data on the specificity of individual CNVs for ASDs and their positive and negative predictive value for an ASD diagnosis are very limited. Whilst some CNVs are highly associated with ASDs, and phenotype and genotype co-segregate within those ASD families, other CNVs are found in people without difficulties. To complicate matters further, some CNVs considered potentially pathogenic in ASD are also associated with other conditions, such as ADHD and schizophrenia (see review by Betancur 2011).

In combination, medical disorders and DNA analysis for CNVs mean that between 20% to 40% of the causes of ASDs may be identifiable through a combination of careful assessment and investigation, where CNV and other genetic analysis is available.

It is generally accepted that unknown non-genetic factors and environmental factors are also important in the aetiology of ASDs. Identifying these factors will be of critical importance in the future. The most high-profile and discredited claim of an environmental 'cause' of ASD in recent years relates to the MMR (measles, mumps and rubella) vaccine. The claims deterred some parents from vaccinating their children, and vaccination rates have still not fully recovered, despite very clear research evidence and epidemiological data demonstrating no association between the MMR vaccine and ASDs.

Common presentations and characteristics of children with ASDs

Children with an ASD have a wide range of clinical presentations. It is essential to have an awareness of the typical and more subtle clinical features of ASDs; these can be elicited through a detailed neurodevelopmental and current functioning history, starting with the newborn period. Parents who have or know a child with an ASD diagnosis may voice their concerns about development and behaviour, and these should always be taken seriously.

Young children with ASDs

You may find that parents report the following:

- **Temperament:** Infants may be unusually quiet and placid or, conversely, irritable and difficult to pick up and carry around, or put down, for any significant period.
- **Visual behaviour:** Infants or children may have reduced looking at their parents' and others' faces.
- **Feeding:** Children may be very difficult to feed, refuse bottles and be difficult to wean. They may be distressed by the taste of certain milks, the colour or texture of food, or the sensation of a spoon in their mouths or food around their lips. Some children spit out textured food, delaying the introduction of solid foods. Some children with ASD present through feeding clinics.

- **Speech and/or language difficulties:** This may be speech delay (single words >24mo, phrase speech >33mo) or unclear articulation, and/or there may be concerns about the way language is used, for example echolalia or stereotyped speech (use of phrases copied from others in their daily language to a greater degree than in typically developing children). Repetitive language, or requests for parents to say a phrase repeatedly, may be reported; parents may have to say or do something in a particular way. There may be loss of previously acquired language skills (regression). Some parents report their children using words or phrase speech, and then losing speech rapidly, or saying words once then never again. For these children, a very careful history is required to differentiate ASD from childhood disintegrative disorder (which is characterized by typical development during the first 2 years followed by a catastrophic loss of skills that are not regained, accompanied by seizures and other difficulties).
- **Social interaction:** Parents may report that their child does not interact with them in a socially reciprocal way as expected, or show much interest in them at all. Parental accounts are often striking, and comparisons with siblings' and other children's 'superior' social skills are naturally made. While many children with ASDs may look at their parents, they modulate their eye contact less well than expected, and do not use it (or use it less) to engage/disengage with others, or to reference objects and establish shared attention. People who are less familiar with ASDs frequently comment that 'he or she looks at you', suggesting that, because eye contact is 'present', this interaction is normal. There may be reduced or no pointing to distant objects, and reduced or no following of an adult pointing to something, as well as less integration with looking at the object and back to the person (joint attention). Children with ASDs use fewer facial expressions and gestures in communication (nodding and/or shaking the head, waving, or others). Interpreting children's mood may be difficult as their non-verbal communication might not show how they feel; parents may report mood changing abruptly. The integration of verbal and non-verbal communication skills such as social use of eye gaze with vocalization and non-verbal communication is important to observe in structured or formal settings such as in the classroom, and in informal settings such as in the playground.
- **Play:** Children with ASDs are commonly less interested than peers in social games (e.g. peek-a-boo) or engaging with their parents in play. They are less likely to bring and show toys or books, or play socially, than typically developing children. They may play alone and be relatively uninterested in being with other children; others may play superficially with other children, for example standing near them, but engaging in less to-and-fro play than their same-age peers. While children might play with parents or older children when items are brought to them, they initiate social contact less than other children. The above behaviours should be seen in the context of the highly social nature of infants and young children: observing the social communication abilities and social nature of typically developing same-age children in the home, and nursery or school visits, can be very helpful in maintaining one's own 'calibration' of typical social development.
- **Rigid behaviour:** Children with ASDs frequently have particular ways of going about everyday activities. They may prefer toys and other items to be in a certain place, and may become more distressed than expected if things are moved, or if the home environment changes. Children may collect or hoard unusual items, or show considerable interest in unusual items.
- **Sensory behaviours:** Children with ASDs can display behaviours in response to sensory stimuli, relating to the smell, taste, sound, sight or feel of objects. Children may engage

in repetitive sensory behaviours in inappropriate circumstances, for example stroking a stranger's hair or clothes in public. Children often engage in repetitive motor mannerisms such as spinning around, rocking, bouncing up and down on their toes, flapping their hands or materials, or flicking their fingers. They may show unusual and usually brief stiff postures with their hands or bodies. Some sensory behaviours have a 'function' for children (for instance, some are calming or used to express enjoyment); others are shown in response to negative situations. Identifying whether sensory behaviours are positive or negative for some children can be challenging.

Some of the characteristics described above (especially sensory behaviours and repetitive interests) are common in the typically developing population, and should not be overinterpreted in children without significant social communication difficulties.

Case vignette 2

A 3-year-old female presents because her parents are concerned about her language development. She spoke using single words at age 18 months, but soon afterwards stopped using words she had previously learned; she has now regained most of these words. She does use words to request and she points at objects, but rarely looks at her parents when she does this. She plays with a range of toys, but tends to use the toys in the same way each time. She prefers to play alone, and is less interested in other children than expected. She does play with her mother, but only when she brings toys or books to her; her father finds it difficult to engage with her except in rough and tumble play. She screams when taken to the shoe shop, and does not like places with public address systems. She is a fussy eater and hates being messy.

Older children with ASD

Older children with ASD frequently show the same behaviours described above, but features change with age. While disordered development may have been present in the early years, many children still only come to the attention of professionals at school age, when their social communication difficulties become more obvious. Children with ASDs often find that although they are able to interact socially to some degree, they understand the subtleties of social relationships less well than their peers. This frequently results in difficulties with social interactions, and may lead to limited friendships, or very brief friendships that end as a result of misunderstandings. Children struggle further in peer relationships as the social demands of mid-childhood increase. Children's need for routine, or their obsessions or interests, may become a focus in the classroom. Similarly, motor behaviours and sensory interests may persist in the classroom and interfere with learning.

Older children frequently develop non-compliance with parents and school staff. Young people may pursue their own interests to the exclusion of others, and of other activities. Difficulties with change often become pronounced, at a time when change and adaptation is a frequent need of daily life. All these areas can lead to conflict at home and in an educational environment and require appropriate autism-specific support.

> ### Case vignette 3
>
> A 9-year-old female presents because her parents are concerned about her progress at school, and her social relationships. She has been considered bright, but is falling behind her peers academically. Whilst she has never played with children as much as her sister, there have recently been arguments with peers in the playground. She has never had a 'best friend'. She is very interested in horses: she has over 50 model horses that she keeps immaculate, but does not play with in an imaginary way. School staff report that she is a quiet and generally well-behaved member of the class. As she has become older, however, they have identified that she is different from her peers. Academically, they are puzzled about her relatively slow progress. Sometimes, she does not seems to pick up verbal instructions and complete tasks as quickly as others.

Assessment

Diagnosing ASD

National guidance (see NICE 2011a,b) suggests that an ASD-trained multidisciplinary team including a paediatrician or child psychiatrist, who may work with a clinical or educational psychologist, speech and language therapist and/or occupational therapist, should make an ASD diagnosis. Whilst not always used, tools such as the Social Communication Questionnaire (SCQ) and standardized assessments (interviews and observation tools) are useful aids to diagnosis (Berument et al. 1999). A combination of the following assessments is used by some teams to make a diagnosis:

- a neurodevelopmental history
- parental interview (e.g. the Autism Diagnostic Interview – ADI-R; Le Couteur et al. 2003) and
- observational assessment (e.g. the Autism Diagnostic Observational Schedule – ADOS; Lord et al. 2000).

Whilst all children should have a neurodevelopmental and current functioning history, not all assessments require the use of standardized tools in diagnosis – although they are often helpful. It is very useful to put information about a child's social communication ability and their repetitive behaviours in the context of language and overall cognitive ability (which means that having a multidisciplinary team with the capacity to measure language and cognitive ability is very valuable). Obtaining the views of others who know the child well, and observing current functioning in more than one environment (e.g. school and home), is good practice. Whilst this can be time-consuming, it is likely to increase the reliability of a diagnosis and it helps in the formulation of appropriate educational placement and management advice.

In recent years, guidance about diagnosis has been produced. In the UK in 2003, the National Autism Plan for Children gave guidance about the diagnosis and management of children under the age of 5 years (see http://www.rcpsych.ac.uk/PDF/NAExecSum.pdf). In 2011, NICE produced its guidance about the assessment of children with ASDs (NICE 2011a), which includes the early signs of ASDs; comprehensive, evidence-based guidance about diagnostic good practice for the assessment of children of all ages; lists of differential diagnoses, comorbidities and coexisting conditions; and early signs of ASD. A quick reference guide (NICE 2011b) has also been published. NICE is currently producing guidance about the management of ASD, and publication is anticipated in 2013.

Examination

Children with ASD are generally healthy. A physical examination can reveal signs of a previously undiagnosed medical condition associated with ASD (see above). A neurological and dysmorphism examination and an inspection of the child's skin with a Wood's light should be carried out. It is good practice to formally assess hearing and/or vision before diagnosis and any time after if there is parental concern.

Investigations

1. Blood should be sent for fragile X and chromosome/array testing in those children with learning disability and/or dysmorphic features. Historically, the positive yield from fragile X and karyotyping results is very low in children with ASDs.

2. As karyotyping is replaced by array-comparative genomic hybridization testing, clinicians will be able to investigate CNVs associated with ASDs. As array-comparative genomic hybridization testing becomes more common, clinicians will need to understand the significance of the test results, as many more potentially relevant genetic abnormalities will be identified than through karyotyping. Paediatricians and child psychiatrists involved in seeing children with ASDs will need to become familiar with the rapidly moving world of ASD genetics. In the shorter term, more families will need to see clinical geneticists for interpretation of results.

3. Electroencephalography and brain magnetic resonance imaging and additional blood/urine metabolic screening tests should be performed only if there is a specific rationale following the clinical history or examination. For example, M-methyl-CpG binding protein (MECP2) deletion should be sought in females with autism and clinical features of Rett syndrome, or a history of regression.

4. In about one-quarter of all young children with ASD there is a history of early developmental regression (most commonly occurring in the child's second year of life, affecting speech). Early language regression does not require investigation when it is recognized as being part of a broader ASD picture. However, children with motor skill regression, or regression of any skills after the age of 3 years, do require very careful assessment, and investigation may be necessary.

Differential diagnosis

With increasing numbers of children referred regarding a possible diagnosis of ASD, careful multidisciplinary assessment, which includes observation in at least two different environments, and consideration of other diagnoses (or no diagnosis) are more important than ever.

Some groups of children continue to cause diagnostic uncertainty for assessment teams because of the association of ASDs with a range of other difficulties that children may present with. Identifying that the presenting difficulty is part of a broader neurodevelopmental disorder can be challenging.

Comorbidity and additional disorders

In recent years, large studies have identified that additional difficulties or diagnoses are very common in children with ASD. Sleep and feeding difficulties are very common and often top the list of issues that parents find challenging. Psychiatric disorders are common, with anxiety and depression highly prevalent in the teenage years. ADHD is common in ASD, and around 50% of children are affected. Some children will definitely benefit from medication for ADHD but it is less effective than when used in ADHD alone. Table 27.2 below shows some of the comorbidities and additional problems associated with ASD.

Table 27.2 Comorbidities and additional disorders (adapted from NICE guidance 2011a)

Mental health and behavioural problem	ADHD; anxiety disorder; specific phobias; mood disorder (depression); oppositional defiant disorder; tics, Tourette syndrome; obsessive–compulsive disorder; self-injury
Neurodevelopmental problems and disorders	Disordered development; intellectual disability; specific learning difficulties (e.g. dyslexia, dyscalculia); motor coordination problems (dyspraxia or developmental coordination disorder); speech and language disorder
Functional problems and disorders	Feeding problems (including dietary restriction, and potentially malnutrition); sleep difficulties (sleep latency, remaining asleep) enuresis; encopresis; constipation; visual impairment; hearing impairment

ADHD, attention-deficit–hyperactivity disorder.

Other conditions associated with ASD include the following:

- **Social anxiety or extreme shyness:** A careful history and observation should determine whether or not a child has ASD. Home videos from a familiar setting with familiar people can be helpful.
- **Selective mutism:** A careful history and observation of social interest and non-verbal communication are usually helpful.
- **Pathological demand avoidance:** ASD assessment teams see children with this label infrequently. This is a controversial term, and is considered by many to be an unhelpful diagnosis. Conceptually, most children with pathological demand avoidance meet the criteria for ASD, and an ASD diagnosis is more helpful to parents and local professionals as it leads to better understanding of the child's needs.
- **Psychosocial deprivation:** This can also lead to an ASD-type picture. However, follow-up studies of young children from Romanian orphanages showed that children's social communication profiles improved with better care and became more typical in their teenage years. In some cases, however, lifelong difficulties did persist, particularly for those in prolonged institutionalized care.

Family history and recurrence of ASD within families

ASDs frequently run in families. Therefore, it is essential to obtain three generations of family history and obtain information about the early development and current functioning of siblings, parents, uncles and aunts, and grandparents. Questions should focus on social communication difficulties, learning disability, mental health disorders as well as diagnosed ASDs in relatives. Some members of the family may have relatively mild ASD-related social communication difficulties and repetitive domain difficulties (such as rigidity), termed 'broader autism phenotype' (BAP). BAP is not a 'diagnosis' in psychiatric classification. It may be suspected based on information provided and/or on meeting the family member.

Identifying that the diagnosed child has another medical condition associated with ASD may affect the chances of those parents having another child with ASD. In families in which a medical disorder is identified, parents probably have around a 1% chance of having another child with ASD (i.e. the population rate). When no 'medical cause' of ASD is identified, and parents have one child with autism/ASD, research shows clinicians should give parents a generic '5% to 10% chance, of having another child with ASD'. In reality, this recurrence rate may be higher or lower for individual families.

Parents should be offered genetic counselling through regional clinical genetics services if they wish to further discuss the chances of their having another child with ASD.

Diagnosing ASDs in children with severe learning disability

One area of controversy in the UK has been the extent to which children (in particular young children) with severe learning disability should be diagnosed with ASD. Some clinicians believe that these children's social communication and repetitive difficulties relate to their learning disability, not to ASD itself; this is of course complicated, as 50% of children with ASD have a below average IQ, and some children have a very low IQ and ability. One helpful strategy is to identify the child's social communication ability and repetitive behaviours and put these in the context of the child's language and cognitive ability. Thus, their developmental age equivalents in all these areas can be compared with their chronological age, and relative areas of strength and weakness identified.

Case vignette 4

A 4-year-old male does not speak, and shows little interest in people, or communicating; he spends hours playing repetitively. His developmental ability is similar to that of an 8-month-old infant.

Placing this child's social communication skills in the context of an 8-month-old infant is helpful as infants at this age are typically very socially interested in others, are already skilled in verbal and non-verbal communication and, while they may have particular items they prefer and are repetitive with, they explore a range of objects. This child's social and communication skills are therefore out of keeping with his cognitive level and a diagnosis of ASD should be considered.

Dual diagnosis

Some clinicians and parents question the value of making a second neurodevelopmental diagnosis when one exists already. Down syndrome is an example of such a disorder in which an affected child might also meet ASD diagnostic criteria. Increasingly, clinicians, parents and educational staff are seeing the value of an ASD diagnosis when a child meets ASD criteria, as this helps people understand the differences between that child and other children with the 'first diagnosis'. Identifying ASD has the benefit of facilitating access to ASD-specific services and appropriate management strategies and interventions.

Understanding parents' perspectives

As with other types of disability, it is always necessary to explore parental perspectives about the diagnosis and its effect on the child and family. Parents' opinions may influence clinical decision making in many ways. Some parents may be reluctant to pursue the diagnostic process because they are concerned about 'labelling' their child; parents may later come to accept that a diagnosis is needed to gain support and services. As ever, clinicians should work with parents in the best interests of the whole family, unless it impacts on parents or professionals being able to meet the needs of the child.

Very occasionally, parents may seek an ASD diagnosis when this is not appropriate, in an understandable effort to gain support for their child. Extremely rarely, parents seek a diagnosis as part of fabricated disability. These are both very challenging situations and involvement of the multiagency team is needed to explore the reasons behind parental behaviour, and in order to identify which agencies need to be involved to support parents and ensure the child's welfare.

Challenging diagnoses and situations

Many clinical teams that provide autism assessments for preschool and school-aged children are now very experienced and are confident in their diagnostic skills. However, some children present particular challenges to diagnostic teams. It is sometimes necessary to reassess a child when doubts remain or when there is disagreement between parents and professionals about a child's diagnosis and/or management. Clinicians should at this point consider carefully if all the required assessments have been done and, if not, arrange for these to be completed. The key for professionals is to openly discuss uncertainties, share concerns and refer to colleagues for a second opinion where necessary. It can be helpful to consider 'If ASD is not the cause of this child's difficulties, then what is?'. On very rare occasions, following local and second assessments, parents and professionals may continue to disagree about whether an ASD diagnosis is warranted or not. In this situation, referral to another clinical team is rarely helpful. Clinicians should decide what is in the best interests of the child and try to work with parents to achieve this with the relevant local professionals.

Discussing diagnosis with parents and children

The news that their child has ASD can come as a shock to some parents, and may cause distress. For other parents it is confirmation of something they have 'known' for some time; it comes as something of a relief from uncertainty. The information giving should occur with both parents together (where appropriate), in a quiet place, and when support is available to parents. Support from a designated member of the multidisciplinary team should remain available afterwards if needed.

Some parents, in particular parents of teenage children, are happy for health staff to talk to the young person about the diagnosis; professionals should work with parents to decide how to share the news with the young person, at a level appropriate to their cognitive abilities. Other parents prefer to explain to their child about their difficulties at a time of their choosing. Usually the time for this becomes obvious, as there is a need to explain why they are different in some way to other children. Some parents prefer to explain differences qualitatively, rather than using the term ASD; there is no right or wrong approach. School staff need information about diagnosis so that appropriate educational provision can be made available. Children in mainstream schooling may want to tell people they spend considerable time with about the diagnosis, so misunderstandings and potentially difficult situations with peers can be explained appropriately.

Following diagnosis, parents need to understand ASD, the severity of their child's ASD, and their child's cognitive and language abilities more comprehensively. For many parents, the knowledge that their child has little interest in relating to them (and may never do so), and may understand little of what has been said to them, is upsetting and sometimes difficult to manage. Most parents welcome post-diagnosis support provided by a member of the multidisciplinary team, a health visitor, general practitioner or local voluntary group; support may not be desired immediately. Providing information in the form of leaflets (for example the Early Support ASD booklet, provided by the Department for Education and Skills, available at www.education. gov.uk/publications/eOrderingDownload/ES12-2010.pdf) and website addresses for local and national ASD resources is useful, as are reading materials and reading lists. Proactively expressing caution to all parents about Internet sites that claim 'cure' and 'miracle results' is appropriate.

For most parents, diagnosis is the beginning of a new journey with their child, learning how to access appropriate health, education and social care support. The multidisciplinary team should support parents in this through liaison with other agencies including education and social care, as needed. Claims for Disability Living Allowance should be advocated and appropriately supported.

Prognosis

ASD is a lifelong condition. It has a highly variable clinical course throughout childhood and the teenage years. In general, difficulties become less pronounced through childhood, but adolescence can be a particularly difficult time for young people with ASD, with concerns about mental health arising (most commonly, anxiety and depression). Very few longitudinal studies of prognosis have been undertaken – those that are available focus on autism as it was conceptualized when adults were diagnosed in the 1960s to 1980s, rather than ASD, as we know it today. Many adults with ASDs require lifelong full-time care. Longitudinal data from autism cohorts suggest that around 15% of adults with autism will live independent lives, whereas

15% to 20% will live alone with community support. Verbal and overall cognitive ability are the most useful predictors of ability to live independently as an adult. These very limited data will be superseded in coming years, but it will require studies of the research cohorts of the 1990s and 2000s to shed light on the 'outcomes' of children with the full range of difficulties on the autism spectrum as diagnosed using DSM-IV/ICD-10 ASD criteria.

Educational placement and liaison

One of the main outcomes for the assessment of children with ASD is informing educational placement and identifying strategies that should be used in the classroom. Some examples in which specific educational recommendations that can be promoted are given below:

- A 5-year-old male in mainstream school with previously undiagnosed ASD has an IQ of 58; this may well result in a change in his educational placement to a school with appropriate resources and educational strategies to meet his needs.
- Identifying ADHD in a young child with ASD is vital, so that medication can be commenced, to help the child to concentrate on his or her school work.
- Finding that a child with autism has average performance ability, but verbal understanding in the learning disability range, helps people understand that the child has an uneven profile of ability, and that instructions need to be differentiated within a mainstream classroom.
- Showing that a 9-year-old female with Asperger syndrome has overall average ability, but a processing speed and working memory ability at the borderline of learning disability range, explains why she is slower than expected in completing school work and homework, and why she underachieves compared with her overall ability (see Case vignette 3).

Liaising with a child's educational psychologist (if he or she has been seen by this service) and with his or her classroom teachers, learning support assistants, and the special educational needs coordinator at school is extremely useful. It is important that clinicians do not advise upon specific educational placements for children as this is an education decision; however, clinicians with considerable experience of ASD are able to suggest appropriate strategies for teaching children with ASD, identify the type of school parents might want to look for and offer advice on specific aspects of schooling that might be important for that individual child.

Educational challenges at specific ages may arise. For example, during children's early education, they initially participate in the Early Years Curriculum, which encourages free-flow play. The lack of a structured environment is enormously challenging for young children with ASD, who struggle to play and organize their play and interact with others.

Some children with significant learning disability are supported appropriately in primary school, to access the curriculum. However, for many children, moving to a secondary school educational placement which has particular experience of teaching children with ASDs and learning disability may be appropriate.

Transition from primary to secondary school is a particularly challenging time for children with ASDs.

Some useful questions (for clinicians or parents) to ask mainstream school staff on visits include the following:

- Has the school taught a child with ASD before? How did that go?
- Is there access to ASD advisory teachers? Is there a peripatetic specialist teaching service that visits the school to assess the child and provide ongoing advice to the class teacher on how to work with the child?
- Are there close links between agencies that promote social and communication skills?
- What resources will the school have to put in place the advice given around managing ASD and working with an individual child?
- Who will be responsible for differentiating the curriculum for the child?
- Is additional support needed within the school to meet the child's needs?
- Are quiet areas accessible within the school?
- Is there a use of time-out cards?
- Are mentors available for individual children?
- How is transition from one establishment to another supported?

The National Autistic Society (http://www.autism.org.uk/) has useful information about individual schools, and how children with ASD can be supported to access the curriculum and achieve their potential.

Treatment approach

The main goals of treatment are to improve social communicative functioning and cognition, to reduce anxiety and the impact of repetitive behaviours on learning and to improve behaviour generally and reduce comorbidity. A detailed description of potential interventions and medications and their effectiveness is beyond the scope of this chapter. A comprehensive review of interventions and medications is available at http://clinicalevidence.bmj.com/ceweb/conditions/.../0322_background.jsp.

Interventions

There is some evidence that 'early intervention' for children with ASD improves parent–child interaction, language outcomes and cognition. Comparative studies between interventions have not been reported and therefore there is little evidence about which interventions are best for particular children. In some educational settings, specific ASD teaching approaches are used, whilst in others a more generic teaching approach is used; as ever, the appropriate provision is dependent on the individual child. Health teams will also often have a role in identifying how ASD and cognitive ability will affect learning.

There are many intervention programmes for ASD, and there is little evidence that one of these approaches is better than another. Interventions are often delivered at home and at school and are time-consuming (up to 40 hours per week); they are expensive when undertaken by trained specialists. Funding for programmes is not always provided by statutory agencies. Robust studies about the effectiveness of some interventions are scarce; some children make little progress whilst others make considerable progress. Studies identifying which children are most likely to benefit from a particular approach is a research priority. Data about children's long-term outcome following interventions are lacking.

As with all treatment/intervention plans, potential negatives must be considered. These include the wider costs of interventions (which may not necessarily be funded through local services: parents undertake some interventions in the home). It is necessary to balance the direct financial costs, indirect costs (such as through possible lost earnings) and the impact on relationships within the family (other siblings/spouse) against the potential improvements in developmental progress and eventual outcome.

In future, there may be a role for new medications to treat aspects of ASD, or coexisting conditions (for example anxiety). New products are being developed following some evidence that ASD may be a synaptic disorder (many potentially pathogenic ASD CNVs are associated with synapse function). It is not clear which aspects of the ASD phenotype will be targeted with such drugs, and careful clinical trials will be needed to investigate their positive and adverse effects.

Interventions commonly used in the UK

- **Intensive interaction** aims to establish the early reciprocal interaction skills, communicative intent, initiating and requesting behaviours that children with ASD do not naturally have.
- **Parent-mediated intervention** such as **Early Bird or Cygnet** programmes sponsored by the National Autistic Society. Parent training programmes aim to help parents better understand their child and interact with them to improve developmental outcome. These provide parental support as well as giving parents a toolkit to help them begin to analyse their child's behaviours and help develop their communication and interaction skills.
- **Early Intensive Behavioural Intervention (EIBI) and Applied Behaviour Analysis (ABA)** are aimed at young children who may benefit from a structured programme involving cue, learned response and reward to improve learning. Some studies have shown an improvement in cognitive ability, but limited change in interaction and spontaneous communication skills.
- **'More Than Words'** (Hanen parent programme) is designed to help young children improve their social communication.
- **Treatment and Education of Autistic and related Communication handicapped Children (TEACCH)** is a structured programme that aims to improve developmental skills and thus enable children to learn. It is based on the premise that most children with autism are strong visual learners and that structure helps them to understand what is going to happen, thus reducing anxiety and promoting comprehension.
- **Picture Exchange Communication System (PECS)** is a communication system to assist children to spontaneously initiate requests and communicate their wants and needs using pictures/photographs of familiar objects (see Chapter 13).
- **Child's Talk** is a programme that aims to identify which strategies result in a particular child becoming more engaged, and communicative.
- **Early Start Denver Model** is a new developmental intervention approach that shows benefits in randomized trials.
- **Signing** is rarely used successfully with children with autism as it is an abstract approach and it is difficult for children who struggle to make sense of gesture and body language to grasp the communicative value of an arbitrary hand movement.

- Social stories are widely used to help children with ASDs to develop greater social under-standing. They take a picture format and give a short description of an event, with specific information about what to expect and why and how the individual should respond.
- SPELL is the framework used in schools run by the National Autistic Society. The acronym stands for Structure (modifying the environment and processes), Positive (approaches and expectations), Empathy (seeing the world from the perspective of a person with ASD), Low arousal (calm, ordered, predictable settings, giving time to process information), Links (between child, parents and professionals).
- Other interventions: There is no robust research evidence that nutritional supplements or the gluten and/or casein exclusion diet in particular improves features of ASDs; however, some parents think exclusion diets are effective for their child and pursue these. It is impor-tant to support parents and children to ensure that the child maintains good nutrition and a healthy weight; advice from a paediatric dietitian is advisable.

It is important for clinicians to advise parents that some interventions or medications may cause harm. Websites of mainstream autism charities or parent groups often contain information that appraise the evidence and provide expert opinion (see Research Autism website at http://www.researchautism.net/). Clinicians should advise parents to interpret anecdotal reports of effectiveness with caution.

Most funded interventions for children with ASD take an eclectic approach using elements of some or many of the above therapies. Some children with ASD are supported in mainstream schools through using these interventions, and others require placement in more specialist educational settings. The Research Autism website provides reviews on which interventions have been subject to scientific research and testing.

Medication

- ADHD symptoms in ASD require treatment; ADHD is seen as part of the child's ASD. Medication trials are appropriate, but medications are frequently less effective than in chil-dren with ADHD alone.
- Depression and anxiety require treatment through cognitive behaviour therapy (there is emerging evidence of effectiveness for some children). In children who do not respond, selective serotonin reuptake inhibitors have a treatment role.
- Irritability, challenging behaviour or aggression can be treated with risperidone; trials show some positive effects, but significant side effects such as weight gain or intolerance occur in many children.
- Some paediatricians refer to child and adolescent mental health services to assess the need for medication and supervision of that medication as regards effectiveness and adverse effects.

References

Baird G, Simonoff E, Pickles A et al. (2006) Prevalence of disorders of the autism spectrum in a population cohort of children in South Thames: the Special Needs and Autism Project (SNAP). *Lancet* 368: 210–5. http://dx.doi.org/10.1016/S0140-6736(06)69041-7

Berument SK, Rutter M, Lord C, Pickles A, Bailey A (1999) Autism screening questionnaire: diagnostic validity. *Br J Psychiatry* 175: 444–51. http://dx.doi.org/10.1192/bjp.175.5.444

Betancur C (2011) Etiological heterogeneity in autism spectrum disorders: more than 100 genetic and genomic disorders and still counting. *Brain Res* 1380: 42–77. http://dx.doi.org/10.1016/j.brainres.2010.11.078

Kim YS, Leventhal BL, Koh YJ et al. (2011) Prevalence of autism spectrum disorders in a total population sample. *Am J Psychiatry* 168: 904–12. http://dx.doi.org/10.1176/appi.ajp.2011.10101532

Le Couteur A, Lord C, Rutter M (2003) *The Autism Diagnostic Interview-Revised (ADI-R)*. Los Angeles, CA: Western Psychological Services.

Lord C, Risi S, Lambrecht L et al. (2000) The autism diagnostic observation schedule-generic: a standard measure of social and communication deficits associated with the spectrum of autism. *J Autism Dev Disord* 30: 205–23. http://dx.doi.org/10.1023/A:1005592401947

NICE (2011a) *Autism: Recognition, Referral and Diagnosis of Children and Young People on the Autism Spectrum*. London: RCOG Press. Available at: http://www.nice.org.uk/nicemedia/live/13572/56424/56424.pdf (accessed 1 November 2011).

NICE (2011b) *Quick Reference Guide. Autism: Recognition, Referral and Diagnosis of Children and Young People on the Autism Spectrum*. London: National Institute for Health and Clinical Excellence. Available at: http://www.nice.org.uk/nicemedia/live/13572/56431/56431.pdf (accessed 1 November 2011).

Further reading

Abrahams BS, Geschwind DH (2008) Advances in autism genetics: on the threshold of a new neurobiology. *Nat Rev Genet* 9: 341–55. http://dx.doi.org/10.1038/nrg2346

Amaral D, Geschwind D, Dawson G (eds) (2011) *Autism Spectrum Disorders*. New York: Oxford University Press.

Blenner S, Reddy A, Augustyn M (2011) Diagnosis and management of autism in childhood. *BMJ* 343: d6238. http://dx.doi.org/10.1136/bmj.d6238

Boelte S, Hallmayer J (eds) (2011) *International Experts Answer Questions on ASD*. Oxford: Hogrefe.

Websites

American Psychiatric Association DSM-5: http://www.dsm5.org/

Clinical Evidence: http://clinicalevidence.bmj.com/ceweb/conditions/.../0322_background.jsp

Research Autism (up to date information about interventions): http://www.researchautism.net/

UK National Autistic Society: http://www.autism.org.uk/

WHO ICD-11: http://www.who.int/classifications/icd/revision/en/index.html

28
Attention difficulties

Val Harpin

Case vignette

Ashley is 7 years old. He lives with his mother, his 11-year-old half-brother, his 4-year-old sister and a new infant. Ashley's mother feels she has always struggled with his behaviour. Now his teacher is complaining to her every day and Ashley has been sent home from school six times this term following episodes of 'silly and dangerous behaviour' in school. He seems 'quite bright' but is well below average in his academic achievement. His attention is very poor except when playing on his PlayStation. His school special educational needs coordinator has asked Ashley's mother to see their general practitioner to request further assessment.

Yesterday, he set fire to his grandmother's carpet and his mother turned up at the general practitioner surgery in a panic.

Learning points

- There are many causes of attention difficulties and a thorough history will help clarify the possible causes.
- You also need to ask about impulsivity and activity levels.
- Attention-deficit–hyperactivity disorder (ADHD) is a possible diagnosis.
- It is important to see if Ashley's behaviour changes in different environments.

Differential diagnosis

There are many reasons why a child may be having difficulty concentrating and present with difficult behaviour. Some possibilities to consider are shown in Fig. 28.1.

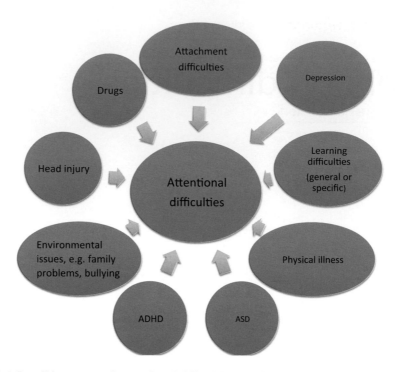

Figure 28.1 Possible causes of attentional difficulties. ADHD, attention-deficit–hyperactivity disorder; ASD, autism spectrum disorder.

Core features of hyperkinetic disorder/attention-deficit–hyperactivity disorder

Children and young people with hyperkinetic disorder (HKD)/ADHD present with

- inattention
- hyperactivity
- impulsivity.

Symptoms must be

- present before 7 years of age (this may change in DSM-5), although there is almost always evidence that they will have been there earlier
- present in more than one situation
- inappropriate for the age, sex and cognitive ability of the child

AND

- impair the child's education and/or social functioning.

How are the symptoms expressed?

The symptoms of ADHD change as the child gets older. See Table 28.1 for an outline of the key features of ADHD and their associated problems that occur within different age ranges.

Table 28.1 Key features of ADHD and common associated problems at different ages

Age	Features	Associated problems
Toddler 1–3y	Temperamental variation Hyperactive and flits between activities Limited social adaptation Less positive parent–child interaction	
Preschool 3–5y	Reduced play intensity and duration Marked hyperactivity	Developmental deficits Oppositional defiant behaviour Problems of social adaptation with family and peers
Primary school 5–11y	Distractability Motor restlessness Impulsive and disruptive behaviour	Specific learning disorders Aggressive behaviour Low self-esteem Repetition of classes Rejection by peers Impaired family relationships
Secondary school 12–17y	Persistent inattention and impulsivity Reduction of motor restlessness Difficulty planning and organizing, starting tasks and sustaining effort	Aggressive, antisocial and delinquent behaviour Alcohol and drug problems Emotional problems Accidents

ADHD is a complex developmental disorder which has been described throughout history and within medical journals since George Still first wrote about children with a 'morbid defect of moral control' in 1902 (Still 1902). The symptoms of inattention, hyperactivity and impulsivity cluster in a consistent group of individuals. Prevalence is estimated to be 3% to 5% in school-age children, with around 1% fulfilling the more stringent criteria for HKD. The symptoms of ADHD are of similar prevalence across geographical and cultural boundaries, but the degree of impairment they are perceived as causing may vary.

Aetiology

Genetics is the major factor governing whether or not a child has ADHD. It has been demonstrated using twin studies that there is between 54% and 98% heritability. *Environment* also plays a part: particular issues include maternal depression and frequent changes of carer with lack of attachment. There appears to be an interaction between genetics and environment, with environmental factors, unless extreme (e.g. Romanian orphans), maintaining or exacerbating ADHD rather than causing it.

Central nervous system injury is another contributing factor and ADHD is seen more frequently following:

- perinatal problems and preterm birth
- antenatal insults (e.g. fetal alcohol syndrome or intrauterine exposure to cigarettes and drugs)
- brain injury, especially with frontal lobe damage
- encephalitis and meningitis
- hypoxia (e.g. drowning or strangling)
- cerebrovascular accident
- chronic neurological problems (e.g. epilepsy and metabolic problems such as phenylketonuria)
- chromosomal disorders such as Williams syndrome, fragile X syndrome or Down syndrome
- neurofibromatosis and tuberous sclerosis.

It is important to consider ADHD in children with the above difficulties as ADHD symptoms may be causing the child and family major disruption and their quality of life can often be significantly improved with careful treatment.

What is the underlying problem?

The exact deficits in ADHD remain under debate but it is clear that individuals with ADHD have problems with some or all of the following executive functions:

- self-regulation
- sequencing of behaviours
- flexibility of response
- response inhibition
- planning and organization.

Pathology

Unfortunately, there is no black and white test for ADHD. As you will see, diagnosis is a combination of careful history taking, observation and data collection. In a research setting, however, differences in brain volume have been demonstrated, particularly affecting the cerebellum and frontal cortex. Functional magnetic resonance imaging shows diffuse and decreased activity in the brain when individuals with ADHD undertake tasks requiring concentration when compared with individuals without ADHD. There is abnormal handling of neurotransmitters noradrenaline and dopamine, which is supported by the response to medications affecting the release or reuptake of these neurotransmitters.

Assessment

Key questions

- Are the core problems of inattention, hyperactivity and impulsivity present?
- Is the degree of these problems inappropriate in comparison with people at a similar developmental level?
- Have symptoms been evident since before the age of 7? (This may change in DSM-5.)
- Are the symptoms evident in more than one setting, such as the home, school or workplace and other social settings?
- Is there an adverse impact on current development and psychosocial adjustment?
- Is there any evidence of other neurodevelopmental disorders and/or other mental health disorders? If so, this should not be taken as evidence for ADHD or mean that the presence of ADHD is ignored when it coexists with them.
- Is there evidence of associated secondary problems?

History

- What are the current concerns at home, out and about and at school? Ask about
  - specific examples
  - the ability to wait (looking for features of impulsivity)
  - relationships with others, both family and peers
  - the ability to follow rules
  - what the child enjoys and is good at
  - when the family first had concerns.
- Are there any risk factors?
  - antenatal and perinatal details (for risk factors)
  - developmental history including information about infancy such as feeding and temperament
  - previous medical history
  - family medical history of learning, neurological and/or mental health problems
  - also ask about cardiac problems and sudden cardiac deaths in case you decide to offer medication later.
- How is it affecting the child?
  - nursery and school progress
  - family and peer relationships.
- What is the child's current social situation?
  - Have there been changes at home?
  - Is there a history of domestic violence or involvement with social care?

Examination

Are there any associated difficulties such as

- developmental coordination disorder
- undetected hearing or vision problems
- signs of alternative diagnoses (e.g. hyperthyroidism or underlying causes such as neurofi-bromatosis, tuberous sclerosis or chromosomal anomalies)
- the child's mental state, looking for evidence of poor self-esteem, low mood or anxiety?

Also examine the child's growth parameters and cardiovascular system in case medication is indicated later.

Key message

Consider the child's developmental level and any specific difficulties which need to be taken into account when considering attention, such as specific learning difficulties, language disorder or autism spectrum disorder.

Additional information

Observation is really important. Think about how the child behaves in clinic but remember that many children may be hyperactive and flit between activities when faced with the many toys and people in paediatric clinics, and that, on the other hand, even severely affected children can concentrate for short periods of time in unusual situations.

School observation, where the child's behaviour can be seen with other children of the same age, in situations requiring concentration, sitting appropriately and following instructions, is particularly informative. In some services in the UK, structured observations are undertaken by specialist ADHD nurses. Clearly, information from the teacher is also vital.

Psychometric testing would be ideal in all children, but is not realistically available. If general or specific learning difficulties are suspected, it is essential to have some idea of the severity of these difficulties to be able to interpret the symptoms appropriately.

Structured questionnaires are also helpful to gather specific information about core ADHD symptoms and to pick up coexisting mental health or developmental difficulties. They can also demonstrate degree of severity and be used to assess treatment response. The most commonly used questionnaires in the UK currently are the Conners' Questionnaire (Conners et al. 1998) and the Strengths and Difficulties Questionnaire (Goodman 2001).

Investigations are seldom necessary but may be needed to exclude other causes of inattention such as epilepsy, hyperthyroidism, hearing impairment or drugs.

Also consider genetic testing if the child is dysmorphic, and imaging if neurofibromatosis or tuberous sclerosis is suspected.

Comorbid/coexisting conditions

Approximately 80% of individuals with ADHD have at least one comorbid/coexisting problem which needs diagnosing and treating, or at least taking into account. Fig. 28.2 shows the most commonly occurring problems and their estimated frequency.

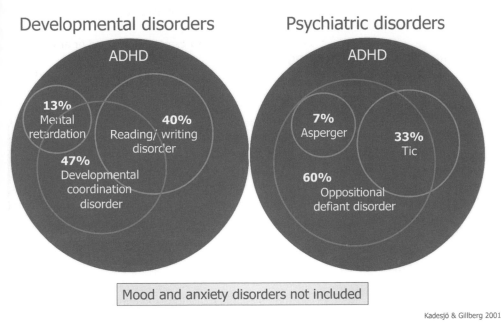

Kadesjö & Gillberg 2001

Figure 28.2 Comorbidity in attention-deficit–hyperactivity disorder (ADHD).

Management

The NICE guidelines (NICE 2008) on the assessment and management of ADHD describe best practice in the UK today.

For all families, children and young people and teachers it is really important to give verbal and written information about ADHD and how to manage it.

When planning further management we need to take into account age, severity of ADHD symptoms, degree of impairment and comorbid problems.

Preschool-age children

It is especially difficult to diagnose ADHD in preschool children. All young children have limited attention and most are very active and impulsive, so developmental norms must be taken into account. If, however, the child definitely has more problems than expected and this cannot be accounted for by other problems such as autism spectrum disorder or learning difficulties, it is important to recognize the problem and support parents appropriately to optimize future development and family relationships.

The mainstay of treatment in this age group is targeted parent management courses. Evidence shows that these should be run by trained facilitators, specific to attentional difficulties, activity levels and impulsivity, and should be around 10 sessions in length. In very severe cases medication may be considered. Evidence suggests, however, that response is likely to be less good and side effects more troublesome than in older children.

School-age children and young people

In most studies the mean age at diagnosis of ADHD is currently between 8 and 9 years. Treatment algorithms require that the clinician decides on the severity of symptoms and impairment. For mild to moderate ADHD, behaviour management is the recommended first-line treatment. Ideally, this will be in the form of group parent management sessions, again dealing specifically with parenting a child with ADHD and lasting 8 to 10 sessions. Sadly, current resource limitations make provision of this degree of support to all families difficult.

In severe ADHD, or when behavioural management has given insufficient improvement, medication is recommended. In severe ADHD medication is usually needed before behavioural management is possible.

Medication (Table 28.2)

Before commencing medication, re-examine the child's cardiovascular system and review any family history of cardiac disease or mental health difficulties.

Methylphenidate was first used to treat hyperactive, inattentive, impulsive children in 1955. It is one of the most researched medications used in childhood. Between 60% and 80% of children with ADHD are helped by methylphenidate. Stimulant medications affect the dopamine pathways in the brain. Some clinicians also use dexamphetamine.

Since 2004, atomoxetine, a noradrenaline reuptake inhibitor, has also been licensed in the UK for use in ADHD.

If these medications are ineffective, always question the diagnosis, but if ADHD is definitely considered to be the problem other medicines or combinations may be tried, but usually under the supervision of a specialist centre.

Table 28.2 Medications used to treat ADHD

Medication	Usual dose range	Length of action	Most common side effects	Advantages
Immediate-release methylphenidate	Start with 5mg twice or three times daily Titrate to maximum of 60mg per day	Up to 4h	Decreased appetite Sleep disturbance Headaches Stomachaches Drowsiness Irritability Tearfulness Mildly increased blood pressure and pulse	Useful for flexibility of dosing and as add-on to lengthen cover in the day
Sustained-release methylphenidate	10 to 108mg	8 to 12h	As for immediate release	Length of action No need for school dosing Improved adherence
Atomoxetine	Start with 0.5mg per kg and increase to maximum of 1.8mg per kg	Some action over the 24h day	Abdominal pain Nausea and vomiting Decreased appetite with associated weight loss Dizziness Slight increases in heart rate and blood pressure	Length of action No need for school dosing

Educational support

Some simple measures in the classroom can be very helpful to the child and teacher.
    These might include the following:

- Sitting the child near the teacher and away from distractions such as the door or windows.
- Giving short clear instructions and targets with small but frequent reinforcements/rewards.
- Pairing the child with a calm child who is an effective learner.
- Addressing any learning problems.

Unstructured times such as break or lunchtime can be a particular challenge, and support at these times may be very helpful indeed and help the child establish supportive peer relationships.
    Overall, at school and at home, most children with ADHD respond best to a well-structured, predictable environment with clear, consistent rules and consequences, both positive and negative, that are realistic, set out beforehand and delivered immediately.

Diet and nutrition

There is no evidence that diet can cause or cure ADHD. It is, however, possible that certain additives and even some healthy foodstuffs can exacerbate hyperactivity. If this is suspected, a careful food diary and nutritionally sound exclusion may be helpful. Low iron levels may also exacerbate difficulties and affect sleep.

Sleep

Many children and young people with ADHD and other developmental difficulties have poor sleep patterns. They often have delayed sleep onset. They describe that they cannot 'switch off'. They may also wake frequently and not be able to self-settle. Parents of children with ADHD cannot leave them awake alone as they may behave impulsively and dangerously. As a result, many children and their carers and siblings are sleep deprived, which affects behaviour and coping mechanisms in the day time. Good sleep hygiene is important. Careful use of ADHD medication may actually give a calm evening and help settling, and for some children melatonin can be very beneficial.

Transition to adult services

By age 25 years we would expect to find 0.6% to 1.2% of adults retaining the full ADHD diagnosis and 2% to 4% of adults to have ADHD in partial remission. This is consistent with population surveys in adult populations that estimate prevalence of ADHD in adults to be between 3% and 4%.

The NICE guidelines (NICE 2008) describe the need for services for diagnosis and ongoing management of ADHD in adults, and services are beginning to develop across the UK.

Table 28.3 Possible problems in children and adults with untreated or poorly treated ADHD

Childhood	Adulthood
School failure	Job failure
Underachievement	Under-employment
Multiple injuries	Fatal car accidents
	Risk taking
	Accidental injuries
Drug experimentation	Drug dependence/abuse
Oppositional defiant disorder	Criminal activity
Conduct disorder	Divorce
Impulsivity	Unwanted pregnancy
Carelessness	Sexually transmitted diseases
	Reckless driving
Repetitive failure	Hopelessness
	Frustration
	Depression
	Anxiety

> ## Key messages
>
> - It is important to consider the child's attention difficulties in relation to their level of learning difficulties.
> - Look for any underlying cause of the child's difficulties.
> - Look for any possible support.
> - Manage comorbities.

References

Conners CK, Park JDA, Sitarenios G, Epstein JN (1998) The Revised Conners' Parent Rating Scale (CPRS-R): factor structure, reliability, and criterion validity. *J Abnorm Child Psychol* 26: 257–68. http://dx.doi.org/10.1023/A:1022602400621

Goodman R (2001) Psychometric properties of the Strengths and Difficulties Questionnaire (SDQ). *J Am Child Adolesc Psychiatry* 40: 1337–45. http://dx.doi.org/10.1097/00004583-200111000-00015

NICE (2008) Attention deficit hyperactivity disorder. Diagnosis and management of ADHD in children, young people and adults [CG72]. Available at: http://guidance.nice.org.uk/CG72/QuickRefGuide/pdf/English (accessed 10 January 2013).

Still G (1902) Some abnormal physical conditions in children: the Goulstonian lectures. *Lancet* 1: 1008–12.

Further reading

Bax M, Gillberg C (2010) *Comorbidities in Developmental Disorders*. London: Mac Keith Press.

Taylor E (2007) *People with Hyperactivity: Understanding and Managing their Problems*. London: Mac Keith Press.

29
Neuromuscular disorders

Anne-Marie Childs

Learning objectives

- To outline the common neuromuscular conditions that present in childhood.
- To recognize symptoms and signs of neuromuscular disorders in children.
- To construct a plan for the investigation and management of a child with a suspected neuromuscular disorder.

Neuromuscular disorders presenting in childhood

The neuromuscular disorders are a group of conditions affecting the peripheral nervous system at any point from the anterior horn cell of the spinal cord to the muscle itself (Fig. 29.1). Overall, these conditions are rare, most are inherited and few have curative treatments. However, early diagnosis and appropriate management is essential for the individual child and their family.

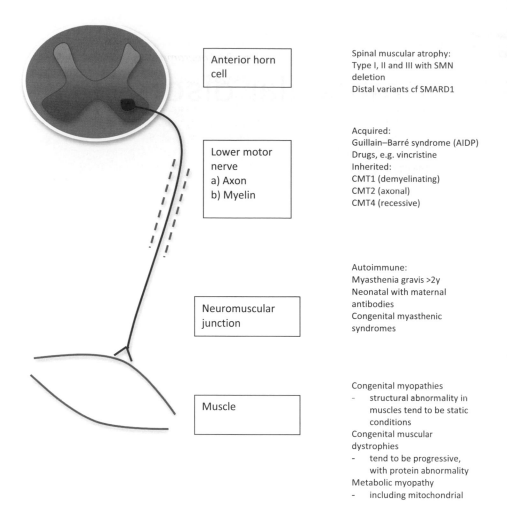

Figure 29.1. Overview of neuromuscular disorder in childhood. SMN, survival of motor neurone; SMARD1, spinal muscular atrophy with respiratory distress type 1; AIDP, acute inflammatory demyelinating polyneuropathy; CMT, Charcot–Marie–Tooth disease.

Symptoms and signs of neuromuscular disorders

The signs and symptoms of neuromuscular disorders will depend on the nature of the underlying disease, that is, which part of the peripheral nervous system is affected (muscle, nerve or neuromuscular junction), the severity of the condition and the age at presentation, with more severe conditions tending to present in younger age groups.

The most common neuromuscular disorders seen in childhood are outlined in Table 29.1.

Table 29.1 Symptoms and signs of neuromuscular disease

Age	Presentation	'Possible' neuromuscular diagnoses
Infancy	Hypotonia Reduced spontaneous movements Bulbar problems – feeding/respiratory Weakness and motor delay Contractures/eye involvement, apnoeas Mixed picture (central and peripheral signs)	SMA type I (usually presents <6mo, rarely at birth) SMA type II (usually presents <2y) Congenital myotonic dystrophy Congenital myopathy CMD (can have CNS involvement) Congenital myasthenic syndrome Transient myasthenia gravis with maternal antibodies Mitochondrial disorders Congenital neuropathies
Early childhood	Motor delay Abnormal gait and posture Frequent falls Reduced exercise tolerance and pain Affected family member Late communication	Duchenne muscular dystrophy SMA type III Congenital myopathy LGMD CMD Congenital myasthenia CMT – usually present later
Late childhood	Abnormal gait Frequent falls Pain/cramps Reduced exercise tolerance Foot deformity Recurrent chest infections Double vision/ptosis	Becker muscular dystrophy CMT SMA type III Congenital myopathies LGMD Facioscapuloperoneal dystrophy Collagen-related dystrophies and other CMD Myasthenia gravis Metabolic myopathies/channelopathies

SMA, spinal muscular atrophy; CMD, congenital muscular dystrophy; CNS, central nervous system; LGMD, limb girdle dystrophies; CMT, Charcot–Marie–Tooth disease.

Key points for assessing infants

- Assessment of infants is not easy, especially if the infant is unwell. Have a low threshold for seeking a second opinion before making judgements (and ordering tests).
- Weakness, judged by observation of antigravity movements in different positions, is the most useful sign suggesting neuromuscular disease. Tendon reflexes are difficult to elicit except at the knee, and tongue fasciculation can be absent in spinal muscular atrophy (SMA).
- Remember that about 80% of floppy infants will have a central problem, not a neuromuscular disorder
- Do not forget Prader–Willi syndrome in a very floppy infant. DNA methylation studies, now widely available, will identify 90% of cases.
- Creatinine kinase is elevated in 'normal' infants in the immediate postnatal period, so defer testing if possible.

- Facial muscles are relatively well preserved in SMA type 1; consider other diagnoses if facial weakness is a prominent feature.

Common neuromuscular disorders presenting in childhood

Dystrophinopathy

The dystrophin-related muscle diseases are still the most common neuromuscular disorders encountered in the UK, with an incidence of 1 in 3500 liveborn males. Duchenne muscular dystrophy and Becker muscular dystrophy were originally described as separate clinical entities, but we now recognize Duchenne and Becker muscular dystrophy as being part of a spectrum of dystrophin-related muscular dystrophy. An intermediate phenotype and a milder form of disease, with pain and cramps but no weakness, can also result from a mutation in the dystrophin gene at Xp21.

The severity of the condition is related to the quantity of functional dystrophin in the muscle and is, to a certain extent, related to the underlying genetic abnormality, with most 'out-of-frame' deletions (those resulting in a reading frameshift) being associated with a more severe Duchenne muscular dystrophy picture and 'in-frame' deletions resulting in a Becker muscular dystrophy phenotype (see Fig. 29.2).

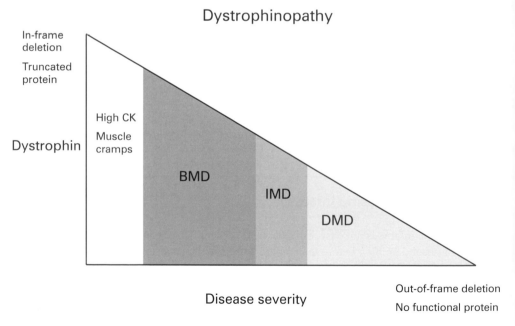

Figure 29.2 Spectrum of dystrophin-related dystrophies. CK, creatine kinase; BMD, Becker muscular dystrophy; IMD, intermediate muscular dystrophy; DMD, Duchenne muscular dystrophy.

There are, however, exceptions to this rule and dystrophin gene testing alone does not allow accurate prognosis. Clinical assessment is very important and further testing with muscle biopsy may be required. Children with Duchenne muscular dystrophy classically present with difficulty running and climbing as toddlers. Only those with significant global delay present with delayed walking (see Chapter 7). The clinical features of the condition are outlined in Table 29.2.

Table 29.2 Comparison of Duchenne and Becker phenotypes

	Duchenne muscular dystrophy	*Becker muscular dystrophy*
Age at presentation	Typically 3–5y Or Second year with global delay (delayed walking)	Variable but later in childhood from 8–13y, unless significant delay
Symptoms at presentation	Difficulty running, odd gait, Gower manoeuvre Fatigue	Reduced exercise tolerance Milder proximal weakness Muscle pain/cramp may be prominent and only feature
Discriminating signs on examination	Unable to hop >7y Unable to hold head up in supine over edge of bed/couch	Able to hop >8y Able to maintain antigravity neck flexion in supine
Other features (Dystrophin expressed in brain/heart/eye)	Associated IQ shift to left Characteristic cognitive profile – difficulty with complex verbal information Increased risk of attentional/behavioural problems	Associated with some IQ difficulties, usually mild, non-progressive Similar cognitive/behavioural profile to *Duchenne muscular dystrophy*
Pattern of progression	Steady decline	Slowly progressive, but often relatively stable in childhood
Loss of ambulation	Untreated (no steroids) mean 10.5y, range 8–13y	Wider variability 17–60y, mean 40y
Survival	Mean now third decade, reduced if early-onset cardiomyopathy	Most have good life expectancy, but early cardiac death occurs
Respiratory impairment	Inevitable in second decade, recurrent infection and hypoventilation, most require ventilator support by 20y	Unusual and mirrors skeletal muscle weakness
Cardiomyopathy	Early ECG change and sinus tachycardia <10y All develop dilated cardiomyopathy in time, some in second decade	Most will develop DCM with time, not related to degree of skeletal muscle weakness

ECG, electrocardiography; DCM, dilated cardiomyopathy.

There is still no definitive treatment for dystrophin-related muscular dystrophy, although there are encouraging phase II clinical trials under way in Duchenne muscular dystrophy. The Treat-NMD website (www.treat-nmd.eu) is a useful resource for keeping up with research developments in Duchenne muscular dystrophy and other neuromuscular disorders.

Management is largely supportive and requires the involvement of a large multidisciplinary team and access to specialist neuromuscular services and advice. The aim, as with all neuromuscular disorders, is to promote independence, inclusion and well-being by offering appropriate support and equipment, minimizing secondary complications and providing timely symptomatic treatments. In 2010, several international groups produced a consensus statement on the 'Standards of Care in Diagnosis and Management of Duchenne Muscular Dystrophy' (Bushby et al. 2010a,b).

Corticoteroids have been shown to improve muscle strength and function in Duchenne muscular dystrophy, although there are still questions as to the best dose regimes and the benefits or otherwise of long-term treatment. Initiation and monitoring of steroid treatment in the UK is done in a standardized manner and led by the neuromuscular centres that are part of the 'North Star' neuromuscular consortium. The long-awaited FOR-DMD study is a randomized double-blind multicentre study that aims to identify the optimal steroid regime.

PRACTICAL POINTS FOR MANAGEMENT OF DYSTROPHIN MUSCULAR DYSTROPHY IN CLINICAL PRACTICE

- A normal creatinine kinase in an ambulant child excludes the diagnosis of Duchenne and Becker muscular dystrophy.
- Males may present with delayed acquisition of communication skills and motor skills.
- A child who has suspected Duchenne muscular dystrophy needs to be referred to a specialist neuromuscular centre for diagnosis and ongoing specialist management.
- Routine DNA testing will pick up 65% to 70% of individuals who have deletion or duplication, but not those with point mutations.
- About 30% of cases are the result of spontaneous mutations.
- Females 'carrying' the mutation may present as 'manifesting carriers' with similar difficulties.
- Mothers who 'carry' the condition (two-thirds of cases) have a 10% to 15% incidence of cardiomyopathy, even in the absence of any other symptoms.
- The local disability/community paediatrician has a key role in management:
  - integrating local and specialist services in health, education and social services
    - updating/supporting parent-held care plans
  - monitoring nutrition and general health
  - providing support/advice for acute medical crises:
    - emergency steroid doses
    - ensuring avoidance of certain anaesthetic agents and alerting to risk of malignant hyperpyrexia (there is an association)
    - fracture management:
      - optimizing vitamin D and bone health
      - ensuring treatment that promotes early mobilization to avoid losing independent mobility
    - respiratory care:
      - facilitating rapid assessment (possible with an open access policy) for respiratory failure and access to suitable support

- encouraging active secretion management and early antibiotic use
- immunization against seasonal influenza
- some units will have paediatric respiratory physiotherapists that offer a home-based outreach service.

Spinal muscular atrophy

There are several different conditions within this category. The most common 'classic' SMA affects 1 in 5000 to 7000 live births. It is an autosomal recessive disease caused by deletion of exons 7 and 8 of the survival motor neurone (*SMN1*) gene, located on chromosome 5q. There is a spectrum of disease that results from the same deletion, as outlined in Fig. 29.3. Those with less severe presentations have a greater number of *SMN2* gene copies. *SMN2* codes for a less functional form of the SMN protein.

Spinal muscular atrophy is characterized by proximal muscle weakness and fasciculation may be present (see Chapter 6 on the floppy infant). The disease is always progressive but the rate of progression varies among individuals. Cognitive abilities are well preserved in all cases. Life expectancy is dependent on the extent of respiratory impairment (secondary to diaphragmatic and respiratory muscle weakness). The ongoing **SMArtnet project** (www.muscular-dystrophy.org/how_we_help_you/for_professionals/clinical_databases) aims to define the natural history by collecting standardized follow-up assessments.

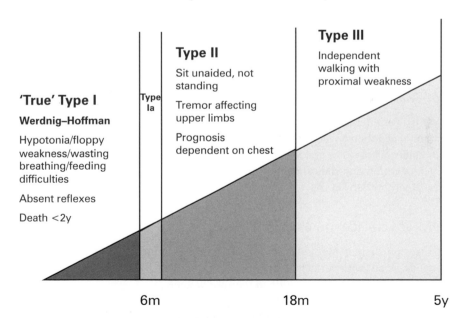

Clinical spectrum in SMA5q

Age at presentation and number of SMN2 copies

Figure 29.3 Spectrum of presentation in spinal muscular atrophy (SMA).

There is no curative treatment for SMA and management principles are similar to those for other neuromuscular disorders. Again, the Treat-NMD website (www.treat-nmd.eu) is a useful source of information on up-to-date research. An international consensus statement on 'Standards of Care' for the management of all types of SMA, was produced in 2007 (Wang et al. 2007). One of the most ethically challenging areas is the management of infants with SMA type 1. Following a series of high-profile cases, a UK workshop was held to consider how to implement the 'Standards of Care' in SMA type 1 (Roper et al. 2010).

KEY POINTS FOR SMA

1   Consider SMA in an infant presenting with a severe chest infection. Do not forget to ask about motor development and to carry out a clinical assessment.
2   A coarse upper limb tremor in a bright child who can sit but does not weight bear is a useful pointer to diagnosis of SMA type II. The tremor is a manifestation of muscle fasciculation.
3   Absent reflexes are a useful early sign but can be present in children with SMA type III.
4   All children should be referred to specialist neuromuscular centres, although discussion and advice may be appropriate for infants with type 1 SMA.
5   Recurrent chest infections are usually the first sign of respiratory difficulties as expiratory muscles are more affected than inspiratory muscles.
    (a)   Secretion clearance is very important and mechanical techniques may be required such as a cough insufflator/exsufflator (cough assist) machine or the use of bilevel positive airway pressure mask ventilation.
    (b)   Watch out for compounding factors such as aspiration, secondary to bulbar weakness. Consider referral to a speech and language therapist and videofluroscopy.
6   Other forms of SMA are rare. There are phenotypes associated with pontocerebellar hypoplasia type II, a form with distal weakness and respiratory distress (spinal muscular atrophy with respiratory distress type 1), as well as others.

Charcot–Marie–Tooth disease

Most inherited peripheral neuropathies present in adult life; the overall incidence is 1 in 5000. Presentation in childhood occurs when the phenotype is particularly severe or on the basis of a positive family history. The genotype–phenotype correlation in the inherited neuropathies is generally poor with many clinical phenotypes resulting from mutations in the same gene and vice versa (Reilly and Shy 2009).

KEY POINTS FOR CHARCOT–MARIE–TOOTH DISEASE

- Most cases of Charcot–Marie–Tooth disease are demyelinating (CMT1) and inherited in dominant fashion, with variable penetrance. The majority of those patients with a positive family history will have a duplication in the *PMP22* gene.
- Axonal variants (CMT2) are rare and can be severe in childhood.
- CMT4, recessive forms, are more prevalent in certain ethnic groups and often have associated features.
- The main symptoms of Charcot–Marie–Tooth disease are
  - foot deformity and poor balance with frequent falls

- reduced exercise tolerance
- muscle/foot pain in absence of weakness
- problems restricted to the lower limbs in the majority of patients, with reduced hand function causing problems only in adult life
- initial pes planus and joint hypermobility, which then evolves into the more classic pattern
- absent tendon reflexes with good muscle power
- congenital dysplasia of the hip is more common.

- Sensory evaluation of children with CMT is difficult. Use the Romberg sign and history. Advise parents about monitoring for injury.
- Diagnosis is usually confirmed by nerve conduction studies and EMG, though this can be difficult in younger children. There is also an 'intermediate' phenotype with demyelination and axonal loss.
- Genetics can be useful in familial cases, though ethical difficulties exist and also funding difficulties for presymptomatic testing.
- Surgical intervention should be considered only after careful multidisciplinary team assessment in a specialist centre.
- Management is supportive. The CMT Association is a useful resource (www.cmt.org.uk/).

Other neuromuscular disorders

A detailed discussion is outside the scope of this text; however, there are some useful points to remember.

1 It is particularly important not to miss 'treatable' conditions such as the myasthenic syndromes, myotonia congenita and other channelopathies.
   (a) Consider myasthenia if there is involvement of extraocular muscles/ptosis.
   (b) Relatively brisk tendon reflexes with a history of fatigue can be a clue to myasthenia.
   (c) Consider channelopathies with fluctuating symptoms or when weakness follows particular triggers such as cold and eating.
2 (a) Scoliosis can be the first presenting symptom of a neuromuscular disorder (see Chapter 11).
   (b) Management of scoliosis will depend on the underlying condition and function of the individual patient.
   (c) Spinal curves due to neuromuscular disorders can progress after puberty. Maintaining standing (including in standing frame) through pubertal growth spurt can minimize the degree of curvature.
   (d) Progression of neuromuscular scoliosis cannot be 'controlled' by a spinal jacket, though one can improve seating and trunk control allowing better upper limb function.
   (e) Treatment is surgical, but should be considered only in specialist neuromuscular centres after careful assessment by a multidisciplinary team.
3 Myopathies associated with spinal rigidity can present with early and relatively silent respiratory failure as a consequence of diaphragmatic weakness disproportionate to other skeletal muscles.
   (a) Symptoms of nocturnal hypoventilation are often non-specific. The patient may have general day-time fatigue, but ask about morning headaches, grogginess and lack of appetite and night-time breathing pattern.

(b) Ask specifically about functional motor skills such as the patient's ability in physical education, climbing stairs, or running for the bus, as ambulation may be relatively normal.

4 If in doubt, refer the patient for specialist neuromuscular assessment.

Diagnostic strategy for suspected neuromuscular disorders

Consider the case of a 2½-year-old male who presents with delayed walking (see Chapter 7).

The first step is a detailed history and examination, as outlined in previous chapters. Following this it should be possible to identify whether the child has an underlying disorder, either central or peripheral. The next steps in investigating a suspected neuromuscular disorder are outlined in Fig. 29.4.

If there is uncertainty about the nature of the disorder, early referral to a specialist centre should take place before tests are ordered. Keep families informed as to the timeframe for investigations and onward referral, but defer providing information about specific neuromuscular conditions until the diagnosis is certain. Ideally, the specialist neuromuscular team should give the diagnosis when members of the multidisciplinary team can provide appropriate support and counselling.

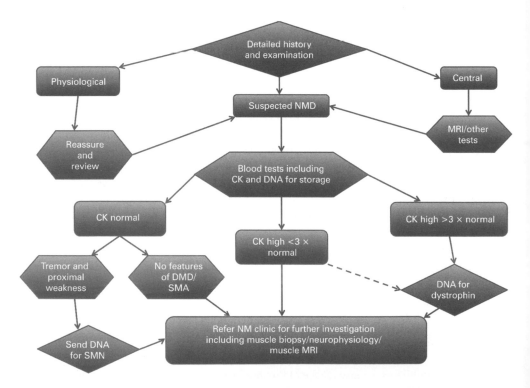

Figure 29.4 Schema for investigation of suspected neuromuscular disorder. NMD, neuromuscular disorder; CK, creatine kinase; DMD, Duchenne muscular dystrophy; SMA, spinal muscular atrophy; SMN, survival motor neurone; NM, neuromuscular.

Key points

- If in doubt refer the patient for specialist neuromuscular assessment.
- Keep families informed as to the timeframe of investigations.
- Keep information general until a specific diagnosis is confirmed.

Key messages

- Neuromuscular disorders, although individually rare, are an important cause of disability and functional impairment in childhood.
- It is important to recognize features that suggest a neuromuscular disorder and to have a structured approach to assessment.
- Despite a lack of curative treatments, making a specific diagnosis is essential for accurate prognosis, ongoing management and genetic counselling regarding the risk of recurrence.
- Neuromuscular disorders are often associated with other problems outside the skeletal muscle which have significant impacts on overall well-being and health (cardiac, respiratory, etc.).
- Management is complex and requires a coordinated multiprofessional approach between the specialist neuromuscular centre and local services.

References

Bushby K, Finkel R, Birnkrandt DJ et al. (2010a) Diagnosis and management of Duchenne muscular dystrophy: part 1; diagnosis, pharmacological and psychosocial management. *Lancet Neurol* 9: 77–93. http://dx.doi.org/10.1016/S1474-4422(09)70271-6

Bushby K, Finkel R, Birnkrandt DJ et al. (2010b) Diagnosis and management of Duchenne muscular dystrophy: part 2; implementation of multidisciplinary care. *Lancet Neurol* 9: 177–89. http://dx.doi.org/10.1016/S1474-4422(09)70272-8

Reilly M, Shy ME (2009) Diagnosis and new treatments in genetic neuropathies. *J Neurol Neurosurg Psychiatry* 80: 1304–14. http://dx.doi.org/10.1136/jnnp.2008.158295

Roper H, Quinlivan R, Workshop Participants (2010) Implementation of 'the Consensus Statement for Standards Care in spinal muscular atrophy' when applied to infants with severe type 1 SMA in the UK. *Arch Dis Child* 95: 845–9. http://dx.doi.org/10.1136/adc.2009.166512

Wang CH, Finkel RS, Bertini ES et al. (2007) Consensus statement for standards of care in spinal muscular atrophy. *J Child Neurol* 22: 1027–49. http://dx.doi.org/10.1177/0883073807305788

Further reading

Websites

Neuromuscular Disease Centre, Washington University: http://neuromuscular.wustl.edu

Treat-NMD: www.treat-neuromusculard.eu

30
Acquired brain injury

Gillian Robinson

An acquired brain injury (ABI) is an injury caused to the brain any time after birth. It has several causes but the broad distinctions are traumatic and non-traumatic.

Learning objectives

- To consider the causes of acquired brain injury and how the site and severity of injury lead to different rehabilitation challenges.
- To identify treatments that help with rehabilitation.
- To understand the long-term difficulties that these children face.
- To identify factors affecting outcome for traumatic brain injury.

Case vignette

Brendan is an 11-year-old boy who was a keen footballer. He was involved in a road traffic accident aged 10 years whilst walking home from school with his mother. This led to mild left-sided weakness and visual field loss, from which he has largely made a good recovery. After some initial difficulties in settling back into primary school, no major concerns were raised. However, Brendan struggled with his football skills and never got back into his team. He has just progressed to high school, and both parents and school have been on the phone saying 'everything is terrible'. When you talk to the school they were unaware of Brendan's previous difficulties.

Learning points

Children can make a good physical recovery and it may be some time before the cognitive impact becomes apparent.

Non-traumatic brain injury is the most common cause of acquired brain injury in childhood, as demonstrated in Table 30.1.

Table 30.1 Causes of acquired brain injury in childhood

	Specific subgroups	Frequency (%)	Per cent of children needing rehabilitation
Traumatic brain injury			
Trauma	Road traffic accident	21	1–2/1000 A&E attendances 5/100 000 ICU admission (mortality of 10%)
	Fall or assault including non-accidental injury, e.g. shaking injury	11	
Non-traumatic brain injury			
Tumour	Direct tumour effects Neurosurgery effects Radiotherapy effects	17	Non-traumatic coma causing ICU admission is 30/100 000 (mortality of 30%)
Stroke		24	
Hypoxic–anoxic brain injury	Cardiac arrest Near drowning Poisoning (e.g. carbon monoxide)	6	
Infections	Meningitis Encephalitis	14	
Encephalopathy		4	
Other		3	

A&E, accident and emergency; ICU, intensive care unit.

Site of injury

The brain is able to make a better recovery from focal damage (e.g. secondary to trauma) than from diffuse damage, such as axonal damage in shaking injuries. Table 30.2 summarizes the difficulties that can be seen as a consequence of different areas of focal damage

Table 30.2 Relationship between area of brain damage and disability

Area	Functional difficulties
Frontal lobe	Planning and organizing(executive functions) Thinking Personality Emotions Behavioural control
Motor cortex (front of cingulate gyrus)	Movement initiation
Sensory cortex (behind cingulate gyrus)	Sensations
Parietal lobe	Perceptions Arithmetic Spelling
Occipital lobe	Vision
Temporal lobe	Memory Understanding language
Cerebellum	Coordination and balance, attention, visual–spatial
Basal ganglia	Coordination
Hippocampus	Memory problems

Severe brain injury: rehabilitation

Early management

During the early stages the aims are to decrease the factors that are contributing to secondary damage, such as hypoxia, raised intracranial pressure and seizures, to allow resolution of oedema and haemorrhage. In addition, attention needs to be given to nutrition and good nursing care. Early management will involve the following:

- Intensive care to manage intracranial pressure including respiratory support.
- Neurosurgery if there is significant intracranial haematoma.
- The management of seizures.
- The prevention of contractures by providing
  - good positioning and splinting
  - early mobilization
  - medications for the control of spasm and evolving dystonia: use baclofen and consider botulinum toxin and intrathecal baclofen.
- The management of agitation by
  - modifying the environment – low stimulation
  - good pain and bowel management
  - occasionally providing propranolol or a stimulant.
- Good nutrition:
  - The development of an appropriate feeding strategy. Remember that gastro-oesophageal reflux and constipation are common.

- Assess bulbar function when appropriate.
- Assess neuroendocrine function as a result of pituitary and hypothalamic damage, particularly thinking about diabetes insipidus.

Medium-term management

At this point medical stability is achieved and ongoing neurological damage becomes apparent. Problems around fatigue and motivation can be significant at this time. During this phase the aims are

- **Medical**
  - To continue to ensure good nutrition.
  - To manage seizures if needed.
  - To consider post-traumatic hydrocephalus (3% of children with contusion or subdural haematoma).
  - To ensure appropriate analgesia, remembering that headaches are common.
  - To assess hearing and vision to understand and ameliorate any deficits.
- **Rehabilitation**
  - Rehabilitation needs to be planned and taken slowly because of fatigue, but with steadily increasing activity.
  - Restore function by therapy, for example physiotherapy to enable sitting, standing and walking.
  - Enable participation, for example through the use of a wheelchair or communication aid.
  - To have a goal-orientated therapy programme, focusing on participation by encouraging the child to say 'I want to . . .' and professionals can then say 'we can help with . . .'
  - To ensure that the child has a method of communication. Communication problems are common – both expressive problems with speech and articulation are easily recognized but more subtle changes in understanding and word finding may be easier to miss; therefore, have a low threshold to consider the need for a communication assessment. Appropriate communication aids can address this and can lead to a more motivated and less frustrated young person.
  - Rehabilitation will be started by a multidisciplinary team in the regional neurology centre. There needs to be good links with local therapy services for effective rehabilitation as the child progresses to the local centre and then home.
- **Education**
  - To assess cognitive difficulties and arrange early and appropriate education.
  - To maintain the links the child or young person has with peers.
  - To help with the phased integration of the child or young person back into school.
- **Family**
  - To support the family as a complete unit. Think about emotional support as the family face the emotional trauma of the effects of the injury as well as practical support to deal with issues around work, finances and having a child in hospital.

Discharge planning – start early

For children with complex difficulties you should organize a multiagency meeting inviting

1   The young person and if appropriate their family.
2   The medical team: both hospital and community.
3   The therapy team including social care and occupational therapy if adaptations are needed.
4   The nursing team including the community nursing team if issues around training or ongoing nursing care are apparent.
5   Staff from the child's school.
6   Social care.
7   A housing representative if the individual is in rented accommodation and adaptations are needed.
8   A lead for continuing care if required.

Ensure that the professionals who attend have completed appropriate assessments and have an understanding of how their services will be budgeted.

Points to consider

- **The home**
  - Adaptations: are any adaptations needed? These can take time to complete.
  - Equipment: what is needed, who is going to provide it and who is going to pay for it?
  - Training: do the parents have any training needs?
- **Education**
  - Is the school aware of the child's accident, current function and if the child is likely to have ongoing functional difficulties?
  - Are any adaptations needed?
  - Have realistic timeframes been set in order to recruit and train any carers?
  - Has funding been applied for?
  - Ensure a phased entry.
  - Is there a plan to catch up on the work the child has missed (if appropriate)?
- **Children's services**
  - Level of therapy and nursing support.
  - Is there agreement about responsibility for the child following discharge?
- **Family**
  - Is there any additional equipment needed for safe transport?
  - Has the family received information about appropriate benefits?
  - Is there ongoing support available to the parents and family?
- **Review**
  - Has a date been set for a regular review of the support package?
  - Is there a clear timeline for discharge planning including home visits of increasing length.
- **Keyworker and lead professional**
  - Appoint a person who will be a link and first point of contact for the family. This person may be, initially, a ward nurse or family support worker; over time and as the child's individual situation progresses responsibility may transfer to the school special needs coordinator. The lead professional will usually be the named consultant paediatrician.

(Council for Disabled Children 2010)

Long-term management

Medical/physical difficulties

Physical difficulties relate to the extent and site of the cerebral damage, and also at times to other injuries that occurred at the time of the accident. Possible medical/physical difficulties include the following:

- Movement difficulties: immediate post-traumatic ataxia is common and often resolves. Ongoing difficulties can include weakness, spasticity, tremor, myoclonus, dystonia through to mild coordination difficulties.
- Sensory problems: subtle visual problems, field defects, hearing loss.
- Epilepsy: the risk of epilepsy increases with the severity of injury. Penetrating injuries, intra-cranial haemorrhages and seizures in the first week after the trauma are known risk factors. The seizures are most commonly focal and they will remit in 50% of cases.
- Continence: loss of bladder or bowel control.
- The development of later-onset endocrine problems, particularly precocious puberty.
- Headache and fatigue.

Cognitive difficulties

Cognitive difficulties may not be immediately obvious as children and parents can be delighted with the child's improving physical skills. In addition, 'allowances are made' as the child has had a serious incident, and there is the hope that the child will improve later. It may take time to appreciate that the child is failing to gain skills – often around 2 to 3 years post injury. Furthermore, in young children some of these skills would not normally be present and it takes until adolescence to see the full impact. Cognitive difficulties include the following:

- A reduced speed of processing of visual and verbal information, meaning that the child needs a longer thinking time and may have slower motor or verbal responses. This can hugely affect a child's life, in particular social relationships and education.
- Poor attention and concentration and high distractibility. Treatment with methylphenidate can improve this.
- Visuoperceptual and spatial problems, which can present with
  - untidy work
  - a decline or difficulties in gaining writing and drawing skills
  - impaired constructional skills
  - poor skills in sports and gymnastics.
- Memory and learning problems, particularly in the ability to learn and retain new information, to integrate this into the existing knowledge base and to generalize what has been learnt to new situations.
- Higher-level language difficulties so that children may have problems processing complex and abstract ideas, making inferences or understanding ambiguity.
- Problems with executive skills such as goal setting, systematic planning and initiating.
- Problems with organizing and executing plans to reach the desired goal. There may be difficulties in evaluating the viability of goals and monitoring progress.

Behavioural difficulties

Even prior to the injury this group of children appear to have more behavioural difficulties than their peers, largely around impulsivity and attention, which may well contribute to the initial accident. After the injury behavioural difficulties are around three times as common in children with severe head injury. Behavioural difficulties include the following:

* Poor attention and concentration.
* Increased irritability, anger and temper tantrums. In the first year post injury this is associated with social class and pre-injury problems and family functioning. By 2 years post injury it relates to injury severity.
* Disinhibited behaviour which can be verbal, physical and, very occasionally, sexual. This causes the greatest concerns for families and teachers.
* Lethargy and inertia.

Emotional difficulties

* Depression may occur as the child adjusts to his or her new level of function, for example the effect of physical difficulties, loss of academic potential and loss of friendships as a consequence of the brain injury. Clearly, the family's response will impact on this.
* Anxiety may also occur and is often related to loss of skills and to children feeling that they are less able to cope with school or life in general. This is often against a background where they are expected to catch up and keep up with their school work.
* Post-traumatic stress disorder due to memory of the accident in which they may not have been the only victim.
* Grief where an accident involves the loss of significant others.

Interaction of impairments

In order to understand the impact of an injury on a child there are multiple factors to take into account:

* premorbid personality
* family strengths and difficulties
* injury and severity
* sequelae – physical, sensory, cognitive and emotional
* having a well-resourced local rehabilitation team.

Traumatic brain injury

Traumatic brain injury is the most common cause of death in childhood, causing 30% of deaths in children aged 0 to 5 years and 70% in children aged 5 to 15 years. It is more common in males (3–4:1). Although most accidents occur in the home, they rarely cause serious brain injury, which is more commonly due to traffic accidents, assault or falls.

Factors that affect outcome include the following:

- *The severity of the injury (see Table 30.3)*
  The injury may be caused by direct trauma leading to fracture, laceration, contusion or shearing. It can also be caused by indirect trauma secondary to ischaemic brain damage, extra- or subdural blood or raised intracranial pressure.
- *Duration since the injury*
  There can be improvement until 2 years following the injury, though most of the recovery occurs in the first 6 months.
- *Age at time of injury*
  In the past we thought that younger children 'did better' as there is more plasticity in younger brains, so that the brain is better able to 're-wire' itself by altering dendritic synapses, which can lead to areas taking on other functions. Against this is the ongoing process of development in younger children. Often after head injury, skills that have been learned can be maintained, but learning new skills post injury can be difficult for some children. This means, for injuries occurring early in childhood, that there are many core skills to gain. The rate of gain is key: is the child able to make a year's progress every year? Clearly, if the rate of gain is slightly slower over many years the impact is significant. This could well explain why children can make good physical recoveries but can struggle with language and even more so with cognitive skills that would be less developed at the time of injury for children in early childhood.
- *Premorbid difficulties*
  Thirty per cent of children with head injuries have pre-existing learning difficulties, which may well predispose the child to having an accident.

Table 30.3 Classifying injury severity

	Loss of consciousness	Post-traumatic amnesia	Frequency
Mild	<15min	<1h	200/100 000
Moderate	15min–6h	1–24h	
Severe	6–48h	24h–7d	5/100 000
Very severe	>48h	>7d	mortality on ICU approximately 10%

ICU, intensive care unit.

Minor brain injury

Minor brain injury can lead to longer-term sequelae even when there is no demonstrable brain damage. The most commonly reported symptom is fatigue but others include

- physical difficulties – headaches and dizziness
- cognitive difficulties – attention, memory planning, organizing, concentration and word-finding problems

- emotional and behavioural difficulties – irritability.

In the case of mild head injury, these difficulties usually last around 2 weeks but can go on for up to 3 months. Following moderate head injuries, similar problems continue for up to 6 to 9 months. Understanding and a paced approached to living are the most practical solutions.

Key messages

- In both traumatic and non-traumatic brain injury the impact of the injury may take a long time to be recognized.
- Unrecognized learning difficulties are common and can often be dealt with informally in a supportive primary school.
- The impact of the brain injury may not be immediately revealed, as is demonstrated, for example, in the case vignette, which describes a child who is no longer in the school football team because of problems with motor, vision and attention skills.
- High school requires a greater level of planning and organizational skills.
- Good communication is key to supporting children, particularly at the time of transitions.
- The home environment may be a positive or negative factor in recovery.

References

Council for Disabled Children (2010). Guidelines on the discharge from hospital of children and young people with high support needs. Available at: http://www.ncb.org.uk/cdc/TertiaryCareFINALmk3.pdf (accessed 1 November 2012).

Further reading

Forsyth R (2010) Back to the future: rehabilitation of children after brain injury. *Arch Dis Child* 95: 554–9. http://dx.doi.org/10.1136/adc.2009.161083

Macgregor D, Kulkarni A, Dirks P et al. (2007) *Head Injury in Childhood and Adolescence*. London: Mac Keith Press.

Middleton JA (2001) Brain injury in children and adolescents. *Adv Psychiatr Treat* 7: 257–65. http://dx.doi.org/10.1192/apt.7.4.257

NICE (2007) Head injury: Triage, Assessment, Investigation and Early Management of Head Injury in Infants, Children and Adults [CG56]. Available at: www.nice.org.uk/cg56 (accessed 10 January 2013).

Websites

Child Brain Injury Trust: http://www.childbraininjurytrust.org.uk

Headway: www.headway.org.uk

31

Spinal cord disorders and hydrocephalus in children

Arnab Seal

Learning objectives

- To understand the functional effects of congenital malformation or acquired damage at various spinal levels.
- To know how to assess and manage spinal dysraphism and neural tube defects (NTDs).
- To know how to assess and manage children with acquired spinal injury.

Anatomy

The spinal cord connects the brain with the peripheral nervous system. Understanding the anatomy of the spinal connections can help with diagnosis and therapy of spinal cord disorders (Fig. 31.1).

The afferent nerves of the peripheral nervous system carry information from the skin, joints, muscle and visceral organs to the spinal cord. The ascending columns of nerve fibres relay the information to various regions of the brain which process and modulate the information. In turn, the brain sends efferent signals down through the descending tracts to the anterior horn cells (AHCs) in the spinal cord. The AHCs form the efferent nerves which carry instructions to the periphery. The vast majority of fibres in the ascending and descending tracts cross the midline at various levels (contralateral supply). Some afferent nerves carrying pain and temperature cross over at their level of entry to the spinal cord. Other fibres carrying touch and proprioception cross after reaching the brainstem. A small proportion of descending nerve tracts from the brain remain uncrossed and supply AHCs on the same side (ipsilateral supply), but the vast majority cross in the brainstem to the lateral corticospinal tracts. Therefore, there is a combination of crossed and uncrossed nerve tracts at the spinal level resulting in bilateral innervation of both afferent and efferent pathways. In addition to ascending and descending tracts, there are some connections at the spinal level between the afferent and efferent fibres, which form the basis for the spinal reflex.

The spinal cord is housed in a bony canal (vertebral canal) formed by intercalating vertebrae which form the spinal column. The body of the vertebrae lie in front of the spinal cord, the lateral arches to the side and the spinal processes to the back. The spinal cord is covered by meninges and in the centre has a fluid-filled canal, the spinal canal. The spinal canal communicates upwards with the fourth ventricle of the brain above the foramen magnum. The ascending, descending and intraspinal tracts are organized as shown in Fig. 31.1. An understanding of the organization and function of the tracts is helpful in working out the likely clinical effects of any cord lesion and, conversely, allows a clinical estimation of the level of lesion.

The spinal cord terminates in the cauda equina (horse's tail), comprising a bunch of nerve fibres, each of which leaves through the spinal foramina lower down. The cord terminates at the L3 level in infants but is at a higher L1/L2 level in adults. This difference happens because the spine grows faster and for a longer period than the spinal cord. Any congenital condition tethering the cord to the spine can lead to a gradual traction on the spinal cord tracts as the child grows, resulting in spinal symptoms.

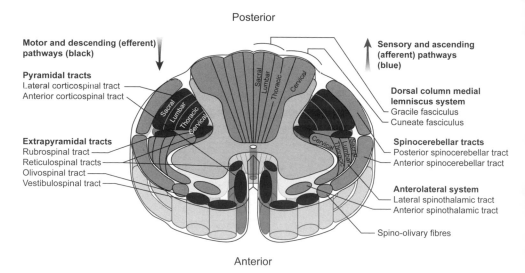

Figure 31.1 Spinal cord section showing ascending sensory (blue) and descending motor (black) tracts.

Signs and symptoms of spinal cord dysfunction

The clinical symptoms of any spinal cord lesion (Table 31.1) are dependent on

1   the spinal level;
2   whether it is affecting the whole cross-section of the cord or only a part of it;
3   whether it is an acute presentation (stage of 'spinal shock' for first few days);
4   the underlying cause.

Table 31.1 Clinical symptoms and signs of spinal cord lesions

Extramedullary lesion and external compression, e.g. neuroblastoma (extradural) or neurofibroma (intradural)	UMN paralysis below level of lesion; may have LMN signs at level of lesion; respiratory muscles affected in high cervical lesion Loss of pain and temperature below level Sparing of touch, vibration, proprioception (posterior column) Late bladder/bowel involvement Vertebral and radicular pain common at level of lesion
Intramedullary lesion and Syringomyelia	Arm weakness and wasting (LMN) and leg stiffness (UMN) in cervical/thoracic lesions Can have LMN lower limb weakness in low-level lesions Early bladder/bowel dysfunction Variable sensory loss (pain/temperature) Funicular pain from spinothalamic tract irritation; sharp jabbing or ill defined, burning; especially when supine
Complete cord lesion, e.g. traumatic transection Transverse myelitis	UMN paralysis below level Sensory loss below level (can demonstrate sensory level) Neuropathic bladder/bowel
Hemicord lesion (Brown-Séquard syndrome)	Ipsilateral: UMN paralysis and loss of vibration/position sense Contralateral: loss of pain/temperature sensation
Cauda equina syndrome	Radicular pain and sensory changes below hip Asymmetrical LMN weakness in lower limbs Bladder/bowel disturbance
Acute spinal shock	Flaccid paralysis below lesion Sensory loss below lesion Reflexes absent or reduced Loss of bladder/bowel control

UMN, upper motor neurone; LMN, lower motor neurone.

Causes of spinal cord dysfunction

There are various causes for spinal cord dysfunction in children (Table 31.2).

Table 31.2 Causes and examples of spinal cord dysfunction in children

Aetiology	Examples
Congenital	Tethered cord Neural tube defects/myelomeningocele/lipomyelomeningocele Dermal sinus tracts Diastematomyelia Syringomyelia
Compression	Extramedullary/intramedullary Examples: Vertebral collapse from infiltration (neuroblastoma, leukaemia, eosinophilic granuloma) causing extramedullary compression Intramedullary astrocytoma
Trauma	Birth injury Road traffic accident Non-accidental injury Spinal cord injury without radiological abnormalities
Infective/ inflammatory	Transverse myelitis Poliomyelitis
Growth/tumours	Intraspinal tumours/metastasis Infiltrative disorders
Vascular insult	Infarction, e.g. from vertebral artery dissection
Demyelinating	Multiple sclerosis Post-infective Autoimmune
Degenerative	Motor neurone disease Genetic disorders, e.g. spinocerebellar degenerations
Metabolic	Vitamin E deficiency Subacute combined degeneration (vitamin B12 deficiency)

Most paediatric neurodisability practitioners would expect to encounter children and young people with NTDs (e.g. spina bifida and myelomeningocele) and sequelae of acquired spinal cord injury. The other conditions are rare and are often jointly managed with paediatric neurologists or other subspecialists. This chapter will cover only NTDs, but the general management principles hold well in most of the other conditions.

Neural tube defects

NTDs are amongst the most common birth defects. The prevalence has dropped in the UK from around 3.6 per 1000 live births in 1964 to less than 1 per 1000 live births in 2004 (Morris and Wald 2007). This is attributed to a combination of screening and preconception folate supplementation. Antenatal exposure to some antiepileptic drugs, especially valproate, can increase the risk of NTD.

NTD is a broad term encompassing a heterogeneous group of congenital spinal anomalies that result from defective closure of the neural tube early in fetal life. The upper and lower ends of the neural tube close last and these tend to be common sites of the anomalies. The NTDs can be open or closed. The 'open' lesions include anencephaly, encephalocele and spina bifida manifesta. 'Closed' lesions include causes of closed spinal dysraphism (Table 31.3).

Case vignette

Aaron initially presented to his paediatrician at the age of 9 months with a deviation of the proximal natal cleft and a small swelling on the right side of the cleft. An ultrasound scan of the mass suggested a fatty swelling and a lumbar radiography revealed spina bifida at L3 to L5 level. Clinically, Aaron was well; he had normal lower limb neurological examination, normal bowel and bladder function, and normal head circumference. Aaron walked at the age of 14 months but at 18 months was noted to have started limping on the right side with an emerging foot equinus deformity. Magnetic resonance imaging (MRI) showed a fibro-fatty mass which extended to the spinal cord, with the lower end of the cord embedded in the mass. Neurosurgical opinion advised against surgery at this stage due to the risk of further cord and/or nerve damage. Aaron was monitored clinically and over the next 5 years he developed a more pronounced foot drop requiring splints, but he did not develop any other significant motor, sensory or bladder/bowel symptoms. He toilet trained successfully at the age of 4 years though he still wets the bed occasionally at night.

Learning point

- Sometimes the dangers associated with intervention are significant and may worsen clinical and functional ability.

Open NTDs are visible at birth and are often picked up on antenatal ultrasound. There are frequently associated spinal cord and brain abnormalities resulting in neurodeficit and craniospinal deformity. Anencephaly occurs when the forebrain fails to form. It is a lethal condition and live-born infants do not survive beyond a few hours. Encephalocele or encephalomyeloceles are protrusion of a part of the meninges and sometimes brain through a skull defect. Spina bifida manifesta is caused by the meninges or spinal cord protruding through a defect in the posterior spine (meningocele/myelomeningocele).

For practical purposes, closed NTDs are the conditions described as closed spinal dysraphism. Spinal dysraphism is the term used to describe conditions in which the spinal column fails to form properly. The spinal dysraphisms are also classified as being open or closed.

Table 31.3 Types of spinal dysraphism

Open spinal dysraphism	Closed spinal dysraphism
Spina bifida manifesta/cystica/aperta	Spina bifida occulta
	Lipomeningocele/lipomyelomeningocele
	Diastematomyelia (split cord)
	Thickened filum terminale
	Dermal sinus

Closed spinal dysraphism is a defect in which the spinal cord and meninges do not herniate through the back. Often there is a clinical mark on the skin over the spine, for example a tuft of hair, fatty lump, deviated natal cleft or a birthmark. The incidence of spina bifida occulta is high (~10%) and it is usually asymptomatic and incidentally recognized on routine radiography. However, it can be associated with conditions that could lead to neurological problems including thickened filum terminale, lipoma, split cord and dermal sinus. Many of these conditions, with the exception of the dermal sinus, can have a tethered cord. As the child grows, the spinal cord and nerves are stretched causing spinal dysfunction, which initially can be subtle but may progress to permanent damage. The symptoms can comprise problems with leg movement, bladder and bowel control, lower back pain and spinal deformity. The presentation may be delayed until adulthood. It is important to diagnose and intervene as early as possible to minimize functional loss.

Spina bifida cystica presents as a sac or cyst, rather like a large blister on the back, covered by a thin layer of skin or membrane. There are two forms depending on whether there is involvement of the spinal cord in the herniation. **Meningocele** is where the sac contains only meninges with cerebrospinal fluid (CSF) and is a less severe and less common variety. There can be some spinal abnormalities but these are usually not severe. **Myelomeningocele** is the most severe and more common variety (Fig. 31.2). The herniation consists of spinal tissue and nerves in addition to meninges and CSF. The spinal cord is damaged and deformed and as a result there is always some degree of paralysis and sensory loss below the level of the lesion. The ascending tracts carrying sensory information and the descending tracts providing motor control are disrupted. The tracts controlling bladder and bowel function are usually affected as the nerves leave near the bottom of the spinal cord and result in neuropathic bladder and bowel. Higher and larger lesions are likely to have more severe neurodeficit. Hydrocephalus is present in 80% to 90% of cases and usually requires shunting.

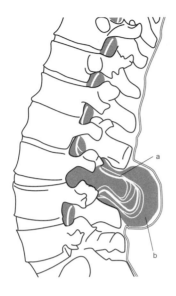

Figure 31.2 Spinal cord with lumbar meningomyelocele. a, Cerebrospinal fluid with a meningeal covering forming the sac. b, Deformed spinal cord and nerve roots protruding into the sac.

Antenatal screening

All pregnancies in the UK are offered the 'triple test', which is a blood test for alpha-fetoprotein (AFP), beta-human chorionic gonadotrophin and oestriol, and fetal ultrasonography, which will show if there is a spinal discontinuity. A raised AFP can be associated with incomplete closure of the spinal canal. Together, the tests have a sensitivity of 70% as a marker of a chromosomal abnormality in the unborn infant. Fetal ultrasonography is aimed particularly at assessing the development of the spinal cord and canal to exclude spina bifida.

When spina bifida is detected, individuals make choices according to the degree of the anomaly. Some fetuses may have such severe malformations that the parents elect to discontinue the pregnancy. If the pregnancy continues, regular antenatal monitoring and planned atraumatic delivery in a hospital with access to paediatric neurosurgery is preferred. With increased expertise in fetal MRI, some specialist units are performing fetal surgery to close the defect. Infants born with the defect need careful evaluation of motor deficits, sensory deficits, bladder and bowel involvement, diaphragm involvement, hydrocephalus and any associated congenital malformations. Current practice favours early closure of the defect and shunting the hydrocephalus. A multidisciplinary team approach is essential to ensure good-quality care.

Management of bladder, bowel and continence

Management of bladder, bowel and continence is important and early involvement of specialists is essential. A neuropathic bladder may not empty completely, increasing the risk of infection and backpressure changes in the kidneys. Some neuropathic bladders may be of small capacity and be hyperexcitable, causing significant urgency and continence problems. From birth children should be monitored for infection, kidney function, blood pressure and with renal tract imaging. Urodynamic studies are helpful in identifying pressure changes in the urinary tract and help in formulating appropriate management decisions. Regular bladder emptying with clean intermittent catheterization should be instituted early by training parents and carers. A balanced diet, good fluid intake, avoiding caffeinated drinks and (in the long term) alcohol and controlling any constipation are recommended. For small hyperexcitable bladders, oxybutynin orally or botulinum toxin injected into the bladder wall can help symptomatically. Surgical options such as bladder augmentation, creating an alternative conduit for catheterization (Mitrofanoff procedure) or artificial urinary sphincter insertion can be considered in selected situations.

Bowel symptoms comprise constipation, soiling and faecal incontinence. Laxatives, suppositories and enemas should be used as necessary in conjunction with toileting advice to ensure regular bowel emptying. As there is reduced bowel sensation, children should be encouraged to have a regular 'toilet time' when they sit on the toilet and aid evacuation by coughing, laughing and gently putting pressure on the abdomen. In some instances bowel emptying can be enhanced by developing the spinal anal reflex, which is brought on by stroking the perianal skin. For persistent problems with constipation and faecal incontinence, surgery can be considered to create an access stoma or a permanent conduit for delivering antegrade continence enemas (ACE procedure). This allows a good degree of personal control over the bowel symptoms in older children and adults.

Other associated problems

Pressure sores can be a difficult problem and are best prevented. Management includes preventative advice (Table 31.4) with early treatment and advice from tissue viability experts. The higher incidence of obesity and spinal curvatures contributes further to the risk of chronic pressure sores. Other skin problems include latex allergy from repeated exposure and it is advisable for these children to avoid all latex products from birth.

Table 31.4 Pressure sore prevention advice

Lift or shift your bottom from your chair every 20 minutes.
Change the position of your legs at the same time.
Check your skin all over at least once a day (twice is better).
If you are wet or soiled, the quicker you clean up and change, the better.
Take care when transferring from your wheelchair.
Eat a good balanced diet with lots of fruit and vegetables, and drink plenty of clear fluids.

Sexual dysfunction is common in young people with spina bifida. It can affect their sex lives, relationships and fertility. Judicious use of oral medication, injections, specialist equipment and surgical implants can address a number of these problems. The Association for Spina Bifida and Hydrocephalus (www.shinecharity.org.uk) has excellent information leaflets for affected men and women.

COMORBIDITIES

Children and young people with spina bifida are at increased risk of brain malformations, in particular the Chiari II malformation resulting in herniation of the cerebellar tonsils across the foramen magnum. Learning disability, coordination difficulties and attention problems are more common. Poor self-esteem and depression are reported in teenagers and young people with spina bifida and can often lead to challenging behaviours.

In spite of the complex multisystem problems, spina bifida is a non-progressive illness and most affected children and young people report a good quality of life. Any clinical deterioration should raise suspicion of a shunt malfunction, tethered cord, worsening kidney problems or syrinx formation. Appropriate craniospinal imaging and blood investigations should identify the cause, which in most cases can be remedied.

Hydrocephalus

Hydrocephalus is a condition in which there is abnormal accumulation of CSF within the ventricles of the brain. The incidence of early-onset hydrocephalus in developed countries is between 0.5 and 1.0 per 1000 live births, with preterm birth, congenital onset and spina bifida being the main causes. In developing countries infective causes predominate.

CSF is formed by the choroid plexuses in the lateral ventricles of the brain. The fluid travels through the ventricular system and reaches the basal cisterns through the foramina of Luschka and Magendie in the fourth ventricle. From here, it is absorbed into the venous sinuses through the arachnoid granulations. Hydrocephalus can be caused by excessive production of CSF (rare) or by a disruption to the flow or absorption of the CSF (see Table 31.5). Obstructions within the ventricular system are called 'closed' or 'internal' hydrocephalus and usually have a small fourth ventricle (e.g. in aqueduct stenosis). On the other hand, an 'open' or 'external' hydro-cephalus has an enlarged fourth ventricle and is caused by a failure to absorb the CSF through the arachnoid granulations or poor CSF flow through the basal cisterns. Rising CSF pressure can cause permeation across the ependymal lining into the periventricular white matter, causing tissue damage and gliosis. Unchecked, the rapid rise in CSF pressure can lead to tentorial or uncal herniation resulting in coning and, in some instances, death.

Case vignette

Five-month-old Daisy is referred by her health visitor with a head circumference which has increased to the 98th centile from being on the 75th centile at birth. She was born at term by a difficult delivery requiring forceps. Her parents noticed a head tilt to the right starting in the first few weeks of birth, which was thought to be a 'sternomastoid tumour'. They report Daisy to be a happy girl who is developing normally. Examination shows Daisy to have a moderate head tilt to the right, which her parents say has got worse. Her anterior fontanelle feels full and there are some prominent temporal veins. She has a full range of eye movement and no obvious 'sun setting' of the eyes. Neurological examination and fundus examination are normal. Her head circumference plots on the 98th centile, her father's on the 50th and her mother's on the 91st. An initial ultrasound scan shows a moderate hydrocephalus with a large third ventricle but poor views of the fourth ventricle. MRI of the brain confirms the hydrocephalus and reveals a right posterior fossa tumour involving the right cerebellum. Daisy underwent successful tumour surgery and had a ventriculoperitoneal shunt insertion.

Learning point

- Tumours in the posterior fossa can cause hydrocephalus by compressing the fourth ventricle and blocking CSF flow.

Table 31.5 Causes of hydrocephalus

Internal/closed/non-communicating	External/open/communicating
Congenital aqueduct stenosis	Intraventricular haemorrhage (usually in
Genetic causes like X-linked hydrocephalus	preterm infants)
Tumours and space-occupying lesions	Spina bifida
Congenital infections, e.g. cytomegalovirus,	Arnold–Chiari malformations
toxoplasmosis	Achondroplasia
	Pus/debris from meningitis
	Sinus venous thrombosis

Clinical symptoms and signs (Table 31.6)

Infants present with enlargement of the head with separation of the sutures and a bulging anterior fontanelle. Often there is downwards gaze (sun setting) and prominent forehead veins. In older children, in whom the sutures are closed, symptoms of raised intracranial pressure (ICP) such as persistent early morning occipital headache, nausea and vomiting may be presenting features.

Table 31.6 Clinical symptoms and signs of hydrocephalus

Infants	Subacute	Acute
Increasing head size,	Drowsiness	Drowsiness
crossing centiles upwards	Early morning occipital	Confusion
Irritable shrill cry	headache	Seizures (especially tonic)
Vomiting/poor feeding	Nausea and vomiting	Papilloedema
'Sun setting' of eyes	Diplopia/new strabismus	Increased blood pressure
Bulging anterior fontanelle	Papilloedema	and slow pulse (late sign)
Prominent forehead veins	Declining attention, behaviour	Unequal pupils
Delayed development	Poor memory and school	Autonomic dysfunction
Increased tone	performance	
Seizures	Change in personality	
	Clumsiness/unsteady gait	
	Developmental delay	
	Urinary incontinence	

Cranial imaging (ultrasonography/computed tomography/MRI) confirms the diagnosis and further tests may be required (e.g. congenital infection screen) to determine the underlying cause.

Comorbidities in the form of learning disability, cerebral palsy and epilepsy are common and most children are affected by one or more of these conditions. Delayed developmental milestones and precocious puberty are also more common.

Hydrocephalus is usually treated by relieving the pressure in the ventricular system by one of the following methods (the neurosurgical team will recommend the most appropriate):

- Inserting a ventriculoperitoneal shunt connecting the lateral ventricle to the peritoneal cavity. The shunt comprises a plastic tube with a built-in one-way valve which allows the CSF to drain into the peritoneal cavity and be absorbed.
- An endoscopic third ventriculostomy can be performed in non-communicating hydrocephalus. The process involves using a neuroendoscope to make a hole in the roof of the third ventricle, which creates a communication between the third ventricle and the basal cisterns.
- Recurrent spinal taps or CSF drainage through an access device may provide a temporary solution in post-haemorrhagic hydrocephalus of newborn infants, until the need for a more permanent device becomes evident.

Shunt systems can experience a number of complications including

- mechanical failure (breakage)
- infection
- obstructions
- the need to lengthen or replace the catheter as the child grows
- some complications can lead to over-draining or under-draining.
  - Over-draining occurs when the shunt allows CSF to drain from the ventricles more quickly than it is produced, resulting in ventricular collapse with slit-like ventricles (slit ventricle syndrome), with or without subdural haemorrhage. A collapsed slit-like ventricle may not expand easily and often has high CSF pressures, thus producing symptoms of raised ICP.
  - Under-draining occurs when CSF is not removed quickly enough, causing chronic high pressure and symptoms of hydrocephalus.

Twenty-four- or 48-hour CSF pressure monitoring, neuroimaging and radiographs of the shunt (shunt series) can usually identify the nature of any mechanical shunt problem.

Shunt infections can produce symptoms of raised ICP, low-grade fever, neck or abdominal pain, and redness and/or tenderness along the shunt tract. Appropriate investigations include tapping the shunt for a CSF sample, blood cultures, blood count and C-reactive protein.

When there is reason to suspect that a shunt system is not functioning properly (e.g. sleepiness, change in behaviour, escalation of seizures, headache or vomiting) a neurosurgical opinion should be sought immediately, appropriate investigations arranged and the child placed under regular neuro-observations. When shunt complications occur, the shunt system usually requires some type of revision.

Key messages

- Spinal malformations often have an external marker such as a tuft of hair.
- A tethered cord can develop progressive signs in childhood as the child grows.
- An enlarging head size crossing centiles is hydrocephalus until proven otherwise.
- An early torticollis can be a sign of a posterior fossa tumour/lesion.
- Carers of a child with a shunt for hydrocephalus should be given clear instructions of symptoms that may suggest shunt malfunction; professionals should have a low threshold for suspicion of shunt problems and seek neurosurgical advice.

Reference

Morris JK, Wald NJ (2007) Prevalence of neural tube defect pregnancies in England and Wales from 1964 to 2004. *J Med Screen* 14: 55–9. DOI: 10.1258/096914107781261945

Further reading

The Association for Spina Bifida And Hydrocephalus, Europe's largest support group for individuals with spina bifida and hydrocephalus: www.shinecharity.org.uk

32
Musculoskeletal conditions

Arnab Seal and Anne M Kelly

> **Learning objectives**
>
> - To be familiar with common musculoskeletal conditions including
>   - clinical features
>   - underlying cause
>   - differential diagnosis
>   - to be able to identify and monitor associations and complications.
> - To be able to assess and manage minor abnormalities of gait.

Achondroplasia

Achondroplasia occurs in 1 out of 15 000 to 25 000 live births and is associated with increasing paternal age. It is the most common non-lethal form of skeletal dysplasia which results in disproportionate short stature.

Genetics

Achondroplasia is inherited as an autosomal dominant trait but 80% of cases are due to new mutations. It is caused by a point mutation in the fibroblast growth factor receptor 3 or *FGFR3* gene. The initial diagnosis is usually made prenatally or in the newborn period by a skeletal survey and appropriate genetic testing.

Clinical features

- Disproportionate short stature.
- Megalencephaly (may be true megalencephaly but can also be arrested hydrocephalus).

- A prominent forehead with frontal bossing.
- Midface hypoplasia with dental malocclusion.
- Rhizomelic (proximal) shortening of the arms and legs.
- A normal trunk length.
- Prominent lumbar lordosis and joint laxity leading to a waddling gait.
- Bowlegs.
- Trident hand configuration (a gap between the middle and ring fingers).
- Normal intelligence with possible minor deficit in visuospatial tasks.

In children and young adults with achondroplasia a number of serious complications should be monitored:

- Cervicomedullary compression can occur from kinking of the cervical cord or atlantoaxial instability or foramen magnum stenosis. Cord compression in infancy may present with severe hypotonia and/or apnoeas. Older children presenting with brisk or asymmetrical reflexes, pain, ataxia, incontinence and apnoea should raise concern regarding cervical cord compression, which can lead to sudden respiratory arrest. Treatment involves cervical decompression.
- Recurrent otitis media and glue ear can occur with resultant hearing loss.
- Obstructive sleep apnoea is common and should be looked for.
- Arrested or progressive hydrocephalus; may need shunting.
- Spinal stenosis can cause compression symptoms; may need lumbar laminectomy.

Management

- Monitor growth and head circumference using specific charts for achondroplasia.
- Monitor development.
- Enquire about sleep and sleep apnoea and consider a sleep study.
- Refer to orthodontics when necessary.
- Manage middle ear infections and concerns about hearing loss.

The usefulness of growth hormone therapy is debated. Significant advances have been made in surgical limb lengthening operations but it can take years to achieve optimal results. The short limbs can cause functional problems which require appropriate adaptations in the home and school to promote independence (e.g. lower light switches, adapted bicycle, adapted toilets, foot rest for seating, etc.). Most children with achondroplasia have normal intelligence and normal life expectancy and lead productive lives.

Osteogenesis imperfecta

Osteogenesis imperfecta is an inherited connective tissue disorder that occurs in 1 in 20 000 live births. It is characterized by 'brittle' bones causing easy fractures, lax joints, poor dentition, blue sclera and wormian bones that are seen on a skull radiographs.

Genetics

It is caused by a defect in the gene that produces type 1 collagen. There are many genetic variants and most of the variants are transmitted in an autosomal dominant manner. The most widely used classification of osteogenesis imperfecta is based on clinical and radiological features (Adapted Sillence Classification) and describes four main types, though further types are now being described. Diagnosis is confirmed by collagen synthesis analysis from fibroblast cultures obtained by skin biopsy.

Clinical features

- Bone fragility is on a spectrum from mild disease with only mild bone fragility, such as in type 1, through to severe life-threatening bone fragility with limb deformity, scoliosis and severe chest deformity, which is usually incompatible with life (as in type 2). The progression of the bone disease varies according to type, with some types (e.g. type 4) improving with increasing age.
- Lax joints.
- Poor dentition.
- Blue sclera.
- Risk of developing sensorineural hearing loss later in childhood.

Management

- Monitor bone density using dual X-ray absorptiometry.
- Bisphosphonates such as pamidronate can be helpful in increasing bone density and reducing fracture frequency, especially in younger children with more severe forms of the disorder. Many children in the UK are now enrolled on regular intravenous infusion programmes.

Arthrogryposis

Arthrogryposis or arthrogryposis multiplex congenita occurs in 1 in 3000 live births and comprises a group of heterogeneous non-progressive conditions clinically characterized by multiple joint contractures found throughout the body at birth. The contractures are believed to arise following decreased fetal movements (fetal akinesia).

Cause

- Fetal abnormalities such as neurogenic disorders, muscle disorders or connective tissue abnormalities.
- Maternal disorders such as infection, drugs, trauma, high fever or other maternal illnesses.
- Uterine crowding causing mechanical limitations to movement such as bicornuate uterus, twins, large fibroids or oligohydramnios.

Clinical features

- Multiple joint contractures and scoliosis.
- Polyhydramnios.
- Pulmonary hypoplasia.
- Micrognathia.
- Ocular hypertelorism.
- Short umbilical cord.

Management

Investigations to be considered include creatinine kinase, congenital infections screen, viral cultures, nerve studies, neuroimaging, ophthalmology for retinal conditions, chromosome or array-comparative genomic hybridization studies, skin fibroblast and muscle biopsy.

A genetic opinion and family counselling should be considered. Recurrence risk depends on whether the contractures are extrinsically or intrinsically derived. Extrinsically derived contractures (i.e. due to uterine crowding) have a low recurrence risk and better prognosis, whereas the recurrence risk and outcome for intrinsically derived contractures depends on aetiology.

No completely successful approach to treat arthrogryposis has been found. Goals include lower limb alignment and establishment of stability for ambulation, and enhancing upper limb function for self-care. Usually, early institution of physiotherapy is beneficial, especially in the case of the inherited distal arthrogryposes. Sadly, recurrence of deformities following stretching is common, and surgery is often indicated. Splinting combined with physiotherapy appears preferable to repeated casting. If surgery is contemplated, early (age 3–12mo) one-stage (bone and tendon transfer) surgery should be considered. There needs to be an active therapy programme planned after surgical treatment.

The lifespan of affected individuals depends on the disease severity, associated malformations and the underlying cause. Infants with limb involvement, scoliosis and central nervous system dysfunction are often ventilator dependent in infancy and often die in the first year of life.

Minor gait problems

Parents often report concerns about their child's gait (Fig. 32.1) including

- in-toeing (a)
- out-toeing (c)
- flat feet
- knock knees.

Virtually all of these minor issues resolve in time without any intervention. Remember to check the family history for similar gait problems or any signs or symptoms of acquired bone disease (e.g. rickets).

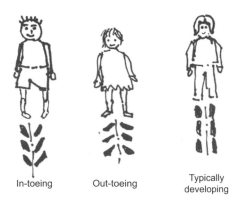

In-toeing   Out-toeing   Typically
                                       developing

Figure 32.1 Problems with a child's gait.

In-toeing

Refers to the child walking with one or both feet medially rotated (pigeon toed), as in Fig. 32.1. Causes include the following:

- Femoral anteversion: the femoral neck is anteverted (twisted forwards) causing the lower limb to turn inwards. This increases the range of internal rotation from 50 to 55 degrees to 90 degrees (see Fig. 32.2). External rotation is correspondingly reduced. The child stands with 'strabismic patellae' and runs awkwardly, catching their toes. They find it comfortable to sit in a 'W' position.
- Medial tibial torsion: outward bowing of the tibia associated with medial tibial torsion. This usually resolves by the age of 3 to 4 years. Rickets and Blount disease should be considered and excluded.
- Metatarsus varus: adduction of the forefoot in relation to the hind foot. A vertical crease is seen medially. It resolves by the age of 8 years. No intervention is required unless adduction cannot be corrected by passive repositioning, or there are neurological signs.

Out-toeing

This is less common than in-toeing. The feet are rotated outwards due to outward rotation of the femoral neck in relation to the shaft. This has the effect of increasing the range of external rotation to 90 degrees and reducing internal rotation. The condition self-corrects with growth, usually by the age of 2 years.

Bowlegs (genu varum)

Bowlegs is common in children under the age of 2 years as they walk with their knees flexed (see Fig. 32.3). This apparent bowing disappears when the child is laid supine and the knees are pushed back. Measure the intercondylar distance between the knees with the child standing with feet placed together. This should be less than 8cm to 10cm.

How to assess for femoral anteversion, tibial torsion or metatarus adductus

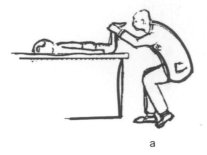

a

Place the child prone and flex his or her knees. Note whether the feet are straight or at an angle. If they are at an angle is this because of a tibial component (tibial torsion) or a foot abnormality (metatarsus varus)?

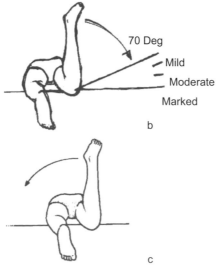

b

Assess whether there is any femoral anteversion by assessing internal rotation. If the child has femoral anteversion this is increased

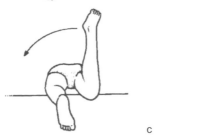

c

Continue and check external rotation; this can be decreased in femoral anteversion

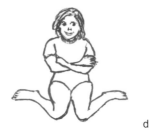

d

Often you will notice that these children 'W-sit'

Figure 32.2 Assessment of femoral anteversion, tibial torsion and metatarsus varus.

If bowing persists in children more than 2 years or in a child with pigmented skin, suspect rickets, particularly in the presence of others symptoms such as general misery, reluctance to walk and swollen metaphyses.

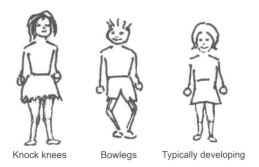

Knock knees   Bowlegs   Typically developing

Figure 32.3 Genu varum and genu valgum.

Genu valgum (knock knees)

This is present in many children between the age of 3 and 5 years. An intermalleolar distance of less than 10cm (distance between medial malleoli measured with child standing with knees touching) should correct without the need for intervention. Remember to consider rickets again.

Pes planus (flat feet)

All children are flat footed before the age of 3 years, as the medial arch does not begin to develop until after this age and it is not fully developed until at least the child's sixth birthday.

Flat feet are due to lax ligaments between the small bones of the foot. This laxity causes the arch to 'fall' when the child stands up, giving rise to the term 'fallen arches'. The arches, however, may be seen when the child is sitting.

No treatment is needed unless the child complains of foot, ankle or knee pain or poor balance. Refer the child to an orthotist, who may advise the use of arch supports and exercises. No restriction on activities is needed. Properly fitted footwear with ankle support is needed, particularly if the ankles go into valgus. Flat feet are pathological only if the foot is rigid or painful and the medial arch cannot be restored when standing on tiptoe.

Key messages

- The vast majority of gait concerns in young children are innocent and require reassurance and no further referral.
- Red flag signs would be associated faltering growth, motor delay, painful joints and groups in which vitamin D deficiency may be more common as a result of dietary, cultural or lifestyle choices.

Joint hypermobility

Presentation

Children's joints all have an increased range of mobility compared with an adult, and this gradually reduces with age. It is therefore difficult to give a prevalence figure for hypermobility, but studies suggest that it is between 2% and 30%.

Joint hypermobility is associated with hypotonia and can present in early childhood with delayed motor milestones (average age of walking is 15mo). In older children the most common complaints are joint pain (74%), gait difficulties (10%) and back pain (6%). In 20% of cases there is a history of recurrent sprains.

Children with joint hypermobility often find schooling difficult as a result of clumsiness leading to difficulties with handwriting (40%) and physical education activities (50%). A significant proportion of children with hypermobility miss time from school because of their difficulties.

In addition to the joint problems, children can also have problems with constipation, soiling and hernias. Adults with the condition have higher rates of depression, anxiety and chronic pain difficulties. In 60% of cases there is a family history of similar difficulties.

See Chapter 6 on the detailed history and relevant clinical features to look for on examination of a child with hypotonia.

Assessment

A clinical examination is required to assess if there is an underlying disorder. Features seen in recognised conditions are highlighted in Table 32.1.

Table 32.1 Differential diagnoses of hypermobility

	Clinical presentation	*Investigation*
Benign	Hypermobility, arthralgia Normal skin and body form	Rule out other causes. Consider Beighton criteria, but validity in children not established
Marfan syndrome	Long thin fingers and limbs Arm span greater than height Kyphoscoliosis Pectus excavatum High arched palate Lens subluxation Aneurysm formation	Clinical diagnosis (check list) If suspicion then ophthalmology and echocardiogram helpful Genetic tests may be helpful, especially if clinically unsure
Stickler syndrome	Flattened facial appearance Visual problems – high myopia Hearing loss – may be progressive Cleft palate	Gene testing – COL2, 9 and 11
Ehlers–Danlos syndrome	Skin elasticity and bruising Aneurysm formation and dissection Kyphoscoliosis (seven subtypes)	Clinical diagnosis DNA studies

	Clinical presentation	Investigation
Osteogenesis imperfecta	Repeated fractures with minimal trauma Blue sclerae Hearing loss Possible family history as autosomal dominant	Skin biopsy
Williams syndrome	Developmental impairment Depressed nasal bridge with upturned nose Big smile with widely spaced teeth 'Cocktail party' personality	FISH test
Down syndrome	Hypotonia Dysmorphic facial features Learning difficulties	Chromosome study for trisomy 21
Prader–Willi syndrome	May present with neonatal hypotonia Feeding difficulties Breathing problems may occur Characteristic facies	Chromosome study requesting detailed examination of 15q

See Chapter 33 for further information on some of above conditions. FISH, fluorescente in situ hybridization.

Joint hypermobility is assessed on the Beighton score (maximum of 9 points). Validity of the Beighton score in children younger than 6 years is not established.

- Passive apposition of the thumb to the flexor aspect of the forearm (1 point for each hand).
- Passive hyperextension of the fingers so that they lie parallel with the extensor aspect of the forearm (1 point for each hand).
- The ability to hyperextend the elbow beyond neutral (1 point for each joint).
- The ability to hyperextend the knee 10 degrees beyond neutral (1 point for each joint).
- The ability to have the knees straight and be able to place palms on floor (1 point).

References

Adib N, Davies K, Grahame R et al. (2005) Joint hypermobility syndrome in childhood. A not so benign multisystem disorder? *Rheumatology* 44: 744–50. http://dx.doi.org/10.1093/rheumatology/keh557

Cheung MS, Glorieux FH (2008) Osteogenesis imperfecta: update on presentation and management. *Rev Endocr Metab Disord* 9: 153–60. http://dx.doi.org/10.1007/s11154-008-9074-4

Website

Children with Achondroplasia: www.mangen.co.uk/media/22099/achon_boy_phr.pdf

The Hypermobility Syndrome Association: www.hypermobility.org

Joint Hypermobility Syndrome: www.dwp.gov.uk/publications/specialist-guides/medical-conditions/a-z-of-medical-conditions/joint-hypermobility-syndrome/

Section 11

Genetics

33
Genetic conditions

Mohnish Suri and Anne M Kelly

Learning objectives

- To have an approach to assessing a child with dysmorphic features.
- To recognize the phenotypes of common genetic disorders causing childhood disability.
- To understand the genetic mechanisms of these conditions.
- To recognize the issues around breaking the news of the diagnosis to families including sibling recurrence risks.
- To recognize and manage the commonly associated medical problems.
- To know the differential diagnosis for each of these conditions.

Overview (Table 33.1)

Table 33.1 Genetic disorders causing disability

Disorder	Example
Chromosomal aneuploidy	Down syndrome
Chromosomal microdeletion	22q11.2 microdeletion syndrome
Chromosomal microduplication	17p11.2 microduplication syndrome (Potocki–Lupski syndrome)
Single gene disorders	Fragile X syndrome Neurofibromatosis type 1 Tuberous sclerosis Noonan syndrome (mutations in several different genes)
Abnormal imprinting (epigenetic disorders)	Angelman syndrome Prader–Willi syndrome

Genetic assessment of a child with developmental delay (Fig. 33.1)

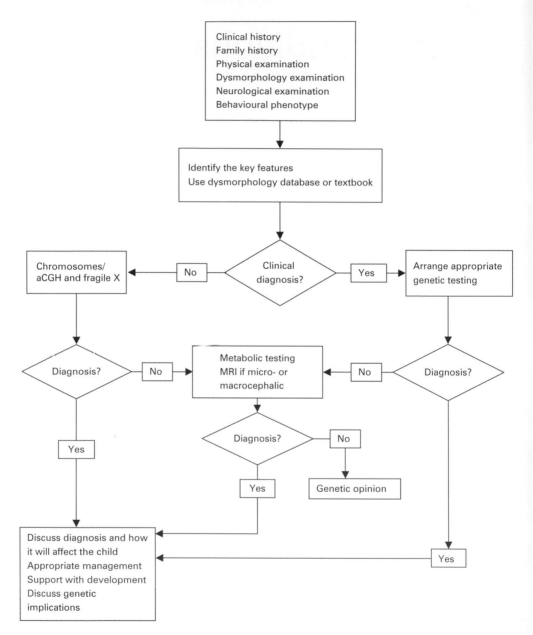

Figure 33.1 Flowchart for genetic evaluation. aCGH, array-comparative genomic hybridization; MRI, magnetic resonance imaging.

Key questions

- Are there any congenital abnormalities?
- Is there any family history of note?
- Is there abnormal body or head growth?
- Are there any dysmorphic features?
- Are there any clues in the child's behaviour (behavioural phenotype)?

History

- Parents' concerns
- Developmental history
- Vision and hearing
- Unusual behaviours
- Health in pregnancy
  - Conception – any infertility treatments?
  - Maternal illness (diabetes, viral infections, phenylketonuria)
  - Drugs – prescribed
  - Non-prescribed drugs/alcohol
  - Antenatal scans – were there any abnormalities?
  - Any invasive antenatal tests (amniocentesis, chorionic villus sampling)?
  - Intrauterine growth

Past medical history

- Congenital abnormalities in other systems

Family history – three generations

- Consanguinity
- Recurrent miscarriages
- Learning difficulties

Dysmorphological examination

- Growth parameters – including head circumference

General appearance

- Facial appearance
- Skin – look for pigmentary skin anomalies (examine skin under Wood's light), haemangiomas and hamartomas
- Hair
- Body proportions, skeletal asymmetry

Limbs, hands and feet

- Proportion
- Palmar creases
- Syndactyly and clinodactyly
- Nails

Head

- Face and head shape, craniofacial asymmetry
- Neck – shortening, webbing
- Eyes – size, spacing, angulation and abnormalities
- Ears – position and structural abnormalities
- Mouth and oral cavity – clefting or pseuodoclefting, other abnormalities, particularly of tongue, teeth and palate, gum hyperplasia

Systems examination (Table 33.2)

- Cardiac abnormalities
- Hepatosplenomegaly
- Neurological abnormalities
- Spine, e.g. gibbus
- Genital abnormality

Development

- Assess degree of delay
- Social interaction
- Any stereotyped behaviours seen?

Behavioural phenotype (Table 33.3)

Certain genetic diagnoses are associated with patterns of behaviour and using this information helps to identify specific syndrome diagnoses, for example typical hand movements in Rett syndrome.

Table 33.2 Examination findings and examples of associated syndromes

Feature	Examples of syndromes
Major malformation	Williams Noonan CHARGE Cornelia de Lange
Growth problems	22q11.2 Albright hereditary osteodystrophy Sotos Cockayne Fetal alcohol
Hypotonia	Down Prader–Willi Zellweger Myopathies
Hypertonia	Smith–Lemli–Opitz Hunter Menkes Trisomy 4p
Microcephaly	Angelman Cornelia de Lange Fetal alcohol Congenital infection
Macrocephaly	Achondroplasia Mucopolysaccharidoses Sotos
Face – 'flat midface'	Down Apert Achondroplasia Stickler
Face -asymmetric	Goldenhar Beckwith–Wiedemann Russell–Silver
Webbed neck	Turner Noonan
Abnormal thumb	Apert Holt–Oram Rubinstein–Taybi
Polydactyly	Bardet–Biedl Ellis–van Creveld syndrome Trisomy 13
Syndactyly	Apert Oculo-dento-digital dysplasia Saethre–Chotzen
Single palmar crease	Down Smith–Lemli–Opitz Cornelia de Lange
Nail anomalies	Adams–Oliver Nail–patella Coffin–Siris

Table 33.3 Behavioural phenotypes seen in syndromes with learning disability

Syndrome	Behavioural phenotype
Fragile X	Autism Hand flapping Attention difficulties and impulsivity Obsessive–compulsive behaviours Emotional lability
Williams	Infants have an interest in faces Children are socially engaging and socially disinhibited ('cocktail party' behaviour) Conversation is loquacious with stereotyped and repetitive phrases Empathetic but fail to recognize social cues Attention-deficit–hyperactivity disorder Anxiety disorders
Prader–Willi	Insatiable appetite with food seeking/hoarding Obsessive–compulsive features Aspects of autism Lying and blame shifting
Angelman	'Happy' affect with bouts of frequent laughter unrelated to context Sociable and inquisitive Hyperactivity Stereotypies, e.g. hand flapping, tongue thrusting and chewing movements Absent or limited expressive language Attraction to water or shiny objects
Rett	Stereotypic hand movements, e.g. wringing or mouthing Irregular respirations Social withdrawal during phase of regression; interested later, but with little or no speech Spontaneous outbursts of laughing or crying, including in sleep Reduced response to pain Teeth grinding
Lesch–Nyhan	Self-mutilating behaviours, characterized by lip and finger biting Facial grimacing Involuntary writhing and repetitive movements of the arms and legs
Smith–Magenis	Disrupted sleep Engaging personality Outbursts of aggression and anxiety Self-injury, including biting, hitting, hair pulling, head banging and skin picking Repetitive self-hugging Compulsively licking their fingers and flipping pages of books and magazines ('lick and flick' behaviour) Insertion of foreign bodies into ears and nose

Genetic testing

Chromosome analysis or standard karyotyping (analysis of G-banded chromosomes; Fig. 33.2) is a technique to produce a visible karyotype by staining condensed chromosomes, e.g. to detect Down syndrome.

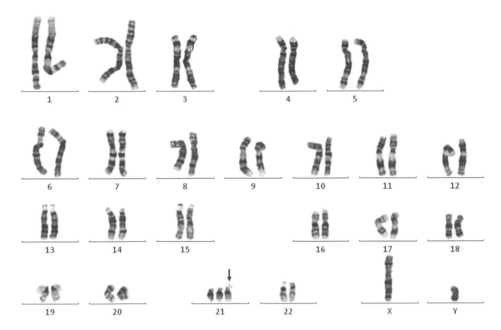

Figure 33.2 G-banded karyotype of a male infant with free-standing trisomy 21 (karyotype 47,XY,+21). The additional copy of chromosome 21 is marked with an arrow. Photograph courtesy of Nottingham Regional Cytogenetics Service.

Fluorescence in situ hybridization (FISH) is used to detect and localize the presence or absence of specific DNA sequences on chromosomes. FISH uses fluorescent probes that bind only to those parts of the chromosome with which they show a high degree of sequence complementarity. Fluorescence microscopy can be used to find out if the fluorescent probe has bound to its target sequence, for example the 7q11.23 region in patients with suspected Williams syndrome, or if the target sequence has moved to another chromosome (e.g. subtelomeric rearrangement).

Southern blot analysis is a technique that breaks up chromosomes into fragments using a restriction enzyme and then separates them by electrophoresis. This enables sections of different lengths to be identified, e.g. fragile X syndrome for which the technique measures the length of the *FMR1* gene region containing the CGG repeat stretch. It is then possible to estimate the length of the CGG repeat.

Multiplex ligation-dependent probe amplification (MLPA) is a method to detect copy number variation in genomic sequences. It can be used to test for a number of different specific micro-deletions or microduplications.

Microarray-comparative genomic hybridization (array-CGH) is another technique to detect genomic copy number variation at a higher resolution than standard karyotyping. DNA from a test sample and normal reference sample are labelled using different fluorophores and allowed to hybridize with probes dotted onto a slide. The probes represent most of the known genes as well as non-coding regions of the genome (Fig. 33.3). The fluorescence intensity of the test sample and of the reference DNA is then measured for each probe on the slide. It is then possible to calculate the ratio between them and identify a copy number change (deletion or duplication) of some of the probes, and thus determine whether the patient has a deletion or duplication at a particular location in the genome.

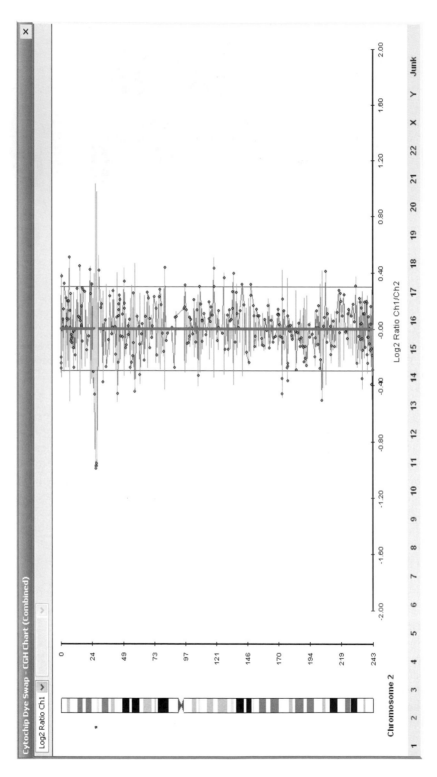

Figure 33.3 Result of array-CGH for a patient showing a deletion of two probes located at 2p23.3.

This is a very sensitive test. It identifies a genetic cause of learning difficulty in around 6% of those who have previously had a normal standard karyotype. This form of testing may have other implications for the child and wider family as a previously unknown abnormality, such as the deletion of a cancer gene, could be identified. Parental DNA samples are required to interpret the results of the array-CGH test in a child. The family needs to understand these implications before commencing this testing.

Because of its high diagnostic yield, array-CGH is replacing standard karyotyping as the first-line investigation in children with developmental delay, learning difficulties and dysmorphic features in some cytogenetics laboratories.

Indications for referral to geneticist

Two or more of the following problems:

- moderate to profound developmental delay
- growth problems – proportionate or disproportionate short stature or overgrowth
- macrocephaly or microcephaly
- facial dysmorphism
- two or more minor congenital anomalies (e.g. single palmar crease, clinodactyly)
- one or more major congenital anomaly (e.g. cleft lip or palate, congenital heart disease)
- abnormal neurology
- significant hearing loss or visual impairment
- parental consanguinity
- family history of learning difficulties or neurological problems.

Recurrence risk and possible prenatal testing or pre-implantation genetic diagnosis

Interpret complex genetics results

Genetic diagnosis is less likely to be made if there are mild learning difficulties and no dysmorphic features.

Down syndrome

Down syndrome is the most common genetic cause of learning disability, affecting 1:700 to 1:1000 live births. It was first described in the medical literature by Langdon Down in 1866. In 1959, Lejeune discovered the association of trisomy 21 with Down syndrome.

Down syndrome is associated with an increased risk of congenital malformations and medical complications affecting all systems, although it appears to confer protection from developing solid organ tumours (except testicular cancer) and atherosclerosis. Regular assessment and monitoring plays an important role in prevention and management of the potential medical and mental health issues commonly seen in children and adults with Down syndrome. Breaking the news to a family that their child has Down syndrome must be done in a supportive, positive and honest manner, providing the family with adequate information without overburdening them.

Genetics

There are three main types of chromosomal anomalies seen in Down syndrome. It is important to recognize each of these to provide accurate genetic counselling regarding recurrence, although this does not influence the severity of the phenotypic manifestation in the affected child.

Standard or regular trisomy 21 (95%): All cells have an extra free-standing chromosome 21. This is the most common type. In 90% of cases it is due to maternally derived meiotic non-disjunction; the rest are attributed to paternally derived meiotic non-disjunction.

Parental karyotypes do not need to be checked in patients with Down syndrome with standard trisomy 21.

The risk of standard trisomy 21 in a pregnancy increases with increasing maternal age. If a woman has a Down syndrome pregnancy at the age of 20 years her risk of having another affected pregnancy is 0.62% higher than her age-related risk, whereas a woman who has a Down syndrome pregnancy at the age of 40 years has virtually the same risk of having another affected child as her age-related risk (Morris et al. 2005).

Translocation (3%): This occurs when an additional copy of the long arm of chromosome 21 is translocated onto another chromosome, most commonly chromosome 14, but also 13, 15, 21 or 22. In three-quarters of cases this is a de novo occurrence, but in about one-quarter of cases either parent could be a carrier of a balanced translocation. Confirming parental karyotype is important in order to be able to offer families accurate estimates of recurrence risk. If the translocation is maternally derived the risk is 10% to 15%, but if it is paternally derived the risk is less than 1%. The recurrence risk is 100% if one of the parents carries a balanced translocation between the long arms of chromosome 21.

Mosaicism (2%): This usually occurs as a result of a postconception mitotic non-disjunction event. Hence, not all cell lines have the extra chromosome 21, and it may be associated with a milder phenotype. It is not thought to be related to parental age and recurrence risk is low.

All children with Down syndrome should have a standard karyotype analysis to confirm the diagnosis and to determine the sibling recurrence risk. The cytogenetics laboratory should be informed if the possibility of mosaic Down syndrome is being considered so that the karyotype can be checked in 30 metaphases. This is able to detect mosaicism for trisomy 21 with 95% confidence.

Assessment and management

The outcomes for children with Down syndrome have improved considerably in the last 20 years owing to vigilant early assessment and intervention, particularly with the correction of the cardiac anomalies and screening and correction for hearing and visual impairments. The median lifespan increased from 25 years in 1983 to 49 years in 1997.

A better understanding of the specific developmental and learning profile of children with Down syndrome has resulted in improved educational and employment outcomes.

Antenatal management

The diagnosis of Down syndrome is often made antenatally as part of the screening process for congenital anomalies. The present guidance is that all women are offered combined screening tests for Down syndrome at 11 to 13 weeks of pregnancy with nuchal translucency scanning and measurement of serum-free beta-human chorionic gonadotrophin (hCG) and pregnancy-associated plasma protein A (PAPP-A). This will detect in excess of 85% of affected pregnancies. Where these tests give a high risk of the infant being affected with Down syndrome, the woman can be offered chorionic villus sampling (up to 15 weeks' gestation) or amniocentesis (after 15 weeks) to check fetal karyotype.

It is important for all professionals involved in screening to be able to talk to the parents in a sensitive manner. Many parents may wish to continue with the pregnancy. It is desirable for a paediatrician to support parents through this period. In addition, it is important to plan for the birth in an appropriate unit if early surgical intervention is likely to be required for any major congenital malformation such as congenital heart disease or duodenal atresia.

Newborn period

At birth the diagnosis is suspected on the basis of physical features. Very rarely, particularly if the infant is well or in cases of mosaicism, the diagnosis is not made until much later when medical complications arise, for example secondary to feeding difficulties or cardiovascular problems.

It is crucial to inform the parents as soon as the diagnosis is suspected by an experienced paediatrician. It is important that, at the time of breaking the news, the mother is supported by her partner or extended family. If possible, special arrangements should be made for the partner to stay overnight in the hospital; this helps enormously in the adjustment process. A preliminary chromosomal diagnosis can usually be confirmed within 24 to 48 hours by FISH analysis; further detailed chromosomal analysis may take up to 2 weeks.

Good-quality written information on Down syndrome for parents and extended families is available from the Down Syndrome Association and the Early Support Pack.

Physical features

Facial (Fig. 33.4)

- Brachycephaly
- Eyes
  - up-slanting palpebral fissures
  - epicanthic folds
  - Brushfield spots
- Flat facial profile
- Small ears with small or absent lobes
- Hypotonia with joint laxity
- Diastasis recti

- Small penis in males
- Poor Moro reflex
- Excess skin over the back of the neck
- Single palmar crease
- Fifth finger clinodactyly
- Sandal gap

All patients with Down syndrome have at least four of these features and 89% have six or more of these features (Hall 1964).

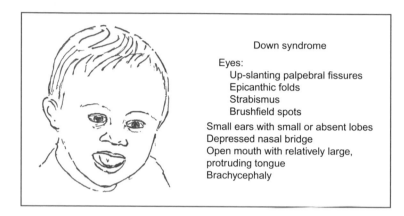

Down syndrome

Eyes:
    Up-slanting palpebral fissures
    Epicanthic folds
    Strabismus
    Brushfield spots
Small ears with small or absent lobes
Depressed nasal bridge
Open mouth with relatively large,
protruding tongue
Brachycephaly

Figure 33.4 Down syndrome.

Screening at diagnosis

- Cardiovascular – clinical examination and electrocardiography; echocardiography within 6 weeks
- Vision – clinical examination including red reflex
- Hearing – Newborn Hearing Screen
- Thyroid-stimulating hormone – blood spot

Differential diagnosis

Clearly, other conditions can have similar features to Down syndrome and these need to be considered if the karyotype returns as normal (Table 33.4).

Table 33.4 Differential diagnosis for Down syndrome. Each causes hypotonia and facial features of Down syndrome with a normal standard karyotype

Diagnosis	Features	Investigation
Prader–Willi syndrome	Lethargy Hypogonadism Initial failure to thrive followed later by obesity	Methylation-specific MLPA (MS-MLPA)
Zellweger syndrome	Hepatomegaly Seizures Chondrodysplasia punctata in patellar region	Very long-chain fatty acids
Smith–Magenis syndrome (17p11.2 deletion)	Sleep problems Self-injurious behaviours	FISH analysis and *RAI1* mutation analysis
Kleefstra syndrome (9q34.3 deletion)	Obesity Microcephaly Speech problems	FISH analysis and *EHMT1* mutation analysis

MLPA, multiplex ligation-dependent probe amplification; FISH, fluorescence in situ hybridization.

Childhood

DEVELOPMENT AND LEARNING

The developmental milestones are delayed; however, there is a wide variation in development. A useful brief guide is included in the Down syndrome-specific parent-held child health record inserts. These can be viewed and ordered through the Down Syndrome Medical Interest Group website (www.dsmig.org.uk).

In addition, Early Support has produced a 'Developmental journal for infants and children with Down syndrome'. This is a particularly useful resource for portage workers and early years educational settings and can be downloaded at www.education.gov.uk

There has been much research on the learning styles and needs of children with Down syndrome. A useful resource is the website of Down Syndrome Education International (www.dseinternational.org).

BEHAVIOURAL PHENOTYPE

Most children (75–85%) do not have an associated neurobehavioural problem. Although many parents express concerns, it is important to consider contributory factors for behavioural challenges including medical, psychosocial and environmental reasons. The behavioural phenotypes commonly present atypically. The common behavioural phenotypes are impulsivity, hyperactiviy, attention-deficit–hyperactivity disorder, autism and mood disorders.

Issues to consider at annual review for children with Down syndrome

Children and adults with Down syndrome are at risk of developing a range of medical complications (Table 33.5). They should be reviewed at least yearly by a paediatrician and later in adulthood by their general practitioner. It is important to recognize that clinical presentations can be atypical, and diagnostic overshadowing is common.

The history and examination should focus on the commonly associated medical complications as listed in Table 33.6, making enquiries in relation to each of the specific systems as listed below, in addition to any developmental and behavioural issues.

Table 33.5 Commonly associated medical complications

	Disorder and prevalence	Recommended surveillance	Recommended intervention
Growth	Short stature Faltering growth Obesity Specific nutritional deficiencies	*0–2y* Monitor weight and length frequently, at least every 2mo *2–18y* Monitor weight and height at least yearly Use Down syndrome specific growth charts	Rule out and treat possible medical causes Involve speech therapist to assess feeding skills Dietetic advice
Eyes	Congenital cataract Infant glaucoma Nystagmus (10%) Blocked nasolacrimal duct Strabismus Blepharitis (30%) Refractive errors (50%) Accommodation errors Keratoconus and cataract due to ageing (four times more common than in the typically developing population)	*Birth* Check for cataracts, glaucoma and visual behaviour *6wk–1y* Check visual behaviour/ squints Blocked nasolacrimal duct *18mo–5y* Yearly formal orthoptic review for refractive errors Ophthalmological review *5y to adulthood* If vision considered normal then 2-yearly review for refractive errors. In adulthood check cataracts/Keratoconus	Initial paediatric review If concerns refer to ophthalmologist Testing by dynamic retinoscopy methods is preferable Early use of bifocals Ensure proper fitting glasses Involve teachers for the visually impaired Surveillance can be provided by good high street opticians
Hearing	Hearing loss (50%) Congenital sensorineural deafness Recurrent otitis media Conductive hearing loss Mixed hearing loss Ear wax	*Birth* Newborn hearing screen *6mo–5y* Yearly formal audiological assessment including hearing, impedance, otoscopy *5y to adulthood* If normal, continue two yearly formal audiological review	Early referral to ENT for possible grommet insertion. This can be technically difficult Important to consider early intervention with hearing aids, particularly the BAHA soft band for children less than 8y of age and a BAHA for older children Involve teachers for the hearing impaired

	Disorder and prevalence	Recommended surveillance	Recommended intervention
Thyroid	Hypothyroidism (5–15%). Incidence increases with age Hyperthyroidism Transient elevation of TSH Presence of thyroid antibodies without presence of thyroid disease (30%)	*Birth* Newborn spot screening test (Guthrie testing)

At 12mo and 3–3y 6mo Thyroid function test Thyroid antibodies

3y 6mo to adulthood If venous sample, two yearly thyroid function test If capillary sample for TSH only, yearly sample | If TSH 6–10U/L and FT4 is normal, treatment is not necessarily warranted. Monitor closely

If TSH≥10U/L initiate treatment with thyroxine

TSH can be raised in intercurrent illness. Important to repeat

The presence of thyroid antibodies do not necessarily indicate presence of thyroid disease |
| Cardiac | Congenital heart disease (50–60%) Pulmonary hypertension Subacute bacterial endocarditis

Mitral valve prolapse (46%) Aortic regurgitation (17%) | *Birth to 2wk* Clinical examination and ECG If abnormal refer for specialist cardiological opinion and ECHO If normal refer for specialist cardiological opinion and ECHO within first 6wk

6wk to adult If normal scan, continue to monitor for pulmonary hypertension In adolescence and adulthood monitor for mitral valve prolapse and aortic regurgitation | Early surgical intervention at less than 4–6 months has a better outcome Affected children are more prone to pulmonary vascular disease secondary to respiratory infections and upper airway obstruction. RSV immunization should be offered to children less than 6mo at the start of the RSV season with haemodynamically significant acyanotic congenital heart disease |
Sleep-related breathing disorders	Obstructive sleep apnoea (58%)	*6mo onwards* Screening is controversial Important to enquire about sleep-related breathing disorders at each visit	If symptoms present, initially screen with overnight pulse oximetry. If abnormal seek ENT opinion If normal but persistent symptoms seek advice from respiratory specialist or organize specialist assessment
Autoimmune disorders	Coeliac (4–11%)	Screening for coeliac is controversial because of lack of evidence of improved outcome for treating asymptomatic coeliac disease	Investigate and treat actively if symptomatic
Dental care	Dental caries Gingivitis Bruxism	*6mo onwards* Referral to dentist	Important to provide advice early on regarding good oral hygiene Special tooth brushes Chlorhexidine and fluoride gel can be useful

Table 33.5 (Continued)

	Disorder and prevalence	Recommended surveillance	Recommended intervention
Behaviour	Autism (5–7%) Oppositional defiant disorder Vulnerability Hyperactivity Impulsivity	*Birth onwards* Support and listen to families concerns at each visit	Early behavioural intervention is important Autism may present atypically
Infections	Impaired immunity Respiratory tract infections Staphylococcal folliculitis	*Birth onwards* Enquire about general health at each visit, particularly if poor growth and development	Ensure primary immunisations May need booster for pneumococcal immunization Advise yearly seasonal 'flu' vaccination Consider referral to specialist for difficult/recurrent chest infections Consider use of regular prophylactic antibiotics if recurrent chest infections Chorhexidine handwash is useful for treating recurrent folliculitis
Sexual health	Increased vulnerability	*School age onwards* Discuss at each visit	Provide early advice on appropriate social behaviours, discouraging indiscriminate affectionate behaviours
	Managing periods	*9y to 10y onwards* Discuss at each visit	Period pain can lead to behavioural challenges Consider early referral to community family planning clinics for use of contraception, not as a contraceptive, but to manage periods

ENT, ear, nose and throat; BAHA, bone-anchored hearing aid; TSH; thyroid-stimulating hormone; ECG, electrocardiogram; ECHO, echocardiogram; RSV, respiratory syncytial virus.

Table 33.6 Other medical conditions that are more commonly seen in Down syndrome

Neurological	*Respiratory disorders*
Epilepsy	Increased respiratory infections
Infantile spasms	Sleep-related breathing disorders
Late-onset myoclonic epilepsy	Acquired tracheobronchomalacia (usually in the
Reflex startle epilepsy	presence of congenital heart disease)
Autonomic dysfunction	Bronchiectasis
Non-specific basal ganglia abnormalities	Pulmonary hypoplasia
Moyamoya disease (risk of stroke)	Lung anomalies, e.g. presence of cysts
Cervical spine instability	
Delayed closure of anterior fontanelle	*Autoimmune disorders*
	Diabetes mellitus
Dermatological	Juvenile rheumatoid arthritis
Alopecia areata 8.8%	Hepatitis
Seborrhoeic dermatitis	Vitiligo
Fungal infections	
Cutis marmorata	*Orthopaedic*
Acrocyanosis	Hypermobility
	Pes planus
Blood disorders	Hip subluxation/dislocation
Acute myeloid leukaemia	Patellar instability
Acute lymphoblastic leukaemia	
Polycythaemia	

Cervical spine disorders

Children and young people with Down syndrome are at risk of neurological disorders as a consequence of an increased incidence of cervical spine disorders. Cervical spine disorders incorporate arthropathies and craniovertebral instability including atlantoaxial subluxation. The main contributory factors are hypotonia in the young, resulting in craniovertebral instability, and in the older person the preterm degenerative processes resulting in arthropathy.

The presentation of atlantoaxial subluxation can be acute, chronic or acute on chronic. The common symptoms are abnormal head and neck posture, neck pain, deterioration of gait and/or motor coordination. Investigations to confirm the diagnosis are plain lateral radiography of the cervical neck in both full flexion and extension. This can be a challenge to obtain! A normal X-ray does not completely rule out the problem. If there is a high suspicion of a cervical spine disorder, a timely neurosurgical opinion should be sought.

Screening is not considered to be predictive of which individuals are at risk of developing a myelopathy; 30% of young people with an increased atlantodens interval can be asymptomatic and surgery can be detrimental.

The current recommendations are as follows:

1 Parents should be routinely made aware of the signs and symptoms.
2 There is no absolute contraindication to participate in gymnastics and trampolining. The British Gymnastics Society has sensible practical advice on its website (www.british-gymnastics.org).
3 To have a low threshold to evaluate and investigate any concerns around cervical spine instability.
4 Timely treatment in a centre of expertise results in relatively good outcomes.

Transition to adult services

It is crucial to support the young person and family in planning for transition to adult services. It is important to provide the family and general practitioner with clear information regarding the young person's current needs and a plan for life-long medical surveillance, as outlined above, and potential problems, e.g. mitral valve prolapse or mental health problems. Very often the local learning disability teams will take a lead in providing a service for young people in adult life.

The median age at death in those with Down syndrome increased from 25 years in 1983 to 49 years in 1997. Death certificates of individuals with Down syndrome are more likely to list congenital heart disease, dementia, hypothyroidism and leukaemia (Yang et al. 2002).

Support organization

The Down Syndrome Association provides excellent support materials and links for families on a wide range of issues, including health, education and social support (see www.down-syndrome.org.uk).

The Down Syndrome Medical Interest Group is a network of healthcare professionals from the UK and the Republic of Ireland whose aim is to share and disseminate information about the medical aspects of Down syndrome (see www.dsmig.org.uk).

Key messages

- Down syndrome is the most common genetic cause of learning difficulties.
- Breaking the news to parents regarding the diagnosis of Down syndrome must be done in a sensitive and informative manner.
- Down syndrome is associated with increased risk of congenital malformations and medical complications affecting all systems; the medical presentation may be atypical.
- With improved health care and support the average lifespan is now at least 49 years.
- Most children with Down syndrome are educated in a mainstream school setting. Children with Down syndrome benefit from having information presented in a visual manner. *Down Syndrome Education International* is a useful resource.
- The Down Syndrome Medical Interest Group UK website (www.dsmig.org.uk) provides information on 'best practice' medical care for people with Down syndrome in the UK and Ireland.

Fragile X syndrome

Fragile X syndrome is the most common cause of inherited intellectual disability. A recent neo-natal screening study revealed a prevalence of 1 in 5161 in males (Coffee et al. 2009).

Genetics

The gene responsible for fragile X syndrome is called *FMR1* and it is located at Xq27.3. Almost all patients with fragile X syndrome have an expansion of a CGG trinucleotide repeat in the untranslated region of this gene. This leads to methylation of its promoter gene, and therefore transcriptional silencing of the gene. Inactivation of the *FMR1* gene results in loss of its protein product, which is called FMRP. This is involved in the regulation of transport and translation of some mRNAs in neuronal dendrites that affect synaptic plasticity, which is central to learning and memory.

Normal allele:	5 to 55 CGG repeats (of which grey zone 45–55 repeats)
Premutation alleles:	56 to 200 CGG repeats
Full mutation alleles:	>200 CGG repeats

Normal *FMR1* alleles do not show significant variation in their repeat size. Once the number of repeats starts to increase, there is further meiotic instability in both the male and female, result-ing in further expansion. Only in the female germline can this expand to a full mutation. The risk of a premutation allele expanding to a full mutation in the female germline is dependent on its size; the risk with 55 to 59 CGG repeats expanding to a full mutation is 3% to 4%, whereas alleles with more than 100 repeats will almost always expand to a full mutation.

Testing is by polymerase chain reaction (PCR), followed by Southern blot analysis.

Fragile X syndrome in males

Clinical phenotype

- Long, narrow face with tall forehead, large anteverted ears and a prominent jaw (Fig. 33.5)
- Global developmental delay – particularly speech and language delay
- Moderate to severe learning difficulties
- Hypotonia
- Seizures
- Accelerated growth in childhood
- Macro-orchidism in postpubertal males.

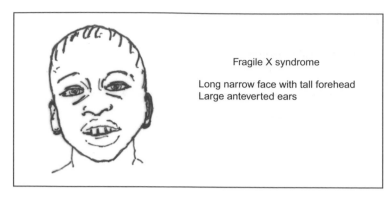

Fragile X syndrome

Long narrow face with tall forehead
Large anteverted ears

Figure 33.5 Fragile X syndrome.

Behavioural phenotype

- Autism (60% of males with full mutation) (Harris et al. 2008)
- Gaze avoidance
- Hand flapping
- Attention difficulties and impulsivity
- Obsessive–compulsive behaviours
- Emotional lability

Other difficulties

- Vision – strabismus, refractive errors
- Hearing – recurrent otitis media
- Dental malocclusion
- Joint hypermobility

Fragile X syndrome in females

Only one-third of all females with a full mutation have clinical problems. These can range from mild learning difficulties or behavioural problems to a phenotype that is similar in severity to affected males with fragile X syndrome. The variable phenotype in females with a full mutation is due to skewed X chromosome inactivation (Martinez et al. 2005).

Problems in fragile X carriers

FRAGILE X-ASSOCIATED TREMOR/ATAXIA SYNDROME (FXTAS)

Around 40% of males and 8% of females with fragile X syndrome over the age of 50 years develop this neurodegenerative disorder. The main clinical features of this condition are intention tremor, gait ataxia, parkinsonism, moderate to severe short-term memory deficiency and difficulties with executive function (Hagerman and Hagerman 2004).

PRETERM OVARIAN INSUFFICIENCY

This occurs in 20% of female carriers.

PSYCHIATRIC PROBLEMS

These can be seen in children and adults and include mood and anxiety disorders and, in males, social avoidance.

DIFFERENTIAL DIAGNOSIS

Children who have features suggesting fragile X syndrome but whose DNA analysis is reported to be normal need re-evaluation and investigation as outlined in Table 33.7.

Table 33.7 Differential diagnosis of fragile X syndrome in males

Diagnosis	Features	Investigation
Idiopathic autistic spectrum disorder	Social communication disorder	Clinical diagnosis
Sotos syndrome	Excessive growth with advanced bone age Developmental delay	NSD1 gene mutation analysis
Prader–Willi syndrome	Hypotonia and poor feeding in infancy Hyperphagia and obesity Hypogonadism	Methylation-specific MLPA (MS-MLPA)
FG syndrome	Hypotonia Macrocephaly Learning difficulties Agenesis of the corpus callosum	Genetically heterogeneous. Common mutation in MED12 gene

MLPA, multiplex ligation-dependent probe amplification.

Issues to consider at annual review for children with fragile X syndrome

At all ages consider the following:

- **History**
  - Development; in particular of communication, including social communication
  - Educational progress and support
  - Behaviour, in particular attention and impulsivity
  - Dental health
- **Examination**
  - Growth

Screening

Vision, hearing, cardiac and skeletal screening are recommended during childhood as children with fragile X syndrome are more likely to have difficulties in these areas than typically developing children. The recommended screening is shown in Table 33.8.

Table 33.8 Fragile X syndrome-specific screening

Age	Examination to be performed once during this period
Infancy	Vision Hearing Cardiac Skeletal assessment for hypermobility Arrange genetic counselling for family
1–5y	Vision Hearing
5–11y	Vision Hearing Cardiac examination Skeletal assessment for hypermobility
11y and over	Vision Hearing Cardiac examination Skeletal assessment for hypermobility Assess testicular volume

Source: Hersh and Saul (2011).

Support organization

The Fragile X Society: www.fragilex.org.uk

Key messages

- All male and female patients with unexplained developmental delay or learning difficulties should undergo molecular diagnostic testing for fragile X syndrome, as should all children diagnosed with autism or autism spectrum disorder.
- Parents of males with fragile X syndrome, females with full mutations and children of both sexes who carry premutations or grey zone alleles should be referred to the clinical geneticist for genetic advice, discussion of the options for prenatal testing where relevant and for family studies.

Neurofibromatosis type 1

Neurofibromatosis type 1 (NF1) is one of the most frequently encountered genetic disorders in paediatric practice with a birth incidence of 1 in 2500 to 3000. It is diagnosed on the basis of clinical criteria which are summarised in Table 33.9.

Table 33.9 Diagnostic criteria for neurofibromatosis type 1

	Age at onset
Six or more café-au-lait macules (Fig. 33.6)	2y
Two or more cutaneous/subcutaneous neurofibromas or one plexiform neurofibroma	Early childhood Increase in size at puberty
Freckling in the axilla, neck or groin	5y
Optic pathway glioma	Early childhood
Two or more Lisch nodules (iris hamartomas) on slit-lamp examination	50% by 5y 75% by 15y
Sphenoid wing dysplasia or dysplasia or thinning of the long bone cortex	
A first-degree relative with neurofibromatosis type 1	

The patient should have two or more of the above features.
Source: Anon (1988).

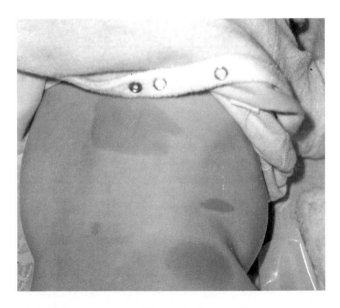

Figure 33.6 Cutaneous features of neurofibromatosis type 1.

Genetics

Neurofibromatosis type 1 is a clinical diagnosis. Genetic confirmation of the diagnosis by *NF1* mutation analysis is available on a diagnostic basis but is expensive because of the large size of the gene (59 exons) and a very large mutational spectrum. It is indicated if parents are likely to want to consider having a prenatal test for NF1 in a pregnancy (this is infrequently requested by families) or pre-implantation genetic diagnosis. In more severely affected children with NF1 it can be useful to test for a whole gene deletion of the *NF1* gene by multiplex ligation-dependent probe amplification (MLPA), as this may provide some prognostic information for the family.

Neurofibromatosis type 1 is inherited in an autosomal dominant manner and is caused by mutations in the *NF1* gene at 17q11.2. There is complete penetrance by the age of about 5 to 6 years but NF1 can show quite marked intrafamilial variability of expression.

In 50% of patients with NF1 this condition is the result of a new mutation in one copy of the *NF1* gene while the remaining 50% inherit the condition from an affected parent. Both parents of an affected child should be carefully examined for the clinical features of NF1 including examination of the skin under Wood's light to look for faint café-au-lait patches, as the condition can show quite marked intrafamilial variability of expression. If one parent is affected with NF1 there will be a 50% (1 in 2) chance of this condition recurring in all of their future pregnancies. If neither parent is affected with NF1 the recurrence risk of this condition in the parent's next pregnancy is less than 1% (1 in 100).

Deletion of whole NF1 gene

About 5% of patients with NF1 are heterozygous for a 1.4-Mb deletion at 17q11.2 that results in deletion of the whole *NF1* gene. These patients have a more severe phenotype. They are more likely to have learning and attention difficulties, dysmorphic features, tall stature, large hands and feet, hypotonia, joint laxity and scoliosis. They also have a significantly increased chance of developing subcutaneous, plexiform and spinal neurofibromas and malignant peripheral nerve sheath tumours.

NF1 – Noonan phenotype or Watson syndrome

Some children with NF1 have Noonan-like facies (ptosis, hypertelorism, down-slanting palpebral fissures, and low-set, posteriorly rotated ears). Most of these patients have mutations in the *NF1* gene. They present with multiple café-au-lait patches, Noonan-like facies, pulmonary stenosis, short stature and learning difficulties.

NF1 complications

These can be divided into four groups for counselling purposes (Huson et al. 1989).

CENTRAL NERVOUS SYSTEM

- Learning difficulties – around 30% are usually mild to moderate, but 3% are severe.
- Attention difficulties
- Macrocephaly
- Unidentified bright objects seen by 60% of children due to spongiform myelinopathy in the basal ganglia, optic tracts, brainstem or cerebellum. These usually resolve with age but can also be seen by adults with NF1. Their clinical significance is unclear.

CENTRAL NERVOUS SYSTEM TUMOURS AND MALIGNANT TUMOURS (4–5% OF PATIENTS)

- Optic glioma – 15% of children prior to 6 years. Presentations include loss of vision, proptosis and precocious puberty.
- Other central nervous system tumours (e.g. astrocytoma)
- Rhabdomyosarcoma
- Malignant peripheral nerve sheath tumour – lifetime risk of 5.9% to 10.3% with a median age at diagnosis of 42.1 years (McCaughan et al. 2007).

COMPLICATIONS THAT DEVELOP IN CHILDHOOD AND CAUSE LIFELONG MORBIDITY (8–9% OF CHILDREN)

- Severe plexiform neurofibromas of the head and neck, usually evident by 18 months to 2 years.
- Scoliosis severe enough to require surgery (5% of children).
- Severe pseudoarthrosis.

TREATABLE COMPLICATIONS THAT CAN DEVELOP AT ANY AGE (16% OF PATIENTS)

- Aqueduct stenosis
- Epilepsy (4% of patients)
- Spinal and visceral neurofibromas
- Phaeochromocytomas
- Renal artery stenosis

DIFFERENTIAL DIAGNOSIS

For children who have features suggesting neurofibromatosis but who fail to fulfill diagnostic criteria, alternative diagnoses need to be considered. The clinical features and diagnostic testing are outlined in Table 33.10.

Table 33.10 Differential diagnosis of neurofibromatosis type 1

Diagnosis	Features	Testing
Legius syndrome	Family history (autosomal dominant) Multiple café-au-lait patches Axillary freckling Macrocephaly and learning difficulties But do not develop Lisch nodules, osseous lesions typical of NF1, neurofibromas or CNS tumours (Messiaen et al. 2009)	Mutations in the *SPRED1* gene
Segmental neurofibromatosis	Café-au-lait patches Axillary freckling Subcutaneous neurofibromas Restricted to one area	Somatic mosaic for an NF1 gene mutation (Ruggieri and Huson 2001)
Neurofibromatosis type 2 (NF2)	Family history of vestibular schwannomas or meningiomas Multiple café-au-lait spots (sometimes) but no Lisch nodules or axillary freckling	Magnetic resonance imaging showing bilateral vestibular schwannomas NF2 mutation analysis will identify a mutation in 65% of patients
Hereditary non-polyposis colorectal cancer due to biallelic mismatch repair gene mutations	Multiple café-au-lait patches Malignancies: haematological (leukaemia, lymphoma); brain tumours (glioblastoma, astrocytoma); gastrointestinal Wilms tumour or neuroblastoma	*MLH1, MSH2, MSH6* and *PMS2* mutation analysis (immunohistochemistry on tumour tissue used to prioritize genetic testing) Clinical criteria used to identify suitable candidate family for genetic testing
LEOPARD syndrome	Lentigines (dark, <5mm on trunk and face) ECG abnormalities Ocular hypertelorism Pulmonary stenosis Abnormal genitalia Retardation of growth Deafness	Genetically heterogeneous disorder Can be caused by heterozygous mutations in the *PTPN1, BRAF* and *RAF1* genes

NF1, neurofibromatosis type 1; CNS, central nervous system; ECG, electrocardiography.

Issues to consider at an annual review for children with NF1

- **History**
  - Progress with learning/development
  - Visual symptoms
  - Headaches
  - Behaviour, in particular attention and concentration
  - Educational progress
  - Seizures
- **Examination**
  - Weight, height, head circumference
  - Pubertal staging
  - Skin – neurofibromas

- Blood pressure
- Fundoscopy and visual fields by confrontation (further visual screening is outlined in Table 33.11)
- Scoliosis

Table 33.11 Schedule for formal visual assessment in neurofibromatosis type 1

Age	Assessment
3y	Visual acuity + ophthalmology assessment of fundi
5y	Colour vision + ophthalmology assessment of fundi
8y	Visual fields + ophthalmology assessment of fundi

Regular brain MRI is not currently recommended in children with NF1 to screen for optic glioma (Ferner et al. 2007).

Ensure that parents understand the diagnosis and talk to the child about this as he or she progresses into puberty.

Support organization

The Neuro Foundation is the working name of the Neurofibromatosis Association. It has excellent information for schools (www.nfauk.org).

Williams syndrome

Williams syndrome is a chromosomal microdeletion syndrome. It has a birth incidence of 1 in 10 000 to 1 in 20 000.

Genetics

Around 95% of patients with Williams syndrome have a heterozygous 1.5-Mb deletion at 7q11.23 with most of the remaining cases having a larger 1.84-Mb deletion affecting the same chromosomal segment (Bayes 2003). The deleted region is estimated to contain 25 to 30 genes including the elastin gene (*ELN*), which is thought to be the cause of the cardiovascular and connective tissue abnormalities seen in Williams syndrome.

The genetic diagnosis of Williams syndrome is made by FISH analysis using a probe that contains the sequence of the *ELN* gene. Most instances arise sporadically. FISH analysis of the parents of a child with a confirmed diagnosis of Willams syndrome is not recommended unless one parent has some features of Williams syndrome. The recurrence risk of Williams syndrome in the parent's next pregnancy is likely to be very small but parents can be offered a prenatal test (chorionic villus sampling or amniocentesis with FISH analysis using the *ELN* probe) for reassurance.

Features of Williams syndrome

- Developmental delay
  - Initially speech and language is delayed, although in time a good expressive vocabulary is developed
  - Mild to moderate intellectual disability (full-range IQ: mean 55, range 40–100)
  - Verbal IQ scores are higher than average performance IQ scores
  - Poor visuospatial skills
- Typical facial appearance, which becomes more prominent with age (Fig 33.7)
  - Periorbital fullness with epicanthic folds, a stellate or lacy iris pattern
  - Flat midface with depressed nasal bridge
  - Anteverted nares
  - Long, relatively smooth philtrum
  - Full cheeks
  - Wide mouth with thick lips
- Behavioural phenotype
  - Infants have an interest in faces
  - Children are socially engaging and socially disinhibited
  - Conversation is loquacious with stereotyped and repetitive phrases
  - Empathetic but fail to recognize social cues
  - Attention-deficit–hyperactivity disorder
  - Anxiety disorders (Morris 2010)
- Arteriopathy/vasculopathy
  - Supravalvular aortic stenosis – seen in older children and can progress
  - Peripheral pulmonary artery stenosis – seen most commonly in infancy and can resolve
  - Other vessels can be affected – aorta, coronary and renal artery
- Hypercalcaemia (10–15%) or hypercalciuria (30%). Usually resolve during the second year of life but can recur in older patients
- Failure to thrive in infancy
- Short stature
- Connective tissue abnormalities
  - Soft, stretchy skin
  - Joint laxity
  - Inguinal or umbilical hernia
  - Bladder diverticulae and rectal prolapse
- Visual problems – strabismus and hypermetropia
- Hearing problems – hyperacusis and recurrent otitis media
- Dental problems – malocclusion, microdontia and enamel hypoplasia

Complications

- Hypertension (Eronen et al. 2002, Collins et al. 2010)
- Vesicoureteric reflux and single kidney
- Nocturnal enuresis
- Constipation
- Coeliac disease
- Precocious puberty

Differential diagnosis

Children who have features suggesting Williams syndrome but whose DNA analysis is reported to be normal need re-evaluation and investigation as outlined in Table 33.12.

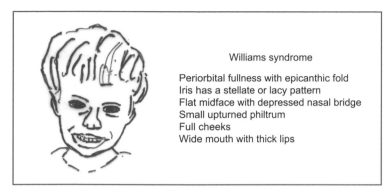

Williams syndrome

Periorbital fullness with epicanthic fold
Iris has a stellate or lacy pattern
Flat midface with depressed nasal bridge
Small upturned philtrum
Full cheeks
Wide mouth with thick lips

Figure 33.7 Williams syndrome.

Table 33.12 Differential diagnosis of Williams syndrome

Diagnosis	Features	Genetics
Alagille syndrome	Peripheral pulmonary artery stenosis Facial features – prominent forehead, deep-set eyes, anteverted ears and a prominent chin Chronic liver disease Vertebral anomalies	Autosomal dominant Mutations or deletions of the *JAG1* gene or mutations of the *NOTCH2* gene
Noonan syndrome	Facial features – ptosis, hypertelorism, down-slanting palpebral fissures and low-set, posteriorly rotated ears Webbing of the neck Pectus excavatum Valvular pulmonary stenosis Hypertrophic cardiomyopathy Cryptorchidism	Autosomal dominant Mutations in several different genes

Annual review

HISTORY

- Feeding
- Bowel habit
- Urinary tract symptoms
- Hypothyroid symptoms
- Dental health – seeing dentist
- Development/learning

EXAMINATION

- Growth – on Williams growth chart (Martin et al. 2007)
- Signs of puberty in childhood
- Blood pressure
- Cardiovascular system (every 2y)
- Spine

SCREENING

As children with Williams syndrome are more likely to have difficulties with hearing, vision, calcium metabolism and coeliac disease, screening is advised as detailed in Table 33.13.

Table 33.13 Screening in Williams syndrome

Screening	Diagnosis	Age (y)								
		0–1	1	3	5	7	9	11	13	15
Cardiac assessment[a]										
Hearing										
Vision										
Serum calcium										
Urine calcium–creatinine ratio										
Thyroid function test										
Renal ultrasound										
Coeliac screening										

Grey shading indicates routine screening. Dark grey shading indicates screening if the child is hypercalcaemic.
[a]Cardiac assessment should consist of four-limb blood pressure and echocardiogram.

The American Academy of Pediatrics (2001) has published a diagnostic checklist for Williams syndrome and guidelines for the health supervision of children with this condition. Expert opinion management guidelines for patients with Williams syndrome have also been published recently (Pober 2010).

Support organization

The Williams Syndrome Foundation (www.williams-syndrome.org.uk) has developed clinical guidelines for the management of affected individuals and these can be downloaded from its website (www.williams-syndrome.org.uk/about/guidelines/guidelines.html).

> **Top tip**
>
> It is important for children with Williams syndrome not to receive multivitamin prepara-
> tions, as most such preparations contain vitamin D, which can have a deleterious effect
> on the hypercalcaemia and hypercalciuria of Williams syndrome.

Angelman syndrome

Angelman syndrome is a severe neurodevelopmental disorder that has an incidence of 1 in
10 000 to 1 in 20 000.

Genetics

There is a variety of molecular mechanisms affecting the maternally imprinted region on the
long arm of chromosome 15 (15q11–q13). All these mechanisms result in loss of expression
of the maternally inherited copy of the *UBE3A* gene, which is located in this region. This gene
shows tissue-specific imprinting with only the maternally inherited allele being expressed in the
brain (particularly the hippocampus and Purkinje cells of the cerebellum).

Table 33.14 Gene defect and frequency in Angelman syndrome

Genetic defect	Frequency (%)	Effect on maternal UBE3A gene
Microdeletion of 5 to 7 Mb in maternal copy (the majority is de novo)	70–75	Absent
Paternal uniparental disomy for chromosome 15	3–7	Two paternal copies but no maternal copy
Imprinting defect	2–3	Maternal copy of *UBE3A* has paternal imprint
Mutation in maternally inherited copy of *UBE3A* gene (80% de novo)	10	No functional copy
Unknown	10	

Investigation

Standard karyotype and methylation pattern analysis at 15q11–q13 (using methylation-specific
multiplex ligation-dependent probe amplification) are the initial tests recommended for the
diagnosis of this condition. This can be followed by further genetic testing that can identify the
specific defect in order for geneticists to understand the mode of inheritance and therefore the
recurrence risk (Table 33.14). Prenatal testing can be performed.

The electroencephalogram has characteristic abnormalities and can help to make the diagnosis, even in children without seizures.

Clinical features

- Severe global developmental delay
- Absent or severely limited speech
  - Most can understand simple commands
  - A few can use Makaton to communicate
- Ataxia or tremulous movements of the limbs
  - Most patients are able to walk (mean age of 4y)
  - Gait is slow, stiff and ataxic with raised arms held flexed at the elbows and wrists
- Epilepsy
  - 90% of patients, onset between 1 and 5 years
  - Febrile and afebrile seizures
  - Many different seizure types, including generalized and focal onset
  - 60% with multiple seizure types (Thibert et al. 2009)
- Acquired microcephaly
- Dysmorphic facial features (Fig. 33.8)
  - Brachycephaly
  - Deep-set eyes
  - Wide mouth with widely spaced teeth
  - Prominent jaw
- Behavioural phenotype
  - Happy, smiling demeanour with paroxysms of laughter
  - Hyperactivity and short attention span
  - Frequent hand flapping
  - Tongue thrusting and excessive chewing or mouthing behaviours
  - A fascination for water and reflective surfaces
  - Disturbed sleeping pattern
- Feeding difficulties in infancy
- Drooling
- Scoliosis

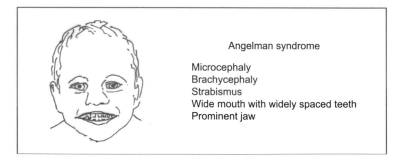

Angelman syndrome

Microcephaly
Brachycephaly
Strabismus
Wide mouth with widely spaced teeth
Prominent jaw

Figure 33.8 Angelman syndrome.

Differential diagnosis

Children who have features suggesting Angelman syndrome but whose genetic analysis is reported to be normal need re-evaluation and investigation as outlined in Table 33.15.

Table 33.15 Differential diagnosis of Angelman syndrome

Diagnosis	Feature	Genetics
Chromosomal disorders		
Inverted duplications of chromosome 15	Hypotonia Severe developmental delay Absent or limited speech Epilepsy, often infantile spasms Behavioural problems	Mosaicism for a supernumary marker chromosome resulting in tetrasomy for the 15q11–q13 region
22q13.3 deletion (Phelan–McDermid syndrome)	Severe expressive language delay Normal or excessive growth	
Single gene disorders		
Rett syndrome	Females Normal development until 6–9mo Acquired microcephaly Loss of hand skills with hand stereotypies Social withdrawal with autistic features Seizures	X-linked dominant Locus Xq28 Gene *MECP2* and *FOXG1*
CDKL5 mutations	Seizures – onset in early infancy Hypotonia Hand stereotypies Autistic features Scoliosis	X-linked disorder Locus Xp22 Gene *CDKL5*
Mowat–Wilson syndrome	Dysmorphic facial features Microcephaly Epilepsy Constipation/Hirschsprung disease	Autosomal dominant Locus 2q22.3 Gene *ZEB2 (ZFHX1B, SIP1)*
Christianson syndrome	Usually affects males Seizures Hands have long thin fingers with stereotypies Cerebellar and brainstem atrophy on MRI	X-linked dominant Locus Xq26.3 Gene *SLC9A6*
Pitt–Hopkins syndrome	Microcephaly Absent or limited speech Dysmorphic facies with coarse features Seizures Ataxic gait Episodes of hyperventilation and apnoea beginning between 3 and 8y of age Happy, placid personality	Autosomal dominant Locus 18q21.1 Gene *TCF4*

Diagnosis	Feature	Genetics
MEF2C deletion/ mutations	Hypotonia Absent speech Hand stereotypies Episodes of hyperventilation and apnoea Epilepsy Subtle facial dysmorphism Corpus callosum anomalies or ventricular dilatation on MRI	Autosomal dominant Locus 5q14 Gene *MEF2C*
Methylene tetrahydrofolate reductase deficiency	Microcephaly Seizures Stroke Psychiatric problems Ataxic gait Increased plasma homocysteine levels, homocystinuria	Autosomal recessive Locus 1p36.3 Gene *MTHFR*
ATR-X syndrome	Males affected Absent or limited speech Hypotonia in infancy followed by spasticity Microcephaly Facial dysmorphism Genital anomalies	X-linked recessive Locus Xq21.1 Gene *ATRX*
Gurrieri syndrome	Early-onset seizures Absent speech Keratoconus Skeletal dysplasia	Autosomal recessive Locus unknown Gene unknown
Mitochondrial disorders	Poor growth Muscle weakness Multiple systems involved Loss of skills	Plasma lactate as screening test CSF lactate
Multifactorial disorders		
Autism spectrum disorder	May have normal early development Lack of social interest Poor non-verbal skills Stereotypies Restricted range of activities	Clinical diagnosis
Lennox–Gastaut syndrome	Multiple seizure types unresponsive to treatment	EEG

Note: all of these conditions cause severe developmental delay. MRI, magnetic resonance imaging; ATR-X, alpha-thalassaemia mental retardation syndrome X-linked; CSF, cerebrospinal fluid; EEG, electroencephalography. Source: Williams et al. (2001).

Issues to consider at annual review for child with Angelman syndrome

- **History**
  - General health
  - Seizures
  - Feeding
  - Developmental progress
  - Hearing (formal assessment at diagnosis)
  - Vision (formal assessment at diagnosis)
  - Nursery/school
  - Behaviour and sleep
- **Examination**
  - Growth
  - Cardiovascular system
  - Contractures
  - Scoliosis
- **Management**
  - The child needs to be under the care of a physiotherapist and a speech and language therapist.
  - Epilepsy. The most frequently prescribed anticonvulsants agents in Angelman syndrome are sodium valproate and clonazepam, but lamotrigine and levetiracetam may have similar efficacy (Thibert et al. 2009).

Support group

The Angelman Syndrome Support Education and Research Trust (ASSERT) is the support group for the families and carers of affected individuals with Angleman syndrome in the UK (www. angelmanuk.org/).

Prader–Willi syndrome

Prader–Willi syndrome is a complex neurobehavioural disorder that has a birth incidence of 1 in 10 000 to 1 in 15 000.

Genetics

Prader–Willi syndrome is caused by several different molecular mechanisms that result in loss of expression of paternally expressed genes on the long arm of chromosome 15 (15q11–q13). There are a number of genes in this region that are imprinted, with several being expressed only from the paternally inherited allele (Table 33.16). Loss of the expression of the paternally inherited copies of the *SNRPN, NDN* and *SNORD116* sno–RNA cluster is thought to be the cause of Prader–Willi syndrome (Duker et al. 2010).

Table 33.16 Gene defect and frequency in Prader-Willi syndrome

Genetic defect	Frequency	Effect on paternally expressed genes at 15q11–q13
Paternal microdeletion 15q11–q13	70–75%	Absent
Paternal larger deletion including 15q11–q13	1–1.5%	Absent
Maternal uniparental disomy for chromosome 15	25%	Two maternal copies No paternal copy
Imprinting defect at 15q11–q13	1%	Functionally inactive as they have a maternal imprint

All children with suspected Prader–Willi syndrome should undergo standard karyotyping and diagnostic genetic testing by MS-MLPA. They should be referred to a clinical geneticist for additional investigations to work out the underlying molecular mechanism and for a discussion about recurrence risk and prenatal diagnosis with the parents.

Clinical features

NEONATAL PERIOD

- Severe hypotonia associated with a history of reduced fetal movements
- Reduced spontaneous arousal
- Weak cry and poor suck with feeding difficulties
- Preserved deep tendon reflexes
- Hypogonadism (Cassidy and Driscoll 2009)

> **Top tip**
>
> All neonates with severe, persistent and unexplained hypotonia should undergo standard karyotyping to look for an underlying chromosomal disorder such as Down syndrome and molecular genetic analysis (MS-MLPA) for the diagnosis of Prader–Willi syndrome.

Infants and children

- Hypotonia
- Learning difficulties. 80% have low to normal intelligence or mild learning difficulties and 20% have moderate learning difficulties. The academic performance of children with Prader–Willi syndrome is poor for their cognitive ability. They appear to have relative strength in reading, good visuospatial skills, and good long-term memory but difficulties with mathematics, sequential processing and poor short-term memory. They can be surprisingly proficient at jigsaws and word puzzles.
- Facial dysmorphism (see Fig. 33.9)
  - Bifrontal narrowing

- Almond-shaped eyes
- Narrow nasal bridge
- Thin upper lip with downturned angles of the mouth
- Hypopigmentation of the skin and hair (the microdeletion results in loss of the one copy of the *P* gene, which is responsible for autosomal recessive tyrosinase-positive oculocutaneous albinism)
- Small hands and feet
- Hypogonadism
  - Seen in both males and females
  - Males – unilateral or bilateral cryptorchidism (80–90%) with scrotal hypoplasia with small testes and small penis
  - Females – hypoplastic labia majora and minora
- Puberty
  - Delayed and incomplete pubertal development in both sexes
  - Preterm adrenarche has been reported in 15% to 20% of patients
  - Precocious puberty in about 4%
  - Most males (and probably most females) are infertile
- Feeding and growth
  - Feeding difficulties in the first 2 years of life
  - From 2 years old an excessive appetite (hyperphagia)
  - Severe obesity developing between 1 and 4 years of age
  - Short stature
- Behavioural phenotype
  - Temper tantrums
  - Stubbornness
  - Manipulative behaviours
  - Obsessive–compulsive behaviour
  - Social communication difficulties
  - High pain threshold and, frequently, skin-picking resulting in infected skin wounds and scarring
  - Food-seeking behaviour and food-hoarding behaviour is common in childhood, as is a high threshold for vomiting. This can lead to morbid obesity, which is the major cause of morbidity and mortality in Prader–Willi syndrome
  - 10% to 20% of adults develop a major psychosis

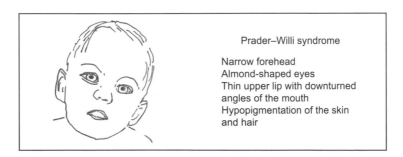

Prader–Willi syndrome

Narrow forehead
Almond-shaped eyes
Thin upper lip with downturned angles of the mouth
Hypopigmentation of the skin and hair

Figure 33.9 Prader–Willi syndrome.

Differential diagnosis

Children who have features suggesting Prader-Willi syndrome but whose genetic analysis is reported to be normal need re-evaluation and investigation as outlined in Table 33.17.

Table 33.17 Differential diagnosis of Prader–Willi syndrome in children with learning difficulties and obesity

Syndrome	Features	Defect and testing
Temple	Neonatal hypotonia Macrocephaly with arrested hydrocephalus Precocious puberty	Maternal uniparental disomy for chromosome 14 Specific MS-MLPA test

Fragile X	A subset of patients present with:
	    hyperphagia
	    obesity
	    pubertal delay with hypogonadism
	    autistic features
		CGG repeat expansion in *FMR1* gene
		Molecular diagnostic test

Bardet–Biedl	Postaxial polydactyly Renal anomalies Cone–rod dystrophy by 7–10y	Autosomal recessive 14 different genes
Cohen	Microcephaly Distinctive facial features Intermittent neutropenia High myopia Retinal dystrophy by 10y	Autosomal recessive Mutations in *COH1* gene at 8q22
Alstrom	Cone–rod dystrophy Sensorineural hearing loss Dilated cardiomyopathy	Autosomal recessive Mutations in the *ALMS1* gene at 2p23.1
Borjeson–Forssman–Lehmann	Males (most frequently) Epilepsy Coarse facial features Short stature Microcephaly Pubertal delay	X-linked recessive Mutations in the *PHF6* gene at Xq26.3
Monogenic obesity due to mutations in *SIM1* gene	Early-onset obesity Few other difficulties	Mutations in the *SIM1* gene at 6q16.3
Deletion 6q16	Dysmorphic features Small hands and feet	Loss of one copy of *SIM1* gene Array-CGH
Diploid–triploid mosaicism	Skeletal asymmetry Partial syndactyly of fourth and fifth fingers Pigmentary skin anomalies on Wood's light examination	Blood karyotype may be normal – need to check karyotype in cultured skin fibroblasts
1p36 microdeletion	Distinctive facies Epilepsy – common	Microdeletion at 1p36 Diagnosis by FISH analysis or array-CGH

MS, methylation specific; MLPA, multiplex ligation-dependent probe amplification. CGH, comparative genomic hybridization; FISH, fluorescence in situ hybridization.

Management

Children with Prader-Willi syndrome have difficulties with eating, growth and puberty which need to be managed as outlined in Table 33.18.

Table 33.18 Specific medical issues and their management in Prader–Willi syndrome

Issue	Management
Obesity	Involve a dietitian Low-calorie diet Ensure vitamin and calcium content of diet Encourage 30min of exercise a day
Food-scavenging behaviour	Put locks on kitchen cupboards and the fridge Make sure that the whole family, school and neighbours are educated in the situation Psychology support
Short stature	Refer to endocrinology Indication for growth hormone treatment
Cryptorchidism	Refer to paediatric urology
Delayed puberty	Refer to endocrinology for treatment
Obstructive sleep apnoea	Overnight oximetry Further sleep studies Refer to ear, nose and throat specialist for an opinion on the upper airway Respiratory physician to consider non-invasive ventilation
Diabetes mellitus	Refer to endocrinology for a special diet and oral hypoglycaemic agents

Other problems

- Strabismus, refractive error
- Thick, viscous saliva that can predispose to dental caries
- Difficulties in controlling temperature during minor illness
- Scoliosis
- Excessive daytime sleepiness and central or obstructive sleep apnoea
- Complications of obesity
  - Increased risk of type 2 diabetes mellitus
  - Increased risk of hypertension
  - Thrombophlebitis and chronic leg oedema
  - Sleep apnoea
- Osteoporosis

Growth hormone

Prader–Willi syndrome is a licensed indication for growth hormone treatment. Trials of growth hormone treatment in children with Prader–Willi syndrome have shown an increase in language and cognitive skills, improved height velocity with significantly greater adult height, normalization of the facial phenotype and improved mobility. However, deaths have been reported in a few children within the first 9 months of starting growth hormone treatment. These were mostly sudden deaths or deaths linked to respiratory infections or insufficiency (Tauber et al. 2008). It is recommended that children are assessed for obstructive sleep apnoea and respiratory problems before starting growth hormone treatment. A recent study has shown that growth hormone treatment in children with Prader–Willi syndrome begun before the age of 2 years improves body composition by reducing body fat, and improves motor function, height and lipid profile (Carrel et al. 2010). There were no significant adverse events in this group (de Lind van Wijngaarden et al. 2009).

Issues to consider at an annual review for a child with Prader–Willi syndrome

HISTORY

- Weight
  - eating and eating behaviours
  - exercise
- General health
  - chest
  - sleep pattern specifically for obstructive sleep apnoea
  - dental health
- Immunizations – including seasonal influenza immunization
- Learning
- Behaviour

EXAMINATION

- Growth – plotted on Prader–Willi chart (Butler et al. 2011) including body mass index (BMI)
- Acanthosis
- Signs of puberty
- Blood pressure
- Strabismus
- Spine for scoliosis
- Ensure testicles in scrotum

VISION SCREENING

- Orthoptic opinion at 6 months to 1 year
- Visual assessment at 2, 4 and 11 years

Metabolic syndrome

If the child's BMI is above the 91st centile, test for fasting glucose and HBA1c, cholesterol and triglycerides and liver function (assess fatty infiltration of the liver).

Support group

The Prader–Willi Syndrome Association (UK) is the support group for patients with Prader–Willi syndrome and their families and carers (www.pwsa.co.uk). Information about Prader–Willi syndrome for parents and healthcare professionals is also available from www.praderwillisyndrome.org.uk.

22q11.2 microdeletion syndrome (22qDS)

The 22q11.2 microdeletion syndrome is the most frequent interstitial deletion syndrome with an incidence of 1 in 4000 live births (Scambler 2000). It is best considered as a spectrum of phenotypes with the DiGeorge syndrome representing the most severe end, the Shprintzen or velo-cardio-facial syndrome representing the middle, and isolated velopharyngeal insufficiency representing the mildest end of the spectrum (Table 33.19).

Table 33.19 Phenotypes associated with 22q11.2 microdeletion

Syndrome	Distinguishing clinical features
Di George	Severe T-cell immunodeficiency
Velo-cardio-facial (Shprintzen)	Overt or submucous cleft palate No significant immunodeficiency
Isolated velo pharyngeal insufficiency	Isolated velo-pharyngeal difficulties No cleft palate
Isolated congenital heart disease	Isolated cardiac defects
Cardio-facial (Cayler)	Asymmetrical crying facies Associated cardiac defects
Conotruncal anomaly face	Normal IQ

Genetics

22q11.2 microdeletion syndrome is inherited in an autosomal dominant manner and can show non-penetrance or reduced penetrance as well as marked intrafamilial variability of expression.

Most (90%) patients with the 22qDS have a heterozygous 3-Mb deletion that results in loss of about 30 genes. Another 8% have a smaller 1.5-Mb deletion that includes about 24 genes (Lindsay 2001).

Deleted genes include

- *TBX1* gene, which is thought to be responsible for some of the phenotypic features of the 22qDS (Yagi et al. 2003).
- *COMT* gene, which encodes catechol-O-methyltransferase. This is associated with prefrontal cognitive functioning and may contribute to the higher incidence of schizophrenia and other psychiatric disorders in this condition (Gothelf et al. 2008).

All children with suspected 22qDS should undergo standard karyotyping and FISH analysis for the 22q11.2 deletion (see Fig. 33.3). If this condition is strongly suspected but the results of FISH analysis are negative, it may be helpful to look for a partial or complete deletion of the *TBX1* gene by MLPA or other chromosomal microdeletions or microduplications by array-CGH.

Both parents should be tested using FISH analysis. About 10% have an inherited deletion from an asymptomatic or mildly affected parent. The recurrence risk in this family would be 50%. The phenotype of an affected child is difficult to predict, although antenatal scans will give some indication, particularly of a congenital cardiac and renal anomaly. Prenatal testing is available.

Ninety per cent have a de novo deletion. The recurrence risk for an affected sibling is around 1 in 200.

Table 33.20 Clinical features of 22qDS

Sign	Common
Congenital heart disease (75%)	Tetralogy of Fallot Ventricular septal defect Interrupted aortic arch Pulmonary atresia with ventricular septal defect Truncus arteriosus Valvular pulmonary stenosis
Facial dysmorphism (abnormal facies; Fig. 33.10)	Myopathic facies with hypertelorism Small, simple, low-set ears Bulbous nasal tip Small mouth
Immune deficiency (thymic aplasia or hypoplasia) Majority – mild T-cell defects, more so in the neonatal period (McLean-Tooke et al. 2007) Evidence of IgA, IgM and IgG subclass deficiency or specific antibody deficiency	Recurrent infections Increased risk of autoimmune disorders (Gennery et al. 2002)
Cleft palate (50%) (velo-pharyngeal insufficiency)	Cleft/submucous cleft palate (15%) Velopharyngeal insufficiency (11% of patients with Pierre Robin sequence have 22qDS)
Hypocalcaemia (60%)	Usually in the neonatal period but some in childhood Present with seizures Responds well to calcium supplements In the majority it resolves with increasing age

Learning difficulties	Mild to moderate motor delay
	Mean full-scale IQ of 73.48 (range 50–109) (de Smedt et al. 2007)
	Strengths
	    Verbal memory
	    Basic reading
	Difficulties
	    Visuospatial memory
	    Reading comprehension
	    Mathematic reasoning (Jacobson et al. 2010)

Sign	Common
Behaviour problems Psychiatric problems	Attention-deficit–hyperactivity disorder Oppositional defiant behaviour Phobias Anxiety (10–12%) Obsessive–compulsive disorder Depression Autism spectrum disorder Schizophrenia (25–30% of adults) (Gothelf et al. 2008, Fung et al. 2010).

Ig, immunoglobulin.

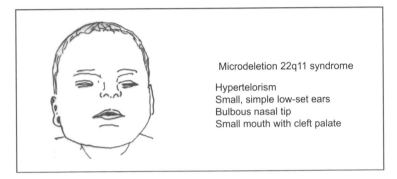

Microdeletion 22q11 syndrome

Hypertelorism
Small, simple low-set ears
Bulbous nasal tip
Small mouth with cleft palate

Figure 33.10 Microdeletion 22q11 syndrome.

In the past the characteristic clinical features resulted in the term CATCH22 for the 22qDS (Table 33.20). However, this term is considered derogatory and is no longer used by health professionals. Nevertheless, the acronym CATCH remains useful for remembering the key features of the 22qDS.

Other medical features include the following:

- hypotonia, feeding difficulties and failure to thrive in infancy
- short stature
- long, slender fingers
- recurrent middle ear infections with conductive hearing loss
- renal anomalies
- minor skeletal anomalies such as talipes or scoliosis.

Differential diagnosis

Children who have features suggesting 22qDS but whose genetic analysis is reported to be normal need re-evaluation and investigation as outlined in Table 33.21.

Table 33.21 Differential diagnosis of the 22qDS in children with congenital heart disease and learning difficulties

Syndrome	Clinical features	Testing
10p13–p14 deletion	Atrial septal defect Otherwise very similar	Array-CGH
Smith–Lemli–Opitz syndrome	Cleft palate Microcephaly Facial dysmorphism Polydactyly Genital anomalies	Autosomal recessive Mutations in the *DHCR7* gene which codes for 7-dehydrocholesterol reductase
CHARGE syndrome	Coloboma Heart abnormalities Atresia of choanae Retardation of growth Genital abnormalities Ears – abnormality of external ear and sensorineural deafness	Autosomal dominant Mutations in *CHD7* gene in 70%
Fetal vitamin A syndrome	Asymmetrical ear anomalies, congenital heart disease, thymic aplasia, hypoparathyroidism, CNS malformations	Antenatal exposure to vitamin A or analogues, e.g. isotretinoin in pregnancy

CGH, comparative genomic hybridization; CNS, central nervous system.

Assessments at diagnosis

CLINICAL EXAMINATION

- Speech and language assessment regarding the safety of swallow
- Ophthalmology opinion
- Audiology opinion
- Calcium
- Full blood count
- Thyroid function
- Immunological studies – prior to live vaccines
- Electrocardiography and echocardiography
- Renal ultrasound to look for renal anomalies

Issues to consider at annual review for child with 22qDS

- History
  - Health
  - Infections
  - Cardiac status
  - Cleft team
  - Eating and growth
  - Development/learning including school support
  - Behaviour

- **Examination**
  - Growth
  - Scoliosis
  - Cardiovascular examination

Screening

Children with 22qDS are more likely to have difficulties with hearing, vision, haematological, immunological and biochemical abnormalities and therefore it is recommended that they are screened as suggested in Table 33.22.

Table 33.22 Screening programme in 22qDS

	Age (y)			
	0–1	1–5	5–11	11+
Ophthalmology		Once		
Audiology	Once	Once		
Full blood count	Yearly	Yearly	Yearly	Yearly
Calcium	Every 3–6mo	Once	Once	Every 2y
Thyroid (thyroid-stimulating hormone)		Once	Once	Once
Immunological evaluation Prior to all live vaccines		Prior to MMR vaccination		

Shading indicates when screening is needed. MMR, measles, mumps and rubella. Source: Bassett et al. (2011).

Support group

The support group for patients and their families and carers with the 22qDS in the UK is called Max Appeal (http://www.maxappeal.org.uk/).

Rett syndrome

Rett syndrome was initially recognized in females by Dr Andreas Rett, an Austrian paediatrician in 1966. This was followed by Professor Bengt Hagberg in 1983, who reported 35 females with a similar constellation of symptoms. Rett syndrome remains a clinical diagnosis. There are associated genetic mutations, most commonly in the *MECP2* gene, but these do not explain all the cases. Rett syndrome affects 1 in every 12 500 female live births.

Rett syndrome in males has been diagnosed, although it is usually fatal, and when found the males have presented with a severe neonatal encephalopathic disorder.

Genetic information

Rett syndrome is caused by mutations in the *MECP2* gene located on the X chromosome (Xq28) and usually arises sporadically. The *MECP2* gene contains instructions for the synthesis of a protein called methyl cytosine binding protein 2 (MeCP2), which is needed for brain development. It acts as one of the many biochemical switches that can either increase gene expression or tell other genes when to turn off and stop producing their own unique proteins.

Mutations in the *FOXG1* gene at 14q13 can cause the congenital variant of Rett syndrome. Mutations in the *CDKL5* gene at Xp22 can also result in a Rett syndrome-like phenotype in girls with early onset and difficult-to-control seizures.

Although most instances of Rett syndrome arise de novo, very rarely the causative *MECP2* gene mutation can be inherited from a phenotypically normal or mildly affected mother. In these cases the mother with the *MECP2* gene mutation is phenotypically normal or mildly affected because of a highly skewed X chromosome inactivation pattern (with the X chromosome carrying the normal copy of the *MECP2* gene remaining active in most cells). The siblings of the affected child in these families have a 50% (1 in 2) chance of being affected with Rett syndrome.

Genetic testing (*MECP2* mutation analysis) allows confirmation of the diagnosis in about 90% of cases with typical Rett syndrome but only in 45% of cases with atypical Rett syndrome.

Diagnostic criteria

Females

MAJOR CRITERIA

- Partial or complete loss of acquired purposeful hand skills
- Partial or complete loss of acquired spoken language
- Gait abnormalities: impaired (dyspraxic) or absence of ability
- Stereotypic hand movements such as hand wringing/squeezing, clapping/tapping, mouthing and washing/rubbing automatisms

EXCLUSION CRITERIA

- Brain injury secondary to trauma (perinatally or postnatally), neurometabolic disease or severe infection that causes neurological problems
- Grossly abnormal psychomotor development in first 6 months of life

SUPPORTIVE CRITERIA (NEUL ET AL. 2010)

- Breathing disturbances when awake
- Bruxism when awake
- Impaired sleep pattern

- Abnormal muscle tone
- Peripheral vasomotor disturbances
- Scoliosis/kyphosis
- Growth retardation
- Small, cold hands and feet
- Inappropriate laughing/screaming spells
- Diminished response to pain
- Intense eye communication – 'eye pointing'

Natural history of Rett syndrome

- Initial normal development at 6 to 18 months
- Developmental arrest or regression at 6 to 30 months
- Usually have accomplished sitting and standing but they do not learn to walk
- Females may initially hold a rattle or block but this skill appears to be lost (some may not have acquired purposeful hand movements)
- Profound difficulties with communication
- Screaming attacks
- Usually well and thriving
- Paroxysmal attacks that may be stereotypies or seizures
- Slowing of head growth, not necessarily microcephalic
- Small hands and feet
- Truncal hypotonia with preserved tendon reflexes, although some females may have spasticity

Stabilization at 2 to 10 years

- Slowing of head circumference, but not necessarily microcephaly
- An early scoliosis can occur (<4y)
- Midline repetitive hand movements (e.g. hand sucking, hand-wringing)
- Variable breathing pattern with episodes of hyperventilation, breath-holding or air gulping. Although it can be, this is usually not an early feature.
- Autistic-like characteristics of
  - repetitive behaviours
  - screaming attacks
  - communication problems

Late motor deterioration – can last for years or decades

- Reduced mobility with rigidity and increased tone – can lead to loss of walking
- Scoliosis
- No further loss of cognition, communication, or hand function
- The majority of females live into adult life

Differential diagnosis

Children who have features suggesting Rett syndrome but who do not fulfil the diagnostic criteria require re-evaluation and investigation as outlined in Table 33.23.

Table 33.23 **Differential diagnosis of Rett syndrome**

Diagnosis	Feature	Genetics
Angelman syndrome	Difficulties from birth Absent or severely limited speech Ataxia or tremulous limb movements Epilepsy Microcephaly Dysmorphic facial features	Standard karyotype and methylation pattern analysis (MS-MLPA) at 15q11–q13
Pitt–Hopkins syndrome	Microcephaly Absent or limited speech Dysmorphic facies with coarse features Seizures Ataxic gait Episodes of hyperventilation and apnoea beginning between 3 and 8y Happy, placid personality	Autosomal dominant Locus 18q21.1 Gene *TCF4*
MEF2C deletion/ mutations	Hypotonia Absent speech Hand stereotypies Episodes of hyperventilation and apnoea Epilepsy Subtle facial dysmorphism Corpus callosum anomalies or ventricular dilatation on MRI	Autosomal dominant Locus 5q14 Gene *MEF2C*
Autism spectrum disorder	May have normal early development Lack of social interest Poor non-verbal skills Stereotypies Restricted range of activities Motor skills not significantly affected	Clinical diagnosis
Cerebral palsy	Difficulties from birth or significant episode of illness Spasticity or movement disorder No repetitive movements Microcephaly	Clinical diagnosis Abnormal MRI
Epileptic encephalopathy	Multiple seizure types that are intractable Cognitive impairment	Abnormal EEG
CDKL5	Severe epilepsy with multiple seizure types Severe learning difficulties Rett syndrome-like features	X-linked dominant Locus Xp22.13 Gene *CDKL5*

MS-MLPA, methylation-specific multiplex ligation-dependent probe amplification; MRI, magnetic resonance imaging; EEG, electroencephalography.

Issues to consider at annual review of a child with Rett syndrome

- **History**
  - General health
    - Stereotypical episodes – these are difficult to diagnose as they could be part of Rett syndrome or they could represent seizures. Assessment by a paediatric neurologist can be helpful.
    - Eating and symptoms of gastro-oesophageal reflux
    - Constipation
  - Dental care
    - Bruxism (teeth grinding) is common
  - Development
    - Mobility
    - Communication
- **Examination**
  - Growth
  - Look for an emerging scoliosis – if present, refer the child to a surgeon who specializes in spinal surgery
- **Screening**
  - Electrocardiography – a prolonged QT interval has been documented

Support group

Rett Syndrome Support UK (www.rettuk.org).

Key messages

- A clinical genetics referral is more likely to yield a diagnosis in children with severe to profound learning difficulties and dysmorphic features than in children with mild to moderate learning difficulties without any facial dysmorphism.
- The diagnosis of Down syndrome is usually made by recognition of the characteristic facial gestalt.
- Neurofibromatosis type 1 (NF1) is a clinical diagnosis.
- The diagnosis of Williams syndrome is usually made by the combination of the characteristic facial gestalt and the typical behavioural profile.
- All molecular mechanisms that cause Angelman syndrome result in loss of expression of the maternally inherited copy of the *UBE3A* gene.
- Hypotonia is a key feature of Prader–Willi syndrome in children.
- The 22q11.2 microdeletion syndrome can result in a wide phenotypic spectrum varying from DiGeorge syndrome to isolated velopharyngeal insufficiency.

References

American Academy of Pediatrics (2001) Health care supervision for children with Williams syndrome. *Pediatrics* 107: 1192–204.

Anon (1988) National Institutes of Health Concensus Development Statement: neurofibromatosis. Bethesda, Md., USA, July 13–15, 1987. *Neurofibromatosis* 1: 172–8.

Bassett AS, McDonald-McDinn DM, Devriendt K et al (2011) Practical guidelines for managing patients with 22q11.2 deletion syndrome. *J Pediatr* 159: 332–9.

Butler MG, Sturich J, Lee J et al (2011) Growth standards of infants with Prader–Willi syndrome. *Pediatrics* 127: 687–95. http://dx.doi.org/10.1542/peds.2010-2736

Carrel AL, Myers SE, Whitman BY, Eickhoff J, Allen DB (2010) Long-term growth hormone therapy changes the natural history of body composition and motor function in children with Prader–Willi syndrome. *J Clin Endocrinol Metab* 95: 1131–6. http://dx.doi.org/10.1210/jc.2009-1389

Cassidy SB, Driscoll DJ (2009) Prader–Willi syndrome. *Eur J Hum Genet* 17: 3–13. http://dx.doi.org/10.1038/ejhg.2008.165

Coffee B, Keith K, Albizua I et al (2009) Incidence of fragile X syndrome by newborn screening for methylated FMR1 DNA. *Am J Hum Genet* 85: 503–14. http://dx.doi.org/10.1016/j.ajhg.2009.09.007

Collins RT, Kaplan P, Somes GW, Rome JJ (2010) Long-term outcomes of patients with cardiovascular abnormalities and Williams syndrome. *Am J Cardiol* 105: 874–8. http://dx.doi.org/10.1016/j.amjcard.2009.10.069

Duker AL, Ballif BC, Bawle EV et al (2010) Paternally inherited microdeletion at 15q11.2 confirms a significant role for the SNORD116 C/D box snoRNA cluster in Prader–Willi syndrome. *Eur J Hum Genet* 18: 1196–201. http://dx.doi.org/10.1038/ejhg.2010.102

Eronen M, Peippo M, Hiippala A et al (2002) Cardiovascular manifestations in 75 patients with Williams syndrome. *J Med Genet* 39: 554–8. http://dx.doi.org/10.1136/jmg.39.8.554

Ferner RE, Huson SM, Thomas N ct al (2007) Guidelines for the diagnosis and management of individuals with neurofibromatosis 1. *J Med Genet* 44: 81–8. http://dx.doi.org/10.1136/jmg.2006.045906

Freeman SB, Taft LF, Dooley KJ et al. (1998) Population-based study of congenital heart defects in Down syndrome. *Am J Med Genet* 80: 213–17. http://dx.doi.org/10.1002/(SICI)1096-8628(19981116)80:3<213::AID-AJMG6>3.0.CO;2-8

Fung WL, McEvilly R, Fong J, Silversides C, Chow E, Bassett A (2010) Elevated prevalence of generalised anxiety disorder in adults with 22q11.2 deletion syndrome. *Am J Psychiatry* 167: 998. http://dx.doi.org/10.1176/appi.ajp.2010.09101463

Gennery AR, Barge D, O'Sullivan JJ, Flood TJ, Abinun M, Cant AJ (2002) Antibody deficiency and autoimmunity in 22q11.2 deletion syndrome. *Arch Dis Child* 86: 422–5. http://dx.doi.org/10.1136/adc.86.6.422

Gothelf D, Schaer M, Eliez S (2008) Genes, brain development and psychiatric phenotypes in velo-cardio-facial syndrome. *Dev Disabil Res Rev* 14: 59–68. http://dx.doi.org/10.1002/ddrr.9

Hagerman PJ, Hagerman RJ (2004) Fragile X-associated tremor/ataxia syndrome (FXTAS). *Ment Retard Dev Disabil Res Rev* 10: 25–30. http://dx.doi.org/10.1002/mrdd.20005

Hall B (1964) Mongolism in newborns. A clinical and cytogenetic study. *Acta Paediatr* 154(Suppl): 1–95.

Harris SW, Hessl D, Goodlin-Jones B et al (2008) Autism profiles of males with fragile X syndrome. *Am J Ment Retard* 113: 427–38. http://dx.doi.org/10.1352/2008.113:427-438

Hersh JH, Saul RA (2011) Health supervision for children with fragile X syndrome. *Pediatrics* 127: 994–1006. http://dx.doi.org/10.1542/peds.2010-3500

Huson SM, Compston DA, Harper PS (1989) A genetic study of von Recklinghausen neurofibromatosis in south east Wales. II. Guidelines for genetic counselling. *J Med Genet* 26: 712–21. http://dx.doi.org/10.1136/jmg.26.11.712

Jacobson C, Shearer J, Habel A, Kane F, Tsakanikos E, Kravariti E (2010) Core neuropsychological characteristics of children and adolescents with 22q11.2 deletion. *J Intellect Disabil Res* 54: 701–13. http://dx.doi.org/10.1111/j.1365-2788.2010.01298.x

de Lind van Wijngaarden RF, Siemensma EP, Festen DA et al (2009) Efficacy and safety of long-term continuous growth hormone treatment in children with Prader–Willi syndrome. *J Clin Endocrinol Metab* 94: 4205–15. http://dx.doi.org/10.1210/jc.2009-0454

Lindsay EA (2001) Chromosomal microdeletions: dissecting del22q11 syndrome. *Nat Rev Genet* 2: 858–68. http://dx.doi.org/10.1038/35098574

McCaughan JA, Holloway SM, Davidson R, Lam WW (2007) Further evidence of the increased risk for malignant peripheral nerve sheath tumour from a Scottish cohort of patients with neurofibromatosis type 1. *J Med Genet* 44: 463–6. http://dx.doi.org/10.1136/jmg.2006.048140

McLean-Tooke A, Spickett GP, Gennery AR (2007) Immunodeficiency and autoimmunity in 22q11.2 deletion syndrome. *Scand J Immunol* 66: 1–7. http://dx.doi.org/10.1111/j.1365-3083.2007.01949.x

Martin ND, Smith WR, Cole TJ, Preece MA (2007) New height, weight and head circumference charts for British children with Williams syndrome. *Arch Dis Child* 92: 598–601. http://dx.doi.org/10.1136/adc.2006.107946

Martinez R, Bonilla-Henao V, Jimenez A et al (2005) Skewed X inactivation of the normal allele in fully mutated female carriers determines the levels of FMRP in blood and the fragile X phenotype. *Mol Diagn* 9: 157–62. http://dx.doi.org/10.2165/00066982-200509030-00006

Messiaen L, Yao S, Brems H et al. (2009) Clinical and mutational spectrum of neurofibromatosis type 1-like syndrome. *JAMA* 302: 2111–18. http://dx.doi.org/10.1001/jama.2009.1663

Morris CA (2010) The behavioral phenotype of Williams syndrome: a recognizable pattern of neurodevelopment. *Am J Med Genet C Semin Med Genet* 154C: 427–31. http://dx.doi.org/10.1002/ajmg.c.30286

Morris JK, Mutton DE, Alberman E (2005) Recurrences of free trisomy 21: analysis of data from the National Down syndrome Cytogenetic Register. *Prenat Diagn* 25: 1120–8. http://dx.doi.org/10.1002/pd.1292

Neul JL, Kaufmann WE, Glaze DG et al.; RettSearch Consortium (2010) Rett syndrome: revised diagnostic criteria and nomenclature. *Ann Neurol* 68: 944–50. http://dx.doi.org/10.1002/ana.22124

Pober BR (2010) Williams–Beuren syndrome. *N Engl J Med* 362: 239–52. http://dx.doi.org/10.1056/NEJMra0903074

Ruggieri M, Huson SM (2001) The clinical and diagnostic implications of mosaicism in the neurofibromatoses. *Neurology* 56: 1433–43. http://dx.doi.org/10.1212/WNL.56.11.1433

Scambler PJ (2000) The 22q11 deletion syndromes. *Hum Mol Genet* 9: 2421–6. http://dx.doi.org/10.1093/hmg/9.16.2421

de Smedt B, Devriendt K, Fryns JP, Vogels A, Gewillig M, Swillen A (2007) Intellectual abilities in a large sample of children with velo-cardio-facial syndrome: an update. *J Intellect Disabil Res* 51: 666–70. http://dx.doi.org/10.1111/j.1365-2788.2007.00955.x

Tauber M, Diene G, Molinas C, Hebert M (2008) Review of 64 cases of death in children with Prader–Willi syndrome (PWS). *Am J Med Genet A* 146: 881–7. http://dx.doi.org/10.1002/ajmg.a.32131.

Thibert RL, Conant KD, Braun EK et al. (2009) Epilepsy in Angelman syndrome: a questionnaire-based assessment of the natural history and current treatment options. *Epilepsia* 50: 2369–76. http://dx.doi.org/10.1111/j.1528-1167.2009.02108.x

Williams CA, Lossie A, Driscoll D (2001) Angelman syndrome: mimicking conditions and phenotypes. *Am J Med Genet* 101: 59–64. http://dx.doi.org/10.1002/ajmg.1316

Yagi H, Furutani Y, Hamada H et al. (2003) Role of TBX1 in human del22q11.2 syndrome. *Lancet* 362: 1366–73. http://dx.doi.org/10.1016/S0140-6736(03)14632-6

Yang Q, Rasmussen SA, Friedman JM (2002) Mortality associated with Down syndrome in the USA from 1983 to 1997: a population-based study. *Lancet* 359: 1019–25. http://dx.doi.org/10.1016/S0140-6736(02)08092-3

Further reading

American Academy of Pediatrics (2001) Health supervision for children with Down syndrome. *Pediatrics* 107: 442–9. http://dx.doi.org/10.1542/peds.107.2.442

Battaglia A (2008) The inv dup (15) or idic (15) syndrome (tetrasomy 15q). *Orphanet J Rare Dis* 3: 30. http://dx.doi.org/10.1186/1750-1172-3-30

Bayes M, Magano LF, Rivera N, Flores R, Perez Jurado LA (2003) Mutational mechanisms of Williams–Beuren syndrome deletions. *Am J Hum Genet* 73: 131–51. http://dx.doi.org/10.1086/376565

Bourgeois JA, Coffey SM, Rivera SM et al (2009) A review of fragile X premutation disorders: expanding the psychiatric perspective. *J Clin Psychiatry* 70: 852–62. http://dx.doi.org/10.4088/JCP.08r04476

Boyd SG, Harden A, Patton MA (1988) The EEG in early diagnosis of the Angelman (happy puppet) syndrome. *Eur J Pediatr* 147: 508–13. http://dx.doi.org/10.1007/BF00441976.

Buiting K (2010) Prader–Willi syndrome and Angelman syndrome. *Am J Med Genet C Semin Med Genet* 154C: 365–76. http://dx.doi.org/10.1002/ajmg.c.30273

Buiting K, Gross S, Lich C, Gillessen-Kaesbach G, El-Maarri O, Horsthemke B (2003) Epimutations in Prader–Willi and Angelman syndromes: a molecular study of 136 patients with an imprinting defect. *Am J Hum Genet* 72: 571–7. http://dx.doi.org/10.1086/367926

Charleton PM, Dennis J, Marder E (2010) Medical management of children with Down syndrome. *Paediatr Child Health* 20: 331–7. http://dx.doi.org/10.1016/j.paed.2010.06.006

Cunningham C (2006) *Down Syndrome: An Introduction for Parents and Carers*, 3rd edition. London: Souvenir.

Dixon N, Kishnani PS, Zimmerman S (2006) Clinical manifestations of hematologic and oncologic disorders in patients with Down syndrome. *Am J Med Genet C Semin Med Genet* 142C: 149–57. http://dx.doi.org/10.1002/ajmg.c.30096

DSMIG UK Guidelines (2012) produced by the DSMIG UK and the proceedings of the meetings at the Down syndrome Medical Interest Group: www.dsmig.org.uk

Flanders L, Tulloch R (2011) Cardiac problems in Down syndrome. *Paediatr Child Health* 21: 25–31. http://dx.doi.org/10.1016/j.paed.2010.09.005

Freeman SB, Bean LH, Allen EG et al. (2008) Ethnicity, sex, and the incidence of congenital heart defects: a report from the National Down syndrome Project. *Genet Med* 10: 173e80. http://dx.doi.org/10.1097/GIM.0b013e3181634867

Gardner RJM, Sutherland GR (2004) *Chromosome Abnormalities and Genetic Counseling*. Oxford: Oxford University Press.

Gillessen-Kaesbach G, Demuth S, Thiele H, Theile U, Lich C, Horsthemke B (1999) A previously unrecognised phenotype characterised by obesity, muscular hypotonia, and ability to speak in patients with Angelman syndrome caused by an imprinting defect. *Eur J Hum Genet* 7: 638–44. http://dx.doi.org/10.1038/sj.ejhg.5200362

Gronskov K, Brondum-Nielsen K, Dedic A, Hjalgrim H (2011) A nonsense mutation in FMR1 causing fragile X syndrome. *Eur J Hum Genet* 19: 489–91. http://dx.doi.org/10.1038/ejhg.2010.223

James R, Kinsey S (2009) Haematological disorders in Down syndrome. *Paediatr Child Health* 19: 377–380. http://dx.doi.org/10.1016/j.paed.2009.04.006

Kent L, Evans J, Paul M, Sharp M (1999) Comorbidity of autistic spectrum disorders in children with Down syndrome. *Dev Med Child Neurol* 41: 153–8. http://dx.doi.org/10.1017/S001216229900033X

Kupferman JC, Druschel CM, Kupchik GS (2009) Increased prevalence of renal and urinary tract anomalies in children with Down syndrome. *Pediatrics* 124: e615. http://dx.doi.org/10.1542/peds.2009-0181

Leno C, Mateo I, Cid C, Berciano J, Sedano C (1998) Autoimmunity in Down's syndrome: another possible mechanism of Moyamoya disease. *Stroke* 29: 868–869. http://dx.doi.org/10.1161/01.STR.29.4.868

Mautner VF, Kluwe L, Friedrich RE et al (2010) Clinical characterisation of 29 neurofibromatosis type-1 patients with molecularly ascertained 1.4 Mb type-1 NF1 deletions. *J Med Genet* 47: 623–30. http://dx.doi.org/10.1136/jmg.2009.075937

McDonald-McGinn DM, Kirschner R, Goldmuntz E et al. (1999) The Philadelphia story: the 22q11.2 deletion: report on 250 patients. *Genet Couns* 10: 11–24.

Miller JL, Couch JA, Schmalfuss I, He G, Liu Y, Driscoll DJ (2007) Intracranial abnormalities detected by three-dimensional magnetic resonance imaging in Prader–Willi syndrome. *Am J Med Genet A* 143: 476–83. http://dx.doi.org/10.1002/ajmg.a.31508

Myers BA, Pueschel SM (1991) Psychiatric disorders in persons with Down syndrome. *J Nerv Ment Dis* 179: 609–13. http://dx.doi.org/10.1097/00005053-199110000-00004

Nolin SL, Brown WT, Glicksman A et al. (2003) Expansion of the fragile X CGG repeat in females with premutation or intermediate alleles. *Am J Hum Genet* 72: 454–64. http://dx.doi.org/10.1086/367713

Nowicki ST, Tassone F, Ono MY et al. (2007) The Prader–Willi phenotype of fragile X syndrome. *J Dev Behav Pediatr* 28: 133–8. http://dx.doi.org/10.1097/01.DBP.0000267563.18952.c9

Ostergaard JR, Sunde L, Okkels H (2005) Neurofibromatosis von Recklinghausen type I phenotype and early onset of cancers in siblings compound heterozygous for mutations in MSH6. *Am J Med Genet A* 139A: 96–105; discussion 96. http://dx.doi.org/10.1002/ajmg.a.30998

Pirozzi F, Tabolacci E, Neri G (2011) The FRAXopathies: definition, overview, and update. *Am J Med Genet A* 155: 1803–16. http://dx.doi.org/10.1002/ajmg.a.34113

Ramsden SC, Clayton-Smith J, Birch R, Buiting K (2010) Practice guidelines for the molecular analysis of Prader–Willi and Angelman syndromes. *BMC Med Genet* 11: 70. http://dx.doi.org/10.1186/1471-2350-11-70

Roizen NJ, Patterson D (2003) Down syndrome. *Lancet* 361: 1281–9. http://dx.doi.org/10.1016/S0140-6736(03)12987-X

Ryan AK, Goodship JA, Wilson DI et al. (1997) Spectrum of clinical features associated with interstitial chromosome 22q11 deletions: a European collaborative study. *J Med Genet* 34: 798–804. http://dx.doi.org/10.1136/jmg.34.10.798

Schieve LA, Boulet SL, Boyle C, Rasmussen SA, Schendel D (2009) Health of children 3 to 17 years of age with Down syndrome in the 1997–2005 National Health Interview Survey. *Pediatrics* 123: e253. http://dx.doi.org/10.1542/peds.2008-1440

Shprintzen RJ (1992) The implications of the diagnosis of Robin sequence. *Cleft Palate Craniofac J* 29: 205–9. http://dx.doi.org/10.1597/1545-1569(1992)029<0205:TIOTDO>2.3.CO;2

Spender Q, Stein A, Dennis J, Reilly S, Percy E, Cave D (1996) An exploration of feeding difficulties in children with Down syndrome. *Dev Med Child Neurol* 38: 681–94. http://dx.doi.org/10.1111/j.1469-8749.1996.tb12138.x

Takahashi K, Kido S, Hoshino K, Ogawa K, Ohashi H, Fukushima Y (1995) Frequency of a 22q11 deletion in patients with conotruncal cardiac malformations: a prospective study. *Eur J Pediatr* 154: 878–81. http://dx.doi.org/10.1007/BF01957496

Van Cleve SN, Cohen WI (2006) Part I: clinical practice guidelines for children with Down syndrome from birth to 12 years. *J Pediatr Health Care* 20: 47–54. http://dx.doi.org/10.1016/j.pedhc.2005.10.004

Van Cleve SN, Cannon S, Cohen WI (2006) Part II: Clinical Practice Guidelines for adolescents and young adults with Down syndrome: 12 to 21 years. *J Pediatr Health Care* 20: 198–205. http://dx.doi.org/10.1016/j.pedhc.2006.02.006

de Vries BB, Halley DJ, Oostra BA, Niermeijer MF (1998) The fragile X syndrome. *J Med Genet* 35: 579–89. http://dx.doi.org/10.1136/jmg.35.7.579

Weijerman ME, Van Furth AM, Van Der Mooren MD et al. (2010) Prevalence of congenital heart defects and persistent pulmonary hypertension of the neonate with Down syndrome. *Eur J Pediatr* 169: 1195–9. http://dx.doi.org/10.1007/s00431-010-1200-0

Section 12

Partnerships with families

34
Talking to families and carers

Arnab Seal

Learning objectives

- To understand the principles of good practice when disclosing difficult news to family members and/or the child.

Effective communication is an important skill for all professionals working with families of children with disabilities. Understanding the principles of good practice, obtaining feedback and learning from experience can help improve your personal practice. For many parents one of life's most significant moments is when they are informed of their child's diagnosis. When performed with skill and sensitivity, it provides an experience for parents that can have a positive impact on future working relationships with professionals. It also impacts on the parents' ability to respond to the immediate situation and share the information effectively with friends and family. The experience often affects parents' future expectations of their child and the bond they develop.

There are a few simple principles of good practice. The Right From The Start (RFTS) initiative is an example of a UK-based initiative that aims to promote good practice at the time news is shared with families of a child's additional needs. This news could relate to concerns about a child's development, a diagnosis of a physical or sensory impairment, learning difficulty or information regarding a child's complex health needs. Honest, transparent communication of this information is critical to developing effective partnerships among parents, health professionals and the child.

Here are some suggested principles and practical tips on how to get it right. These recommendations are non-prescriptive and will need to be adapted to the circumstances depending on:

- setting: hospital/community/family home/other settings
- timing: antenatal diagnosis/diagnosis at birth/older child/evolving diagnosis
- the nature of the disability: physical/sensory/intellectual/behavioural/autism/multiple
- planned events following tests or unplanned and unexpected results.

Principles of good practice

- Do not break bad news in a letter or telephone call.
- Disclosure should be family centred.
- Always have respect for the child and his or her family.
- Communication should be sensitive and empathic.
- Information should be appropriate and accurate.
- Use positive, realistic messages and hope.
- Use a team approach with forward planning.

Practical aspects

Preparation

INVITING THE FAMILY

If you need to contact the family to arrange a meeting, for example after receiving an investigation result, do not do this yourself as you may be forced into an uncomfortable telephone conversation. Ask a secretary or clerk to set up the meeting. Tell them you have received a test result and that you think it would be more helpful to meet up with the family. The meeting should be shortly after the phone call whenever possible as the wait will cause significant anxiety for the family. Certainly try to avoid a Friday phone call for an appointment the next week.

THE SETTING

Meetings should be in a private place with no interruptions (display an 'Engaged' board). It should be in a comfortable room with suitable chairs that can be available for the family to spend time in afterwards to absorb the news. Make sure there are tissues available and, if possible, tea/coffee facilities so you can make the family a drink. If the child is present and needing to be occupied, have suitable toys available.

THE INTERPRETER

Offer an interpreter if English is not the first language of one or both parents (even if one parent has good English). Avoid using a family member/friend for interpreting. Provide written information (if possible in the first language).

THE TEAM

It is important to have a team discussion before disclosure and a team plan for supporting the family afterwards. A second professional, preferably known to family, should be present for any required assistance, for example playing with the child and to support the family during and after disclosure. Keep to a minimum number of professionals involved during disclosure. Make sure appropriate information is handed over afterwards to other relevant teams. Offer debriefing opportunities for all team members.

THE PERSON COMMUNICATING THE NEWS

You must be familiar with the name of the child and, if possible, of family members. You must have all the correct information including notes, results and information regarding condition. Preferably you need to have experience and confidence in breaking difficult news, and have sufficient time to answer all questions the family may have. Seek help and supervision from a senior colleague if necessary. Mobile phones and pagers need to be switched off or handed to someone else.

THE FAMILY

Wherever possible try to see both parents together. If only one parent is available, consider the feasibility of waiting for the other parent. If not, provide the option of another family member or friend to be present.

THE CHILD

Try to keep infants and young children with the parents whenever possible. Make arrangements for younger children to be suitably occupied during the session. In the case of older children, you may need to consider a separate session during which the information can be tailored to the appropriate developmental age and understanding of the child. Discuss with the older child and parent separately who they would like to be present at the session.

The meeting

Start by introducing everybody present. If the child is present then acknowledge and greet him or her appropriately. Use simple, understandable, non-judgemental, non-medical language. Check what parents know already and whether they have had any concerns. Often you can confirm what parents have suspected for a while. Provide face-to-face verbal information, not just a letter or over the phone. Practise active listening. Be aware of your own body language. Be empathic, sensitive and honest. Use the child's name and use language which puts the child first rather than the diagnosis, for example 'infants with Turner syndrome' rather than 'Turner syndrome infants'.

Provide positive realistic messages. This can include describing the support, assistance and interventions that will be available to the child and family. Rather than outlining the worst possible scenario (even if that is the likely outcome), discuss the range of possible outcomes and the percentage of children who are affected by different severity or different clinical aspects of the condition. Avoid making specific predictions or pronouncements about the child's future.

Look out for cues of distress and/or anger. Acknowledge the parents' feelings. Remain calm at all times. Stop if necessary and check whether parents need time for composure. Little information is absorbed by a distressed mind.

It is helpful to check the parents' understanding – you need to be prepared to explain again. Acknowledge parental concerns and also any uncertainties that may exist. Outline a further course of action including any referrals and possible time frames.

INFORMATION AND SUPPORT

Provide a contact number for a designated team member. Provide written information on useful websites for good-quality information. Offer local and/or national support group contacts.

Always provide a follow-up appointment. Communicate with other professionals who are likely to be in contact with the family and/or who can help.

FAMILY MEMBERS

Parents often are unsure of what to tell their other children and other family members. Ask them to be honest and provide clear, simple explanations. Offer to speak to other family members if the family so wish. It is important to explain to siblings that it wasn't their 'fault'. Sometimes children will wonder whether they will also be affected and need reassurance with simple truthful explanations.

Training

Ensure that there is appropriate training of team members and junior staff. Have a team plan of how best practice can be delivered in your own setting. Use peer support and critical reflection to inform and improve practice. A 'Practice checklist' has been included in Appendix XIV 'Disclosing difficult news to families'.

Further reading

Contact a Family (2006) Health Support Pack: Information sheet 9. Available at: www.cafamily.org.uk/media/389235/healthsupportpack.pdf (accessed 2 December 2012).

35
The impact of childhood disability on the family

Lorna Highet, Anne M Kelly and Anne Hall

Much has been written in books and journals on this subject, but spending time with families will quickly reveal some of the reasons why caring for a child with a disability can be difficult. They must adjust to the loss of expectation of bringing up a healthy and typically developing child, and accept a future that can be much less certain – even when they have a diagnosis for their child's difficulties.

This uncertainty can add to the already obvious stresses of having to manage their child's additional physical needs, which require extra time, energy and emotional strength in addition to the financial strain caused by the loss of income and the extra living costs their child generates. Mental health problems can and often do affect carers – particularly those whose children have complex needs. Siblings as well as parents are affected, with the plan for their lives shifted from the anticipated path.

However, in spite of all of these stresses, without wishing to minimize these difficulties or to sound patronizing, parents who have been interviewed for research studies in this area often seek to highlight the joy and love they receive from their child. The response they receive from their child may not only enrich their lives and the lives of those around them but also contributes towards creating a better understanding of the need and benefits of caring for the most vulnerable in our society.

Financial implications of caring for a child with a significant disability

The Joseph Rowntree Foundation has carried out valuable research in this area. Two studies, completed in 1998 and 2000, assessed the costs of caring for a child with a disability and the adjustments families made to meet these added costs (Dobson and Middleton 1998, Dobson et al. 2000). While the standard of living has risen since then, the proportion of income spent on the child with a disability is unlikely to have changed much. In fact, with the recent recession and genuine fall in many families' income, the proportion is likely to have increased, causing even greater hardship within these families.

The extra time required to care for a child with a disability impinges on the time available to care for one's self, partner and other children. There is less time to spend outside the home working, thereby reducing potential family income.

Many carers who try to continue to work struggle to find childcare arrangements that fit with their work requirements and may give up work as a result, leading not only to a loss of income but also to a loss of self-esteem and independence.

There are extra costs involved in caring for a child with a disability. Children with disabilities may have a greater need for items such as clothing, toys, toiletries and nappies. Parents describe a need for more items to occupy and stimulate their children. Many of these items are more expensive than those used by children without disabilities and on average twice as much is spent on items for the child with a disability as on comparable items for a non-disabled sibling.

Family incomes are lower than the national average in many affected families, yet parents in these studies strived to spend enough to meet the needs of their children, spending on average a fifth of their total family income on their child with a disability. In order to achieve this they spent less on themselves and made other savings wherever possible.

The benefits system recognizes the fact that bringing up a child with a severe disability costs more and provides financial help through entitlement to particular benefits, though the level of remuneration is still 50% less than the extra family expenditure needed to care for the child. This problem is exacerbated by many parents not being aware of the full benefit allowance to which they are entitled.

Socio-emotional effects of disability on carers and families

As well as struggling to cope with the added financial costs, families of children with disabilities must confront new and unexpected experiences. Research has shown that parents go through a process of adjusting to a new norm after the child's disability is confirmed. Central to this process of adjustment is the way in which they are informed of the diagnosis (see Chapter 34). This is an important stage as it is often the point from which parents begin to think about their futures and to understand the nature of their child's disability. This process does not happen instantly and the bereavement reaction which occurs in response to the loss of a healthy child may continue alongside it for a considerable period, lasting possibly months or years. For many parents the diagnosis often represents a turning point from which they start to regain some control over both their own and their child's lives. Diagnosis is also crucially important because it is often the gateway to other services, including the entitlement to financial benefits.

A particular difficulty for parents after diagnosis is their growing awareness of the attitudes that many disabled people experience all the time: they can be marginalized and avoided by some people, even by some of their friends and family, resulting in isolation for some families. They need support from their pre-existing networks of family and friends but also the strength to challenge the way in which they and their children are treated by society. The need for extra support is now recognized, but it is often still up to parents to find these sources of support, some of which may be provided by the local council or, alternatively, by groups of parents themselves.

Many parents report that they become used to being stared at in public or the topic of other people's conversations. Yet despite their prominence in public, parents report feeling that they become invisible. They are no longer regarded as an 'ordinary' family, with the same hopes and expectations. While the physical exclusion is hard to deal with, it is the attitudes displayed by society, including that of some professionals, that affect them most and sometimes devastate them – by seeing their child with a disability as being viewed as a 'matter of regret' they feel they are stripped of their family status and denied the same value as 'normal' families. It is therefore not surprising to find that there are higher rates of mental health disorders in carers.

A cross-sectional European study on parenting stress in parents of children with cerebral palsy found very high risk associated with communication difficulties, intellectual impairment and pain in the children (Parkes et al. 2011). However, contrary to expectation, there was no relationship with the severity of motor impairment (as measured by the Gross Motor Function Classification System).

A study in Australia showed a significant positive relationship between maternal psychological problems and caregiving time required per 24 hours (Sawyer et al. 2011). On average, mothers spent 6 hours each weekday and 8.3 hours on weekend days caring for children with cerebral palsy.

Behavioural problems in children with a disability can have an important negative effect on the caregiver's ability to cope and it may be more difficult to access leisure opportunities because of a child's needs and behaviours.

Depressed parents are less sensitive and responsive to their children than non-depressed parents, which may adversely affect their child's development and confidence but also may impact on the care of siblings.

There will be less time for parents to provide for the needs and interests of non-disabled siblings. Some siblings act as carers, impinging on their socio-emotional development; they too need 'time off' from responsibilities and should not be burdened inappropriately.

More complex care is now delivered to children in their homes; although this is advantageous psychologically for the child, it leaves parents with a dual role as parent and carer. They must learn to nurse, position their child, use equipment and administer medicines. Some carers admit to finding these interventions stressful, particularly as they had no expectation of this role.

The pattern of care for children with the most severe disabilities will not change as the child grows up. Their needs are likely to persist and will probably increase rather than diminish with time. This has been described as a 'trap' for these carers, who are frequently mothers. They will not free themselves from this role unless the young person is offered residential care.

Ideally families with a child with a disability should be offered a service that is based on a sensitive and comprehensive assessment of both the child's and his or her family's needs; a service that enables reassessment to be undertaken from time to time, particularly at times of transition; a service that allows families some choice in the provision they have and which makes a formal agreement with the families to deliver an agreed package of services to an acceptable standard.

There is still some way to go before this goal can be achieved. With the current cuts in budgets in government departments including social care, many disabled people are unfortunately finding that services they previously received are being reduced or withdrawn – one can only hope that these changes will be reversed when the country's economic fortunes improve.

References

Dobson B, Middleton S (1998) *Paying to Care: The Cost of Childhood Disability*. York: Joseph Rowntree Foundation.

Dobson B, Middleton S, Beardsworth A (2000) *The Impact of Childhood Disability on Family Life*. York: Joseph Rowntree Foundation.

Parkes J, Caravale B, Marcelli M, Franco F, Colver A (2011) Parenting stress and children with cerebral palsy. *Dev Med Child Neurol* 53: 815–21. http://dx.doi.org/10.1111/j.1469-8749.2011.04014.x

Sawyer MG, Bittman M, La Greca AM et al. (2011) Time demands of caring for children with cerebral palsy: what are the implications for maternal mental health? *Dev Med Child Neurol* 53: 338–43. http://dx.doi.org/10.1111/j.1469-8749.2010.03848.x

Further reading

Baldwin S (1985) *The Cost of Caring: Families with Disabled Children*. London: Routledge & Kegan Paul.

Curran AL, Sharples PM, White C, Knapp M (2001) Time costs of caring for children with severe disabilities compared with caring for children without disabilities. *Dev Med Child Neurol* 43: 529–33. http://dx.doi.org/10.1017/S0012162201000962

Website

Sibs: www.sibs.org.uk

36
Supporting families during the process of adjustment

Gillian Robinson

It is hard for families to hear that their child has difficulties. This is still true when, from our perspective, those difficulties may seem relatively minor. For children with disability to achieve their potential it is important for the families to be able to understand them, meet their needs and encourage them to take the next step. The ability of families to successfully go through this process depends on their own strengths and abilities as well as the abilities of the team members who support them (Fig. 36.1).

Families need to retain control. Gaining an understanding of the child's condition, along with the practical skills to meet their needs, will help with this process. Social support, particularly if provided by the extended family and friends or by professionals, will also enable adjustment.

It is important for professionals to treat parents as equals; we need to respect their knowledge of the child, appreciate their need to understand their child's condition and, later, respect their knowledge of that condition. We must acknowledge the difficulties they face and be willing to engage in dialogue in order to achieve joint decisions on issues of mutual concern.

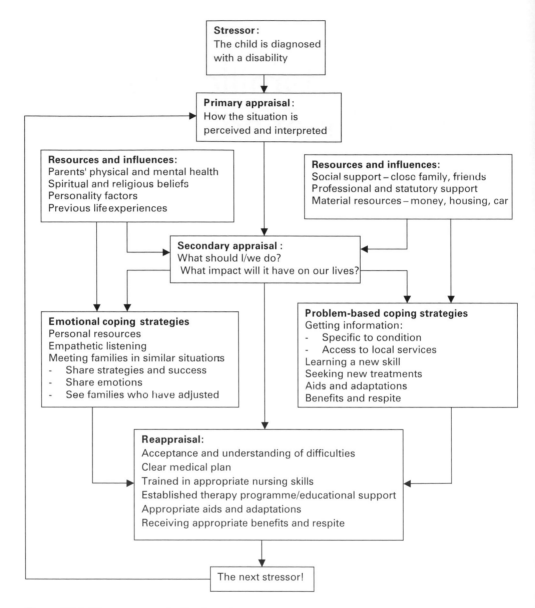

Figure 36.1 The process of adjustment.

Handy hints

Tips for helping families cope with caring for a child with a disability.

- Work with the family and listen to their needs.
- Acknowledge openly to parents that childhood disability impacts on all family members.
- Coordinate appointments where possible.
- Ask about sleep difficulties.
- Review the child's medication regime regularly and consider practical issues such as time of administration.
- Ensure that you are up to date with local sources of support.
- Signpost families to sources of support for issues such as benefits, childcare and employment rights.
- Advocate for access for children with disabilities to play and leisure.
- Advocate for the child and family for provision of short breaks.
- Encourage parents to share the diagnosis with siblings as early as possible, in an honest and age-appropriate way.
- Ask parents to invite siblings to appropriate clinic appointments so that they feel included and are given the opportunity to meet staff and ask questions.
- Ask siblings themselves about how they are finding things at home and at school. If siblings are not present, ask parents how siblings are coping.
- Signpost parents and siblings to Sibs, the UK charity for people who grow up with a disabled brother or sister, and to local support for siblings.

Further reading

Beresford BA (1994) Resources and strategies: how parents cope with the care of a disabled child. *J Child Psychol Psychiatry* 35: 171–209. http://dx.doi.org/10.1111/j.1469-7610.1994.tb01136.x

Davies S, Hall D (2005) 'Contact a Family': professionals and parents in partnership. *Arch Dis Child* 90: 1053–7. http://dx.doi.org/10.1136/adc.2004.070706

Lazarus R, Folkman S (1984) *Stress, Appraisal and Coping*. New York: Springer.

37
Early support

Gillian Robinson

Learning objectives

- To understand the need for early support for families of children affected by any developmental disability.
- To know the range of early years support available (in the UK).

Parents and carers have a key role in supporting their child's development when he or she is younger than 3 years, and this is more so for children with developmental difficulties. With the best support possible, it is possible for outcomes to improve. This can be a very challenging time for families as they will

- have many concerns
- have many appointments
- be taught many new skills such as nursing skills, e.g. managing a gastrostomy tube
- learn therapy skills to aid their child's development
- be coming to terms with the child's additional needs
- need to find time to enjoy being a parent
- need time for themselves.

It is crucial that they receive coordinated training and support from health, education and social care professionals to enable them to confidently and effectively care for their child. Respectful and clear communication between family and professionals and between agencies is key to this progress.

What are the aims of early support (Fig. 37.1)?

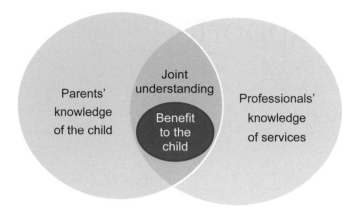

Fig 37.1 Aims of early support.

Effective early support

- is based on respect and good communication
- recognizes that all children and families are different and responds to these different needs
- provides health condition-specific information for families about their child's difficulties
- helps parents and carers of young children with disabilities to understand health, education and social care services so they can appropriately access all available services and make informed choices
- works collaboratively with parents (not forgetting fathers) to clarify goals and to create play-based therapy that can fit around the child and family's routine
- encourages family-held information, which will enable partnership working with all agencies
- promotes and supports inclusion in 'early years' settings including childminders, children's centres and nurseries
- helps families to lead a normal a life as far as possible.

Which children benefit from additional early years support?

- Preterm infants with atypical development or who are at high risk of developmental disabilities.
- Children with genetic diagnoses that will affect development including Down syndrome.
- Infants who leave hospital with significant medical needs.
- Children with significant vision or hearing impairment.
- Children with recognized developmental delay.
- Children with significant communication difficulties including autistic spectrum disorder.
- Children with acquired neurological disorder causing functional impairment.

Who provides early years support?

Services are organized in different ways in different areas. As they are multiagency in nature and 'bespoke for the child', they are complex systems. In some areas early years support services nominate a team member to be the family keyworker. The keyworker can help families to negotiate systems and coordinate care. He or she also provides advice and support to families. Research shows that families who are supported by a keyworker have a greater access to services and that these families feel better supported.

Health

The initial health input may have been from neonatal or general paediatric teams. Once developmental needs have been identified, child development teams will provide ongoing therapy input. In addition, families may be involved with outreach nursing teams.

Education

Education authorities will fund early years workers, teachers (including teachers for the hearing and visually impaired) and educational psychologists to support the additional needs of children under 3 years. Their support can include giving advice about development and behaviour for families and also early years settings. Education staff are also in a good position to offer advice about appropriate local settings, and ensure that there is a smooth transition into that setting. They can advise if a statement of special educational needs will be needed for a child.

Voluntary sector

Voluntary organizations can offer families help based on their own experiences, and therefore have different strengths. Encouraging families to be involved with voluntary agencies for help with specific conditions (e.g. Shine for spina bifida) or for generic help (e.g. Contact a Family) can be invaluable (see Chapter 45). Many families gain huge knowledge about their child's difficulties and they are a great resource not only for their child, but also for professionals who will listen.

Early years support worker

Early years support workers can be funded by health, education and the voluntary sector. They offer support and activities based on play. In some areas workers follow specific programmes such as those based on portage. In all areas this is more effective if there is joint working with specific therapists who can suggest appropriate individualized programmes.

Portage

Portage is a home visiting scheme for preschool children with additional needs. Portage workers can have a wide variety of experience working with families including teachers, nursery nurses, health visitors or members of the voluntary sector. All workers then have additional training from the National Portage Association.

Portage home visitors make weekly or fortnightly visits to families' homes when they initially come to a joint understanding with the parents of a child's abilities by using developmental profiles and checklists. This highlights what children can already do and identifies skills to build on from this point. Parents take the lead in planning the goals relevant to the needs of their child and family. Goals may focus on developing movement, learning, play, communication and participation in the activities of everyday living. Portage workers can then form steps that will help to lead to overall goals.

At each home visit activities to help make the next developmental step are shown to the family and those that the family can practise and enjoy are identified. These activities are based on play grounded in everyday situations to provide fun and success for the child. Each activity may represent a small step towards one of the family's planned goals.

Parents and professionals may use charts or diaries as a reminder of the activity and a record of what happens between visits. This enables families to build a shared record of their child's progress.

Early Support Information and Early Support Pack

Having clear information enables families. The Early Support Pack materials were devised by the Department for Education (England) for families of children with additional needs. Although some information is specific to the England, there is a significant generic component.

The information includes

- A Family File to store all relevant information regarding the child, including the family background, in one place. This acts as a parent-held record.
- Information about how services work and what help and support is available. This includes information regarding health, education, social care, financial entitlements, benefits and voluntary sector organizations.
- Disease-specific information for families (10 different booklets covering the most common developmental conditions including a booklet for conditions associated with complex needs but without an identified diagnosis. 'Contact a family' also have good resources for less frequently encountered conditions)
- Developmental journals for children with
  - learning difficulties without an identified underlying cause
  - visual impairment
  - hearing impairment
  - Down syndrome.

These journals help track and record children's progress, focus on the child's strengths and improve joint working with professionals. The journals are substantial and some families can find them off-putting unless there is professional help in completing them and keeping them up to date.

Further reading

Department of Health (2004) National Service Framework for Children, *Young People and Maternity Services. Disabled Children and Young people and those with Complex Needs*. Available at: www.dh.gov.uk/en/Publicationsandstatistics (accessed 2 December 2012).

National Children's Bureau (2010) *Principles for Engaging with Families*. Available at: www.ncb.org.uk/ecu_network/nqin/resources/engaging_families_principles.aspx (accessed 2 December 2012).

Websites

Early Years Support Programme: www.education.gov.uk/childrenandyoungpeople/sen/earlysupport/resources

National Portage Association: www.portage.org.uk

38
Cultural perspectives

Arnab Seal

Learning objectives

- To understand the influence of cultural factors in the management and outcomes for children with disabilities.
- To recognize the responsibilities of an individual practitioner and those of a service provider to be culturally aware.

Cultural factors can be broadly described as a set of variables related to tradition, knowledge systems, ethnicity and religion, grouped together into a single entity. Cultural factors influence parental beliefs, parenting practices and attitudes towards disability. Even within the population of a single country, there can be substantial differences in ethnic influences, religious practices, customs and belief systems.

Case vignette

Sonia, aged 5 years, has a neurodegenerative disorder with total body involvement, severe learning difficulties, disordered swallowing and seizures. She has been investigated extensively but no specific underlying diagnosis has been made so far. Sonia's parents, Zaheer and Samreen, are of Pakistani origin, Zaheer having grown up in the UK and Samreen coming to the UK after marriage. Both families have their roots in the same community and are distantly related. Sonia's parents are devoted to her and have sought answers from doctors in the UK and Pakistan. On a recent visit to Pakistan they consulted a faith healer, who provided a special charm for Sonia to make things better. Sonia's parents do want another child but are afraid of the risk of recurrence. Deep inside they feel it is their fault that Sonia has an incurable condition and it is a divine retribution for their sins. Sonia lives in an extended family with Zaheer's parents. She enjoys the love, care and attention of cousins, uncles, aunts and grandparents. The family have never considered respite care as an option as they feel any such care need will be met within the family. Zaheer's parents are keen that he has a male heir to carry his name and have recently had a quiet word with the couple. Zaheer is willing to consider this but Samreen is unsure and feels a bit under pressure. She is hoping against hope that the faith charm may just help Sonia turn the corner.

Learning points

* The majority of parents from all cultural backgrounds will try alternative treatments.
* The belief systems and desires of the extended family often play an important role.

Aspects of cultural variations

Language

Language plays an important role within any cultural context. Even though a language may not define a culture, it plays an important role in promoting communication, understanding and trust. This can become a particular issue where one parent, often the mother, who is providing the majority of the care does not speak English and her partner insists on interpreting.

Some children will not have English as their first language or may be exposed to multiple languages at home. This may result in language acquisition delay or difficulties with language form or structure in the initial phase of language acquisition. These delays and/or changes do not imply any significant language problem and tend to resolve over time.

Religious beliefs

Religious beliefs can strongly influence attitudes to disability and the interactions between families and professionals. Examples include the following:

- A religious belief of abortion as sinful can have profound implications on decision making following antenatal diagnosis of a genetic disabling condition.
- Dietary habits, for example exclusion of some food such as pork or non-Halal food by Muslims, need to be considered when providing advice.

Practitioners need to be aware of some aspects of religious beliefs that may have an effect on how families are treated and counselled. Some of these aspects are discussed for four major world religions. We recognize that there is a large number of other religions of equal importance and would advise that you make yourself aware of the relevant religious beliefs as necessary. We also recognize that there are many variations in practice within religions; you would be best advised to use the information here as broad guidance, but check with individual families regarding their own practice.

Christianity

Disability: Christians believe that children and families with a disability should be supported. Western medical causality is generally understood.

Prenatal testing and abortion: This is unacceptable to the Catholic church, but in some specific situations it is viewed as acceptable by Protestant denominations.

End of life: All denominations believe that medication can be used to relieve suffering, even if this decreases the duration of life. Stopping significant life-sustaining treatment, such as ventilation, can be considered with families.

Rituals at death: If a child is dying a minister will come to say prayers of preparation and reconciliation. Either parents or professional staff may wash the body.

Autopsy is acceptable if needed, and should be performed with care and respect.

The funeral is held about a week after death; either burial or cremation is acceptable.

Hinduism

Disability: The belief is that actions in a previous life affect your state in the present life. However, it also places a responsibility on the family and community to act with care and concern towards disabled people or they too would be disadvantaged.

Prenatal testing and abortion: Hinduism is generally opposed to abortion except where it is necessary to save the mother's life.

End of life: The end of life is viewed as the time when a soul makes progress towards liberation. To alter this can affect the progress of the soul and also the lives of the people involved in the act. Having said this, in helping to end a life which is filled with pain, a person is performing a good deed and so fulfilling their moral obligations. Ventilation is viewed as keeping a person artificially alive and therefore altering the course of life, which may be viewed as a bad thing unless healing is possible.

Rituals at death: Relatives gather around the dying person and may put some holy water on the lips of the dying person while singing holy songs and reading holy texts. It is viewed as being better to be conscious at the time of death and therefore pain relief may not be requested. At death, an oil lamp, photograph and the family's favourite deity may be placed at the head of the corpse. Hindu adults would choose to be cremated as they believe this releases the soul, but infants may be buried. The family may choose to wash and embalm the body.

Islam

Disability: Families believe that Allah is aware of the disability and will give them the strength to care for their child.

Prenatal testing and abortion: Muslims regard abortion as wrong and haram (forbidden), but many accept that it may be permitted in certain cases.

End of life: Muslims believe that all human life is sacred because it is given by Allah, and that Allah chooses how long each person will live. Human beings should not interfere in this.

Rituals at death: It is important that the family surrounds the person when dying. Verses from the Qur'an will be recited. Allah should be the last word the person hears. Those around are encouraged to stay calm and pray for the departed. Family members may wash and shroud the deceased. Muslims strive to bury the deceased as soon as possible after death.

An autopsy may be performed, if necessary, but should be done with the utmost respect for the dead.

Judaism

Disability: The disabled are seen as people with a challenge to overcome and the faith community has a responsibility to be compassionate and understanding and to facilitate their needs.

Prenatal testing and abortion: Prenatal testing is acceptable in the first 40 days of pregnancy as it considers the embryo to be of relatively low value during this time. Judiasm does not forbid abortion, but it does not permit abortion on demand. Abortion is permitted only for serious reasons.

End of life: Life is viewed as a gift from God and therefore it is sacred; however, treatments, including ventilation, can be restricted if continuing would cause further distress.

Rituals at death: At death the Kaddish, a funeral prayer, is said. The dead person must not be left alone and must be buried (not cremated) as soon as possible, preferably within 24 hours. The family is viewed as needing time to grieve and it is believed that demonstrating their grief formally helps them to recover from their loss.

Autopsy is viewed as despoiling the body. Orthodox communities feel autopsies should be banned and find them very distressing. It may be permissible if it will help another. The body needs to be buried within 3 days.

Cultural practices

Cultural practices such as marriages between cousins or uncles and nieces can be routine in some communities. There are perceived advantages of social support and economic gain, but there is a higher risk of genetic disorders because of inbreeding within the same genetic pool.

Parenting practices

Different ethnic groups often have different parenting styles. An example of this is sleeping practices. In many cultures children sleep in family beds. Western cultural practices and advice following sudden infant death research is for children to sleep in their own cot, but the family may feel uncomfortable about such an arrangement.

Causality

Parents' beliefs regarding causes of disability, and their ideas about treatment, vary among different cultural groups. Parental belief about disability affects how they approach their child's treatment, interventions and integration into society, which in turn affects the child's development and participation. Parents often hold both biomedical and socio-cultural views at the same time regarding their child's disability, reflecting a duality in beliefs. For example, the parents of a child with hemiplegia may accept that the cause of the disorder is an antenatal stroke, but may also accept that this happened as retribution from the Almighty for their own sins. Some socio-cultural belief systems run deep and can impart long-lasting guilt and/or retribution; for example, a mother being blamed by the father and his family for bearing a child with a disability.

Cultural understanding of disability

Parents may believe that the 'stigma' of disability may compromise social acceptance or may harbour concerns regarding physical disfigurement. This can result in non-compliance with advised treatment, such as gastrostomy placement, or an urge to keep the child within the family, away from the eyes of the world.

Some communities take measures as a collective group. For example, Ashkenazi Jews became aware that within their community children were dying from a progressive neurodegenerative disorder. They worked with geneticists to identify the underlying genetic defect, the testing for which was then offered to the community as a whole so that couples can make informed decisions around parenthood.

Community support

In certain communities individual rights can be considered to be less significant than what is considered good for the community as a whole. In such traditions an individual and family identify themselves primarily as part of a kinship/community with a network of relationships, mutual obligations, support systems and often interlinked religious and economic priorities.

Alternative therapies

Faith in traditional beliefs and trust in the advice of elders and religious leaders can carry more weight than generic advice from the health service. Some of these practices may be potentially harmful or abusive to the child, such as skin 'branding' with hot irons.

Implications for service providers

Training in cultural competency

Staff need to be aware of cultural differences to be able to provide appropriate family-based support. Healthcare professionals also need to recognize that they themselves may have certain unrecognized cultural or religious bias that can affect the quality of care provided. For example, unbiased genetic counselling is difficult for doctors/counsellors who hold certain strong religious beliefs. When such issues are recognized, it is important that other members of the team address it in a supportive fashion.

Use of interpreters

Interpreters are recommended for any consultation in which one or both parents do not speak or understand the language. Sometimes parents are wary of interpreters as they may come from the same community and may breach the family's privacy. Such fears should be explored if a parent declines an interpreter and alternative solutions should be found.

Effect of sex or race of health professionals

Attitudes towards health professionals may also be affected by the sex or race of the service provider. For instance, a male physiotherapist providing home-based therapy for a child may not be acceptable in all cultures if the mother is the only adult available at home. Practitioners should ensure that such factors are identified and relevant individuals, for example community and religious elders, are involved in any planning process to ensure that the package of care is culturally acceptable.

Working collaboratively with families

The child's ability to participate is affected by his personal cultural context (see Chapter 7). Failure to recognize the cultural context can result in failure of individual treatments and community-based rehabilitation programmes. Setting up community-based rehabilitation programmes in developing countries based on the Western model of community services is likely to fail because of the different understandings of the aims and aspirations of the communities they serve.

Rehabilitation is a gradual process that cannot escape cultural factors. Being flexible, empathic and matching one's cultural style to that of the family can create a reassuring sense of congruence, thus enabling sensitive delivery of care. It is important for healthcare professionals to move beyond broad generalizations about cultural differences and instead focus on particular behavioural and social customs relevant to the individual family. An adaptable system which is tailored to the child's individual needs based on disability type, sex, age, education in the context of their family and acceptable cultural practice will be the package of care that will enable the greatest participation.

Key messages

- Cultural beliefs and practices can have a positive or negative effect on the quality of life, opportunities and participation of any child with a disability.
- Traditional beliefs about the cause of chronic illness or disability play a significant role in determining family and community attitudes towards the child with a disability and his or her family. It also influences when, how and why medical input is sought.
- Having a child with a disability can have positive or negative influences, based on cultural expectations of a family/community. For example, deaf parents might wish to have a deaf child or, in some communities, there may be a higher risk of discrimination against a female child with disability.
- The preconceived expectation of a child's life expectancy when he or she has a disability can have an effect on the amount of time, energy and cooperation shown by the family and community.
- There is a higher risk of genetic disorders which may cause disabilities in communities in which consanguinity is an accepted practice.
- Healthcare providers need to be culturally aware and any intervention or package of care needs to be culturally acceptable for it to succeed.

39
Ethical perspectives

Gillian Robinson and Anne M Kelly

Learning objectives

- To understand the principles of ethical decision-making and know how to apply them in practice.
- To recognize that the care of children with disabilities can sometimes present ethical dilemmas and there often is not a right or wrong answer/decision.

It is an accepted tenet of paediatric practice that decisions about medical treatment are made in the best interests of the child. However, for children with disabilities there are additional challenges to consider, as follows:

- Consent is usually given by a proxy for young people aged under 16 – normally this is their parent or a person with parental responsibility. For difficult decisions with long-term consequences, consent should be sought from both parents, if possible.
- Usually families will act in the best interests of the child, but some decisions around the child's care will impact on the whole family and this can sometimes lead parents into some conflict with trying to meet their own and their other children's needs (therefore placing them in a double bind).
- If the child has sufficient intelligence and comprehension to understand the treatment and its implications then he or she is Gillick (Fraser) competent (see also Chapter 46, section on Gillick and Fraser Competence) and can give his or her own consent to treatment without the parents' knowledge. To date, this judgement has been used by young people to gain access to treatment such as the oral contraceptive pill, but not to justify their refusing to have further treatment such as chemotherapy.

- Once over 16 years old, the mental capacity of the young person needs to be assessed under the Mental Capacity Act (2005). In order for someone to have capacity and to be able to give his or her own consent, a young person needs to be able to
  - understand the information relevant to the decision
  - retain that information
  - weigh it up as part of a decision-making process
  - communicate his or her decision.
- For certain young people there are issues around communication. It is important, if possible, to take time and have a familiar adult who can communicate with the young person effectively so that he or she is fully aware of the issues.
- Most of us assume that quality of life for a child with a disability will be lower than that of an able-bodied person. The SPARCLE study (see Chapter 2) demonstrated, however, that the quality of life for children and young people with cerebral palsy were similar to the scores obtained on questioning able-bodied children of the same age.
- Some children with complex disabilities require significant resources. If they become acutely unwell, difficult decisions often need to be made around the appropriateness of admission to paediatric intensive care facilities or invasive care. Balanced against this are the arguments based around the right to life, equality of access, freedom of choice for parents and the dignity of the affected child or young person.

Ethical principles

The four ethical principals of autonomy, beneficence, non-maleficence and justice (Table 39.1) are used when considering how to reach a resolution in an ethical dilemma.

Table 39.1 Ethical principles

Principle	Meaning	Example of ethical dilemma
Autonomy	The patient has the right to refuse or choose their treatment	Families making end of life decisions – parents acting in the best interests of the child?
		Young person with learning difficulties seeking contraception – direct autonomy
Beneficence	Acting in the best interest of the patient	Gastrostomy for a child with unsafe swallow when the family wishes to orally feed
Non-maleficence	First, do no harm	Non-treatment of short seizures in a child with a severe learning disability who has difficulty tolerating antiepileptic medication
Justice	Distribution of scarce health resources, and the decision over who should receive treatment and its extent	Home ventilation

Practical approach to ethical dilemmas

Case vignette

Florence is a 9-month-old female who developed grade 3 hypoxic–ischaemic encepha-lopathy requiring ventilation for the first 3 days of life, having had a difficult home delivery. She is now hypotonic but is just gaining some head control. Her mother has always been keen to feed her orally, but Florence coughs during feeds. Speech and language therapy assessment raises significant concerns about her swallow, and videofluoroscopy studies of swallowing confirms aspiration of thickened liquids. The family still feels that it is safe to feed their daughter orally and will not consent to her being fed enterally through the use of either a nasogastric tube or a gastrostomy tube.

- What is the problem?
  - Is it difficulties with communication? Check the parents' understanding.
  - Is it a professional dilemma about the most appropriate course of action?
  - Is it a child protection issue due to ignorance or a deliberate refusal to meet the child's needs?
  - Is it an ethical problem?
- Try to understand the parents' perspective. Why do they think it is safe to feed orally? What is unacceptable about alternative enteral feeding?

Seek advice

- Consult with colleagues, including a speech and language therapist and a dietitian.
- Search the literature for any useful guidance and evidence of efficacy for the procedure.
- Consult with a senior colleague who may have had experience of a similar case and who can offer advice on how to 'steer a course'.

Discussion of treatment options

- Consider all of the possible options for treatment and their predictable outcomes in terms of autonomy, non-maleficence, beneficence and justice. Discuss these out-comes with the parents and the multidisciplinary team involved with the child.
- Offer a gentle step-by-step plan to move along the course towards the goal, for exam-ple nasogastric feeding on the ward for few days before going home and frequent review by community nursing team.
- Arrange for the family to meet with another family whose child is fed by an alterna-tive route.

If the situation cannot be resolved, consider seeking recourse to the local ethics commit-tee for guidance or legal advice from the hospital trust's legal department on how best to proceed.

> ### Key messages
>
> Acting in the 'best interests of the child' should result in child-centred decisions, but this can be difficult. Other pressures may come to bear on the situation. Child-centred decisions can be achieved only if certain pressures, including parental choice, limited resources and religious choices, are not included as part of the decision-making process.

Further reading

Dickinson H, Parkinson K, Ravens-Sieberer U et al (2007) Self-reported quality of life of 8–12-year-old children with cerebral palsy: a cross-sectional European study (SPARCLE). *Lancet* 369: 2171–8. http://research.ncl.ac.uk/sparcle. http://dx.doi.org/10.1016/S0140-6736(07)61013-7

General Medical Council (2010) *Treatment and Care Towards the End Of Life: Good Practice in Decision Making*. Available at: www.gmc-uk.org/guidance/ethical_guidance/end_of_life_care.asp (accessed 2 December 2012).

Websites

Mental Capacity Act (2005): www.legislation.gov.uk/ukpga

40
Access to leisure activities

Donna Hilton and Jane Williams

Learning objectives

- To understand the importance of leisure activities in promoting health and well-being of children with disabilities.
- To know how to help families access these services.

Impact of chronic illness or disability on participation

It is well known that young people living with a chronic illness or disability may face many different issues related to their stage of development, as well as all of the challenges of adjusting to their health condition. Key issues highlighted include social isolation, stigma of the illness or disability, low self-esteem, loss of independence and privacy and restriction of physical activities.

Even though the Chronically Sick and Disabled Person's Act of 1970 required local authorities to make 'recreational and educational facilities available outside the home', the needs of young people with disabilities were not really considered in the youth service until the 1980s. It remains the case that involvement in mainstream youth clubs for young people with disabilities is still a rarity.

In addition, hospital-based youth work is quite rare and under-researched; however, the evidence that is available suggests that it can be effective in addressing many issues surrounding chronic illness. Peer interaction and access to leisure opportunities are instrumental in aiding young people's development and transition to adulthood.

What young people say they want

Case vignette

Nottingham University Hospitals (NUH) youth service has been running a youth club for 10 years. The club is specifically for young people with a chronic illness or disability. The club was set up as a response to demand from young people and families who had been involved with hospital youth work activities during inpatient stays and/or during school holidays and wanted something of this nature on a regular basis.

A youth forum was set up with a view to taking this project forward and assisted the hospital youth worker in acquiring a venue, buying the equipment, choosing opening days/times and recruiting additional staff to help run the club.

Young people, and their siblings, can take part in activities such as pool, table tennis, computer games, art and craft activities, group games, team-building activities and inclusion sports and youth achievement awards, or have a drink and a chat with peers and the youth work team.

A youth forum is still involved in helping run the club, with previous members now trained as volunteers. The club still attracts over 40 different young people per week, which is a better average than most mainstream youth clubs.

Making a youth club's premises accessible and then expecting young people with disabilities to arrive is never going to happen. The key to any successful work with young people is to have a 'LIP' service in place:

- *Listen* to what young people need and want.
- *Involve* young people in all aspects of meeting those needs.
- *Plan* to make it happen; encourage young people to become whatever it is in them to be.

How can you, as a paediatrician, help?

Case vignette

Alex was 10 years old and about to be excluded from mainstream primary school. He had a diagnosis of autism and was hyperactive. Alex had a weight of 25kg and a body mass index (BMI) of 27. His mother says he had difficulty sleeping and was exhausted. Alex had a younger sister.

Dr Jones suggested that Alex might enjoy some after-school activities. Alex's mother said that all had been tried; he just could not be included with the other children in various local groups, such as football teams. Alex was referred to Positive Moves, a local youth activity group for children with additional needs. Alex reluctantly went along after referral. He enjoyed the sessions and became a regular team member, enjoying trampolining and swimming in particular. His BMI, sleep and school behaviour improved; he was happier. Alex's sister has a special few hours alone with her mother. All were happy – a positive move for all!

This is a scenario that is too familiar in many community paediatric clinics. As a paediatrician you may feel you have no answers.

However, as a paediatrician you can help.

- Approach your local authority and ask what leisure opportunities they have for young people with additional needs. Find out how to advise parents to access these. Several authorities will have a named officer appointed for this purpose.
- If there is no facility, approach the local authority and ask why – we have a role as advocates, too!
- Discuss with your local hospital trust what its youth policy is. Hospital-based youth groups might exist in your area and your patients with chronic illness might be eligible, too.
- Children and young people with additional needs have an entitlement to inclusion and support – this is a service that social care organizations should be providing: approach them.

Leisure opportunities and youth groups

Although it is essential for the needs of young people with disabilities to be met in relation to participation in mainstream activities, some young people living with a chronic illness or disability will not have the confidence to engage in a generic environment. Therefore, specialist provision is essential in aiding their development (Table 40.1).

Table 40.1 Examples of youth work

One-to-one support work	Issues include coping, school, family, health, bullying, self-esteem, bereavement, careers, alcohol awareness, sexual health
Hospital youth club	A twice-weekly facility for young people affected by a chronic illness/disability (and their siblings) to meet together for peer support and activities to help personal and social development
Outdoor education	Day trips to places of interest and challenging activities have helped raise self-esteem and enabled a sense of achievement
Accreditation	Youth achievement awards and open college network courses have enabled patients to gain qualifications and accreditations for life and social skills
Volunteering	The patient volunteer scheme and peer mentoring have been invaluable in extending support for patients and siblings by young people that have 'been there'
Group work	Condition-specific social groups, issue-based support groups, siblings groups, daily drop-in sessions, hospital youth club
Residential programmes	A core ingredient in youth work provision: condition specific, generic, themed (e.g. self-esteem), transition and volunteer training are all examples offered by Nottingham University Hospitals
Sibling support	Group work, youth club, day trips and residential programmes have played a crucial role in supporting siblings
Youth participation	A youth forum, involving young people in conference presentations, planning and evaluation, ensures that patients do have a voice and are actively listened to
Transition	Residential programmes, a transition working group and individual transition plans have been developed, ensuring that young people are supported before, during and after transfer to adult services

Case vignette

Trudy is a 14-year-old female with cerebral palsy (Gross Motor Function Classification System level III). She and her mother attend her annual review with a paediatrician and her mother reports that Trudy has had a change in mood and becomes tearful at times. After discussion, the paediatrician tells Trudy about the hospital youth club and gives information about the local disability sports unit, a team within the county council's community department. Soon Trudy has included herself in the youth club and a wheelchair basketball group. Trudy's family reports a positive change in Trudy.

What is the evidence base?

Reviews have examined the evidence on how services can improve the access of children and young people with disabilities to inclusive and positive activities and the impact this can have on their well-being. It also identifies the most promising directions for future research and development. There is also an argument for disease-specific and non-disease-specific leisure opportunities – both have a place. Positive activities are defined as leisure-time activities outside school hours and taking place in, or being delivered by, children's centres, extended services, youth services, school-based extracurricular activities, play and leisure services, sports and recreation services and the arts.

Key messages

- Children and young people with disabilities appear to have very limited opportunities to access positive activities in their local areas.
- Children and young people with disabilities and their families want more and different things to do so that they can choose where and how they spend their free time.
- Participating in positive activities is associated with positive outcomes in terms of children's health, experiences of enjoyment and achievement and community participation.
- At the same time, children and young people with disabilities report that bullying or fear or bullying spoils their experiences of, or stops them accessing, inclusive activities or using local leisure and recreation facilities.
- Achieving inclusion for children with disabilities requires planning, resources and the active involvement of skilled staff.
- There is scope for children's centres, extended schools and youth services to become more inclusive. Examining service delivery alongside best practice examples would be of benefit.
- Children and young people with disabilities value provision that is designed to facilitate their participation in activities and interaction between children with and without disabilities. However, they also value provision for children or young people with disabilities only.
- Supporting the participation of children and young people with disabilities in positive activities requires much more than making a service inclusive.
- The provision of information about positive activities needs to be improved and some families will need active support to identify and join positive activities provided.

Further reading

Beresford B, Clarke S, Sloper P (2005) *Integrating Services for Disabled Children, Young People and their Families in York: Consulta tion Project*. York: Social Policy Research Unit, University of York.

Brown A (1995) *Group Work*. Aldershot: Ashgate Publishing Ltd.

Davies B (2005) Youth work: a manifesto for our times. *Youth Policy* 88: 5–28.

Harrison R, Wise C (2005) *Working with Young People*. Sage: London

Hilton D, Watson AR, Walmsley P, Jepson S (2004) Youth work in hospital: the impact of a youth worker on the lives of adolescents with chronic conditions. *Paediatric Nursing* 16: 36–9.

Kehily, MJ (ed.) (2007) *Understanding Youth: Perspectives, Identities and Practices*. Sage: London.

National Youth Agency (2007) *The NYA Guide to Youth Work in England*. Leicester: National Youth Agency.

National Youth Agency (2008) *Nottingham University Hospitals Youth Service: A Youth Work 4Health Case Study*. Leicester: National Youth Agency.

Robertson S (2005) *Youth Clubs: Association, Participation, Friendship and Fun!* Dorset: Russell House Publishing.

Thompson B, Taylor H, McConachie R (2000) Promoting inclusive play and leisure opportunities for children with disabilities. *Child Care Pract* 6: 108–23. http://dx.doi.org/10.1080/13575270008413198

Watson AR (2004) Hospital youth work and adolescent support. *Arch Dis Child* 89: 440–2. http://dx.doi.org/10.1136/adc.2002.022855

Yates S, Payne M, Dyson S (2009) Children and young people in hospitals: doing youth work in medical settings. *J Youth Stud* 12: 77–92. http://dx.doi.org/10.1080/13676260802392965

41
Bullying

Gillian Robinson

Sadly, children with special needs are more vulnerable to bullying with up to 90% reporting being bullied. There may be many different reasons for this, including the following:

- Negative attitudes and lack of understanding about disability among others.
- They are seen as different from other children.
- They may find it more difficult to make friends and therefore can be more isolated.
- They may have difficulties informing people about bullying.

Warning signs can include becoming withdrawn, losing belongings or the presence of unexplained bruising. They may become reluctant to go to school or clubs. Their mood might change and they may become anxious, angry or depressed. They may also experience sleeping difficulties.

All children find it hard to talk about bullying, and this is more so for a child with communication difficulties. Asking them about school, who they played with and whether it was fun can sometimes be a 'way in', as well as more specific questions that check whether there is anyone they do not like and the reasons for this. Using pictures, puppets or dolls with non-verbal children may enable them to communicate what has been happening.

Practical strategies to help

In school

It is always good to clear paths of communication with school and a well-used communication book helps with this. If parents are uncertain who to talk to then initially this should be the class teacher, but if the issue persists then the special educational needs coordinator would be the next port of call. The issue may not be resolved with the first contact with school, in which case keeping school well informed about the situation by keeping a diary of incidents with photographs of the injuries can help to understand the situation and to identify appropriate action to take. Parent partnership would also help to support families with managing the issue.

The school should be able to have a named person whom the child can go to if he or she is being bullied. For some children a sign or signal could be better than having to ask to see someone. It is also helpful to be able to have access to a safe place, particularly during unstructured times such as a lunch break. This could be either a quiet or well-supervised area. Buddy schemes or friendship groups can also help.

The child

Social stories about bullying can help children understand what is going on and should emphasise the importance of telling an appropriate adult. These can also be used to enable the child to understand how to behave in different situations, such as in the dinner queue. It can also be helpful to get the child to act out walking away and what he or she could say to the adult if he or she were being bullied. Identifying, with the child, safe and dangerous places (e.g. toilets) on a map of the school can also increase their understanding.

Bullying is, by definition, hurtful and children need to talk about that to someone they trust. It damages self-esteem, and this can be particularly true for children who already have difficulties with communication. Parents spending time with children, telling them it is not their fault, doing activities they enjoy, telling them how much they love them, and specific praise will all help with the child's self-esteem. Excellent resources for families have been produced by Contact a Family and mencap.

Further reading

Contact a Family (2011) Bullying of Children with Disabilities and Special Educational Needs in Schools: Briefing Paper for Parents On the Views and Experiences of Other Parents, Carers and Families. Available at: www.cafamily.org.uk/media/395239/reports_and_research_bullying_of_children_with_disabilities_2011_parents_briefing.pdf (accessed 2 December 2012).

Mencap (2007) Bullying Wrecks Lives. London: Mencap. Available at: http://www.equalpeopleinstoke.org/Libraries/Local/698/Docs/Documents/News/Mencap%20Anti%20Bulllying%20Booklet.pdf (accessed 2 December 2012).

Websites

Contact a Family (leaflet on bullying): www.cafamily.org.uk/media/388418/bullying.pdf

Kidscape: www.kidscape.org.uk

Mencap (easy read fact sheet on bullying): www.mencap.org.uk/sites/default/files/documents/Bullying_factsheet.pdf

Section 13

Frameworks for family support

42
Health services

Gillian Robinson

Learning objective

- To understand the composition and function of child development teams.

The needs of children and families with disability are complex and all unique. This means that there cannot be one ultimate model for working with children and families, as what could be excellent for one family could be inappropriate for another. To try to meet children's and families' needs in the most appropriate manner, there are many different systems around the country, and even more around the world.

Fig. 42.1 summarizes the different services for children with disabilities in the United Kingdom, their major goals and some of the typical inter-relationships. When viewing these complex systems it is clear that effective communication is key to a successful service.

What are child development teams?

Child development teams vary across the country; most commonly, they have the core members of physiotherapist, occupational therapist and speech and language therapist along with a specialist nurse or health visitor and a community paediatrician. In the majority of cases they work from a child development centre that can either be community or hospital based, often depending upon the size of the town or city. The age range of children the team covers again varies over the country, some being preschool teams whereas others cover the whole of childhood until completion of secondary education.

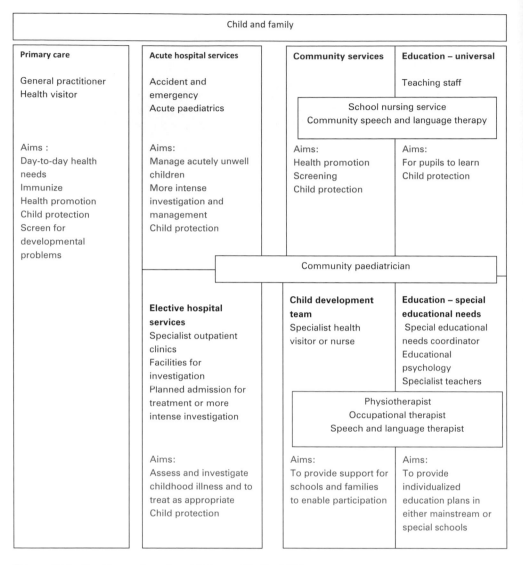

Figure 42.1 Health services for children with disabilities.

What difficulties are assessed by the child development team?

- Learning difficulties
- Global developmental delay
- Cerebral palsy and other motor disorders
- Coordination and fine motor disorders
- Other motor and neurological impairments including spina bifida and children with neuro-muscular disorders
- Autistic spectrum disorders

- Isolated severe language delay
- Visual impairment
- Hearing impairment
- Children with multiple disabilities

Criteria for assessment by the child development team vary between settings. Many teams use the criterion that a child needs to see more than one therapist. This implies that that child has a delay of more than a third of their chronological age in more than one area of development, that is a developmental quotient (DQ) of less than 67%.

What are the aims of the child development team?

The clinical aims of the child development team are to provide the following:

- Assessment and investigation of children with complex disorders and to provide the family with a summary document of the teams' conclusions that is written in language that the family can understand. This enables professionals and families to come to a joint understanding of the child's needs.
- General and condition-specific information that is easily understood by parents and enables families to identify suitable goals for their child. Professionals can then provide coordinated advice to families and schools to help achieve these goals and provide parents, teachers and others with advice and support on management of the child so that he or she can participate fully in life.
- Specialist advice to schools and other agencies.

Operational aims are as follows:

- To be able to provide data on the needs of children in the area and therefore be able to advise on service provision.
- To be involved in monitoring the effectiveness of services including audit.
- To act as a source of information.
- To organize training for professional staff.
- To support effective local surveillance through training of primary care and nursery staff.

What are the key elements to good assessment?

1. An assessment that involves the parents and thinks about the family's needs as a whole. This should include contact with them at home.
2. An assessment initially completed by a multidisciplinary team.
3. A specialist assessment of hearing and vision.
4. Appropriate medical investigations completed including genetic investigations, biochemical screening, neurophysiology and radiology. Onward referral, for example to neurology or genetics colleagues, may be appropriate.

5   Both verbal and written feedback to parents summarizing not only the medical diagnosis but specific functional problems. This needs to be written clearly and without jargon.

6   An action plan, including specific intervention goals for problems the family and professionals have highlighted.

7   A process for coordinating ongoing care, which will usually involve a meeting with all appropriate agencies, to which the family are actively encouraged to contribute.

8   Providing further opportunity for the family to ask questions and at this time attempting to answer questions about prognosis.

9   Ensuring genetic counselling is available if this is appropriate.

10 Ensuring that there is a periodic review system.

11 Including a named keyworker for the family to contact when they are unsure of who to ask for help.

Ongoing care and support

Who does the 'hands on' treatment?

In practice this is done by the parents and carers when the child is young and later by school staff. The child development team has an important role in training parents, nursery, school and other staff dealing with the child and family so that therapeutic approaches can be applied widely and consistently. Therapy staff need to work collaboratively with schools to work out appropriate intervention programmes; this may include contributing to statements of special educational need.

Where should treatment be delivered?

Treatment may be delivered in the child development centre, the home, nursery, local clinic or school. The most effective and efficient setting for the child will change with age. As children are being more often included in mainstream settings there is a need to ensure that appropriate support for staff and adaptations are in place to enable a smooth progression into nursery and school.

Core team members and their roles

Speech and language therapists

Speech and language therapists assess, diagnose and develop programmes of care to help children develop communication skills. They offer support and advice to parents and to other professionals about developing communication that may be verbal (i.e. using speech) or non-verbal, using signs, symbols or communication aids.

A number of children with disability have an ongoing need for speech and language therapy input throughout childhood. This includes at least a quarter of all children with cerebral palsy, children with hearing impairment and many children with severe learning difficulties who require a speech and language programme in conjunction with their other special educational needs.

Speech and language therapists are also involved with helping children with significant feeding problems as they have expertise in assessing chewing and swallowing.

Physiotherapist

A physiotherapist has skills in assessing motor development. They work with families and schools to develop plans to help children learn to control their movements. These are often goals based in order for progress to be assessed. Physiotherapists also teach carers and education staff how to support children in different positions to enable function, improve physical skills and to minimize any secondary difficulties (24h postural management). They also advise, if needed, on how to transfer children between positions and about equipment that helps with mobility.

Occupational therapist

An occupational therapist helps children to participate as much as possible in play and later life skills by therapeutic techniques, environmental adaptations and the use of specialist equipment. Occupational therapists are concerned with difficulties that children have in carrying out the activities of everyday life, for example eating, bathing and dressing. They have particular expertise in assessing hand function, coordination and sensory profiling.

Specialist health visitor

Specialist health visiting staff offer information and support before, during and after additional needs have been identified or a diagnosis is made. They encourage parents/carers to be partners in their child's care and make informed choices. The specialist health visitor helps to coordinate multiagency services around individual children and families.

Extended team members (Table 42.1)

Keyworker

Keyworkers help to coordinate services from different agencies. They may be a separate worker or a nominated team member. A keyworker is a source of support for families. The range of support often includes advice regarding some developmental issues such as behaviour management, sleep, and so on. They are a good resource for families to obtain general information regarding the range of available services across various agencies and also specific information about the diagnosis as relevant. They help to coordinate services and ensure that information about children is shared efficiently. Specific keyworker services are not available in all areas.

Table 42.1 Extended team members

Team member	Support provided
Audiologist	Hearing testing Provision of effective hearing aids Works alongside an audiological physician or ear, nose and throat (ENT) surgeon
Clinical psychologist	Assessment of children with emotional and behavioural difficulties. May be part of paediatric or child and adolescent mental health services team Standardized assessment of cognitive function Supports families in finding and implementing appropriate management strategies for behavioural problems
Community dental services	Specialist dental services with experience and appropriate equipment to manage children with disability. They have access to general anaesthetic lists for treatment if needed
Dietitian	For children with faltering growth or feeding difficulties, dietitians will assess and give advice on nutrition For children with nasogastric or gastrostomy feeding, dietitians draw up a feeding plan which includes the feed type, the volume, the method of administration and any equipment required
Geneticist	Help with diagnosis and management of genetic conditions. Counsel families around recurrence risk, which may include antenatal testing and diagnosis
Educational psychologist	Addresses problems in school around learning difficulties and social or emotional problems. Provides specialist assessments Works with teaching staff and develops plans to optimize the child's learning
Nursing	Community nurses support families with nursing activities at home Specialist nurses, e.g. epilepsy nurse specialists, support families around management of specific conditions like epilepsy
Ophthalmologist	Diagnosis and management of eye defects and diseases
Optometrist or ophthalmic optician	Dispenses and adjusts spectacles and other optical aids
Orthoptist	Skills in assessing sight, strabismus and eye movements Use non-surgical means such as patching to improve vision
Orthotist	Measures, designs, makes, fits, or services braces, splints and special footwear for children with movement difficulties
Paediatric neurologist	Helps in diagnosis and medical management of disorders of the nervous system
Paediatric orthopaedics	Orthopaedic surgeon skilled in management of children and who have skills in managing the orthopaedic consequences of cerebral palsy
Social services occupational therapist	Gives advice on housing adaptations

How do you ensure effective services?

Patient participation

Patient participation is key, both for feedback on present services and also for a vision around how services should be developed. It is important that if patients or parents are involved in service planning they are equal in status to professionals present. Ideally, parents or young people should be paid for attending meetings, just as professionals are. If this is not possible it should be ensured that, at the least, child care is provided.

Interagency planning

It is clearly essential to plan with colleagues from education and social care in order to provide a 'joined-up service'. This planning needs to involve staff with managerial 'clout' who are, preferably, budget holders. Joint commissioning of services can be helpful. An effective partnership with parents, carers, children and families who access the centre is important in delivering a responsive service which meets local needs.

Governance

Governance describes the structures that need to be in place for effective and safe clinical working. It can be challenging for child development teams in view of their multidisciplinary basis. Effective governance is helped by clear management structures – and preferably one for the whole team rather than separate disciplines.

Components of governance include the following:

- **Effective practice**
  - Maintaining purposeful continuing professional development of the whole team.
  - Ensuring that the team is working to national standards both for individual disciplines and the team as a whole.
  - Ensuring that there are methods for implementing central guidance (e.g. NICE guidance or national service frameworks).
  - Developing evidence-based pathways.
- **Risk management**
  - Ensuring that there is appropriate supervision for clinical work, specifically around child protection.
  - Ensuring that there is an effective system to enable learning from compliments and complaints.
  - Encouraging critical incident forms to be completed and acting upon them.
  - Learning from serious case reviews.
- **Audit**
  - For a multiagency team, for example
    - The Audit Commission (www.audit-commission.gov.uk/nationalstudies/localgov/disabledchildren)

- Early Support Programme (http://media.education.gov.uk/assets/files/pdf/e/early%20support%20service%20audit%20tool%202009.pdf)
- For a child development team, for example
  - Measures of Processes of Care (eMPOC) (King et al. 1995)
- For specific disorders, for example
  - Down syndrome – DSMIG guidelines (www.dsmig.org.uk)
  - Autism spectrum disorder – NICE guidelines (www.nice.org.uk)

Appraisal

For appraisal to be effective it should be completed in a reflective and supportive manner. It should review progress in the above areas and allow practitioners to highlight specific and achievable areas for development in the coming 12 months.

Reference

King S, Rosenbaum P, King G (1995) *The Measure of Processes of Care: A Means to Assess Family-Centred Behaviours of Health Care Providers*. Hamilton, ON: McMaster University, Neurodevelopmental Clinical Research Unit. Available at: www.canchild.ca/en/measures/mpoc56_mpoc20.asp (accessed 2 November 2012).

Further reading

British Association for Community Child Health – Child Development and Disability Group (2000) *Standards for Child Development Services: A Guide for Commissioners and Providers*. London: BACCH.

Court Report (1976) *Fit for the Future: The Report of the Committee on Child Health Services*. London: HMSO.

Websites

Association of Educational Psychologists: www.aep.org.uk

British Academy of Childhood Disability: www.bacdis.org.uk

British Psychological Society: www.bps.org.uk

The College of Occupational Therapists: www.cot.org.uk/

Community Practitioners' and Health Visitors' Association: www.unite-cphva.org

Royal College of Speech and Language Therapists: www.rcslt.org

43
Children in hospital

Jane Williams

> **Learning objectives**
>
> - To know that children with disabilities are frequently admitted on to children's wards.
> - To be aware of the difficulties in assessing children with disability presenting with intercurrent illness.
> - To know that it is important to plan for any inevitable admission that may occur.
> - To understand the common problems faced by children with disabilities and their careers in hospital settings.
> - To follow best practice guidelines for any potential admission.

Background

There were 770 000 children with disabilities in the UK in 2009, which equates to 1 in 20 of the childhood population. These children and young people can be admitted with an unplanned medical problem but the vast majority of admissions, particularly in younger children, are secondary to respiratory problems (17%). We know that children with disability, particularly a physical disability, are more prone to respiratory difficulty; hence, this is a common reason for admission for this group of children. Hospital admission data show that behavioural problems and poor seizure control are also common causes for admission.

Studies carried out in Bristol found that children with disabilities make up around 7% of all children admitted to hospital, their length of stay is usually longer and nearly twice the average stay for children with no disability, and 15% are admitted to the intensive care unit (Marsh and Allport submitted).

Reported problems

A recent Care Quality Commission study has also confirmed difficulties with the admission of children with disability to UK hospital wards. This study asked acute trusts to return information about delayed discharge or transfer of care from services for children and young people with disabilities. They found significant delays in discharge for many of the admitted children. The key reasons cited for delayed discharge from hospital were

- hospitals not having arrangements in place to support discharge home
- other acute trust not being prepared to accept referral
- family refusing discharge.

Children with disabilities and their families report a range of difficulties they encounter while accessing hospital-based care. Some of the main issues include the following:

- inadequate training of staff to meet the needs of children and young people with learning disabilities
- inadequate facilities for parents
- families lacking confidence that the staff will be able to understand their child's needs
- some wards having inadequate facilities for nursing and bathing care for children and young people with a disability
- services being disjointed, meaning that different services do not work well together
- children with disabilities and their families not being consulted on how their care is provided
- clinicians and managers providing services which they think the family needs rather than what the family feels is a priority: main problem areas cited were communication, listening and attitudes
- long waiting times for planned admissions and inadequate access to specialist care and urgent/semi-urgent care.

Best practice for unplanned and planned admission to hospital

- Have a prewritten individual Emergency Health Care Plan (EHCP) or passport, describing the child or young person.
- Ensure that this is with the child always – preferably laminate the document.
- Ensure that the local emergency department has some information which is accessible to them should the child attend.
- In the most vulnerable group, inform the ambulance service of their needs (see Chapter 62).
- Review the EHCP with the child, parent and carer at frequent intervals.
- Ensure ease of access for urgent/semi-urgent care.
- All children and young people with disabilities 18 years or younger should have the choice to be admitted and cared for in a paediatric ward and not an adult ward.
- Liaison and close working between community services and hospital services before, during and pre-discharge is essential.

Intercurrent illness

There are many good reasons why it is difficult to assess children with a disability when they present with intercurrent illness. These include

1 There are communication difficulties and the child cannot describe pain.
2 There are motor difficulties so the child cannot point or direct the examiner to the area that hurts.
3 The child's illness means that the traditional findings will be different, for example a child with muscle weakness and a respiratory infection may not cough or have respiratory muscle recession.

The examiner therefore needs to place a higher emphasis on the reported concerns of the main carer and to be aware that the child's response to illness and manifestation of this may differ, for example the child may become more agitated or, alternatively, become more placid or withdrawn when unwell.

The examiner may need to perform some blood investigations to support clinical suspicions earlier than in a child in whom the examiner is more confident of the clinical findings. Alerting more senior staff or accessing an assessment from a doctor who knows the child can be very helpful.

Training for hospital staff

Ensure that the admitting and ward nursing team are aware of the ECHP/passport and have a good understanding of the needs of the child. Appropriate training should be available for paediatric nursing staff to understand and meet the needs of children and young people with learning difficulties, physical difficulties, autism, behavioural difficulties and other complex needs as well as of non-communicating children. Training in diversity, consent and communication needs for those with special needs (e.g. low vision and deafness groups) is also important. Care should be tailored to the needs of the individual child and family as much as possible.

Many areas have developed a 'hospital passport' scheme. These are based on the 'traffic light system':

* red – things you *must know* about me
* amber – things that are *important* to me
* green – my *likes and dislikes*.

The child who has developed a disability as a result of the cause of the admission

Unfortunately, many children who have had an inpatient stay for a range of problems will develop a residual disability. It is important that you plan to discharge those children in this group as early as possible. In addition, understanding and dealing with evolving behavioural, emotional, communication and cognitive needs that have developed is crucial.

Consider the possibility of a life-threatening presentation requiring admission

Discussing with families and the young person where possible how they want to manage a potentially life-threatening admission before the event happens is helpful for all. The emergency department or paediatric intensive care unit is not the best setting to consider whether it is in the child's interest for advanced resuscitation or ventilation. Refer to Chapter 62 on the planning of care for life-limiting and life-threatening conditions.

Further reading

Avis M, Reardon R (2008) Understanding the views of parents of children with special needs about the nursing care their child receives when in hospital: a qualitative study. *J Child Health Care* 12: 7–17. http://dx.doi.org/10.1177/1367493507085615

Mahon M, Kibirige M (2004) Patterns of admissions for children with special needs to the paediatric assessment unit. *Arch Dis Childhood* 89: 165–9. http://dx.doi.org/10.1136/adc.2002.019158

Marsh B, Allport T (submitted) Inpatient Care of the Disabled Child: A Prospective Study of Quality of Care, Parent Satisfaction and Causes and Costs of Delayed Discharge.

Websites

Care Quality Commission: http://www.cqc.org.uk/sites/default/files/media/documents/health_care_for_disabled_children_easy_read.pdf

Council for Disabled Children: www.councilfordisabledchildren.org.uk/

Spotty the Sick Child: www.spottythesickchild.com/

44

Supporting the needs of children and their families

Lorna Highet

Learning objectives

- To know the existing mechanisms for the assessment of family needs and state provided support available in the UK for children and young people with disabilities and their families.
- To understand the provision for children with disabilities, partially or fully looked after by the state in the UK.

Assessment of need

Health, education and voluntary sector staff are encouraged to use mainstream local resources to help support families. To help identify needs the Common Assessment Framework (CAF) has been developed in the UK.

The aim of this framework is to

- ensure that children and young people who have 'additional needs' are identified as early as possible
- provide a simple process for a holistic assessment of children's needs and strengths, taking account of the roles of parents, carers and environmental factors in children's development
- reduce the number of assessments children and young people require by the various agencies
- improve the quality of assessments across all services for children
- support any referrals between different services.

After a CAF has been completed, the multiagency team consisting of the professionals involved with the child has the task of identifying resources that may help the family meet the identified needs and fulfil the actions.

Whilst a CAF process sounds laudable, in practice there are difficulties:

- The framework is long and considerable time is required by the family and professionals in order to complete it.
- The multiagency meetings are costly in terms of professional time.
- The outcome for families is partly dependent on the skills of the worker who completes the CAF and the engagement of the family and professionals.
- Many services continue to complete their own assessments if they feel the CAF as inadequate for their purpose.
- It can sometimes act as a barrier to access to services (e.g. not eligible for a service till CAF has been completed).

Social care provision

Social services have certain statutory responsibilities arising from the Chronically Sick and Disabled Persons Act 1970, the Disabled Persons Act 1986 and the Children Act 1989. These charge social services with the following responsibilities:

- To provide services for children in need.
- To keep a register of children with disabilities – this is primarily to help manage services.
- To ensure services are coordinated.
- To include families in decision making.
- To make provision for respite care, which is often funded from the social care budget.
- To safeguard the welfare of children in respite care, and in health or educational facilities.
- To collaborate with the education authority to assess the needs of school leavers with disabilities (see Chapter 45).
- To provide leisure activities.
- To provide day care facilities.

In addition, social care staff have a working knowledge of the benefits system that is available to support families financially.

Government benefits

Having a child with additional needs is costly for families, in terms of both the time required to care for their needs and also financial costs; therefore, the government provides families with additional benefits. Government benefits vary between countries and will change with every governmental budget. There are now good web-based resources to find out the current situation such as the Contact a Family website (www.cafamily.org.uk/know-your-rights/benefits-and-tax-credits/) and the Directgov website (www.direct.gov.uk/en/MoneyTaxAndBenefits).

The majority of benefits require previous National Insurance contributions. Some benefits are available to all families (universal, non-means tested) but the majority are paid to families on low income with little savings (means tested). It is difficult to get any benefits backdated, so delaying claims will decrease the money the family is likely to receive. At present, asylum seekers are not eligible to apply for government benefits. These benefits are summarised in Table 44.1.

Table 44.1 Government benefits in the United Kingdom

Benefit	Who is it for	Financial criteria
Disability Living Allowance	*Care component* – for children who need extra attention or supervision. It is paid at one of three different rates depending on how much extra care the child needs *Mobility component* – for children who need help with getting around. This is paid at one of two rates depending on the nature/severity of the mobility problems	Non-means tested
Carer's Allowance	Paid to people who care for someone who receives the middle or highest rate of Disability Living Allowance Carer either does not work, or has low income and is not in full-time education	Means tested, not affected by savings
Working Tax Credit	Payable if either partner works for 16h a week or more and have a dependent child or for people with a disability working at least 16h a week. There can sometimes be money towards certain 'approved' childcare costs	Means tested
Child Tax Credit	Do not have to be in work Increased if child receives Disability Living Allowance or is registered blind	Means tested, not affected by savings
Income Support	Families on low income	Means tested
Direct Payments Scheme	Councils make direct payments to people receiving social care services, instead of the council providing the service directly	Non-means tested
Community Care Grant	Help towards one-off costs to ease exceptional pressures	Means tested
Family Fund	Charity which provides grants for specific items to help relieve the stress arising from the day-to-day care of a child under 18 years old who has a severe disability or serious illness	Means tested
Disabled Facilities Grant	One-off payment for adaptations approved by social care occupational therapy	Means tested

Families can get support from their local Citizens Advice Bureau or Welfare Rights Service about the benefits they can claim in their situation. It is even more complex during the transition to adulthood, and a discussion with a social worker who understands the system can be very helpful for families.

Housing

Families that include a child with a disability are less likely to be living in decent accommodation than families with a non-disabled child. They are 50% more likely than other families to live in overcrowded accommodation and to rate their home as being in a poor state of repair. Families with disabled children are more likely than the families of their non-disabled peers to live in rented accommodation.

Common problems include lack of space for living and lack of space for the use and storage of therapy equipment. Parents describe the negative impact that living in unsuitable housing has on their child's well-being and development as well as on their own and that of their other children. One-third of families report difficulties with the location of their home. The location may be unsafe for the child (e.g. situated on busy road), there may be disagreements with neighbours or the area may lack accessible local facilities such as shops or services such as a general practitioner surgery.

Moving, as opposed to adapting the current home, is the preferred option by families for dealing with unsuitable housing. Housing services are run by a wide variety of bodies, including local councils and housing associations, each of which has individual rules about priority. At present, social housing stock is limited and therefore priority is given to homeless families. Medical need is recognized by many housing agencies and letters of support can help families to increase their priority, but ranking of need is complex.

Improvements in a family's housing situation can lead to improvements in the child and family's sense of well-being and confidence, and results in reduced reliance on local services. Unfortunately, it is not always possible to find suitable accommodation that meets all the requirements of the family. In practice, families may wait a very long time until they find something they can accept as being suitable.

Adaptations

Adaptations may be needed to the child's home to enable the child to live as independently as possible. These needs are assessed by occupational therapists working for social care. Potential adaptations can include

- widening doors and installing ramps
- providing or improving access to rooms and facilities, for example by installing a through-floor lift or a chair lift or providing a downstairs bathroom/wet room
- improving or providing a heating system
- adapting heating or lighting controls for remote access.

If the assessment shows that adaptations are needed, local councils have to provide disabled facilities grants to eligible applicants. The level of funding depends on the family's financial circumstances. Families can claim back value added tax on the building work.

Short-term breaks

Short-term break services when administered well can provide significant benefit for both the child and the family. The child can benefit from a different, and hopefully fun, environment which may offer activities that facilitate progress towards greater independence. This arrangement allows the rest of the family an opportunity to spend some time together without their child with a disability taking priority. It allows carers to 'recharge their batteries' and also enables them to have some time to take care of essential tasks. The majority of these services are accessed through social care and places are limited. The family need is assessed and provision is decided by matching need, parental choice and available resource. The types of services that are available include the following:

1 *Day nurseries or family centres*, which can be seen as providing respite care as well as professional input and opportunities for social mixing.
2 *Sitting services* in the child's home. This scheme allows parents to have a few hours off whilst their child is cared for within the home by an experienced carer, enabling them to go out on short trips such as shopping or to attend appointments.
3 *Family twinning*: families who have had experience of disability in the past or who are just interested in helping can be twinned with a family who has a child with a disability. The two families gradually build up a relationship, leading to trips out, overnight stays and possibly longer stays for the child.
4 *Support worker*: teenagers benefit from time with an adult other than their parents to participate in activities such as going to the cinema. This can be facilitated by a support worker.
5 *Specially designated respite care facilities* either in social services, health or 'extended education' facilities. Most facilities can provide either day or overnight care, which is normally on a planned basis but can also be used in an emergency.

Children and young people with disabilities accessing the care system (partially or fully looked after by the state and/or adopted)

Local authorities provide a range of services for children in need affected by disability including the following:

Short breaks: This can include support provided within a child's home, day-time care or leisure activities and occasional overnight stays or regular periods of care with an approved foster carer or in a children's residential unit. These breaks are planned and do not exceed a total of 120 days a year in the UK (see above).

Shared care: This is when a child lives elsewhere than the family home for more than 120 days a year. This is often in a group home setting for children who have complex medical needs (e.g. a child who is home ventilated) or, more commonly, whose behaviour is challenging.

Local authority care: Some young people are in local authority care full time. This may be either on a voluntary basis, for example if the child has significant needs that the family feels unable to meet, or on a statutory basis for child protection purposes. These children can either be in long-term foster placement or in a local authority children's home. Children with disabilities are over-represented in long-term local authority care.

Adoption: The number of children without adverse circumstance or given up for adoption at birth in the UK is now low. The majority of children will have some difficulties; these may be a consequence of genetic conditions (e.g. learning disability), the mother being unable to look after her child, or abuse, or rarely families who do not want to take on the responsibility of raising a child with a disability.

Medical assessment of children in the care system

• Past medical history
• Vision
• Hearing
• Medications, feed regimes if on dietary supplements and allergies
• Immunization status
• Dental health
• Family history
• Growth including head circumference
• General examination including teeth
• Current developmental level using screening tool or current school achievement plus additional support in education
• Emotional status using, for example, the Strengths and Difficulties Questionnaire
• Substance misuse screen when appropriate
• Sexual health

Children in the care system

Children can be moved at short notice and the new carers are unlikely to know the child's needs. Written information that travels with the child should include the following:

• Present difficulties including any allergies
• Underlying diagnosis
• Medication, including feeding regime if on gastrostomy or nasogastric feed
• Known allergies
• Immunization status
• How the child communicates
• Appropriate contact details for further information

Children being placed for adoption

Children being placed for adoption need a summary of their

- medical issues using lay language
- current development
- likely prognosis – highlighting strengths and possible areas of difficulty. This would include the consequence of any abuse they have experienced as well as any underlying medical problems.

If the birth mother is present this may be the only opportunity for

- a full family history of three generations
- establishing whether there was maternal drug or alcohol usage during pregnancy.

What children like to know when older

- What their natural parents looked like – stature, eye and hair colour.
- The story of their mother's pregnancy and their birth, including the time and place.

Further reading

Burns C (2009) *Disabled Children Living Away From Home in Foster Care and Residential Settings*. London: Mac Keith Press.

Children's Workforce Development Council (2009) *The Common Assessment Framework for Children and Young People: A Guide for Practitioners*. Available at: http://education.gov.uk/publications/eOrdering-Download/CAF-Practitioner-Guide.pdf (accessed 2 November 2012).

Joseph Rowntree Foundation (2008) *Housing and Disabled People*. Available at: www.jrf.org.uk/sites/files/jrf/2208.pdf (accessed 2 November 2012).

Websites

British Association for Adoption and Fostering: http://www.baaf.org.uk/info/disability

Contact a Family: www.cafamily.org.uk/families

Directgov: www.direct.gov.uk/en/MoneyTaxAndBenefits

45
Voluntary sector

Christine Lenehan and Amanda Allard

Learning objectives

- To understand the role of the voluntary sector.
- To know the range of organizations/services available and how to access them.

The voluntary sector plays a significant role in the provision of information, services and support for children with disabilities and their families. A number of charities provide funding for treatments or support. Most of these charities will consider applications and request information from professionals in order to tailor the help for the individual child. Providing families with information regarding the various organizations and the type of help these can offer is part of the role of professionals involved as the family 'keyworker'.

A number of national voluntary organizations focus primarily on sharing and promoting good practice and pushing for policy and practice change which benefits children with disabilities, for example the Council for Disabled Children and The Communications Trust. Such organizations can be an important source of information on policy change and practice innovation.

Many charities, whether local or national, focus on a single condition or need. These organizations may run services for families and provide advice and information as well as being a useful source of accessible condition-specific information aimed at parents and children. Contact a Family provides advice and support to families of children with disabilities, whatever their condition, and as part of this role signposts parents to local and national charities that provide support with specific conditions.

A recent trend in the NHS in the UK is for specific services to be contracted out to any willing provider. This has resulted in a number of charities bidding for these contracts and becoming a service provider. This can blur some boundaries and make the role of the voluntary sector more complex.

The following section looks at the different types of support that may be available to families from a range of national and international organizations. Information regarding local voluntary organizations can sometimes be obtained from the Contact a Family website or by contacting a local parent group. The organizations listed below provide a wide variety of services, advice and information relevant to children with disabilities and their carers. They have been grouped based on the type of service that they provide.

Umbrella organizations

The Communication Trust

www.thecommunicationtrust.org.uk
Tel: 0207 843 2526
The purpose of The Communication Trust is to highlight the importance of speech, language and communication across the children's workforce and to enable practitioners to access the best training and expertise to support the communication needs of all children.

There are over 40 voluntary and community groups which contribute to the work of the Trust.

Council for Disabled Children (CDC)

www.councilfordisabledchildren.org.uk
Tel: 0207 843 1900
The CDC undertakes a wide range of roles and activities, which include developing information and resources for parents, young people, public sector professionals and those in the voluntary sector. Whilst the CDC does not give advice directly to parents, it does develop and signpost parents to a number of useful resources. *Disabled Children: A Legal Handbook* is available to view for free on the CDC website.

The CDC coordinates a number of specialist networks; those of most direct interest to parents are the following:

- The National Parent Partnership Network (NPPN) coordinates the network of parent partnership services in England. Parent partnership services are statutory services offering information, advice and support to the parents and carers of children and young people with special educational needs. It is also able to put parents in touch with other local and national organizations. Contact NPPN for the contact details of your local parent partnership service (www.parentpartnership.org.uk, tel: 020 7843 6058).
- The Transition Information Network (TIN) provides information and resources about transition through its website, publications and events. TIN publishes *My Future Choices*, a magazine aimed at young people with disabilities, their families and professionals. It includes articles about transition projects around the UK, interviews with young people with disabilities about their dreams for the future, latest policy and charity news and news about resources and events. TIN also produces a policy e-bulletin *Getting a Life*, which lists the latest policy and practice development affecting young people with disabilities who are in transition (www.transitioninfonetwork.org.uk, tel: 0207 843 6006).

Genetic Alliance UK

www.geneticalliance.org.uk
Tel: 0207 704 3141
The Genetic Alliance UK is a national alliance of patient organizations with a membership of over 130 charities that support children, families and individuals with a genetic disorder. It provides a wide range of information on genetics, including a comprehensive glossary.

National Voices

www.nationalvoices.org.uk
Tel: 0203 176 0738
National Voices is a coalition of national health and social care organizations representing users of health and social care in England.

National Network of Parent Forums (NNPCF)

http://www.nnpcf.org.uk/
Tel: 0773 889 6474
Under the 'Aiming High for Disabled Children' programme, local areas received a grant to set up a forum for the parents of children with disabilities in order that they could better work in partnership with their local authority to develop and provide the kinds of services that they and their children want. The NNPCF was set up to ensure that good practice, knowledge and shared expertise about parent participation continued to grow and strengthen. The NNPCF identifies common priorities, and ensures that information and experiences are shared so that service delivery can be influenced at a national level.

Parents can find out about their local group from the organization's website or by contacting sue.north@cafamily.org.uk.

General support organizations

Contact a Family

www.cafamily.org.uk
Tel: 0207 608 8700
Since 1979, Contact a Family has provided support, advice and information for the families of children with disabilities. It does this in a variety of ways including through the provision of the following.

• A comprehensive A–Z directory of over 400 conditions giving medical information on rare disorders and conditions. For each condition listed, there is information on the symptoms and causes, diagnosis and treatment, inheritance patterns and prenatal diagnosis. Contact details of support groups specific to the condition as well as any other charities or resources specific to those conditions are also given. The directory is available in electronic format on the Contact a Family website or a paperback version can be purchased from the online shop

- Information or advice on any aspect of caring for a child with a disability. This can be accessed by a freephone helpline (0808 808 3555) on weekdays or by e-mail (helpline@ cafamily.org.uk).
- A father's zone, providing information for fathers who have a child with a disability.
- A team of family workers covering some parts of the UK. Family support workers help families with a range of issues that families face when caring for a child with a disability.
- A special educational needs national advice service offering a one-stop shop for parents and carers to get one-to-one personalized advice from experienced special educational needs advisers regarding any concerns about their child's education.

Family lives

http://familylives.org.uk
Tel: 0808 800 2222
Family lives is a national charity that works for, and with, parents with any problems around a range of issues affecting parents and their families from having a new infant, starting a new relationship and disagreements in the family, to issues with teenagers, school, homework, sleep or eating patterns.

Newlife Foundation for Disabled Children

www.newlifecharity.co.uk
Tel: 0800 902 0095
Email: nurses@newlifecharity.org.uk
Newlife Nurses provide families with a gateway to information, grants and care. The charity runs a free, confidential national helpline which supports and informs families, whether they have just been told of their child's disability or need help accessing local services. Families can get help with medical jargon and discuss what questions they should be asking at appointments. In addition, Newlife Foundation offers grants for essential medical equipment. If the statutory health and social care services cannot help, Newlife Nurses can progress a grant for equipment direct from Newlife funds or provide information on grants available nationally from other sources.

Newlife also recognizes the specific needs of terminally ill children who cannot wait for statutory services to respond to their needs. The 'Just Cannot Wait' equipment loan service aims to deliver items from its suite of specialist equipment within 72 hours, from anywhere in the UK.

Newlife also offers an online condition information service dedicated to children with disability due to a range of conditions, including malformations, genetic conditions, preterm birth, injury or cancer. The service has been created by UK professionals to provide families, patients and health professionals with accessible key information that is regularly updated The service holds information or references on over 3000 conditions.

WellChild

www.wellchild.org.uk
Tel: 0845 458 8171
WellChild is the national charity for sick children, including those with serious illness and complex conditions. The charity provides direct care through a team of specialist WellChild

children's nurses and practical support through its Helping Hands scheme of volunteers, and invests in children's health research projects.

Aids and equipment

British Red Cross

www.redcross.org.uk
Tel: 0844 871 1111
The British Red Cross has a volunteer-led medical equipment service that provides wheelchair hire and short-term loans of equipment in almost 1000 outlets in the UK.

Disabled Living Foundation (DLF)

www.dlf.org.uk
Tel: 0845 130 9177
Textphone: 0207 432 8009
DLF gives impartial advice and information on all aspects of daily living equipment for children, including a UK-wide directory of suppliers. The DLF also has a self-assessment, rapid access (SARA) website at www.asksara.org.uk.

Fledglings

www.fledglings.org.uk
Helpline: 0845 458 1124
Fledglings is a national charity which aims to assist the parents and carers of children with disabilites by identifying, sourcing and supplying practical, affordable products to address everyday issues.

MedicAlert

www.medicalert.org.uk
Tel: 0800 581 420 within the UK or 1800 581420 from Ireland
MedicAlert is a charity providing an internationally recognized life-saving identification system for people with hidden medical conditions and allergies, supported by a 24-hour emergency telephone service (from within the London Ambulance Service).

Whizz-Kidz

www.whizz-kidz.org.uk
Tel: 0207 233 6600
Whizz-Kidz provides children and young people who have disabilities with mobility equipment, opportunities to meet and have fun, and training to help them gain skills.

Funding

The Family Fund

www.familyfund.org.uk
Tel: 08449 744 099
Textphone: 01904 658 085
E-mail: info@familyfund.org.uk
The Family Fund helps low income families across the UK who are raising a child or young person with additional complex needs or children and young people with a serious illness.

Families often apply for essential items such as washing machines, but the Fund will take into account requests for any item that will make a real difference to a child and their family, and have funded tennis coaching and holidays in the past.

Turn2Us

www.turn2us.org.uk
Tel: 0808 802 2000
Turn2Us provides a comprehensive online service to help find sources of financial support based on particular needs and circumstances. Its helpline provides free, confidential information given by trained professional advisers on welfare benefits entitlement and applying for grants.

Carers

Carers Trust

www.carers.org
Tel: 0844 800 4361
Carers Trust works to improve support, services and recognition for anyone living with the challenges of caring.

Carers UK

www.carersuk.org
Tel: 0808 808 7777
A UK-wide membership organization run by carers for carers, providing information and advice to all carers.

Crossroads Caring Scotland

www.crossroads-scotland.co.uk
Tel: 0141 226 3793
This organization provides short breaks and practical support for carers in Scotland regardless of the age, disability or illness of the person receiving care.

Education

Independent Parental Special Education Advice (IPSEA)

www.ipsea.org.uk
Advice line: 0800 018 4016
Tribunal helpline: 0845 602 9579
Office: 01799 582 030
IPSEA gives independent advice to parents who are uncertain about, or disagree with, their local educational authority's interpretation of their child's special educational needs.

National Parent Partnership Network (NPPN)

See Council for Disabled Children entry.

SEN National Advice Service

See Contact a Family entry.

Palliative care

Together for Short Lives

www.togetherforshortlives.org.uk
Tel: 0117 989 7820
Together for Short Lives is the new name for ACT & Children's Hospices UK, which merged on 1 October 2011. Its vision is for all children and young people unlikely to reach adulthood and their families to have the best possible care and support in the place of their choice. Together for Short Lives brings together all those involved in children's palliative care, from the children and families themselves to the professionals and organizations who provide the full range of care and support.

Make A Wish Foundation, UK

www.make-a-wish.org.uk
Tel: 01276 40 50 60
Charity granting the wishes of children and young people aged between 3 and 17 years living with life-threatening illnesses.

Bereavement

Child Bereavement Charity

www.childbereavement.org.uk
Tel: 01494 568900
This organization offers support to families and young people who have lost a child. There is a searchable database of support in your area on its website.

Child Death Helpline

www.childdeathhelpline.org.uk
Tel: 0800 282 986
The Child Death Helpline is for adults and young people affected by the death of a child whatever the time period since the death. The Child Death Helpline is staffed by bereaved parents. All volunteers are trained, supervised and supported by professionals within Great Ormond Street Hospital for Children NHS Trust and the Alder Hey Children's NHS Foundation Trust.

Cruse Bereavement Care

www.crusebereavementcare.org.uk
www.rd4u.org.uk (young person's website)
Helpline: 0844 477 9400
Young person's helpline: 0808 808 1677
Cruse Bereavement Care provides a free counselling service for bereaved families, including children and young people, over the telephone or through local offices providing one-to-one support or group work, plus forums for children/young people.

The Compassionate Friends

www.tcf.org.uk
Tel: 0845 123 2304 (NI 028 77 88 016)
This organization has local befrienders who listen to and support all bereaved parents and their immediate families, a helpline staffed by bereaved parents, forums, a website for siblings and a legal helpline.

Young carers

Sibs

www.sibs.org.uk
Tel: 01535 645 453
Sibs provides information and support for the siblings of children with disabilities and information on how their parents can support them. In addition, they provide information and advice for professionals supporting young carers.

Young Carers Net

www.youngcarers.net
c/o Princess Royal Trust for Carers (contact details above)
A website for siblings and young carers with discussion boards and chat rooms (moderated by adults who have been police checked), an 'agony aunt' page for young people's questions plus where to find local young carers' projects around the UK.

46

Legal frameworks for support

Christine Lenehan and Amanda Allard

> **Learning objective**
>
> - To know the legal framework underpinning the rights of children and young people with disabilities in the UK.

Over recent years, the rights and entitlements of children with disabilities and their families have increased. Families often still find many barriers to accessing those rights and entitlements (e.g. environmental and attitudinal) but it is important that those who work with children with disabilities and their families are at least aware of some of the key pieces of legislation and statutory guidance which confer entitlements. Some confer entitlements to education and to support services and others give rights of access.

Principal Acts and statutory guidance that confer service entitlement

- Children Act 1989
- Carers and Disabled Children Act 2000
- Framework for the Assessment of Children in Need and their Families 2000
- Education Act 1996
- Children Act 2004
- Children and Young Persons Act 2008

Principal Acts that give rights of access

- Chronically Sick and Disabled Persons Act 1970
- Equality Act 2010

Acts conferring entitlements

Children Act 1989

This was the starting point for provision of additional support to children with disabilities who were included in the definition of 'children in need'. Under Section 17, children with disabilities are eligible for support under the general duty to safeguard and promote the welfare of children in need through a wide range of services. The mechanism for determining a local authority's obligation to provide social care is via an assessment of need.

Education Act 1996

Whilst education is a fundamental right for all children, there are two primary law duties which guarantee the right to education for children with disabilities. The local authority is required to make a 'statement' following an assessment of the educational needs of children with substantial special educational needs. There follows an absolute duty on the local authority to arrange the provision identified in the statement. Section 19 of the Education Act 1996 requires local authorities to make arrangements for the provision of 'suitable' education at school or otherwise for children who may not for any period receive suitable education. The Act defines 'suitable' as being relevant to the child's age, ability and aptitude and to any special educational needs he or she may have. The government will be legislating to replace 'statements' with an Education, Health and Care Plan from 2014.

Carers and Disabled Children Act 2000

This Act concerns carers' assessments with a view to the provision of services for carers. Section 6(1) provides that a person with parental responsibility for a disabled child has the right to an assessment from the local authority of his or her ability to provide (and to continue to provide) care for the child. The local authority must take that assessment into account when deciding what services, if any, to provide under Section 17 of the Children Act 1989.

Framework for the Assessment of Children in Need and their Families 2000

The nature and extent of the duty to assess the needs of children with disabilities is set out in this statutory guidance. It gives an entitlement to either an initial or a core assessment, the latter being more likely required for children with complex needs or those requiring joint agency working and services from more than one agency.

Children Act 2004

This created a duty on education, health and social care to cooperate in order to promote children's well-being. This duty is essential for children with disabilities as they can only overcome the barriers if these agencies work together.

Children and Young Persons Act 2008

Enacted in April 2011, Section 25 places a legal duty on local authorities in England to provide short breaks. These must include overnight breaks as well as breaks during the day and evening. Families must be given a choice about the type of break and where it takes place, for example in the child's own home, in the community or in a residential setting.

Acts providing rights of access

Chronically Sick and Disabled Persons Act 1970

Section 2 imposes a specific duty to provide a wide range of services if the authority is satisfied that such a service is necessary in order to meet the needs of that disabled person (or child). It is open to the authority to decide if provision of a service is 'necessary' following an assessment. If the authority determines under this Act that a child needs support, then it must legally provide it. Local authorities that determine that support is not required may be challenged in the High Court on an application for judicial review on the basis that the assessment fails to comply with the Assessment Framework 2000.

Equality Act 2010

This created a new legal framework to help achieve equality for children with disabilities and others who have 'protected characteristics'. It replaced the former Disability Discrimination Acts and sets out the types of disability discrimination which may result in 'prohibited conduct'. It covers education and service providers, requiring them to make necessary physical and practical adjustments and to provide auxiliary aids and information in accessible formats. Duties under the Act are anticipatory, continuing and evolving.

Gillick and Fraser competence

In addition to an understanding of entitlements and right of access, anyone working with children with disabilities needs to have an understanding of the Gillick/Fraser competence used in medical law to decide whether a child (16 years or younger) is able to consent to his or her own medical treatment, without the need for parental permission or knowledge. It is important to note that, although Gillick competent children can consent to treatment, any refusal can be overridden.

Although raised initially in the context of contraceptive advice, the Gillick ruling is now an accepted concept in all areas of medical treatment. The Fraser ruling is confined to contraceptive advice and other areas of reproductive health. The age guidelines on when a child is 'Gillick/Fraser competent' are not always appropriate for children with disabilities who have cognitive impairments and learning disability. However, it should never be automatically assumed that such children cannot give informed consent, and health professionals need to work to the Department of Health guidance on whether the child or young person can give consent based on their ability to

- comprehend and retain information material to the decision
- understand the consequences of having or not having the intervention in question
- use and weigh up the information in the decision-making process
- make a voluntary uncoerced decision that remains reasonably consistent.

It is therefore important to give information at a level and in words that the person with a disability can understand, before assuming that he or she cannot give consent.

Further reading

Author (2012) *Support and Aspiration: A New Approach to Special Educational Needs and Disability – Progress and Next Steps*. London: Department for Education.

Broach S (2011) *Cemented to the Floor by law: Respecting Legal Duties in a Time of Cuts*. Available at: www.councilfordisabledchildren.org.uk/resources/our-partners-resources/cemented-to-the-floor-by-law (accessed 24 November 2012).

Broach S, Clements L, Read J (2010) *Disabled Children: A Legal Handbook*. Available at: http://www.lag.org.uk/or to download at www.councilfordisabledchildren.org.uk/resources/cdcs-resources/disabled-children-a-legal-handbook (accessed 24 November 2012).

Department of Health (2001) *Seeking Consent: Working with Children*. Available at: http://www.dh.gov.uk/en/Publicationsandstatistics/Publications/PublicationsPolicyAndGuidance/DH_4007005 (accessed 5 November 2012).

Read J, Clements L, Ruebain D (2006) *Disabled Children and the Law: Research and Good Practice*, 2nd edition. London: Jessica Kingsley Publishers.

47
Education

Gail Treml

Learning objectives

- To understand the general organization of education within the UK.
- To understand the current national curricula assessment regimes.
- To know about the range of special educational needs (SEN) provision and personnel.
- To understand and know what should be included in medical advice to education.

UK education systems

Ninety-three per cent of pupils in the UK attend publicly funded state schools. By law, all children in England and Wales between the ages of 5 and 16 **must** receive a full-time education. In England the compulsory school age will rise to 18, effective in 2013 for 17-year-olds and in 2015 for 18-year-olds. In Northern Ireland, children begin school at the age of 4 years, whilst in Scotland children start school between the ages of 4½ years and 5½ years.

Publicly funded nurseries and preschools are available for a limited number of hours each week for children under the age of 5 years (12.5h/wk is currently funded by the government for preschool children, from the term after the child's third birthday). After the age of 16, students can attend sixth-form colleges or other further education institutions or remain at school.

Curriculum

All of the countries within the UK have national curricula encompassing preschool learning and education up to age 16 years. State schools **must** follow the national curriculum; however, independent schools, including academies and free schools, are not so obliged. The Scottish secondary curriculum has greater breadth across a range of subjects, whereas the English, Welsh and Northern Irish systems provide a greater depth over a smaller range of subjects. Significant numbers of Welsh students are educated either wholly or largely through the medium of Welsh, with lessons in Welsh compulsory for all until age 16. The Northern Irish curriculum includes the Irish language in Irish-speaking schools.

Progress and achievement

Progress and attainment is formally assessed in all four countries within the UK at Key Stages 1, 2 and 3 corresponding to ages 7, 11 and 14 years using SATS tests (standard attainment tests), with each level being subdivided into a, b or c, with c being the highest. By the end of Key Stage 1, most English 7-year-olds are expected to achieve level 2 in maths, English and science. By age 11, most are expected to achieve level 4, and by the end of Key Stage 3, at age 14, most children should achieve level 5. Many children assessed as performing at level 3 can cope with the secondary curriculum, albeit with additional support. Young people with a reading age of 9½ years can access GCSE examinations and attain low grades.

In England and Wales school-age children with severe or complex cognitive difficulties performing well below national expectations are assessed on 'P' (Pivat) scales. These subscales are a set of descriptions recording the achievement of pupils with SEN who are working towards level 1 of the national curriculum. The P-scales, just like national curriculum levels, are split into eight levels with P1 being the lowest and P8 the highest. Levels P1 to P3 are not subject specific, describing early learning and conceptual development.

The English national curriculum review is considering subjects to be taught and content, assessment, tests and national curriculum levels. Implementation is scheduled for 2013.

Special educational needs and legislation

The UK supports the UNESCO Salamanca Statement (1994) adopting the principle of inclusive education, enrolling all children in regular schools, unless there are compelling reasons for doing otherwise. Most children's SEN are met in ordinary (mainstream) school, sometimes with the help of outside specialists or additional support. Local authorities aim for a flexible range of provision able to meet the SEN of individual children.

The law relating to SEN is mainly in Part IV of the Education Act (1996) and accompanying regulations. Section 312 defines children with SEN as 'those having a learning difficulty [the definition of which includes having a disability] which calls for special educational provision'.

A 'learning difficulty' is defined as arising if a child

- has a significantly greater difficulty in learning than the majority of children in the same age group
- has a disability which either prevents or hinders him/her from making use of educational facilities of a kind generally provided for children of the same age group in schools within the area of the local authority[1]
- is under the age of 5 years and is, or would be, if special educational provision was not made, likely to fall within the above categories, when above that age.

But a child

• does not have a learning difficulty simply because English/Welsh is not his/her first language.

The legal definition of disability is *not* the same as that for SEN. The Disability Discrimination Act (DDA 1995), now subsumed into the Equality Act 2010, defines disability as 'a person with a physical or mental impairment which has a substantial long-term adverse effect on their ability to carry out normal day-to-day activities'.

It is therefore possible to be disabled and not have SEN, and vice versa. It is also possible both to be disabled and to have SEN. A medical diagnosis may mean that a child is disabled but that does not necessarily imply SEN. A child's educational needs rather than a medical diagnosis or disability **must** be considered when assessing educational support required in the classroom.

The English SEN Code of Practice (DfE 2001), the SEN Code of Practice for Wales (NAW 2004) and the Code of Practice on the Identification and Assessment of Special Educational Needs (DENI 1996) are similar as they are based on the same legislation. However, they also reflect the slightly different education systems and practice of each country. The UK government has announced legislation that proposes changes to the English SEN system, which will not come into force until 2014.

The above codes of practice provide guidance on how preschool provision, schools, learning authorities, health and social care **must** comply with the law. All professionals and every statutory body **must** have regard to the code; they cannot ignore it. If they depart from it, they **must** have good reason for doing so and be able to demonstrate that their actions are in the best interests of children and young people with SEN.

The codes promote a graded approach to identifying, assessing and providing for SEN. This approach is designed to help children with SEN make adequate progress and access the curriculum. The majority will have their needs met within local mainstream schools at *School Action* or *School Action Plus* (England and Wales) or Stages 1, 2 or 3 (Northern Ireland). *School Action Plus* and Stage 3 occur when education support services or health or social work professionals are asked for advice.

Advice from an educational psychologist, an advisory teacher specializing in a particular area of SEN or a health therapist, or a medical diagnosis and report, could all give ideas as to how to work differently with the child in class. Information on a child's home circumstances might explain changes in a child's behaviour and attitudes to learning that help teachers understand and resolve the situation.

Statutory assessment

Where a child's SEN are such that they cannot be met by a preschool or school from its own resources, a multidisciplinary assessment is indicated. There are detailed statutory requirements covering the decision on whether such an assessment is necessary and the assessment arrangements that may lead to a statement.

Statutory assessment always requires advice from representatives from health, education, social care and from parents. There is a statutory timetable and deadlines for assessment, drafting and finalizing of a *Statement of SEN*. Once a formal request for advice is received, health professionals have a 6-week time limit in which to respond. Health services should have local protocols for ensuring that all relevant health professionals are aware of the request and respond appropriately.

Statements of special educational needs

Statements of SEN are legal documents and are necessary when children have SEN which require educational provision that is additional to or different from that ordinarily available in local mainstream state schools (SEN provision). Statements **must** set out all of the child's SEN and specify all the additional or different provision required. The latest English statistics show that 17.9% of pupils had identified SEN but no statement and 2.7% had statements of SEN (DfE 2011). The majority of children with statements continue to be included in mainstream schools, but some children require SEN specialist provision, which takes a variety of forms, including resourced provision or special units within mainstream schools or, alternatively, special schools.

The Education (Additional Support for Learning) (Scotland) Act 2004 introduced a wider concept of additional support needs to replace the previous SEN system. Additional support needs can arise from any factor which causes a barrier to learning, whether that factor relates to social, emotional, cognitive, linguistic, disability, or family and care circumstances. Supporting Children's Learning: Code of Practice (The Scottish Government 2005) provides statutory guidance.

Coordinated support plans are legal documents for children with additional support needs:

- arising from complex or multiple factors
- requiring a range of support from different services and enduring for 1 year or more
- under the age of 3 years, if the child has additional support needs because of a disability and has been referred by an NHS board.

Health input is required only if requested because a child faces barriers to learning and development caused by health or a disability.

Medical advice

Young children with substantial disabilities are likely to be known to local health and education services before they begin school, and they may have a statement of SEN. However, most children with SEN are first identified after starting school. Schools need to know whether health factors contribute to a child's educational difficulties. Such factors may lead to SEN if they hinder a child in learning or accessing the curriculum.

Some children enter school with previously unidentified mild to moderate health problems such as fluctuating hearing loss, mild speech and language difficulties or developmental coordination disorders which require assessment and input from health professionals but no statement of SEN.

For statutory assessment, the designated medical officer for SEN or an appropriately trained community paediatrician should collect and coordinate the advice from all the relevant health professionals and submit this in a report. The advice may rarely include a report from the child's general practitioner or, more commonly, from the community paediatrician (who will specifically see the child for the purpose of providing this advice), community nurses, therapists, child and adolescent mental health service workers or, when required, from other specialists such as paediatric neurologists, child psychiatrists and psychologists. Parents can submit reports from non-NHS practitioners. The local authority **must** consider such reports in parallel with the advice from NHS professionals.

Writing a good medical report or statement

Medical reports should

- be written in straightforward language, avoiding the use of jargon so as to be clearly understood by parents and other professionals
- where possible use layman's language or explain any specific medical terms that are used
- be supported by clear evidence of all views expressed or comments made
- provide a clear indication of all sources of information used
- avoid subjective descriptions or judgements.

Regulations require that advice **must**

- relate to the educational, medical, psychological or other features that appear relevant to a child's current and future *educational* needs;
- set out how those features *could* affect the child's *educational* needs and the provision that advisers consider is appropriate in the light of those features.

However, advice **must not** be influenced by consideration of the name of a school at which the child might eventually be placed and specific schools **must not** be suggested. The local authority decides placement in the light of preferences or representations made by the parents. Professionals may discuss the child's needs and options *in general* with parents, although discussions and advice **must not** commit the local authority nor pre-empt the parents' preferences. These are matters for the local authority to determine on the basis of its consideration of all the advice received.

Written advice may involve consideration of the following:

- the scope for mainstream education
- the type of school in which the child's needs might best be met – mainstream, special or residential. In practice such directive advice is rarely written by paediatricians: decisions around types of provision are left for discussion between parents and educational staff.

Medical advice should

- include views about any known educational needs which health advisers feel the child may have
- indicate the type of medical or therapeutic support required, derived from the advice of the relevant therapists, which *might* be necessary to overcome or ameliorate the child's difficulties

- indicate clearly the aims and objectives of any future health care provision which needs to be provided or specially commissioned
- if there are no medical factors that appear to affect a child's performance at school, this should be stated in the advice.

Medical advice may include information on

- physical and mental health problems and/or developmental conditions and how they are likely to affect a child's learning ability
- recent reports on hearing and vision
- management of a health condition, especially any health and safety issues (e.g. management of seizures in the classroom, treatment of hypoglycaemic episodes)
- treatment that has or is likely to affect the child's learning ability
- the speech and language, occupational therapy and physiotherapy programmes required.

Advice should set out the likely impact on the child's education of the medical or developmental condition and/or its treatment, including

- managing the condition in the school context
- managing any emotional and behavioural difficulties
- any special aids, equipment or access requirements
- health and safety matters, for example the need for additional supervision during potentially hazardous activities
- the length of time special provision is likely to be necessary where medical problems are considered short term, together with information on how the condition will be monitored
- any non-educational provision such as therapy services and the mechanism for commissioning provision.

Whenever possible, medical and health advice should be discussed with parents prior to submission. Advice should never include issues that have not previously been raised.

Annual reviews

All statements **must** be reviewed annually so as to consider the child's progress over the previous 12 months and whether any amendments need to be made to the description of the child's needs or the SEN provision specified in the statement. It is a way of monitoring and evaluating the continued effectiveness and appropriateness of the statement. It is unlikely that all relevant health professionals will be able to attend all review meetings. If necessary, a written report should be provided instead.

Transition planning

Year 9 annual reviews are particularly important in preparing for moving young people to further education and adult life. All the agencies that may play a major role in a young person's life post school should be involved. For young people with specific disabilities or medical conditions, health services will be of particular importance. The aim of the annual review in Year 9 and subsequent years is to

- review the young person's statement of SEN
- draw up and subsequently review the Transition Plan.

The Transition Plan

The aim of a Transition Plan is to plan coherently for the young person's transition to adult life; it is not just about post-school arrangements (see Chapter 48). It should also consider ongoing school provision. The head teacher must make sure that the Transition Plan is completed after the Year 9 review meeting.

Health professionals involved in the management and care of the young person should provide written advice for Transition Plans. They should provide advice on the services likely to be required and discuss arrangements for transfer to adult healthcare services with the young person, their parents and their general practitioner. They should facilitate any referrals and transfers of records that may be necessary.

Working with education staff

Medical staff will work with a number of education colleagues in supporting children with SEN including the following:

- The SEN coordinator (SENCO): a key professional in all mainstream schools and early years settings. It is mandatory that a school SENCO is a qualified teacher. The SENCO is responsible for coordinating SEN provision including liaison with outside professionals. Some schools choose to designate the SENCO as an Inclusion Manager. Such teachers may have wider responsibilities.
- Educational psychologists work closely with SENCOs and special school staff. They can provide diagnostic and psycho-educational assessments and psychological counselling. They also advise education staff on appropriate teaching techniques, strategies and approaches in relation to individual children with SEN.
- Advisory and support teachers usually specialize in an area of SEN. They may advise on specific equipment, teaching strategies and approaches or work directly with individual children. Local authorities often provide behaviour, learning, autism spectrum disorder and sensory services.
- Portage workers provide planned, home-based educational support for preschool children with SEN. Local authorities usually provide portage services.

Key messages

- Just over 20% of children have some learning difficulty that calls for some special educational provision, but for the vast majority of children their needs can be met from within the resources available in the mainstream classroom.
- 2.7% of children currently have statements of SEN, which is a legal document that sets out the child's educational needs and the resources required including therapy, nursing or specialist teaching to meet these needs.
- Medical advice for statements of SEN should be written in a straightforward language that avoids jargon and clearly sets out the child's health needs, how these impact on learning and the resources needed as regards to the therapy required. Specific statements about types of provision or particular schools should be avoided.

Note

1. 'Local authority' refers to local authorities in England, Scotland and Wales and Education and library boards in Northern Ireland.

References

DDA (1995) *The Disability Discrimination Act 1995*. London: The National Archive. Available at: http://www.legislation.gov.uk/ukpga/1995/50/contents (accessed 10 January 2013).

DENI (Department of Education Northern Ireland) (1996) *Code of Practice on the Identification and Assessment of Special Educational Needs*. Department for Education Northern Ireland. Available at: http://www.deni.gov.uk/the_code_of_practice.pdf (accessed 10 January 2013).

DfE (Department for Education) (2001) *The English Special Educational Needs Code of Practice*. Available at: https://www.education.gov.uk/publications/eOrderingDownload/DfES-0558-2001-2.pdf (accessed 26 November 2012).

DfE (2011) *Statistical First Release. Special Educational Needs in England, January 2011*. Available at: http://www.education.gov.uk/rsgateway/DB/SFR/s001007/sfr14-2011v2.pdf (accessed 26 November 2012).

Eduation Act (1996) *The Eduation Act 1996*. London: The National Archive. Available at: www.legislation.gov.uk/ukpga/1996/56/contents (accessed 10 January 2013).

NAW (National Assemble for Wales) (2004) *Special Educational Needs Code of Practice for Wales*. Llywodraeth Cynullaid Cymru, Welsh Assembly Government. Available online at: http://wales.gov.uk/docs/dcells/publications/120705sencodeofpracticeen.pdf (accessed 10 January 2013).

The Scottish Government (2005) *Supporting Children's Learning: Code of Practice*. Statutory guidance relating to the Education (Additional Support for Learning) (Scotland) Act 2004. Available at: http://www.scotland.gov.uk/Publications/2005/08/15105817/58187 (accessed 26 November 2012).

48
Transition planning: a health perspective

Shiela Puri

Transition is typically defined as 'the purposeful, planned movement of adolescents and young adults with chronic physical and medical conditions from child-centred to adult-oriented health care systems' (Blum et al. 1993: 570). However, it is important to consider the various different phases of transition in a child's and young person's life (Table 48.1) including the transition from good health to ill health and vice versa.

Table 48.1 Phases of transition in a child's life

Transition stage	Health team transition	Educational provision transition	Social support access
Infancy to toddler	Hospital-based services → child development teams and GP	Early years education support services, e.g. portage, children's centres, teachers for the hearing/visually impaired	Outreach/specialist nurses Early support pack DLA often best applied for after age 3–6mo unless care needs much more than expected Family fund
	Age at handover varies in different districts	Discuss referral to education authorities at 12–24mo	
Toddler to childhood	Child development teams (if only for under 5y) ↓ Community-based children's services (usually transition occurs once the child is in a school setting)	Preschool education ↓ Primary school Discuss transition at 30–40mo	At age 2y, if oxygen dependent, can apply for disability parking badge At 3y mobility allowance and free nappies Consider short breaks, referral to social care Convene CAF Housing adaptations

Table 48.1 (Continued)

Transition stage	Health team transition	Educational provision transition	Social support access
Childhood to adolescence	Period of continuity within health; therapy teams may change with change of school Introduce concept of independence and responsibility to self-medicate where appropriate	Primary school ↓ Secondary school Discuss transitions from Year 4 (aged 9y) onwards	Respite care Holiday play schemes Consider short breaks and referral to social care Consider CAF
Adolescence to adulthood Parental care ↓ Assisted living/ independent care	Children's services ↓ adult specialist clinics for defined conditions, e.g. epilepsy specialist Learning disability teams, young adult rehabilitation teams Identify specific health needs and refer to appropriate professional Involve GP Ideally, joint appointments between services and overlap care for a year	Secondary school ↓ Sixth form Further education ↓ Employment Discuss transitions from Year 8; even if in specialist setting Education centred Transitions Review in Year 9 is the responsibility of the head teacher	Involve social care at the time of transition planning Inform families to reapply for DLA before 16th birthday Mental Capacity Act becomes relevant at age 16y. Consider referring to independent mental capacity advocate Aged 17 transition from children's social services to adult social services Consider housing/ assisted living/care arrangements Consider equipment needs, adaptations and environmental control

GP, general practitioner; DLA, Disability Living Allowance; CAF, Common Assessment Framework.

Generally, children receive good care from the local child development services and early years services during the preschool years. The quality of care is usually more variable once the child is at school, but there is access to therapy, specialist services, education, social care and voluntary services, with the community paediatrician keeping an overview and cocoordinating medical care. In the UK, a national initiative, the Common Assessment Framework (CAF), is an attempt to coordinate multiagency care throughout the childhood years (see Chapter 46). Young people with disabilities have a wide variety of needs, and often their medical need comes bottom of the list of priorities for them or their family. However, some young people do have significant ongoing medical needs with multiple problems continuing into adulthood requiring multiple specialists, but it is difficult to find adult consultants or general practitioners (GPs) who feel equipped to take on the role of coordinating the young person's care.

Case vignette

Tom is a 16-year-old young man who has total body cerebral palsy with normal cognition, hearing and vision. Tom is in a wheelchair and attends mainstream school. He uses a communication aid with the help of a forehead laser pointer. Tom would like to go to university to study philosophy and history. Ultimately, he would like to be a teacher and live independently.

Tom is having a carefully planned transition to adult services in which he is an equal partner. He has identified the following critical factors which will make his transition plans successful.

These include

- being treated as an individual;
- good interagency information and liaison;
- keyworker support but not dependency;
- coordinated appointments with minimum disruption to education;
- support for independent living and leisure;
- financial support for equipment and university fees;
- support for access to a university of his choice;
- flexible training and employment as a teacher.

Key issues

During the transition to adult services the common problems young people experience with the UK system are

- no equivalent post in adult services to a community paediatrician, who coordinates health-related care for the young person and family and acts as the 'lead professional';
- lack of knowledge/information among children's services staff about adult services;
- poor coordination and poor information exchange between agencies;
- a higher threshold to access services and support in adult services;
- they are treated differently in adult services – different teams have different approaches;
- they are encouraged to be independent – can may come as a shock to some young people;
- services are not specific for young adults; they are for anyone over the age of 18 years.

Families often find each transition phase to be fraught with anxieties; this is perhaps related to a fear of change and the unknown. The paediatrician and GP are often the only professionals that remain constant throughout the child's life until transfer to adult services. The paediatrician is frequently expected to take on the role of the navigator and facilitator through the various phases of transition, anticipating the challenges and signposting as appropriate. It is important to involve the GP wherever possible, as he or she remains the primary care provider for the young person as he or she moves into adulthood. The transition planning needs to be person specific to the needs of the young person concerned, giving the individual choice and control where possible. In addition to the young person's needs, the needs of the family as a whole must be considered

With improving health care the life expectancy of young people with disabilities has increased considerably; for example, the average lifespan of a person with Down syndrome currently is around 47 years, and for young people with Duchenne muscular dystrophy life expectancy is around 25 years. Technology-dependent children (e.g. tracheostomy- and ventilator-dependent children) are also starting to survive to adulthood. Disabled people, even those with severe multiple problems, often live to the age of 60 years or more. Many women now have their children in their thirties or even forties. Put those two facts together and we have the prospect of parents in their eighties still looking after their disabled offspring. Families often report that once they leave the paediatric services they experience a void in provision. This may partly be attributed to the fact that in current paediatric practice we often work within a medical model and foster a dependency between the parent/carer and the healthcare professional, whereas in young adulthood the emphasis of care needs shifts to one of promoting independence and taking responsibility for one's own health. Although there are some superb examples of disabled young adults living in the community with appropriate support, it is still often unavoidable that parents continue to care for their offspring. An additional issue facing young people with disabilities is a reduction in their package of care with relocation. They may have a good package of support in one area but when moving to another town they often have to renegotiate it and may not get the same deal.

The transition process needs to be a continuous process and not a single specific event for the professional delivering the care and the recipient. A distinction needs to be made between the physical transfer of care to adult services and a well-planned process of transition from childhood to adulthood. In most instances the planned transition to adult services starts at age 14 years (Year 9). Young people and families particularly value having one main person with the right skills and knowledge of children's and adult services who can guide them through the complex transition process.

The importance of transition planning is being increasingly recognized in children affected by a range of disabilities. Research shows that a young person with four-limb cerebral palsy and learning difficulty can lose health rapidly after leaving paediatric services. The cause of this decline is multifactorial and includes the lack of an adult equivalent of a community paediatrician, and often of dedicated health or care provision, and loss of motivation for self-care. However, a number of examples of good practice care models are emerging, particularly for well-defined specific conditions (e.g. young people with physical disabilities and epilepsy). We still have a long way to go before achieving optimal planned transition arrangements with transfer of care to interested colleagues in adult medicine.

Transition 'health plan' checklist

A transition health plan should be used by the young person and health professional together to identify the strengths and specific person-centred needs. The plan should cover

- physical health and well-being (e.g. nutrition, vision, hearing, dental care, pain, etc.)
- physical fitness and coordination (e.g. mobility and postural management)
- neurological status and resulting needs: anticipate needs based on prognosis
- cognitive development and any resultant needs
- communication ability and any resultant needs
- medical management, including medication
- personal care (e.g. personal hygiene, continence, sexual health, health promotion)
- mental health and psychosocial well-being and support, and social skills
- learning, education, pre-vocation and vocational needs
- independence needs (e.g. equipment, environmental adaptations and housing)
- need for specialist carers or any other support
- community participation and independent/supported living arrangements
- leisure needs
- finance arrangements, benefits
- peer support, advocacy needs
- links with other agencies
- information sources

Key messages

- Transition planning is a process and not a single event.
- It should begin long before the actual transfer of care.
- Transition should be purposeful and planned.
- Transition planning involves identifying met and unmet needs.
- Transition planning should be holistic, person centred and needs specific for the young person and family.

Reference

Blum RW, Garell D, Hodgman CH, et al. (1993) Transition from child-centred to adult health-care systems for adolescents with chronic conditions: a position paper for the Society of Adolescent Medicine. *J Adolesc Health* 14: 570–6. http://dx.doi.org/10.1016/1054-139X(93)90143-D

Further reading

Department of Health (2008) *Transitions 'Moving on Well'*. Available at: http://www.dh.gov.uk/en/Publicationsandstatistics/Publications/PublicationsPolicyAndGuidance/DH_083592 (accessed 5 November 2012).

Leeds and York Partnership NHS Foundation Trust (2010) *Traffic Light Hospital Assessment Booklet*. Available at: http://www.leedsmentalhealth.nhs.uk/_documentbank/Traffic_Light_Hospital_Assessment_Including_Discharge__Information_June_2010.pdf?phpMyAdmin=M3W4e1cy%2CYXWyzbOphZOEV my5x3 (accessed 5 November 2012). [A booklet for people with learning difficulties to define their needs during a hospital admission.]

O'Brien R, Rosenbloom L (2009) *Developmental Disability and Ageing*. London: Mac Keith Press.

Websites

Contact a Family (a factsheet about transition for families with disabled young people): www.cafamily.org.uk/media/379939/transitioncurrentlastupdatedfeb2012_final_for_web.pdf (accessed 24 November 2012).

Foundation for People with Learning Disabilities: www.learningdisabilities.org.uk

Transitions Information Network: www.transitioninfonetwork.org.uk

49
Advocacy

Arnab Seal

Learning objective

- To understand the role of advocacy and the importance of speaking up on behalf of children with disabilities and their families.

Advocacy is the act of pleading or arguing and/or offering active support in favour of a cause, idea, or policy. For professionals working with children and young people with disabilities, it is about speaking on their behalf and helping them take part in decisions that affect their lives. Often children are 'invisible' to decision makers. Children and young people with disabilities are even more likely to be spoken down to ('Does he take sugar?' syndrome) because of their perceived disability. Advocacy involves making sure that the rights of children and young people with disabilities are considered, and their views heard, even if this does not lead to their wishes being met by decision makers. Paediatricians and other professionals working with children have a major role in advocacy and raising the profile of issues pertaining to individual children or, where necessary, regarding services for all children with disabilities at a local or national level.

The following case vignette shows how professionals can be advocates and make a difference.

Case vignette

Ralph is a child with Down syndrome who has an inoperable complex cyanotic congenital heart disease. He has had a temporizing operation but his only hope is a heart transplant. Ralph has moderate developmental delay and poor growth. Ralph's parents are keen for him to have the heart transplant but the transplant unit is unsure whether it is appropriate.

Learning points

The ethical issue regarding Ralph's transplantation is whether individuals with disabilities should have equal access to organ transplants. In this instance the availability of organs and the costs of transplant are being weighed up against the (perceived) quality of life and the demands of complying with treatment after heart transplantation. The role of Ralph's paediatrician (often a community paediatrician) is to ensure that the decision taken is in Ralph's best interests and hopefully that the decision fits in with his parents' wishes too. This can be achieved by his parents having an open discussion with the cardiologist regarding what is involved, quality of life issues, and ascertaining their wishes. The relevant teams should be involved in the discussion to aid the decision-making process (see Chapter 39 on ethics regarding beneficence vs. maleficence).

The basic issue of rationing of health care owing to rising costs and falling budgets is likely to increase in the future. It will be important for paediatricians to remain vigilant in this area to ensure that children and young people with disabilities are not being unfairly treated when such decisions are being made. Paediatricians should remain advocates to ensure that the needs and wishes of the child and family are fully considered.

Similar arguments concerning the rights of disabled individuals apply to their access to the intensive care unit, invasive care and specialist services/treatments. Cost implications and quality of life considerations can also affect decisions involving educational support, reproductive rights (e.g. contraception for learning-disabled people), independence (e.g. home adaptations) and issues promoting equal opportunities. In all these situations a balanced and well-informed paediatrician can advocate to achieve the best decisions for the child and the family.

On a broader community scale, the commissioning of services available to children and young people with disabilities, earmarking and ring fencing of funding/resources and legislating to ensure equal opportunities and rights of children and young people with disabilities are all areas where one can be an effective advocate and make a difference. Professional organizations of paediatricians, such as the British Academy of Childhood Disability (BACD) and the Royal College of Paediatrics and Child Health (RCPCH), and a number of other organizations such as The Children's Society, already play a significant role in lobbying decision makers in government and local authorities/organizations (e.g. commissioning groups) regarding key issues affecting children and young people with disabilities.

Key messages

- Advocacy for children and young people with disabilities can improve the life of the child and that of their family.
- Advocacy can enable children and young people with disabilities to have their views heard and to contribute to a complex decision-making process.
- Advocacy can be effective for a range of issues from those pertaining to the individual child to issues affecting the wider population of disabled people (e.g. legislation and government policy affecting children and young people with disabilities).
- There is a need to increase the awareness of the availability of specialist advocacy provision for children and young people with disabilities.
- Professionals working with children with complex health needs such as paediatricians are well placed to act as advocates for children to protect their rights, engage in ethical discussions on their behalf and to ensure they are afforded equal opportunities.

Further reading

Franklin A, Knight, A (The Children's Society) (2011) *Someone on Our Side: Advocacy for Disabled Children and Young People*. Available at: http://www.childrenssociety.org.uk/sites/default/files/tcs/someone_on_our_side_summary.pdf (accessed 5 November 2012).

Section 14

Caring for a child with a disability

50
Feeding problems and growth failure

Anne M Kelly and Helen Harrison

Feeding and growth problems are common in children with neurological impairment because of oral motor impairment and swallowing dysfunction.

Case vignette 1

Helena is 15 months old. She has Turner syndrome and four-limb spastic cerebral palsy. Her birthweight was only 1.33kg at 33 weeks' gestation because of intrauterine growth restriction. She has continued to grow well below the 0.4th centile.

She has feeding difficulties and has been unable to tolerate her milk feeds. She vomits at variable times after feeding. A barium swallow showed severe gastro-oesophaegal reflux (GOR) up to the level of the proximal oesophagus. Helena has oromotor dysfunction with tongue thrusting and difficulty sucking.

The multidisciplinary team of paediatrician, specialist speech and language therapist, paediatric dietitian and community nurse are involved. Feeds were reduced in volume, thickened and a prokinetic agent started (erythromycin) together with an H2 receptor antagonist (ranitidine). Helena continued to vomit, but less frequently than before. She failed, however, to gain weight. She then had a period of nasogastric (NG) feeding but her weight gain still did not improve. She was referred for a percutaneous endoscopic gastrostomy (PEG). A PEG combined with laparoscopic fundoplication was done in view of her severe GOR. Weight gain and linear growth improved post surgery.

Learning points

- NG feeding is only offered as a temporary measure because of the risks associated with NG feeding and its potential for interfering with the establishment of oral feeding.
- A team approach is important in managing children with complex feeding problems.
- Liaison with a paediatric surgeon is important when deciding if a PEG is indicated.

Case vignette 2

Ella is 2 years old. She has four-limb spastic cerebral palsy (CP), GMFCS level IV, secondary to non-accidental brain injury aged 6 weeks. She has epilepsy with frequent seizures and has feeding difficulties. Ella could not tolerate her oral anticonvulsant medication and her weight gain has been poor. She had episodes of distress due to GOR, which were treated with omeprazole. A PEG was inserted but Ella continued to experience episodes of arching and crying. It was unclear whether these episodes were caused by GOR or epileptic seizures, but it was thought that reflux was the more likely cause. EEG was always abnormal. Ella underwent a laparoscopic fundoplication, which she tolerated well. Post surgery the abnormal movements decreased in frequency and virtually ceased. Ella's weight gain improved and her carers were more able to manage her needs.

Background knowledge

The Oxford Feeding Study (Sullivan et al. 2000) demonstrated that feeding problems are common in children with neurological impairment. Based on parental reports, of the 440 children in the study

- 89% of children required help feeding
- 56% choked on eating
- One-third had prolonged feeding times (>3h/d)
- One-third were underweight but more than two-thirds had never had a nutritional assessment;
- Gastrointestinal problems were common:
  - constipation occurred in 59%
  - vomiting in 22%
- 31% of children had had a chest infection in the previous 6 months.

Most (93%) of the children in this study were diagnosed with CP. Almost half were unable to walk, 75% had speech difficulty and more than 25% drooled saliva constantly.

Up to one-third of children with disabilities are significantly undernourished. Feeding impairment is correlated with the severity of the motor deficit. Children with extensive bilateral signs (GMFCS levels IV and V) are more likely to have feeding and articulation problems than those with unilateral involvement. Clues that a child is likely to have oromotor dysfunction can be observed in clinic (Table 50.1). Growth failure is more likely to occur in children with severe disabilities, but effects on growth can still be seen in children with milder mobility deficits. Height, muscle mass, fat stores and bone density are all reduced compared with the same measurements in able-bodied peers. Overall linear growth is reduced, with lower limbs being more affected than upper limbs in children with CP. Mobility and weightbearing are important factors in stimulating growth, and reduced mobility further contributes to this process.

Growth failure occurs mainly because of inadequate food intake resulting from impaired self-feeding and oromotor dysfunction. In addition, poor nutrition leads to other difficulties, as outlined in Table 50.2.

Table 50.1 Typical features of oromotor dysfunction

Poor lip closure
Excessive drooling
Lip retraction
Involuntary biting
Inability to move the tongue laterally and tongue thrusting
Swallowing is uncoordinated and leads to choking and coughing during feeds

Affected children eat slowly and spill more than half of the food that is offered to them. Mothers spend on average 3.5 hours per day feeding their child who has a disability, compared with 0.8 hours for able siblings (Sullivan et al. 2000). Despite these long feed times, children may remain undernourished.

Table 50.2 Effects of undernutrition in children with disabilities

Linear growth failure
Decreased muscle strength, reduced cough reflex, increased risk of aspiration
Decreased cerebral function leading to irritability, reduced motivation and reduced energy to play and learn
Decreased circulation in limbs, causing cold mottled peripheries
Disturbed immune system, risk of infection particularly in chest and urinary tract

Growth failure was, until fairly recently, accepted as an inevitable and irremediable consequence of CP. This belief is no longer acceptable as simple measures such as increasing the calorie density of foods can improve weight gain and function in children with CP. The earlier nutritional management is instituted, the easier it is to reverse nutritional deficits.

How to assess feeding difficulties and growth failure

Establish the current concerns

• Consider current and previous growth measurements.
• Plot the weight and height of the child. Height measurements may be difficult to record accurately depending on the degree of physical disability. Ideally, other measurements such as mid-upper arm circumference or triceps skinfold thickness should be recorded to provide information about body fat stores. There are centiles available for these. Sitting height may also be possible.
• If heights and weights are available, are the centiles fairly closely matched?
• View measurements taken over a period of time. Have measurements tracked the curve of a centile even though it may be only the 0.4th centile? If not, when did growth faltering occur?
• Consider the birth centile: was intrauterine growth restriction present at birth?
• Consider genetic potential too: are parents and other family members small?
• Body mass index (BMI) measurements in children with neurological impairment who have poor weight gain are not helpful but are helpful when they are overweight.

- Measurements are usually plotted on standard centile growth charts (Child Growth Foundation, www.childgrowthfoundation.org) but there are growth charts available which are specific for children with motor impairment secondary to CP. A measurement on the 50th centile on the latter chart plots below the 10th centile on a standard growth chart. These charts are not widely used. Some clinicians believe that using these charts for this group may underplay the degree of undernutrition, and they continue to use standard growth charts.

Feeding history

Gather enough information to build a picture of how the child is fed, how long it takes, what the child is offered and how much is actually consumed. Bear in mind that feeding histories are notoriously inaccurate and carers often overestimate intake.

- Is the child able to indicate when he or she is hungry or thirsty?
- Is the child self-fed or fed by a carer?
- Where is the child fed? On his or her carer's lap/high chair/wheelchair?
- What is offered to the child and how much is taken? Obtain daily fluid volume and quantity of solids (e.g. as teaspoons of solids).
- Which textures are tolerated – smooth or lumpy puree/mashed/chopped up?
- Are there any problems with sucking, swallowing or chewing ability?
- Does the child vomit or are there signs of discomfort during or after feeds (see below)?
- How long is spent trying to feed the child each day?
- Does the child turn away when offered food? Will the child tolerate food placed on his or her lips?
- Does the child accept foods and then spit them out?
- Can the child tolerate his or her teeth being brushed and face being washed?

Diet in children with neurological impairment

- You should request dietetic input. Obtain a food diary to assess the adequacy of the child's diet. Calculate the energy and protein content of the foods along with the intake of iron, calcium, vitamins, especially C and D, and minerals and compare these with recommended daily intakes. This diary information can be used together with the blood levels of iron, calcium and vitamin D. If the diet is deficient in calories, food fortification methods will be advised and/or nutritional supplements.
- Children with neurological impairments consume a diet that is deficient in energy compared with that of their healthy peers. They are also at a higher risk of iron deficiency as their diet is often limited and is often largely based on cow's milk. Meat, fruit and vegetables are often avoided, as they are difficult to eat. If reflux oesophagitis is occurring, this may further exacerbate iron deficiency.
- It important to understand that spasticity in CP does not lead to excessive calorie consumption and affected children do not need a higher energy intake. Energy requirements are in fact far lower than those of unaffected children. Despite this, many children still do not consume enough calories to meet their requirements because of the difficulties described above.

Examination

It is important to ensure that the child is not acutely unwell. Examine the child to assess for

- level of alertness compared with normal state
- hydration: mucous membranes, capillary refill, skin turgor
- pallor suggestive of anaemia
- wasting (e.g. of buttocks)
- abdominal distension (remember constipation)
- respiratory signs: tachypnoea, crackles and wheeze.

Decide if there is reason to be concerned about the weight gain. Management is based upon the severity of the problem and the likely underlying cause in the context of the child's underlying diagnosis.

Investigations to consider in faltering growth

- Full blood count, ferritin, thyroid function, renal function, liver function including albumin and bone screen if nutrition is perceived to be inadequate or there are symptoms of lethargy or pallor. Consider measuring vitamins A, D, E, B12 and folate and also trace elements zinc, copper and selenium if on enteral feeding, although recommendations for the extent and frequency of monitoring have not been agreed.
- Barium swallow if GOR is suspected; chest radiography and videofluoroscopy (VFS) if aspiration is suspected.
- Stools for microscopy to exclude infection, *Helicobacter* antigen and chromatography to exclude malabsorption, if indicated by history.

Management

- Estimating calorie, nutrient and fluid requirements in any child with complex disability is difficult. The requirements are less than normal but there is great individual variation. Knowing the child's rate of growth (weight increase) and oral intake prior to the initiation of feeding strategy can be useful in identifying an initial best-guess regime. This should then be altered according to response. Providing calories in excess of requirement needs to be avoided owing to the risk of excess fat deposition.
- If oral feeding is safe and is to continue, then consider
  - food fortification – enrich the child's diet with added butter, cheese, full-fat milk, cream, etc.
  - increasing the energy density of the food that is offered (e.g. offer a high-calorie milk to infants)
  - adding additional energy supplements in the form of fat emulsions, glucose polymers and combined fat and carbohydrate supplements (e.g. Calogen, Liquigen, Super Soluble Maxijul or Super Soluble Duocal)
  - adding in a nutritional supplement such as a fortified milkshake or juice drink (e.g. Fortini, one or two cartons per day, in addition to existing diet).

- Treat treatable causes: consider using an antireflux milk, adding thickeners to feeds and/or antireflux medication for GOR.
- Treat oral adversity if present with a programme of desensitization (see below).

The difficult to feed child: oral aversion

This is a problem that occurs in children with and without neurological impairment. Prolonged bottlefeeding is likely to have occurred, leading to delay in the introduction of solids. Some children may have had adverse oral experiences, such as ventilation, suction, nasogastric feeding, and so on. Meal times are often lengthy and stressful with parents trying to coax their child to take small volumes of solids. The child may have a history of sensory defensiveness, disliking anything being placed close to the mouth, such as a toothbrush or face flannel.

The child with oral adversity should initially be encouraged to take part in messy play before moving on to offer play with foods such as chocolate buttons and the kind of crisps that melt in the mouth rather than having to be chewed. Gradual desensitization can occur with this retraining, but this process can take a very long time and skilled input from a specialist speech and language therapist may be necessary.

Oral sensorimotor management

This is a therapeutic intervention for children with dysphagia (difficulty eating or swallowing lumpy food), often secondary to neurological impairment, provided by specialist speech and language therapists. Its aims include improving the coordination of the oral motor movements to enhance feeding and promote normal oral sensory experiences during meal times and to improve sensory processing. It can bring about improvements in chewing, tongue lateralization, lip closure, swallowing and spoon feeding, but not drinking. It does not decrease feeding time, improve weight gain or improve airway protection.

Gastro-oesophageal reflux

This is a common problem in children with neurological impairments, with estimates of the frequency ranging from 32% to 75%. Several factors contribute towards this:

- prolonged lying in the supine posture
- raised abdominal pressure from scoliosis and spasticity of abdominal muscles
- lower oesophageal sphincter pressure
- flaccidity of the diaphragm and distortion of the diaphragmatic crura
- oesophageal dysmotility.

Clinically, the child presents with chronic vomiting, dysphagia, oesophagitis, grimacing and neck hyperextension (Sandifer syndrome), excess salivation, food refusal, growth failure and recurrent aspiration.

Investigations for GOR

- If the child vomits frequently after feeding and seems to be in discomfort, a barium swallow should be requested to look for evidence of GOR. The report will indicate if reflux was seen and its severity (graded according to how high up the oesophagus reflux reaches). An oesophageal stricture may be found if the reflux has been severe and persistent.
- An upper gastrointestinal endoscopy may be required to confirm the above findings and perform biopsies.
- Lower oesophageal pH studies are less frequently requested nowadays. They are difficult procedures practically to complete as the probe may be pulled out or fall out. There is less need for this investigation as more often PEGs are initially inserted and antireflux surgery is generally only considered later if GOR symptoms are worse with enteral feeding.

Management of GOR includes

1 Thickening feeds, reducing volumes of milk and increasing solids in the diet.
2 Altering the position of the child during and after feeds in order to keep the child more upright.
3 The use of drugs such as domperidone or erythromycin (to increase gastric emptying), an H2 receptor antagonist (ranitidine) or proton pump inhibitors (omeprazole/lansoprazole).

Aspiration

Aspiration is defined as the entry of foreign material into the airway below the true vocal cords. This can occur in healthy children when the airway protective mechanisms are stressed during laughing, talking, eating or sleeping. In practice, an inconsequential amount of material is aspirated and the child remains well. In children with swallowing difficulties, however, the risk of aspiration is much higher, and this may result in acute or chronic respiratory problems and growth failure. Estimates of the frequency of aspiration in children with neurodisability range from 31% to 97%.

Clinically ascertain if there is a history of dysphagia which may be accompanied by an episode of coughing, choking or colour change. Have there been any chest symptoms or a history of recurrent chest infections? Arrange for the child to be seen by a specialist speech and language therapist. The specialist speech and language therapist may perform cervical auscultation that may lead to a suspicion that aspiration is occurring; however, diagnosis requires a VFS examination that provides dynamic images of the oral, pharyngeal and oesophageal stages of swallowing. The specialist speech and language therapist and radiologist usually jointly undertake the examination. The child is fed a variety of food textures mixed with barium while the process of swallowing is filmed from the anteroposterior and lateral view with the focus on the oropharynx and oesophagus. Views are not obtained of the lower oesophagus or stomach. Commonly observed abnormalities seen include

- swallow delay
- food residue after swallows
- pharyngeal dysmotility

- upper airway penetration without aspiration
- aspiration into the tracheobronchial tree.

These abnormalities occur with specific textures of foods. Aspiration is more common with thin liquids and is termed silent because of the absence of coughing or choking. VFS may not always identify aspiration because of its intermittent nature. If aspiration is still suspected, then other investigations or repeating the VFS may be required.

If the child's swallow is deemed unsafe as aspiration occurs with both solids and liquids, then oral feeding should be stopped immediately and an alternative route (e.g. nasogastric feeding) should be instituted. If aspiration occurs only with liquids then the child can still be offered some solids orally but drinks must be given by another route, usually via a PEG.

Nasogastric feeding

A short trial can be very useful to assess the effects on weight gain by offering a known volume of feed of fixed calorie content. It can also be instituted acutely if a VFS study demonstrates an unsafe swallow making oral feeding unsafe.

Beware that feeding enterally may exacerbate or unmask gastro-oesophageal reflux because of the increased pressure of the feed delivery. Prolonged nasogastric feeding also interferes with the swallowing process and suppresses normal oral feeding, making it hard to re-establish oral feeding after the tube is withdrawn. It is uncomfortable, and unsightly for the child and parent, and it may cause erosion of the nasal and oesophageal mucosae. Therefore, nasogastric feeding should only be done for a period of weeks before proceeding either to gastrostomy or recommencing oral feeds.

Gastrostomy feeding

The earlier this is instituted, the better the result for growth. However, it is preferable not to abandon oral feeding completely as feeding a child even only very small amounts orally can have beneficial social and emotional effects on the child and his or her carers.

Issues to consider when thinking of referring a child for gastrostomy feeding include the following:

- Undernutrition: This is the most common indication for gastrostomy referral, followed by limited fluid intake and difficulty giving medications. Other indications include unsafe swallow and aspiration with associated chest disease.
- It is generally a safe procedure and complications are usually easily managed. The indications and potential benefits of PEG feeding must be carefully explained to carers.
- It is an effective way of improving nutritional status, and this in itself leads to other gains, including overall improvement in general health and developmental progress.
- The child must be followed up in the long term to monitor weight gain as the child may become overweight and the volume of feed may need to be reduced or the feed altered to provide a less energy-dense formula. Children can still grow if fed with low-energy,

high-fibre and micronutrient-complete feeds that provide less than 75% of the estimated average requirements.

Most gastrostomies are now inserted percutaneously under endoscopic control (PEG) under a brief general anaesthetic. This does not require a laparotomy and tubes can be changed without an anaesthetic. The tubes are more comfortable and they are very difficult to dislodge, unlike nasogastric tubes. They are also much less obtrusive and as such are more acceptable to carers.

Common minor problems that may be encountered are described in Table 50.3 and most can be managed with good general care and topical treatments. Fewer complications occur following Freka tube placement, and it is usual for this type to be changed to a button-type gastrostomy device, which lies flush with the child's abdomen, 8 to 12 weeks after initial insertion.

PEG feeding is usually a quicker method of feeding, freeing the child and carer to spend more time on other activities. Other health gains have been noted post PEG insertion, and these include

- reduction in drooling and secretions
- decreased vomiting
- decreased constipation
- developmental progress following the improved nutritional state of the child.

Vomiting due to GOR, however, may worsen post PEG, and if this fails to respond to medical management and alterations in the feed delivery from bolus to continuous pump feeding then referral for a fundoplication may be indicated.

'Dumping syndrome' can occur post PEG and causes epigastric pain, nausea and sweating as blood pools around the stomach as the feed enters the small intestine. It is difficult to recognize but dietary management such as increasing the frequency of feeds or the osmolarity of the feed may help.

Fundoplication

A PEG was often combined with a Nissen fundoplication, an antireflux procedure, if the clinical history and 24-hour oesophageal pH studies suggested severe reflux. This procedure has an appreciable morbidity and mortality risk. This approach has been changed in recent years as research has indicated that many children do not require an antireflux procedure after a PEG has been sited. If it is required, it can now be performed laparoscopically rather than through an open incision, thus leading to much quicker recovery and a reduced incidence of complications.

Table 50.3 Common problems with percutaneous endoscopic gastronomies

Problem	Possible cause	Prevention and treatment
Infection	Contamination at time of insertion Poor hygiene when using tube	Assess patient and amount of exudate at site If patient is well and mild response, keep area dry and clean Consider using soframycin as topical antibiotic If worse, test pH of exudate. If acid is caused by a leak of gastric contents, neutralize acid with oral antacid (H2 blocker) and protect skin with barrier cream and dressing Consider 5d course of flucloxacillin if moderate exudate greater than 5d or cellulitis Swab if not improving Prevention: keep site clean and dry. Cleanse daily with cooled boiled water or mild soap and water. Leave gastrostomy site uncovered until healed
Over-granulation (mild)	Friction caused by rubbing from clothing or seat belt Ill-fitting tube	Ensure tube is securely taped to skin Position tube above or to side of stoma Change tube for better fit
'Wet' stoma site	Overgranulation	Keep dry Use non-woven gauze not cotton wool balls to clean Apply mild topical steroid cream (use ointment if skin is dry) Proceed to topical moderate steroid if no better Use silver nitrate only if experienced with its use
Leaking stoma site – Leakage of gastric contents	Stoma site stretched by tube being pulled	Test pH with litmus paper Neutralize with ranitidine or omeprazole, if acid, to protect skin Use paraffin on skin or Cavilon spray Orabase topically provides a barrier Ensure tube correctly positioned – above or to side of stoma, not tucked in pants
Blocked tube	Not flushed adequately after feed or medication Multiple medicines given together Prone to blocking after omeprazole given via tube	Flushes: use 1–2ml in infants 5–10ml in children 30ml in adults If blocked, try push-stop technique to shift. Use small syringe and 10ml water Use soda water or 10ml of 8.4% bicarbonate – leave in situ for 15min, if blockage due to omeprazole Do not use Coca-Cola, lemonade, lemon or pineapple squash to unblock tube as they are acidic. Alternatively, use Clogzapper
Leak from tube	Tube split due to trauma	Flush tube with blackcurrant squash, holding white tissue around tube to detect leak. If confirmed, refer to ward/specialist team
Tube fallen out	Balloon deflated in button or balloon type tube	Check tube or button is correctly positioned, if loose or looks more prominent, check volume of water in balloon. Re-inflate with correct volume Stoma can reduce in size quickly or close over within 12h of tube being out if tube inserted less than 4wk prior Insert new balloon gastrostomy tube/button of same French size. If not possible, insert 10–15cm of same or smaller sized Foley catheter and inflate balloon, then tape tube securely. If Foley not available, try nasogastric tube or refer to ward

> ## Key messages when considering oral feeding in children with neurological impairment
>
> - Dysphagia is common.
> - Weight gain is a good measure of oral feeding. If there are difficulties with oral feeding, undernutrition may result, which will become apparent in early infancy.
> - Those fed orally have slower weight gain and a higher incidence of growth failure than those fed via gastrostomy.
> - Feeding history is important but it is often misleading.
> - Feeding time is, however, a reliable measure of the severity of the feeding impairment. If feeding time is greater than 3 hours per day, consider alternative enteral feeding.
> - GOR is very common and can adversely affect oral feeding, growth and chest symptoms.
> - Aspiration is a common complication of dysphagia and it can occur silently.
> - It is important to offer small amounts of food daily, as this maintains the pleasure of eating for the child and recognises the social benefit of the family eating together.
> - Chronic lung disease is the most common sequela of aspiration.

Obesity

Definitions

- Overweight: BMI greater than the 91st centile.
- Obese: BMI greater than the 98th centile.
- Extreme obesity: BMI greater than the 99.6th centile.

Waist circumference centiles can be used to assess body fat.

As well as seeing children with severe growth failure, you will also be referred children who are grossly overweight. This is not only because we are currently experiencing an epidemic of obesity in the UK, but also because the risk of obesity is much higher (almost double) amongst children with physical disability and/or learning disability. This often occurs as a result of a combination of factors including

- impaired mobility
- reduced motivation
- reduced suitable opportunities for exercise
- need for extra supervision, time and equipment
- food is often used a reward by carers
- high-calorie foods are often offered as part of the usual diet
- requirements are overestimated.

Among children aged 2 to 15 years who are neurodevelopmentally healthy, the proportion who are obese has increased from 10.9% in 1995 to 18.0% in 2005 among males, and from 12.0% to 18.1% among females (Reilly and Dorosty 1999).

Some children with disability on supplemental feeding can put on excessive weight if they are fed the quantity of calories based on 'normal' calculations, as the caloric requirement for children with impaired mobility is considerably lower than normal.

The energy requirement calculation using measured height provides a good example of this difference:

- 15kcal/cm in children without motor dysfunction
- 14kcal/cm in children with motor impairment but who are ambulatory
- 11kcal/cm in children who are non-ambulatory

Growth in children with CP and impaired mobility who are on supplementary feeds needs to be monitored using appropriate charts for their grade of mobility. Adjustments to feed volumes need to be carefully made to ensure that fluid requirements are not compromised. There is a range of products available to ensure that the fluid and caloric needs can be adequately met depending on each individual child's requirement.

Some children with particular syndromes and conditions are at an even higher risk of becoming obese. These conditions include

- myelomeningocele
- Down syndrome
- Prader–Willi syndrome
- osteogenesis imperfecta
- overgrowth syndromes such as Beckwith–Wiedemann syndrome
- Duchenne muscular dystrophy
- some types of dwarfism.

Children with Prader–Willi syndrome develop overeating in childhood. In order to prevent these children from becoming obese, calorie intake should be reduced to 60% to 70% of the recommended daily intake (RDI), unless the child is on growth hormone.

Children with myelomeningocele similarly require a reduction in their calorie intake by 50%, and those with Down syndrome should be offered an intake of 85% to 90% of their RDI.

Consequences of obesity include

- reduced mobility (e.g. difficulty transferring)
- reduced self-care and self-esteem (e.g. washing, dressing and toileting problems)
- an increased burden to the carer
- a greater need for equipment (e.g. hoisting)
- health risks such as
  - cardiovascular disease – hyperlipidaemia, hypertension
  - respiratory compromise
  - sleep apnoea
  - type 2 diabetes
  - fatty liver
  - joint symptoms.

Management

Prevention of obesity is much better than cure as there is no cure currently available.
If the child is orally fed then prevention must be promoted early on.

* Encourage healthy eating habits: eating at regular meal times, rather than eating and drinking constantly.
* Encourage the family to eat together at meal times.
* Advise on a healthy diet for the child with a wide range of foods including plenty of fruit and vegetables.
* Encourage a reduction in the amount of sugar and fat in the child's diet (i.e. the amount of fizzy drinks, crisps, chips, etc.).
* Promote activity and exercise that is adapted to the child's level of function and ability. Encourage activity as part of the family's routine, for example walking the dog, going out on bicycles at the weekend. Some families are motivated to find solutions for their non-ambulant child such, as riding an adapted bicycle or attending swimming sessions for the disabled.
* Physical sports at school are to be encouraged: some young people play rugby, basketball, etc., or adaptations of these games.
* Advise against the use of food as a reward.
* Use star charts with younger children to encourage them to stick to their activity and/or diet, if cognitively able enough.
* Advise parents and carers to reduce the amount of television and screen time that the child is allowed, to a maximum of 1 to 2 hours per day if this is part of the child's daily routine.

References

Reilly JJ, Dorosty AR (1999) Epidemic of obesity in UK children. *Lancet* 354: 1874–5. http://dx.doi.org/10.1016/S0140-6736(99)04555-9

Sullivan PB, Lambert B, Rose M et al. (2000) Prevalence and severity of feeding and nutritional problems in children with neurological impairment: Oxford Feeding Study. *Dev Med Child Neurol* 42: 674–80. http://dx.doi.org/10.1017/S0012162200001249

Further reading

Andrew MJ, Parr JR, Sullivan PB (2011) Feeding difficulties in children with cerebral palsy. *Arch Dis Child Educ Pract Ed* 97: 222–9. http://dx.doi.org/10.1136/archdischild-2011–300914

Bandini LG, Puelzl-Quinn H, Morelli JA, Fukagawa NK (1995) Estimation of energy requirements in persons with severe central nervous system impairment. *J Pediatr* 126: 828–32. http://dx.doi.org/10.1016/S0022–3476(95)70423-X

Clark M, Harris R, Jolleff N, Price K, Neville BG (2010) Worster–Drought syndrome: poorly recognized despite severe and persistent difficulties with feeding and speech. *Dev Med Child Neurol* 52: 27–32. http://dx.doi.org/10.1111/j.1469–8749.2009.03475.x

Craig GM, Carr LJ, Cass H et al. (2006) Medical, surgical, and health outcomes of gastrostomy feeding. *Dev Med Child Neurol* 48: 353–60. http://dx.doi.org/10.1017/S0012162206000776

Day SM, Strauss DJ, Vachon PJ et al. (2007) Growth patterns in a population of children and adolescents with cerebral palsy. *Dev Med Child Neurol* 49: 167–71. http://dx.doi.org/10.1111/j.1469–8749.2007.00167.x

Morton RE, Bonas R, Fourie B et al. (1993) Videofluoroscopy in the assessment of feeding disorders of children with neurological problems. *Dev Med Child Neurol* 35: 388–95. http://dx.doi.org/10.1111/j.1469–8749.1993.tb11659.x

Reyes AL, Cash AJ, Green SH et al. (1993) Gastro-oesophageal reflux in children with cerebral palsy. *Child Care Health Dev* 19: 109–18. http://dx.doi.org/10.1111/j.1365–2214.1993.tb00718.x

Rudolf MCJ, Hochberg Z, Speiser P (2005) Perspectives on the development of international consensus on childhood obesity. *Arch Dis Child* 90: 994–6. http://dx.doi.org/10.1136/adc.2005.075762

Stallings VA, Cronk CE, Zemel BS, Charney EB (1995) Body composition in children with spastic quadriplegic cerebral palsy. *J Pediatr* 126: 833–9. http://dx.doi.org/10.1016/S0022–3476(95)70424–8

Sullivan PB, Juszczak E, Lambert BR, Rose M, Ford-Adams ME, Johnson A (2002) Impact of feeding problems on nutritional intake and growth: Oxford Feeding Study II. *Dev Med Child Neurol* 44: 461–7. http://dx.doi.org/10.1111/j.1469–8749.2002.tb00307.x

Sullivan PB, Juszczak E, Bachlet AM et al. (2004) Impact of gastrostomy tube feeding on the quality of life of carers of children with cerebral palsy. *Dev Med Child Neurol* 46: 796–800. http://dx.doi.org/10.1111/j.1469–8749.2004.tb00443.x

Sullivan PB, Juszczak E, Bachlet AM et al. (2005) Gastrostomy tube feeding in children with cerebral palsy: a prospective, longitudinal study. *Dev Med Child Neurol* 47: 77–85. http://dx.doi.org/10.1017/S0012162205000162

Sullivan PB, Alder N, Bachlet AM et al. (2006) Gastrostomy feeding in cerebral palsy: too much of a good thing? *Dev Med Child Neurol* 48: 877–82. http://dx.doi.org/10.1017/S0012162206001927

Vernon-Roberts A, Wells J, Grant H et al. (2010) Gastrostomy feeding in cerebral palsy: enough and no more. *Dev Med Child Neurol* 52: 1099–105. http://dx.doi.org/10.1111/j.1469–8749.2010.03789.x

51
Drooling

Anne M Kelly

Drooling is abnormal in children after the age of 18 months, although it is seen intermittently in typically developing children until the age of 3 years. It is commonly seen in children with neurological impairment, most commonly in cerebral palsy (CP), with the prevalence among children with spastic quadriplegic CP (SQCP) being 30% to 53%.

Causes

The major cause is neurological impairment leading to poor lip closure secondary to oromotor difficulties and impaired swallowing of oral secretions. Do consider other factors which may contribute to the problem including

- dental problems
- ear, nose and throat problems (e.g. adenotonsillar hypertrophy)
- medications – particularly clobazam and clonazepam
- intercurrent respiratory illness (upper and/or lower) can also increase secretions.

Assessment

Assess the severity of the problem and the impact on the child's quality of life caused by the discomfort of inflamed lips and chin and frequently soaked bibs and clothing.

Examination

- Posture
- Dental health
- Ear, nose and throat examination

- Neurology: observe the child's swallow whilst drinking and feeding, if possible with a speech and language therapist.

Management

Ensure that any treatable causes, such as poor dental care, have been resolved. Check that the child has a good posture and is appropriately seated at meal times. Consider

- **Oromotor exercises** for children who can give attention and whose families are motivated.
- **An intraoral device** for older children with mild to moderate problems. These devices are modified braces which encourage lip, tongue and palatal movement. They are not suitable for any child who may aspirate.

Medical options

- **Hyoscine patch (topical):** This is sited behind the ear or under the angle of the jaw and should be changed every 2 to 3 days. This has been the most commonly used treatment but it is often not well tolerated owing to skin irritation at the patch site.
  Dose:
  - A child under 8 years should use only half a patch.
  - A child over 8 years should use one patch.
- **Glycopyrronium bromide (oral):** This is often better tolerated than hyoscine skin patches.
  Dose:
  - A child weighing less than 15kg: start 0.25mg daily.
  - A child weighing 15–25kg: start 0.5mg daily.
  - A child weighing more than 25kg: start 1mg once or twice daily.
  Doses can then be increased slowly to a maximum of 0.04mg/kg/day in three doses.
- **Trihexiphenidyl – benzhexol hydrochloride (oral):** This can be particularly helpful if the child has an underlying diagnosis of a dystonia
  Dose:
  - Start 0.5mg (infant) to 1mg (child) once daily for a week.
  - Increase by 0.5mg to 1mg twice daily for a week.
  - Increase by 0.5mg to 1mg alternate dose each week to a maximum of 2mg three times a day.
- **Ipratropium bromide:** This is more often used for asthma treatment but, as it is a derivative of atropine, it also dries one's mouth.
  Inhaled dose via spacer:
  - 20mcg tds for children under the age of 6 years.
  - 20mcg to 40mcg for children over the age of 6 years three times a day
- **Botulinum toxin A:** This can be injected into the salivary gland and the benefit may last between 1 and 6 months. This is offered in some tertiary centres under ultrasound guidance.
- **Surgical options:** There are a variety of approaches, for example submandibular duct repositioning, which have a range of benefits. However, the effects may only be temporary and a resultant dry mouth may lead to difficulties with oral hygiene.

Further reading

Fairhurst CBR, Cockerill H (2011) Management of drooling in children. *Arch Dis Child Educ Pract Ed* 96: 25–30. http://dx.doi.org/10.1136/adc.2007.129478

52
Tracheostomy and airway support

Anne M Kelly

A small but growing number of children who require some mechanical aid with breathing (long-term ventilation [LTV]) are now cared for in the community. This will include children

- who have a tracheostomy (22% of the total), who are at the severest end of the spectrum, some of whom require ventilation for 24 hours (<10%)
- who require non-invasive mask ventilation (NIV) to deliver some positive end-expiratory pressure overnight (75%)
- who require negative pressure ventilation
- who require tracheostomy and phrenic nerve pacing (Wallis et al. 2011).

Tracheostomy

A tracheostomy is created by insertion of a flanged tube into the trachea via an incision between the second and third tracheal rings. The tube's component parts are as follows:

- The inner cannula: this is the 'sleeve' inside the tracheostomy tube that can be removed for cleaning.
- The neck plate (flange): this is the site for ties. It prevents movement and skin breakdown secondary to pressure points.
- The obturator: this is a guide for positioning the actual tracheostomy tube.
- The cuff: this is inflated with air to fill the empty space, preventing aspiration and potential air leak around the cannula. Cuffed tracheal tubes are used predominantly in those requiring mechanical ventilation with high pressures. For those requiring only nocturnal ventilation, the cuff can be deflated during the day.

A tracheostomy provides an airway that bypasses the epiglottis. Tubes generally need changing weekly in paediatric patients. Decannulation refers to permanent removal of the tube, which will lead to closure of the stoma spontaneously within hours or days.

Insertion of a tracheostomy tube enables the child to receive airway support from a mechanical ventilator or a continuous positive airway pressure (CPAP) machine. CPAP delivers a constant flow of pressurized air throughout the breathing cycle, resulting in increased mean airway pressure and functional residual capacity, but it does not alter tidal volume. It 'splints' the airway open, preventing collapse. Bilevel or biphasic positive airway pressure (BPAP or BiPAP as it is sometimes referred to) provides two different levels of pressure: higher pressure during inspiration (IPAP) to improve tidal volume and a lower pressure during exhalation (EPAP) to increase mean airway pressure and functional residual capacity. BPAP can also be set to provide 'backup breaths' to maintain a certain minimum number of breaths per minute.

A tracheostomy tube enables delivery of humidified air or oxygen and provides access for direct airway suction. If ventilator support is not required, then a humidifying device can be attached to the tracheostomy tube. A speaking valve may be attached to the tracheostomy tube in the older child to allow more air to flow through the vocal cords to allow voice production.

The risks associated with a tracheostomy include

- an increased risk of chest infections
- impaired development of speech
- humidification problems
- accidental dislodgement or obstruction of the tube, which may or may not disconnect from the ventilator
- failure of the alarm system when attached to the ventilator;

Tracheostomy can also be considered unsightly.

Mask ventilation

This is sometimes referred to as 'non-invasive ventilation' (NIV) as the mask provides ventilation without the need for a tracheostomy. NIV is increasingly used for children who can breathe independently during most of the day but need some assistance when they are sleeping. It can be delivered via a number of different interfaces such as a nasal mask, nasal prongs, helmet or facial mask. No surgical procedure is needed. It does not have the potential for affecting speech and language development, unlike a tracheostomy, and there is less risk of respiratory infections.

When to use invasive and non-invasive ventilation

If ventilation is needed for 24 hours, tracheostomy is preferred, and it is also preferred during the child's first year of life. In some cases, mask ventilation has been started very early (at age 2wk) if hypoventilation is less severe. Alternating between nasal and orofacial masks every 3 days may minimize midface hypoplasia, which is a serious long-term complication related to the daily compression of the mask on the face. To reduce this risk, it is important not to seal the mask too tight. Customized silicone masks can be helpful. Facial masks are avoided as long as possible in children because of the potential risk of aspiration.

There were over 900 children as of 2010 who are receiving LTV in the UK. The vast majority of these children are cared for at home (91%) (Wallis et al. 2011).

The most common reasons for LTV are

* neuromuscular disease (43%)
* chronic respiratory disease (37%)
* central nervous system disease (18%).

The number of children requiring LTV has increased almost 10-fold since 1999 (Edwards et al. 2004). Much of the increase is due to greater use of non-invasive masks overnight to assist ventilation in children with neuromuscular disease.

Some of these children will have a package of care funded by the National Health Service which will provide nursing support from children's community nursing teams. Those on ventilators require additional support and carers provided by the continuing care team or equivalent. This support will include some overnight care provided by trained staff, depending on local resources and budget. Carers will require training in resuscitation, as will those who support the child in school.

Paediatric follow-up is usually provided by a variety of paediatricians from the specialties including from the neurology, respiratory, paediatric intensive care unit and community teams.

References

Edwards EA, O'Toole M, Wallis C (2004) Sending children home on tracheostomy dependent ventilation: pitfalls and outcomes. *Arch Dis Child* 89: 251–5. http://dx.doi.org/10.1136/adc.2003.028316

Wallis C, Paton JY, Beaton S (2011) Children on long-term ventilatory support: 10 years of progress. *Arch Dis Child* 96: 998–1002. http://dx.doi.org/10.1136/adc.2010.192864

53
Pain in children with complex needs

Arnab Seal

Learning objectives

- To know how to recognize pain and assess pain severity in children who have complex needs, learning disability and communication difficulty.
- To know the common causes and sources of pain and discomfort in children with complex needs.
- To be able to manage the cause of pain and provide appropriate pain relief.

Prevalence

Pain is common in children with neuromuscular and neurodevelopmental problems such as CP. Chronic pain is frequent in children with moderate to severe CP with a prevalence of approximately 60% at any given time. Adult studies suggest that 66% to 94% of adults with CP experience chronic pain. Chronic pain and discomfort reduce a child's participation in everyday activities, hinder sleep and lower quality of life. Older children self-report more pain, but this does not seem to be related to the severity of impairment. Proxy reports by parents in children with communication difficulties and/or cognitive impairment show a much higher reporting of pain, with the severity and frequency of pain relating to severity of impairment, seizures, presence of a gastrostomy and parental unemployment.

Case vignette

Anne is a 12-year-old female with total-body cerebral palsy (CP) with mild visual impairment and moderate hearing impairment. She was born preterm at 25 weeks' gestation. She has moderate to severe cognitive delay and her communication is limited. She recognizes people who are close to her and will smile and laugh during activities she enjoys. Anne's parents have recently become concerned with Anne's behaviour. She seems more irritable, is pulling her hair, head banging and is sometimes hitting her carers. There has been no change to her routines and care. A careful examination does not reveal any obvious reason for the behavioural change or any obvious source of pain. Anne's parents and teachers were requested to maintain a diary of the behaviours and any possible precipitants. Over a 2-month period it becomes clear that the behaviour change is most prominent in the week prior to Anne's periods, which had started 6 months previously. She was prescribed regular mefenamic acid for the premenstrual week and parents maintained a Paediatric Pain Profile (PPP). Anne's behaviour improved along with the pain profile scores but it was difficult for parents to determine when to start the medication as Anne's periods were irregular. Parents were advised to use the PPP summary charts to determine the day Anne was starting to experience discomfort. If there was no other obvious source of discomfort, then they would assume it was likely to be premenstrual pain and start the medication.

Learning point

Pain can often result in challenging behaviour in children with severe disability.

Why is pain so poorly recognized?

Recognizing pain can be challenging in children who are unable to self-report. Children experiencing chronic pain may not show behavioural signs to indicate pain as they have often learnt to live with the pain. Therefore, if you do not ask or look for it, you will not always know. Some children with developmental problems may also have a higher pain threshold and their response to pain may not be indicative of the pain severity. Irrespective of the reasons for under-recognition, the pain is very real and needs to be identified and alleviated.

Discomfort is not synonymous with pain. Pain can cause discomfort but there are a large number of other causes of discomfort, for example itching, nausea, ill-fitting clothes, a cold bed, dark room, and so on. Discomfort may not be painful but can be equally annoying and intolerable. When faced with any child displaying pain-related behaviour, it is important to consider discomfort as the cause. Sometimes the problem is minor and easily correctable and can be identified using a practical and common-sense approach rather than a medical one.

When should you suspect pain or discomfort in a non-communicating child?

A non-communicating child usually communicates pain, discomfort and distress by changes in behaviour. Common behaviours include excessive crying, irritability, change in personality and being 'not him- or herself'. Some children will display self-injurious behaviour (SIB) such as head banging and hair pulling. Parents can often identify specific patterns in their child which alert them to pain. Wincing or crying during everyday handling may give clues regarding the source of pain, for example hip pain.

How can pain be identified and measured in children?

There are a number of instruments which have been used for pain identification and for gradation of pain severity (Table 53.1). Some of the tools are used for acute periprocedural/perioperative pain assessment and some are for use in other settings. The assessments used for non-communicating children are primarily behavioural tools because reliable physiological tools are not available and would be difficult to implement in everyday practice. The Paediatric Pain Profile is a tool which can be used by caregivers in all settings and increases in reliability with repeated and regular use by the same caregiver. A detailed discussion is outside the scope of this book and the interested reader is directed to the Royal College of Paediatrics and Child Health and Royal College of Nursing (2009) approved guideline 'The recognition and assessment of acute pain in children', which has a section on assessing pain in children with cognitive impairment.

Table 53.1 Validated tools for pain assessment in children with a disability

	All settings	Perioperative
Children able to self-report	FACES Pain Rating Scale (Fig. 53.1) Colour Analogue Scale	FACES Pain Rating Scale Colour Analogue Scale
Non-communicating children with cognitive impairment	PPP Valid 1–18y NCCPC-R Valid 3–19y	FLACC Valid 4–18y NCCPC-PV Valid 3–19y

PPP, Paediatric Pain Profile; NCCPC-R, Non-Communicating Children's Pain Checklist – Revised; FLACC, Face, Legs, Activity, Cry, Consolability; NCCPC-PV, Non-Communicating Children's Pain Checklist – Postoperative Version.

Wong-Baker FACES™ Pain Rating Scale Instructions For Usage

Explain to the person that each face is for a person who has no pain (hurt) or some, or a lot of pain.

Face 0 doesn't hurt at all. Face 2 hurts just a little bit. Face 4 hurts a little bit more. Face 6 hurts even more. Face 8 hurts a whole lot. Face 10 hurts as much as you can imagine, although you don't have to be crying to have this worst pain.

Ask the person to choose the face that best describes how much pain he has.

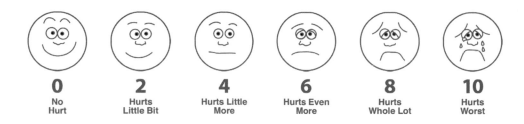

0	**2**	**4**	**6**	**8**	**10**
No Hurt	Hurts Little Bit	Hurts Little More	Hurts Even More	Hurts Whole Lot	Hurts Worst

©1983 Wong-Baker FACES™ Foundation. Used with permission.

Figure 53.1 Wong-Baker FACES Pain Rating Scale. © 1983 Wong-Baker FACES™ Foundation. Used with permission.

Common causes and management of pain and discomfort

When a child self-reports pain, further assessment of the site, cause and severity should be undertaken using validated tools. Management involves relevant investigations, pain relief and treatment of underlying cause. In non-communicating children the problem is more complex as often the source of pain and/or discomfort is unclear. Taking a detailed history and considering different possibilities with parents can sometimes identify the problem. A thorough examination with appropriate exposure, looking for all possible causes (Table 53.2), is recommended. The common causes to specifically look for include gastro-oesophageal reflux, constipation, otitis, dental pain, hip pain, bone pain, menstrual pain and spasticity. If the picture remains unclear, then a pain diary over a few weeks may be quite useful. Pain relief should be offered depending on the severity of pain. Occasionally, symptomatic and empirical treatments can be considered after a full discussion with parents regarding possible benefits and adverse effects.

Table 53.2 Common causes and management of pain in children with disabilities

Causes	Management of cause of pain
Musculoskeletal Spasticity, contractures, deformities Hip subluxation/dislocation Scoliosis Ill-fitting orthoses, shoes, wheelchair, bed Pressure points (hip/spine/others)	For spasticity: 24h postural care Analgesics (paracetamol, ibuprofen) Physiotherapy/hydrotherapy/careful exercise Oral muscle relaxants such as baclofen Intrathecal baclofen Surgery (soft tissue releases, joint surgery, spasticity surgery)
Trauma Accidental injury Hairline fractures/bone pain Muscle sprain Consider child abuse	Radiography, dual energy X-ray absorptiometry scans; consider bisphosphonates for poor bone mineralization
Gastrointestinal Gastro-oesophageal reflux/gastritis Trapped wind Fundoplication with antegrade peristalsis Gut dysmotility/irritable bowel syndrome Constipation/fissure Gastrostomy-related problems Feed-related problems, e.g. intolerance, volume, timing, etc. Feed aspiration	Antireflux treatment/positioning 'Winding' the gastrostomy; peppermint cordial Active bowel management for constipation using regular laxatives Food diary may help; hypoallergenic feed trial Feeding regime management in consultation with child, parent and dietitian Videofluoroscopy to assess aspiration. Thickening of fluids
Infections/inflammation Otitis Sore throat Chronic nasal congestion Urine infection Ingrowing toenail Pressure sores Dental pain Sinus pain	Analgesics as indicated Check ears; antibiotics and local lignocaine ear drops as indicated Check throat; local anaesthetic spray Normal saline nose drops and steroid nasal spray as indicated for congestion Check urine dipstick Refer podiatry; wide shoes Protect pressure areas, use second skin Regular dental checks and care Decongestants for sinus congestion
Neurological Headache/migraine Central neurogenic pain Shunt malfunction/shunt block Hypersensitivity to touch/allodynia	Family history of migraine? Chronic analgesic headache Investigate shunt system
Discomfort Itching (eczema/lice/scabies) Nausea Ill-fitting clothes, shoes, equipment Poorly controlled epilepsy Medication side effects Vasomotor instability/poor perfusion Excessive sweating Premenstrual tension/period pains Poor sleep Anxiety (separation/other causes)	A detailed history considering all the possibilities taken from parents and regular caregivers can often 'light a bulb' as to what the cause is. When identified, treating the underlying cause and/or empirical treatment can be successful

Pain relief options

The first line in pain relief is adequate doses of paracetamol and local analgesics as appropriate (e.g. anaesthetic creams, drops and sprays). Ibuprofen alone or in combination with paracetamol is stronger. Codeine and other non-steroidal anti-inflammatory drugs such as diclofenac sodium can be used for moderate to severe pain. For uncontrolled pain and postoperative or acute pain, opioids and patient/parent-controlled analgesia (PCA) should be provided. For chronic unrelenting severe pain, opioid patches, local blocks and the services of a children's chronic pain team, where available, should be considered. Neuropathic pain often responds to pregabalin, gabapentin, some anticonvulsants (carbamazepine) or amitriptyline. The biology of pain is closely linked with psychological factors and psychological support is often very useful. Alternatives to medicines include physiotherapy, transcutaneous electrical nerve stimulation, massage, acupuncture and osteopathy, all of which can have a role in specific situations. Psychological factors, depression, 'memory of pain' and family dynamics play an important role in chronic pain. Encouraging participation, family support and cognitive behavioural therapy (CBT) can be helpful in these situations.

Key messages

- Children with neuromuscular and neurodevelopmental conditions such as CP frequently experience pain.
- Non-communicating children are at high risk of under-recognized and undertreated pain.
- Being vigilant and anticipating pain and discomfort should be an important part of daily care.
- Children's self-reporting is preferred wherever possible. Where it is not possible, use validated tools appropriate to the setting, for example the Paediatric Pain Profile.
- Ask these questions of the child or parent (as appropriate) during your consultation:
  - How *much* bodily pain or discomfort have you/your child had since last seen?
  - How *often* have you/your child had bodily pain or discomfort since last seen?
- When acute or recurrent pain is present, re-evaluate the patient at regular intervals using a validated tool. Using a pain diary can be useful.
- Parents and/or a regular caregiver will be aware of any unique markers of pain in individual children. Listen to them.
- Be aware that language, ethnicity and culture may influence the expression and assessment of pain.
- Be aware that discomfort without pain can present with the same behaviour patterns as pain. Remember this when looking for a cause and when treating.

Reference

Royal College of Paediatrics and Child Health and Royal College of Nursing (2009) *The Recognition and Assessment of Acute Pain in Children.* Available at: http://www.rcn.org.uk/__data/assets/pdf_file/0004/269185/003542.pdf (accessed 6 November 2012).

Websites

Paediatric Pain Profile: www.ppprofile.org.uk

Wong-Baker FACES Foundation: www.wongbakerfaces.org

54
Sleep disorders

Arnab Seal

Learning objectives

- To know the common reasons for sleep disturbance in children with complex needs.
- To understand the principles of management of these common sleep disorders.

The amount of sleep a child will need changes throughout childhood. See Table 54.1 for sleep requirements at difference ages.

Table 54.1 Average sleep requirements at various ages

Age	Amount of sleep required
Term-born infant	16–18h
1y	15h
2y	13–14h
4y	12h
10y	8–10h
Mid-adolescence	8.5h
Later adolescence	7–8h

Factors affecting sleep

- Environment
  - A dimly lit quiet place without any distractions helps.
- Child factors
  - A consistent bedtime routine, for example bath, story and going to bed when calm, but awake with the child going to sleep by him- or herself.
  - Avoid factors leading to sleep associations such as drinking milk or being cuddled.
- Parent reaction
  - Parents need to allow the child to self-settle and fall asleep independently.
  - For a child who will not settle and for night waking, parents should wait a few minutes before going in to see if the child settles spontaneously. Then check on the child in a 'robot-like' manner, that is without positive reinforcements (smile, cuddle, milk) or negative reinforcements (scolding), and leave the room. Repeat as necessary until the child settles. Inadequate sleep has a number of negative effects on the child and family members (Table 54.2).

Table 54.2 Consequences of poor sleep

Day-time sleepiness and fatigue
Mood changes and irritability
Cognitive impairment leading to poor school performance
Attention difficulties
Poor memory
Reduced motivation
Increased reaction time leading to increased risk of accidents
Increased stimulant intake, e.g. caffeine (particularly the parent)
Impaired family functioning and impaired relationships
Increased risk-taking behaviours

Sleep problems in children with a disability

Sleep problems are very common and affect 60% to 80% of children with complex needs. This high prevalence is because of a combination of psychological, physiological and environmental factors. The most common sleep problems in the general population are also common in children with complex needs. Therefore, the first line of management is ensuring good sleep hygiene, boundary setting and simple behaviour modification techniques. There are a number of reasons for the high prevalence of sleep problems in children with complex needs (Table 54.3), but often there is an intrinsic sleep regulation problem as well.

Table 54.3 Impact of disability on sleep

Health difficulties
- Physical problems, e.g. spasticity or hypotonia (turning, positioning, reflux), muscle cramps, feeding pumps bleeping, epilepsy (seizures), incontinence, etc.
- Respiratory problems, e.g. obstructive sleep apnoea, chronic wheeze/aspiration
- Pain or discomfort, e.g. hip pain, itching from eczema
- Medication may interfere with natural sleep cycles, e.g. methylphenidate
- Prolonged hospitalization in infancy may not have allowed the establishment of a regular sleep pattern

Consequence of disability
- Rituals around bedtime in children with ASD and LD can be inimical to good bedtime routine
- LD and poor memory may result in the child never learning to sleep in their own bed
- Sensory processing problems in ASD and LD may cause extreme sensitivity to environmental factors, e.g. hot/cold, light, colour, noise, texture of bed clothes, etc.
- Sleep–wake cycle (circadian rhythm) disruption is common in all developmental disorders, but particularly visual impairment
- Children may be hyperactive and unable to 'shut down', e.g. ADHD.

Poor sleep routines
- Parents may never have established a good bedtime routine because the demands of caring were simply too tiring
- Parental anxiety may lead to overprotectiveness, co-sleeping or overstimulation
- Overtired children are often hyperactive, leading to a cycle of decline. They are often very irritable and overemotional and difficult to manage
- Underlying psychological factors may disrupt sleep, e.g. night-time fears, nightmares
- Common problems which can affect all children, such as attention seeking (curtain calls), coming into the parents' bed, hunger/thirst, soggy nappy, nightmares, etc.

ASD, autism spectrum disorder; LD, learning disability; ADHD, attention-deficit–hyperactivity disorder.

Assessment of a disordered sleep pattern

A careful history should be taken that includes the following:

- Sleep:
  - Bedtime routine including who is present when the child settles to sleep.
  - Any sleep associations such as drinks, dummy, music.
  - Factors disturbing sleep:
    - pain including gastro-oesophageal reflux
    - cough
    - sleep apnoea.
- The child's disability – in particular thinking about communication
- General health
- Medications
- Household:
  - Who the child sleeps with and why
  - Family dynamics – who is involved with the bedtime routine?

Using a structured approach such as a *Sleep Questionnaire* (an example is provided in Appendix XI) face to face with the carer often results in the carer themself identifying the problem. The questionnaire can often be used to build on parents' motivation when they recognize the effect it has had on their personal and family life.

A *Sleep Diary* (an example is provided in Appendix XII and an example of a completed *Sleep Log* is provided in Appendix XIII) completed for at least 2 weeks can identify patterns of waking and contributory factors. It is important to ask parents to do a 24-hour recall at a set time every day, as longer periods of recall are unreliable.

Sleep disorders

Behavioural insomnia of childhood

The most common sleep problem is the 'bedtime struggle' caused by either an inadequate bedtime routine and/or a sleep association. The management strategy is to provide a good bedtime routine, often called 'sleep hygiene', which involves the following:

- A bedtime at the same time each evening.
- Cueing the child 5 minutes before the bedtime routine starts, allowing activities to be completed. For children with communication difficulties an object of reference such as a pillow or blanket can be used.
- A routine that, once started, should be kept in the child's own sleeping environment (not allowing the child to return downstairs to watch the television), which should be quiet and calm.
- Routine bathing and changing, which should start 30 minutes before sleep time.
- A bedtime story, wishing 'goodnight' and leaving the room.
- Leaving the room with the child awake in the cot or bed so that he or she learns to fall asleep alone.
- Dimmed lights.

The child may initially cry, but loving carers with firm and consistent boundaries will give the child a secure message that this is a safe place to sleep. Avoid the following:

- television or video games in the bedroom
- lots of toys in the bedroom: children do not know if it is playtime or sleep time
- sending the child to the bedroom as a punishment.

Sleep associations

Sleep associations are common and often go unrecognized unless looked for specifically. These are objects or conditions a child associates with falling asleep, such as a dummy, watching television, rocking by parents, the parent lying next to the child, a bottle of milk, and so on. This then becomes a learnt behaviour and the child expects the same parental response every night and if he or she wakes up at night.

Parents will often complain about night-time waking, and it is only when you take the history that it becomes clear that there are sleep associations. There is no point in trying to tackle the night-time waking until the process of self-settling is secure. Sorting out the evening can often lead to a full night's sleep, and these techniques are applied at a time when the parents are more than able to apply them consistently (i.e. in the evening and not in the middle of the night, if possible). The same techniques are applicable to night-time waking episodes.

Management strategies

- **Controlled crying technique:** Leave the child to cry for 3 to 5 minutes and then go in. Talk to the child calmly until he or she stops screaming, say 'goodnight' and leave. Parents may need to do this repeatedly until the child settles. Initially, this may take hours depending on how entrenched the behaviour is. This is difficult for parents but usually works within a week with a consistent approach.
- **Graded leaving approach:** For parents wanting a gentler approach, start sitting beside the bed and then gradually move the chair away towards the door every 3 days until out of the room. Replace presence with voice reassurance. This is a more gentle approach but takes a great deal longer.
- **Night-time bed invaders:** If a child comes into the parent's bed then he or she should be taken back to his or her own bed every time. The parent needs to remain impassive ('robot parent'), not provide any positive (eye contact or hugs/kisses) or negative (getting cross) reinforcements.

It usually takes between 3 days and 3 weeks of consistent management for a good sleep routine to be restored. Warn parents about this before they start so that they can prepare for it. A shorter trial may lead to failure and disappointment.

Top tips for setting a sleep routine

- Make sure bedtime is calm.
- Ensure that everyone involved in the sleep routine is in agreement.
- Carers need to decide when they are ready to implement the programme.
- Recruit help – a night's rest or day-time help from extended family can help.
- Warn the neighbours if appropriate!
- Remember: it will get worse before it gets better.

Parasomnias

Parasomnias are undesirable physical phenomena that occur usually during arousal or transition from rapid eye movement (REM) and non-REM sleep.

Night terrors are characterized by an onset that is usually within 1 to 3 hours of falling asleep. The child usually looks frightened and can have their eyes wide open. There may be associated sweating and the whole episode lasts between 5 and 30 minutes. The child is not awake during these episodes even though their eyes may be wide open. There is no recall of the events and quite often there is evidence of autonomic arousal and automatic behaviours. Commonly, it is a self-limiting disorder which disappears by 7 to 8 years of age. In some children it can be a regular occurrence and, even though the child is not aware of the process, it can disrupt family life. Management consists of reassurance regarding the benign nature of the disorder and asking parents not to wake the child. In troublesome cases partly arousing the child 15 to 30 minutes before the expected time of the night terrors can abort the attack.

Sleep-walking and *sleep-talking* are relatively common parasomnias. They usually occur between the ages of 3 and 13 years and spontaneously resolve. The episodes usually last between 5 and 15 minutes. There is a positive family history in a first-degree relative in 60% of cases. Usually the condition is benign but in certain instances there is a risk of injury.

Management strategy

Insufficient sleep, stress, anxiety, drugs and alcohol may act as precipitating factors for all parasomnias. Addressing the sleep deprivation can often resolve the problem.

Circadian rhythm disorders

Our 'body clock' is situated in the suprachiasmatic nucleus and controls the sleep–wake cycle or circadian rhythm. It is influenced by daylight and melatonin release from the pineal gland. Disorders of the sleep–wake cycle can occur by routine, for example night-shift work or pushing back normal bedtime, causing delayed sleep-phase syndrome (e.g. as in teenagers who are busy with computers/television/games at bedtime). Some children with developmental problems, particularly visual impairment, are at higher risk of circadian disorders.

Management strategies

- Ensuring good sleep hygiene.
- Removing all distractions.
- Bringing forward the sleep time by 30 minutes every third day.
- Melatonin may help in some situations, especially if visual impairment is present.

Paroxysmal movement disorders in sleep

Rhythmic movement disorder

In some children rhythmic movements occur during falling off to sleep or during any stage of sleep. It is relatively common and has a prevalence of 2%. It is more common in children with developmental problems and learning difficulties. The movements can involve any part of the body and usually have a frequency between 0.5 and 2 movements per second. The movements are repetitive and stereotyped. In some children they can present as head banging, head rolling, body rolling or body thrusting movements. The urge tends to be worse, or may appear exclusively, in the evenings and at night.

MANAGEMENT STRATEGY

- Padding cot sides for safety when necessary.
- Reassuring parents regarding the benign nature of the condition.

Restless leg syndrome and periodic limb movement disorder

Restless leg syndrome and periodic limb movement disorder are related conditions which are often under-recognized. They have a prevalence of around 2% in the population. Although most of these conditions start after adolescence, about a third of them start during childhood. The conditions are characterized by involuntary twitches or jerks of the legs (occasionally arms) which cause partial awakening and sleep disruption, often leading to chronic sleep deprivation. The child's description of the event is often as 'bugs or spiders crawling over my legs', itching, burning or 'energy in my legs'.

MANAGEMENT STRATEGY

- Identifying and treating any iron deficiency.
- Tackling any sleep deprivation.
- Consider medication – gabapentin, clonazepam or dopamine antagonists may help.

Teeth grinding or bruxism

Teeth grinding affects 5% of the population. It is normally present in infancy but the more troublesome variety begins in late childhood or adolescence. Precipitants include anxiety, stress, teeth malocclusion and occasionally drugs, alcohol, stimulants and allergies. Children with developmental disorders are more likely to suffer from this. The condition tends to be self-limiting but, if persistent, can cause damage to the teeth and musculoskeletal pain around the head and neck areas.

MANAGEMENT STRATEGY

- Treat any pain.
- Refer the patient to a dentist for dental shields if there are concerns about attrition of the teeth.

Sleep-related breathing disorders

Sleep-related breathing disorders are common and predominantly consist of snoring and obstructive sleep apnoea. Only a small proportion of snorers have obstructive sleep apnoea. The most common cause in children is adenotonsillar hypertrophy.

Clinical features of obstructive sleep apnoea include snoring in a typically irregular crescendo–decrescendo pattern. Other symptoms include mouth breathing, snorting, gasps, sweating, paradoxical ribcage movement, restlessness, frequent awakenings and witnessed apnoeic episodes. There may be associated unusual sleep postures such as extended neck position. Some children may also present with failure to thrive. Children older than 5 years usually have the above symptoms and can additionally present with enuresis, behaviour problems, poor attention span and poor school performance. Day-time sleepiness can also be a feature, particularly in obese children. In extreme cases there may be cor pulmonale with progressive pulmonary hypertension.

Risk factors for obstructive sleep apnoea

- Down syndrome
- Neuromuscular diseases
- Craniofacial malformations
- Pierre Robin syndrome
- Achondroplasia
- Severe obesity including Prader–Willi syndrome
- Mucopolysaccharidoses
- Central hypoventilation syndromes

Management strategies

- Appropriate sleep studies such as overnight pulse oximetry, capnography, actigraphy and sleep studies (polysomnography). This may require referral to a sleep laboratory.
- Treatment of the underlying cause, for example craniofacial malformation, obesity, and so on.
- Treatment of nasal congestion.
- If the problem is cause by adenotonsillar hypertrophy, consider surgery.
- In symptomatic children with persistent symptoms consider non-invasive ventilation.

Specific sleep issues for children with physical disabilities

- Positioning
  - Some children with increased muscle tone have muscle spasms at night and benefit from baclofen.
  - It is important for children with hypertonia or hypotonia from any cause to be well positioned for sleep. Use of sleep systems can provide gentle supportive positioning. They may be recommended for children with asymmetry of spine and hips. Maintaining a good position at night helps prevent or slow down shortening of muscles and joint deformity. Sleep systems are particularly helpful for those who are more likely to move into an abnormal uncomfortable position and are unable to move back to a position of comfort.
  - Some children with physical disabilities may develop a fear of separation as they may be unable to get up and reach their carer should they need to. Having a bell or alarm which a child can use to call carers may reassure the child and help him or her to settle more easily.

- Frequent checks at night may make a child feel reassured but may also lead to the child becoming dependent on that attention. Some families find the use of an infant monitor or intercoms reassuring, to know that the child can be heard.
- **Overnight pump feeds**
  - Children on pump feeds can be fed through the day, at night or with a combination of day-time and night-time feeds. Night feeds are usually given as an overnight continuous feed with the use of a feeding pump.
  - Night-time feeding is an individual choice. In most children night-time feeds are convenient, well tolerated and can be the right choice. If a child's sleep is interrupted by the feeds or if he has difficulty tolerating the feed, or becomes very wet, then a different feeding regime should be looked at. Discussion with the child's dietitian, taking into account lifestyle and day-time activities, can help in selecting the right regime of feeds without affecting sleep.
  - Problems of reflux during night feeds can be prevented to some extent by raising the head end of the bed or by using a specially adapted bed that can be tipped. Some children may also benefit from using medication to control reflux.
  - Trapped wind may cause pain and discomfort and may interfere with overnight feeds. Using antireflux measures along with 'winding' the gastrostomy tube may help. The body usually adapts to night-time feeding over a period of time.
  - The main problem tends to be feed pumps alarming and waking up the child and other family members. Sometimes a parent has to get up to check the pump or turn it off. This can be avoided by ensuring that the feed finishes at a more convenient time.
- Children with cerebral palsy or other physical difficulties often have other **associated difficulties** which can affect sleep, such as epilepsy, visual impairment and learning disability
  - **Associated visual/hearing impairments**
    - For children with visual and/or hearing impairment it is important to have and maintain a good bedtime routine so that the child is aware of what is going to happen. This can be done using 'objects of reference' to mark the start of each stage. For example, an object used in the bath (sponge) can be associated with bath time, a cushion to represent being in bed, and so on.
    - Some children with visual impairment may respond well to oral melatonin.
  - **Associated epilepsy**
    - Poor seizure control is known to cause disturbed sleep.
    - Having a good night's sleep is vital for children with epilepsy as lack of sleep may increase seizures in some children.
    - Use of a seizure alarm is controversial. The risk of sudden unexplained death in epilepsy should be discussed in full with families where children have high-risk factors. The advantages and disadvantages of monitoring also need to be discussed.

Specific issues for children with autism spectrum disorders and/or learning disabilities

Sleep disturbance is common in children affected by autism spectrum disorders (ASDs) and/ or learning disability. The following advice can be provided to the carers of affected children.

- **Have a set routine and visual timetable:** The child should have a set bedtime routine and follow it every day including at weekends and during holidays if possible, as children with ASD and/or learning disability find it hard to accept changes to routines. A visual/picture timetable may be useful as it shows clearly what the evening routine is. For example the routine could be as follows:
  - Teatime–toilet–activity–bath–clean teeth–toilet–bedtime.
  - This visual timetable could be placed somewhere that is easily accessed by the child and placed on a Velcro strip. Each step has a symbol and the child can remove the symbol and put it in an envelope as he or she finishes each step. These symbols can be made using the computer program Boardmaker, either at home or in the local library, or alternatively photographs can be used.
- **Provide the child with a social story:** A 'social story' can help children with ASD to understand the 'social rules' regarding sleep. For example, the story can include the concepts that everyone needs to sleep, of where to sleep, when to get up, and so on. A speech and language therapist or teacher may help carers develop a social story that is specific to a child.
- **Provide objects of reference:** These are everyday objects that can help a child with learning disability or ASD to communicate his or her needs/choices, particularly if the child is non-verbal. For example, a photo of the child's bed/bedroom or a certain blanket or cuddly toy could be introduced to indicate bedtime. With consistent use over time, the child will use that object to indicate that he or she wants to go to bed, or will realize that this object indicates what is happening next.
- **Continence:** The child should be encouraged to use the toilet during the evening before bed to reduce the chance of a wet or soiled nappy. Actively look for and manage constipation.
- **Winding/calming down:** 'Winding down' should start an hour before bedtime with turning off the television, switching off any stimulating music, avoiding lively play, and dimming the lights.
- **Temperature:** The bedroom should be kept at a constant temperature that is comfortable for the child. Using a room thermostat or a room thermometer as a guide can help.
- **Relaxation techniques:** Massage and/or relaxation music can be helpful in reducing any child's activity levels but this depends on the child's individual sensitivity.
- **Food and allergies:** A lot of sugar (e.g. sweets), caffeine (e.g. fizzy drinks) or additives (e.g. colourings in food/drink) should be avoided, especially before bed, as these may affect sleep.

Top tips for children's bedrooms

- Wherever possible the child should have their own bedroom and the following points need to be considered.

HEARING/NOISE

- Consider using thick carpets that deaden noises.
- Shut the bedroom door.
- Have the child's bedroom in a quieter part of the house. Consider noises from the bathroom and the position of the bed; avoid it being near pipes.
- A 'white noise', for example humming or a radio tuned out, may help.

VISION

- Use plain neutral or pastel colours that are not too intense or loud.
- Avoid visual displays on the walls.
- Keep the room clutter free: remove toys/television/PlayStation/Wii, and so on.
- Use the bedroom only for sleep – not for play.
- Use blackout blinds/curtains/shutters to block out the light.
- If the child is frightened of the dark, introduce a night light.
- If 'switch flicking' is a problem then remove the light bulb or consider having the switch moved to outside the bedroom door.

SMELL/TASTE

- Use odourless non-toxic paints/wallpaper paste.
- Avoid strong-smelling air fresheners and cleaning materials.

BED

- Would cot sides help? For 'climbers', a mattress on the floor with a safety gate at the door can be the best option.
- Make sure there is a good mattress cover.
- You can also get waterproof duvet covers.

TOUCH

- If the child likes deep pressure when being touched then think about heavy-weighted blankets that are tightly tucked in.
- If the child is hypersensitive to touch then have lighter bedding with a smooth surface.

Use of melatonin and other medication

Melatonin is a natural hormone which is involved in regulating the sleep–wake cycle. It can be helpful in sleep initiation and maintaining sleep in children with complex needs. It is unlicensed in children but has been used for a number of years with a good safety profile. Controlled-release melatonin can be used in children with predominant problems with sleep fragmentation (repeated awakenings) and early-morning awakenings. Various preparations (capsule, controlled release tablet, liquid) are available. Doses vary from as little as 0.3mg to 10mg and are given around 30 minutes before bedtime. Standard-release capsules and controlled-release capsules can be opened and mixed with normal-temperature or cold food to improve compliance. A mixture of controlled-release and standard-release preparations is sometimes successful. Melatonin should always be used in conjunction with good sleep hygiene measures. Another useful agent which can be tried is low-dose clonidine at bedtime. Sedatives such as chloral hydrate are best avoided but can be used with caution for a short period (3–5 days) to reset a disrupted sleep routine.

Further reading

Gringras P (2008) When to use drugs to help sleep. *Arch Dis Child* 93: 976–81. http://dx.doi.org/10.1136/adc.2007.128728

Gringras P, Gamble C, Jones AP et al. (MENDS Study Group) (2012) Melatonin for sleep problems in children with neurodevelopmental disorders: randomised double masked placebo controlled trial. *BMJ* 345: e6664. http://dx.doi.org/10.1136/bmj.e6664

Royal College of Paediatric and Child Health Working Party on Sleep Physiology and Respiratory Control Disorders in Childhood (2008) Standards for Services for Children with Disorders of Sleep Physiology. Available at: www.bprs.co.uk/documents/RCPCH_sleep_resp_cont_disorders.pdf (accessed 9 January 2013).

Stores G (2001) *A Clinical Guide to Sleep Disorders in Children and Adolescents*. Cambridge: Cambridge University Press.

Stores G (2009) Aspects of parasomnias in childhood and adolescence. *Arch Dis Child* 94: 63–9. http://dx.doi.org/10.1136/adc.2007.131631

Stores G, Wiggs L (2001) *Sleep Disturbance in Children and Adolescents with Disorders of Development*. London: Mac Keith Press.

Wiggs L (2009) Behavioural aspects of children's sleep. *Arch Dis Child* 94: 59–62. http://dx.doi.org/10.1136/adc.2007.125278

55
Continence

Gillian Robinson

Learning objectives

- To know how to assess and manage continence issues in children with disabilities.
- To be able to provide practical advice to parents and other professionals regarding continence issues in children with disabilities.

Key questions

- Can the child be continent? Is there any neurological/medical/surgical abnormality affecting sphincter control?
- Is the child functionally ready for bladder and bowel control?
  - Does the child know when he or she is wet or dirty?
  - Can the child be dry for an hour?
- Can they cooperate and communicate?
  - Does the child understand one-part commands, for example, 'Can you pass me the ball?'.
- Are there appropriate and accessible toileting facilities?
- Will the child have any physical difficulty in using the toilet?

Continence assessment

Bowels

Make sure the child is not constipated and if the child is, then treat this first. If the family are unclear then keeping a diary for a week can help (as shown in Table 55.1).

- Use the Bristol stool chart: anything harder than a sausage (grade 4) is abnormal.
- What is the frequency?
- What is the size: small (rabbit droppings), medium or large (blocking the toilet)?
- IS there any pain or withholding (jiggling on the spot) or any blood?
- Are there any symptoms suggesting overflow, for example offensive-smelling diarrhoea over which the child has not control?
- If the child is constipated, determine the age at onset.

Table 55.1 Continence assessment diary

Day	Bowels (record 7 days)			Bladder (record 3 days)	
Time	Type (Bristol stool chart)	Size Small (S) Medium (M) Large (L)	Where? Toilet (T) Pants or pad (P)	Size Small (S) Medium (M) Large (L)	Where? Toilet (T) Pants or pad (P)

Fluid intake

Does the child drink five to six glasses of fluids a day?
Good fluid intake is

4 to 8 years	1000ml to 1400ml per day
9 to 13 years	1400ml to 2100ml per day
14 to 18 years	2100ml to 3000ml per day

Past history

- The age at which the child passed meconium (if late, investigate)
- Constipation
- Urinary tract infections
- Any pica.

Development

- Is the child developmentally ready (around a cognitive level of 2 to 3 years)?
- Does the child have a way to communicate wet or dirty?

Emotional factors

- Are there any emotional or behavioural risk factors such as bullying, bereavement, neglect, abuse, friction between parent and child or challenging behaviour?
- Are any punitive measures taken when accidents occur?

Family history

- What was the age at which parents and siblings were dry, particularly at night?

Social situation

- Are there appropriately adapted toilets that are close by in all settings?
- Are there any family upheavals such as separation or financial difficulties?
- Is the child in different households with different rules, for example separated parents?

Examination

- Abdomen
  - faecal loading
  - palpable bladder
- Genitalia – any abnormality
- Anus
  - position of anus
  - anal abnormalities (fissure or skin tag at 12 o'clock may indicate a healed fissure)
  - anal tone – patulous anus? Soiling?
- Legs –any abnormal neurology including reflexes
- Spine – any markers for spina bifida occulta such as midline birth marks or lumps.

Investigation

Unless there are abnormal signs a routine investigation is not indicated.

Constipation

Constipation is a common problem and its causes and presentation can vary with the developmental stage of the child (Table 55.2). Clearly, in the disabled population this may not be at typical ages for a variety of reasons which are explained in Table 55.3.

Table 55.2 Causes of constipation during childhood developmental stages

Developmental stage	Problem	Causes
Infant	Diet and fluids	Poor feeding Milk intolerance
Toddler	Diet Perianal pain Oppositional behaviour	Food fads Food intolerance Anal fissure
Preschool	Learned avoidance – withholding stool	If + urine consider neuropathic bladder Stool withholding – behaviour Poor compliance
School age	Faecal retention	Poor compliance Behaviour problem School problems including bullying

Table 55.3 Specific developmental conditions with higher risk of continence problems

Condition	Problem
Spina bifida	Neuropathic bowels
Cerebral palsy Neuromuscular diseases	Decreased voluntary movement – particularly abdominal muscles Decreased fluid intake and food with low fibre content Possibly of disordered autonomic function; slow bowel
Autism	Rigidities about bowel habit, e.g. wants to have nappy on to open bowels, will only pass in a chosen place, etc.
Learning difficulty	Inability to learn toileting routine
Williams syndrome	Hypercalcaemia, hypercalciuria, dehydration

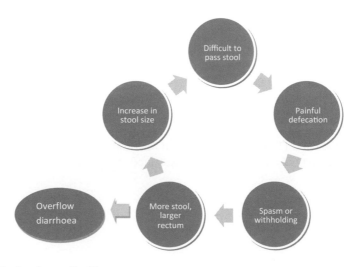

Figure 55.1 Cycle of constipation.

Principles of care

- Talk to the family about childhood constipation (see Fig. 55.1).
- Discuss the need for regular treatment that is ongoing for a number of months or years. Stopping treatment early can lead to a 're-accumulation' of the problem, while persisting with treatment will slowly allow resolution of rectal distension and return of gut muscle tone.
- Always consider if the child needs a 'clearance' regimen at the start.
- Families need support in finding the correct dose – time spent on weekly or fortnightly telephone calls can pay long-term dividends.
- Try not to change maintenance treatment more than weekly or you will never be sure what the effect of the previous change was. A management plan is shown in Figure 55.2.

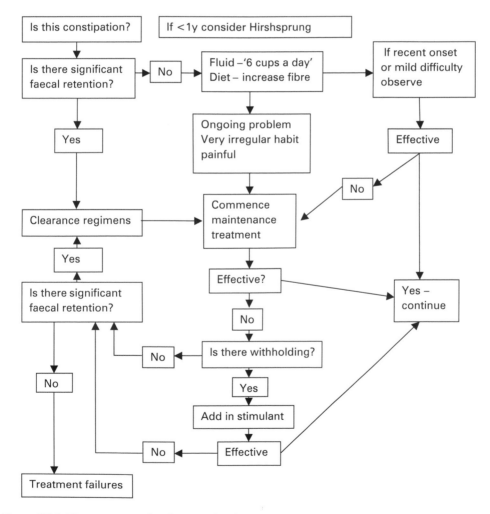

Figure 55.2 Management plan for constipation.

Faecal impaction: clearance regimens

If there is faecal loading then this needs to be cleared if you are going to have success. If the child passes occasional massive stools it might be worth waiting for this before starting treatment, as this will decrease the amount of treatment needed and mess created.

ORAL TREATMENT

Oral treatment is likely to precipitate overflow diarrhoea and this needs to be explained to the family – it is going to get worse before it gets better. Going back into pull-ups or nappies during this period may help.

Movicol paediatric plain sachets contain polyethylene glycol, which is usually effective in a bowel clearance regimen. Preferably, this can be taken orally or via gastrostomy, but a nasogastric route is also possible. Treatment must continue until the stool is a smooth gravy consistency for 24 hours. Stool that is granular or has lumps implies that there continues to be a faecal mass which is being eroded by the passing diarrhoea. The maximum duration is for this treatment is 7 days (NICE 2010a).

SUPPOSITORIES AND ENEMAS

The advantage of a rectal route for treatment is that it decreases the amount of loose stool and allows more control of stooling; however, thought should be given to how acceptable this is as a treatment method. Different treatment options include

- bisacodyl suppositories
- sodium citrate – Micolette or Relaxit microlax enema
- phosphate enema.

MANUAL EVACUATION

This method of treatment can be used when all else fails.

Maintenance treatment

Treatment needs to be regular and ongoing to keep the rectum clear, or the problem merely recurs. Most parents do not want their children on ongoing treatment, so this needs to be explained and encouraged. If the rectum is regularly emptied, then the rectal size will usually steadily decrease, and with it the need for treatment.

BEHAVIOUR

It is helpful for the parents to establish regular times when the child will sit on the toilet for 5 minutes, when 'success' is most likely; this is usually 20 minutes after breakfast or the evening meal. A number of children can achieve regular 'potting' with this method without being toilet trained.

ORAL MEDICATION

Softeners can be used that will soften the stool and make it more comfortable to pass; for example, polyethylene glycol – Movicol paediatric (most effective), docusate sodium and lactulose.

Stimulants that can be used include sodium picosulphate (very effective and the child needs to take only a small volume), docusate sodium and senna. Stimulant laxatives are given once a day with the aim of achieving a regular and predictable bowel action. Usually senna is given in the evenings to increase the chance of a stool 12 hours later, whereas picosulphate appears to have a rather more rapid action.

RECTAL TREATMENTS

SUPPOSITORIES

- Bisacodyl
- glycerine.

Rectal treatments are not popular with children or parents; however, for children with ongoing soiling for many years they can allow the child to be clean for the first time, and then everyone feels they are worthwhile. Rectal treatments also have a role in children with neuropathic bowels, as they stimulate reflex action and the child can become clean.

ENEMAS

- Microlette
- Phosphate

Stopping treatment

The rule of thumb is that you need to treat the child for the same length of time as the preceding duration of the problem. A weaning dose should be tried every 3 to 6 months, but if constipation returns then promptly return to treatment. In the case of children with neurodevelopmental disorders, the underlying difficulties often persist and therefore you should anticipate ongoing treatment.

Treatment failure

- Poor compliance: The child or the child's parents or carer may refuse to comply with toilet sitting, medications, or clean-out procedures, undermining the fundamental principles of most treatment protocols. Sometimes parents may be reluctant to administer long-term medication and may stop the treatment.
- Abdominal radiography does not have a role in the initial assessment of constipation. It can occasionally be useful to determine if the problem is overflow or constipation, particularly if the child has been on faecal softeners for some time, in which case abdominal examination becomes less reliable. Demonstrating to families the loaded colon can also be helpful when compliance is an issue. Every radiograph needs adequate justification.

- If the constipation does not respond to treatment after 6 months then consider taking bloods to check for calcium, thyroid function and coeliac screen to exclude rarer causes.
- Consider abuse.
- Peristeen is an anal irrigation system that can be used at home, either self-administered or administered by a parent. It uses an anal catheter to introduce lukewarm tap water into the rectum. The user sits on the toilet while the water is pumped into the rectum. The water is then emptied from the bowel, along with the stools, into the toilet. This takes around 30 minutes and needs to be done approximately every other day. This system can be useful, particularly when predictability of bowel movements becomes important (e.g. a teenager who wants to be able to control his or her bowels).
- If all of the above fail, refer the patient for paediatric surgical assessment. Possible treatment options include anal dilatation, internal anal myectomy, intrasphincteric botulinum toxin injections and antegrade continence enema (ACE or Malone) stoma.

> **Top tips**
>
> - Treat early and treat sufficiently.
> - If you are going to succeed the rectum needs to be fully emptied.
> - Make sure the child is drinking plenty of fluids.
> - Explain to the child and parents about the long-term nature of treatment.

Soiling

Key questions

- Is this overflow?
- How is the family managing the soiling? Is the child getting attention for inappropriate behaviours?
- Is this deliberate encopresis (usually full stool in pants or clearly inappropriate place)?

Management

- **Explanation:**
  - If the problem is overflow, explain to the child's carers that soiling is an inevitable consequence of an overfull rectum. The rectum continues to contract on the stool which leads to a reflex relaxation of the internal sphincter. This leads to liquid stool leaking out of the anus. The child has no control over this and is not to blame or lazy.
- **Medication:**
  - Treat any concomitant constipation.
- **Toileting:**
  - All activities around continence must be in the bathroom.
  - Regular 'pottying' or sitting on the toilet for 5 minutes should take place around 20 minutes after breakfast or the evening meal. The child should sit in a comfortable posture.

Sometimes a step will help.
- Focus on toilet sitting and have reward charts or stickers for this.
- The cleaning up process should be without fuss. Older and more able children should be involved in the clean-up process. For example, putting solid stool down the toilet, 'the first wipe', or putting the soiled underwear into a bucket can help encourage cleanliness.
- The subtle availability of 'incontinence rescue packs' at school should be provided.
- Celebrations for stool in the toilet.

- Other thoughts:
  - A social story about toileting may help (e.g. see: http://kidscandream.webs.com).
  - 'Sneaky Poo' is a narrative therapy involving a story for families about how a character called Sneaky Poo comes to attack the child and cause them problems. This externalizes the problem from the child and offers the opportunity for the family to unite to beat Sneaky Poo (see www.narrativetherapylibrary.com/img/ps/spoo2.pdf). Families will usually need support to implement this therapy.

Encopresis and smearing

Encopresis comprises deliberate passage of stool in an inappropriate place.

- **Try to understand why:**
  - Is it deliberate – a form of protest?
  - Doe the child dislike the sensation of a soiled nappy?
  - Does the child like the sensation of a warm stool on his or her hands?
- **Management:**
  - Completing a bladder and bowel chart may help to understand why the problem is occurring.
  - As for soiling, ensure that there is minimal fuss about the tidying-up process.
  - Try to establish a regular bowel pattern with regular toileting sitting so that the stool goes in the toilet. Stimulants may help with this.
  - If it is 'exploratory play', particularly at night, a popper vest or all-in-one swimsuit over the pad and/or a back-fastening sleepsuit (Houdini suit) will make it much more difficult.
  - Ask for help from psychology.

Day-time wetting management

- **Is the child ready?**
  - Is the child developmentally ready (around a 2- to 3y functional level)?
  - Does the child have awareness of bladder sensation?
  - Complete a bladder and bowel diary: the child needs to by dry for at least an hour.
  - If the child was previously dry, perform a urinalysis.
- **Sensible steps**
  - If there is any associated constipation, treat it.
  - Ensure that there is adequate fluid intake: six glasses a day – but no fizzy drinks (ask the family to write down every time a full glass of fluid is drunk within a period of 2d).
  - Ensure that there is minimal fuss about the clean-up process and ensure emergency clothing at school.

- Are there any issues around toilets, particularly at school?
- Is clothing easy to remove? Consider elasticated waist bands.
- Make sure the child stays on the toilet until his or her bladder is empty. Teach the child double micturition ('trying to wee again after you have finished').
- **Management**
  - Give the child a reward for toilet sitting or passing urine on the toilet, using reward charts or stickers.
  - Consider regular toileting every hour. When this is achieved, then increase by 10-minute increments (you can buy vibrating reminder watches to help with this).
  - If there is marked frequency and urgency then consider oxybutynin.
  - Consider a body-worn moisture alarm.
  - For males with 'inaccurate aim', a ping pong ball in the toilet they need to try to 'sink' can help.
  - Excellent information for families is available from the Education and Resources for Improving Childhood continence (ERIC) website (www.eric.org.uk).

Night-time wetting (nocturnal enuresis)

- **Is the child ready?**
  - Bedwetting is common; it is not the child's fault and punitive measures should not be used.
  - Is the child developmentally ready to be dry at night? Remember that 20% of typically developing 4-year-olds and 8% of 9-year-olds will not be dry. Typically developing children would not be treated until 7 years of age and functioning around that level is probably a useful marker for children with learning difficulties.
  - Progress will not be made with a child in pads.
  - Assess the child or young person's readiness and progress:
    - How many nights a week does bedwetting occur?
    - How many times a night does bedwetting occur?
    - Does there seem to be a large amount of urine?
    - At what times of night does the bedwetting occur?
    - Does the child or young person wake up after bedwetting?
- **Sensible steps:**
  - Make it easy to change bedding by using a waterproof mattress and duvet covers.
  - Ensure sufficient fluids: six glasses a day, but none in the hour prior to bed time.
  - Reward charts should be used for actions within the child's control. For example, drinking and toileting during the day should be rewarded, rather than dry nights, which are beyond the child's control.
  - Discuss with the parents that waking and lifting does not lead to dryness.
  - Discuss night-time sleep arrangements and access to a toilet.
- **Treatment:**
  - *Moisture alarm*: 70% of children improve with use of a moisture alarm but the family needs to be motivated as it involves waking up the house and changing bedding in the middle of the night.
  - **Medication:**
    - desmopressin (synthetic vasopressin) – short-term improvement, often not sustained
    - oxybutynin (anticholineric)

- imipramine (tricyclic antidepressant)
- see NICE guidance on nocturnal enuresis (NICE 2010b).

Excellent information is also available for families from the ERIC website (www.eric.org.uk).

References

Clayden GS, Keshtgar AD, Carcani-Rathwell I, Abhyankar A (2005) The management of chronic constipation and related faecal incontinence in childhood. *Arch Dis Child Educ Pract Ed* 90: ep58-ep67. http://dx.doi.org/10.1136/adc.2004.066019

NICE (2010a) *Constipation in Children and Young People*. Available at: www.nice.org.uk/nicemedia/live/12993/48754/48754.pdf (accessed 7 November 2012).

NICE (2010b) *Nocturnal Enuresis: The Management of Bedwetting in Children and Young People*. Available at: ww.nice.org.uk/nicemedia/live/13246/51382.pdf (accessed 25 November 2012).

Further reading

DLF (Disabled Living Foundation) (2005) *Choosing Children's Daily Living Equipment*. Available at: www.dlf.org.uk/factsheets/Choosing_childrens_daily_living_equipment.pdf (accessed 7 November 2012).

Websites

Education Resources for Improving Childhood continence (ERIC): http://www.eric.org.uk/

Tough going (parent and family information along with the local pathway): www.refhelp.scot.nhs.uk/dmdocuments/Paediatric_GI/guidelines%20for%20management%20of%20idiopathic%20childhood%20constipation.pdf (accessed 13 December 2012).

56
Bathing

Gillian Robinson

Equipment required for bathing that is assessed by occupational therapy includes

- low-tech aids such as a non-slip mat, foam support, grab rails or bath board (a board that sits on the edges of a bath and allows a shower to be used)
- facilities for changing
- supportive bath seats for children without stable sitting
- hoists for larger children to get in and out of the bath
- showers, which may be easier to use in a wet room, particularly for older children.

Bath time

- Have a warm bathroom.
- Tell children what is about to happen. For children with limited communication, using an object of reference such as a bath sponge, which is shown to the child before bathing, can help.
- For children with increased tone, being held in a flexed posture or having a seat that helps the child to be in a flexed posture will help.
- Bath time is a great time for play and learning:
  - The child may be more able in water and can enjoy grasping toys.
  - Talking and singing at bath time helps with vocabulary.
  - Simple bath toys include plastic jugs and empty bottles and containers.
- A laminated card prompting young people about how to bathe can help build independence.

Further reading

DLF (Disabled Living Foundation) (2005) *Choosing Children's Daily Living Equipment*. Available at: www.dlf.org.uk/factsheets/Choosing_childrens_daily_living_equipment.pdf (accessed 7 November 2012).

57
Oral hygiene

Gillian Robinson

Oral hygiene is a greater problem for children with disabilities for the following reasons:

- The underlying condition can increase problems with oral health, for example mouth breathing in Down syndrome and gastro-oesophageal reflux leading to oral abrasion in cerebral palsy.
- Medications in syrup form and high-energy feeds increase dental caries.
- Difficulties in carers performing good oral hygiene owing to either physical factors, such as bite reflex in cerebral palsy, or communication or behavioural problems such as autistic spectrum disorder.
- Teeth grinding resulting in attrition.
- Difficulties in accessing appropriate dental care.

Consequences of poor oral hygiene include

- dental pain, which can also present as self-injurious behaviour
- difficulties in eating and speaking
- social integration can be inhibited
- a poor self-image.

How to help with good oral hygiene

- Avoid oral hypersensitivity: encourage a programme that involves the touching of face and lips, particularly for children who are not orally fed.
- Ensure good hydration.
- Encourage good dietary habits: low amounts of processed sugar.
- Use sugar-free medications.
- Advise on the appropriate use of fluoride: this can be in the local water supply or, if not, advice on the use of fluoride supplements should be given.

- From 6 years of age children should use an adult variety of fluoridated toothpaste.
- Position the child well before teeth brushing in a flexed posture, particularly with the neck flexed.
- A soft toothbrush and toothpaste should be provided for the child to brush his or her teeth at least once a day. Some children, particularly children with cerebral palsy, find electric toothbrushes easier.
- The dentist may apply fissure sealants.
- For severe teeth grinding dental guards can help, but compliance can be an issue.

Tips for reluctant teeth brushers

- Tell the child that you are going to brush their teeth and use the toothbrush as a visual clue.
- Have brief sessions of teeth brushing.
- Having a mirror so the young person can see what is going on can be helpful.
- Use distractions such as music and videos.
- Try to have two carers, one to clean the teeth and the other to hold the person's hands to prevent interference (e.g. clapping game).
- If the child is learning to brush their teeth a 'cartoon checklist' of different stages can be used as a prompt.
- Use of chlorhexidine mouthwash or spray over short periods can be beneficial.

Dental treatment

If the local family dentist is struggling to meet the child's needs then using a specialist dental service who has more experience, specific equipment (e.g. a device to tip the wheelchair) and longer appointment slots can help. For treatment, sedation or general anaesthetic may well be needed. Guidelines on this topic have been written by the British Society for Disability and Oral Health and are available online (BSDOH 2001).

Reference

BSDOH (British Society for Disability and Oral Health) (2001) *Clinical Guidelines and Integrated Care Pathways for the Oral Health Care of People with Learning Disabilities*. Available at: www.bsdh.org.uk/guidelines/Dianatru.pdf (accessed 7 November 2012).

58
Dressing

Gillian Robinson

Helping with dressing skills does take time and patience. It helps the child not only with learning dressing skills, but also body awareness, balance, movement and language, if you talk to them whilst dressing (e.g. put your arm down here).

Choosing clothes

- Choose loose-fitting comfortable clothes with wide neck and arm holes.
- Avoid fiddly fastenings such as buttons: use garments with elastic and Velcro instead. You can change a button to Velcro without this being obvious if you sew the button onto the top flap of clothing. For cuffs you can use elastic so that the cuff does not need to be undone.
- Avoid slippery garments.
- If there are zips, a loop of ribbon or a curtain ring can help make this easier to pull.
- Tube socks are easier than ones with heels.
- Have a label to identify the back or have clothes that have a design on the front.
- Mark the inside border of each shoe with a permanent marker and teach the child that these must go together.

Before starting to dress

- Ensure that the child is in a good position:
  - If the child has cerebral palsy, do not lie them down flat to get dressed as this will increase their tone. Use a flexed posture either by placing a pillow under the child's head and keeping the hips and knees flexed, or by lying the child over a parent's knee, with the child face down.
  - If the child's sitting is not stable, then sit behind the child, if necessary stabilizing their hips, or use a wall or corner to help the child sit.
  - If the child is sitting on a chair make sure their feet are on the floor.

- If the child has one affected limb, put the clothes on that limb first.
- Have a mirror so that the child can see what is happening and also so he or she can identify his or her own mistakes and correct them.

Teaching dressing

- Do not hurry the child.
- Success is important: break down dressing into small steps and praise for achieving a step.
- Tackle one step at a time and give help where needed with the other steps of the task.
- Encourage the child to do as much as he or she can for themselves.
- Follow a consistent sequence and technique when dressing:
  - Clothes can be placed in a pile in the order in which they need to be put on.
  - Follow the same technique for each garment, for example a T-shirt is put over the head first and then the arms are put through the sleeves.
  - There are two main techniques:
    - *Backward chaining*, in which the adult begins the task, with the child doing only the last step. Gradually the adult does less as the child is able to do more of the task themselves. This way the child always gets the reward of finishing the task. For example, the adult puts the T-shirt over the child's head and helps them to get their arms through the holes. The child then pulls down the T-shirt at the front.
    - *Forward chaining*, in which the child starts the task (e.g. putting the T-shirt over their head), and the adult helps with the later stages that the child needs help with (e.g. putting their arms through the sleeves). The child needs to be motivated to begin the task themselves.

59
Optimizing participation: the role of assistive technology

Benita Powrie

Assistive technology is a broad term that applies to all devices designed to enable people with disabilities (WHO 2001). These range from simple jar openers to sophisticated communication aids with integrated computers or extensive home modifications with automated environmental controls. Assistive devices can play a significant role in optimizing the participation of young people with complex disabilities in all aspects of life (Chantry and Dunford 2010, Murchland and Parkyn 2010).

Independence in all activities, even if technically possible, is not necessarily desirable. Independently completing self-care tasks can consume a lot of time and energy that could be used for preferred occupations which contribute more to overall quality of life. The emphasis should therefore be on enhancing participation in activities valued by the young person and family (Salminen 2008, Chantry and Dunford 2010).

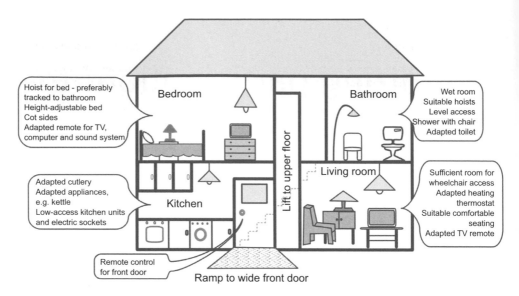

Hoist for bed - preferably tracked to bathroom
Height-adjustable bed
Cot sides
Adapted remote for TV, computer and sound system

Bedroom

Bathroom

Wet room
Suitable hoists
Level access
Shower with chair
Adapted toilet

Adapted cutlery
Adapted appliances, e.g. kettle
Low-access kitchen units and electric sockets

Kitchen

Lift to upper floor

Living room

Sufficient room for wheelchair access
Adapted heating thermostat
Suitable comfortable seating
Adapted TV remote

Remote control for front door

Ramp to wide front door

Figure 59.1 Range of aids and adaptations to enable participation.

There are a huge range of aids and adaptations, from cheap items that all families can afford to very expensive and technical pieces of equipment (Fig. 59.1 and Table 59.1). It is important for the correct choices to be made, and this often requires a team of professionals with appropriate skills and experience.

Case vignette

Peter is 15 years old and in Year 10 at his local high school, where he is performing well academically, especially in his favourite subjects of history and science. At home, he likes to relax in his room, watching horror movies and listening to thrash metal music. He enjoys attending gigs as often as possible, and is writing his own lyrics and music. He has joined a film-making club, where he prefers directing to acting. He also enjoys cooking, specializing in soups and cakes. Peter competes with Luke, his younger brother, on PlayStation sports games and chases his younger sister with his remote control car.

Peter has dystonic cerebral palsy. He has some voluntary head and eye movement, but no functional control of his limbs or trunk and no speech. He uses a head switch to control his powerchair, his communication aid with integrated computer, and devices such as the Powerlink™, which enables mains-powered items such as food processors to be switch operated. His environmental control unit controls all his bedroom equipment, including DVD, television, stereo, fan and lamp, with a switch and scanner. His adapted remote-control car is operated by motion-sensitive switches mounted on a hat. His home and car are fully modified so that he has full access and his family can support his needs safely. His multidisciplinary, multiagency team is working together with him and his family to ensure that his needs are being met as he grows and develops.

Table 59.1 Common appliances/adaptations that improve function and participation

	Example	*Staff involved in advice*
Home	Level access or appropriate lifts Widened doorways Turning room for wheelchair Electric sockets at appropriate height Automatic front door opener with camera Environmental controls, e.g. adapted iPod to operate lighting, temperature, television and curtains	Occupational therapy Rehabilitation engineer Architect Builder
School	Level access or appropriate lifts Sufficient space for wheelchair Height-adjustable tables Appropriate hygiene facilities Adapted computer to record classwork	Teaching Occupational therapy Rehabilitation engineer
Mobility and seating	Walking aids Powered wheelchairs Manual wheelchairs Adapted cars	Wheelchair services Physiotherapy Occupational therapy Independent living centres
Communication	Communication aids, either paper or computer based Adapted computers to enable writing and texting Switch-operated mobile phones Mobile phone applications for communication	Speech and language therapy Occupational therapy
Toileting	Toilet support seats and frames Changing plinths Toilet with automatic bidet and drying facility	Occupational therapy
Bathing	Bath supports, seats or hammocks Hoists and tracking (to take child to bedroom) Adjustable height for baths and basins Shower with shower chair in wet room	Occupational therapy
Eating	Adapted cutlery Eating systems, e.g. Neater Eater	Occupational therapy
Food preparation	Kitchen adapted utensils – jar openers, kettle tipper, rocker knife Switch-operated unit for food processors Height-adjustable sink and cook-top	Occupational therapy
Leisure	E-books PlayStation switch adaptor Remote-control car with head movement switch Computer with adapted controls and software Switch-adapted toys Music-making equipment, e.g. Soundbeam	Occupational therapy

How to make assistive technology work

Assistive technology provision for children with complex needs works best when all of the agencies involved with the child work together in an integrated process with clear multiagency planning around provision, set-up, training and support (McCarty and Morress 2009). This is becoming increasingly important as technology advances, which enables the use of mainstream products and also one base product to access many devices (van Woerden 2006, Vanderheiden 2007).

It is important to balance the likely gains in using assistive technology with the possible costs involved, and to ensure that all efforts are made to promote positive outcomes.

Assessment needs to include

- Identification of aspirations, values and priorities of the young person and family.
- Clearly identified goals.
- A focus on participation, not just independence.
- Multiprofessional and multiagency input as appropriate.
- Planning around provision, set-up, training and support.
- Balancing the anticipated benefits against the cost of the equipment and effort required to use it.
- Clarification regarding who has financial liability for insurance, servicing and replacement of equipment.
- Support provided to access charity funding for technology not available through statutory bodies (Desch et al. 2008, McCarty and Morress 2009).

Support needs to include

- Ensuring that everyone is trained; children with disabilities are likely to have had less access to technology and therefore will be less confident (Desch et al. 2008).
- Maintenance that is easy and quick for families to access.
- Regular backup and maintenance to avoid breakdowns, which would have implications ranging from inconvenience, such as the inability to contribute to a lesson, to catastrophic, such as physical harm, or loss of vital coursework.
- Regular reviews to ensure that equipment is still appropriate.

Assistive technology to support carers

Assisting young people with daily care tasks is physically demanding and over time it can have a serious impact on carer health and well-being (Raina et al. 2005). Home modifications and specialist equipment are critical in supporting young people and their families. Many families initially resist equipment for many reasons. They may still be coming to terms with their child's disability, and having a through-floor lift in the middle of the living room, or ceiling track hoist in the bathroom, may feel too clinical and confronting (Heywood 2005). Hoisting with equipment can be slow and impersonal so parents often prefer to lift and carry their child much longer than their professional support team would like, and the child may also prefer this (Østensjø et al. 2005). These issues need to be addressed with sensitivity, respecting the family's preferences and supporting them through any changes (Shepherd et al. 2007). A family's recognition of the need for equipment often arises suddenly, as a result of carer injury or other health problems. It is important that professionals are proactive in identifying and anticipating needs as expensive and bulky equipment or adaptions will not be immediately available.

Problems with assistive technology

It needs to be recognized that assistive technology can also be a major source of frustration and disappointment, leading expensive equipment to be abandoned.

Common problems include

- unreliable performance
- lack of confidence and competence in operation
- unmet expectations
- inappropriate provision (Copley and Ziviani 2004, Desch et al. 2008)
- increased isolation owing to withdrawal of valued human assistance (Gatward 2004)
- Person-centred assessment, support and partnership working will avoid or minimise these problems, and ensure that assistive technology provision supports children and young people to reach their full potential.

Key messages

- Assistive technology can increase participation in all aspects of daily life.
- Assistive technology must be centred on the values and priorities of the person.
- Outcome measurements should focus on participation rather than independence.
- Integrated multiagency working will promote more efficient and effective equipment provision.
- Ongoing successful use of equipment relies on follow-up, training, backup and maintenance.
- Assistive technology supports carer well being, but requires sensitive introduction.

References

Chantry J, Dunford C (2010) How do computer assistive technologies enhance participation in childhood occupations for children with multiple and complex disabilities? A review of the literature. *Br J Occup Ther* 73: 351–68. http://dx.doi.org/10.4276/030802210X12813483277107

Copley J, Ziviani J (2004) Barriers to the use of assistive technology for children with multiple disabilities. *Occup Ther Int* 11: 229–43. http://dx.doi.org/10.1002/oti.213

Desch LW, Gaebler-Spira D, Council on Children With Disabilities (2008) Prescribing assistive-technology systems: focus on children with impaired communication. *Pediatrics* 121: 1271–80. http://dx.doi.org/10.1542/peds.2008–0695

Gatward J (2004) Electronic assistive technology: benefits for all? *Housing, Care and Support* 7: 13–17. http://dx.doi.org/10.1108/14608790200400026

Heywood F (2005) Adaptation: altering the house to restore the home. *Housing Stud* 20: 531–547. http://dx.doi.org/10.1080/02673030500114409

McCarty E, Morress C (2009) Establishing access to technology: an evaluation and intervention model to increase participation of children with cerebral palsy. *Phys Med Rehabil Clin N Am* 20: 523–34. http://dx.doi.org/10.1016/j.pmr.2009.05.001

Murchland S, Parkyn H (2010) Using assistive devices for schoolwork: the experiences of children with disabilities. *Disabil Rehabil Assist Technol* 5: 438–47. http://dx.doi.org/10.3109/17483107.2010.481773

Østensjø S, Carlberg EB, Vøllestad NK (2005) The use and impact of assistive devices and other environmental modifications on everyday activities and care in young children with cerebral palsy. *Disabil Rehabil* 27: 849–61. http://dx.doi.org/10.1080/09638280400018619

Raina P, O'Donnell M, Rosenbaum P et al. (2005) The health and well-being of caregivers of children with cerebral palsy. *Pediatrics* 115: e626–36. http://dx.doi.org/10.1542/peds.2004–1689

Salminen A-L (2008) European research related to assistive technology for disabled children. *Technol Disabil* 20: 173–8.

Shepherd A, Stewart H, Murchland S (2007) Mothers' perceptions of the introduction of a hoist into the family home of children with physical disabilities. *Disabil Rehabil Assist Technol* 2: 117–25. http://dx.doi.org/10.1080/17483100601174293

Vanderheiden GC (2007) Redefining assistive technology, accessibility and disability based on recent technological advances. *J Technol Hum Serv* 25: 147–58. http://dx.doi.org/10.1300/J017v25n01_10

van Woerden, K (2006) Mainstream developments in ICT: why are they important for assistive technology? *Technol Disabil* 18: 15–18.

WHO (World Health Organization) (2001) *International Classification of Functioning, Disability and Health.* Geneva: World Health Organization. Available at: http://www.who.int/classifications/icf/en/ (accessed 7 November 2012).

Further reading

Disabled Living Foundation (2005) *Choosing Children's Daily Living Equipment.* Available at: www.dlf.org.uk/factsheets/Choosing_childrens_daily_living_equipment.pdf (accessed 7 November 2012).

Judge S, Robertson Z, Hawley M, Enderby P (2009) Speech-driven environmental control systems – a qualitative analysis of users' perceptions. *Disabil Rehabil Assist Technol* 4: 151–7. http://dx.doi.org/10.1080/17483100802715100

60
Puberty

Anne M Kelly

Learning objectives

- To understand the issues surrounding puberty, sexuality and reproduction in children and young people with disabilities.
- To know how to manage pubertal disorders and contraception needs in children with disabilities.
- To understand the importance of sex education for children and young people with disabilities and to know where to access relevant training material.

The parents or carers of children with a disability may have concerns about the onset of puberty for the following reasons:

- the timing of onset
- the timing of menarche and worries around managing periods
- the need for contraception
- the risk of sexual abuse
- the risk of unplanned pregnancy
- the risk of sexually transmitted infections.

In the UK, the onset of puberty in children occurs between the age of 8 years 6 months and 13 years in females and between 9 and 14 years in males. While precocious puberty is more common in females with neurological abnormalities such as hydrocephalus, menarche occurs at a similar time in most females with learning disabilities as in those females without neurological disability. Pubertal onset occurs slightly earlier in Caucasian females who have cerebral palsy, but menarche is a little later, with a median age of 14 years compared with 12.8 years in the typically developing population. Menarche also tends to occur slightly later in females who have a diagnosis of autism.

Parents may express some of the following concerns in relation to menstruation.

* Worries around behaviour related to pad usage or the physical difficulties involved in changing.
* Difficulty interpreting the fluctuations in mood, the level of discomfort and presence of other symptoms related to periods because of the difficulties communicating with their daughter.

Health staff should be aware that

* Menorrhagia can cause or contribute towards iron deficiency and may even lead to severe anaemia.
* Medication used in this group can cause irregular periods. Anticonvulsants such as sodium valproate may increase the rate of clearance of oestrogen by induction of the hepatic P-450 system. Antipsychotic agents such as risperidone can cause hyperprolactinaemia, which is associated with menstrual disturbance.

Menstrual management and contraception

Useful strategies for menstrual management include the following:

* Analgesia for dysmenorrhoea such as paracetamol, ibuprofen, mefanamic acid.
* Menorrhagia or irregular periods can be managed by regulating the menstrual cycle which, at the same time, will reduce menstrual losses. The following interventions can help achieve this:
  * *The combined oral contraceptive pill* (OCP). Extended or continuous regimens will reduce or stop menstruation. Risks include
    - An increased embolic risk in patients with reduced mobility and wheelchair use.
    - Possible interactions with other medications such as anticonvulsants (e.g. sodium valproate). This will reduce the efficacy of the contraceptive.
    - There are still concerns about the increased risk of breast and cervical cancer.
  * *Depot preparation of medroxyprogesterone acetate* (Depo-Provera injections, 150mg every 12 weeks given intramuscularly). This intervention is used particularly in the learning-disabled female in whom the risk of unprotected intercourse is high and the OCP is not suitable because it may not be taken reliably. Possible long-term effects include reduction in bone mineral density. Bone health in the disabled is of concern as there are multiple factors that may adversely affect it. These include:
    - Reduced weightbearing exercise because of limited mobility or wheelchair use.
    - Poor vitamin D levels because of poor diet, lack of exposure to sunlight and use of some anticonvulsants which adversely affect levels.
    - Reduced calcium intake caused by feeding difficulties. Calcium and vitamin D intake must be monitored whilst on Depo-Provera and supplements provided together with oestrogen replacement if necessary.

- *Progestogen-only pill (POP) or implantable device.* Both of these may be associated with irregular bleeding and weight gain. Implantable devices are rarely used. Norethisterone 5mg is a commonly prescribed POP. It can be used continuously to suppress menstruation. POP efficacy is reduced by enzyme-inducing drugs such as carbamazepine.
- *Levonorgestrel-releasing intrauterine system* (Mirena coil). This device provides good contraception for up to 5 years with very low risks of uterine perforation, infection or transient irregular bleeding. Periods are reduced but not eliminated. A general anaesthetic is likely to be required for insertion; therefore, this intervention is not often considered.
- *Surgery:*
  - Endometrial ablation: This is an invasive form of surgery, will require a general anaesthetic and may need to be repeated. It has no contraceptive effect.
  - Hysterectomy: This is major surgery and will cause permanent sterility. It is rarely necessary and would be considered only when medical treatment has failed for persistent and distressing symptoms. Consent for surgery requires approval of a High Court judge, as consent cannot be taken from parents alone. Historically, sterilization of young women with learning disabilities was carried out on eugenic grounds. This is now considered to be unethical.

The reasons underlying requests should be carefully explored before recommending an intervention. Input should be considered only if the presenting problem is severe enough to cause significant distress to the young person after all the usual educational and symptomatic approaches have been tried.

> ## Key messages regarding menstruation and contraception
>
> - There are no long-term interventions that exist to completely suppress menstruation without the possibility of adverse consequences.
> - Referral on to a gynaecologist with a special interest in managing these issues in young females with a disability may be required to provide an expert opinion for carers.
> - In practice, relatively few young people require medical intervention. For the majority, education provided by parents, teachers, special school nursing staff and the learning disability nursing team is sufficient to reassure young people and their parents.

Precocious puberty

Precocious and early puberty are defined as true puberty with onset before the age of 8 years in females and 9 years in males. Precocious puberty is relatively common in females (1 in 1000), in whom it is usually idiopathic, and uncommon in males, in whom there is a much higher chance of pathology.

Early and precocious puberty may occur in association with central nervous system (CNS) disorders such as

- myelomeningocele (spina bifida) and hydrocephalus

- severe cerebral palsy
- following on from periventricular haemorrhage related to preterm birth.

Twenty per cent of females with myelomeningocele experience accelerated pubertal maturation because of increased gonadotrophin secretion, possibly resulting from non-physiological variations in intracranial pressure. Those who experienced early surges in pressure are more likely to be affected.

Young people with a condition associated with early puberty should have their pubertal status and growth closely monitored in order to detect early pubertal changes. Arm span can be used to measure growth instead of linear growth, as height is likely to be inaccurate in wheelchair users.

Precocious puberty in a socially immature female with a disability is a challenge because of the obvious physical and emotional changes that it engenders. Treatment when needed is with gonadotrophin-releasing hormone analogue (e.g. goserelin) given as a depot injection subcutaneously. This blocks pubertal development and can be used to halt puberty. This will reduce the potential distress in the child and parent related to fears about early menstruation, physical maturation and sexual vulnerability.

Fertility

Fertility in females with myelomeningocele is generally preserved but is reduced in males. Affected females have a 5% risk of having children with neural tube defects but this risk can be reduced by 50% by providing folate supplementation for at least 3 months before and during the first month of pregnancy. The need for pre-pregnancy counselling for such females is obvious and should not be overlooked because of incorrect preconceptions that fertility is low and that the chances of such an occurrence are therefore slim. The other option is to offer 4mg of folate daily to females of childbearing age with this condition, routinely.

Delayed puberty and primary amenorrhoea

Delayed puberty is defined as the absence of secondary sexual characteristics beyond the age at which 95% of children of that sex and culture have begun sexual maturation. For females this occurs at the age of 12 years and for males, 14 years. Typically, females begin with breast budding at the age of 11 years, menstruate by 13 years and finish growing by 15 years. Males start later, at around 12 years of age, with increase in penis and testicular size, and reach their final height by 17 years or even later.

Primary amenorrhoea is defined as the absence of menses by the age of 16 in the presence of normal growth and secondary sexual characteristics (Table 60.1). There has been a secular trend of an earlier onset of menarche in the UK for several years.

Delayed puberty is common, with more males being affected than females. It is much less of a concern amongst the parents of children with special needs and fewer referrals arise in relation to this problem. Parents are often grateful that their child remains prepubertal for a while longer and is therefore spared the effects of the hormonal and consequent physical changes, including menstruation in females. If the onset of puberty is delayed, it is the associated growth failure that often occurs which is flagged up initially.

Delayed puberty most commonly occurs as a result of inadequate gonadal steroid secretion which, in turn, is most often caused by defective gonadotropin secretion from the anterior pituitary owing to defective gonadotrophin-releasing hormone (GnRH) production from the hypothalamus. This is the underlying mechanism in constitutional delay that is often familial. Other causes of delayed puberty include

- endocrine disorders such as hypothyroidism or hypopituitarism
- intracranial pathology such as septo-optic dysplasia
- syndromes associated with growth failure and pubertal delay such as Turner syndrome
- growth failure because of systemic factors, for example chronic ill health, undernutrition as a result of feeding difficulties, neglect or other factors.

Investigations to assess pubertal status would be required and these include

- full blood count, ferritin, renal and liver function, thyroid function tests, follicle-stimulating hormone, luteinizing hormone, oestradiol, testosterone, prolactin, bone age, karyotype
- pelvic ultrasound in females to assess uterine size and ovarian development
- possible referral on to paediatric endocrinology for further assessment and opinion on management.

Table 60.1 Causes of primary amenorrhoea

Causes of primary amenorrhoea	Proportion of all cases (%)
Chromosomal abnormalities causing gonadal dysgenesis, e.g. Turners syndrome	50
Hypothalamic hypogonadism	20
Absence of the uterus, cervix and/or vagina	15
Transverse vaginal septum or imperforate hymen	5
Pituitary disease	5
Other causes	5

Sexuality

Attitudes have changed significantly since the 1960s, when society and the parents of children with disabilities took a preventative attitude towards the provision of sex education to young people with disabilities. Parents and healthcare professionals were overly pessimistic about the potential for children with disabilities to enjoy intimacy and sexuality in their relationships. They often perceived these young people as asexual and childlike and therefore in need of constant protection. Conversely, some parts of society held the view that young people with disabilities had uncontrollable sexual urges that therefore needed to be controlled in some way. Concern too was raised about the capacity of learning-disabled adults to care for children resulting from any pregnancies, as well as the increased likelihood of disabilities amongst the children from these relationships.

There has been a profound shift in attitudes towards young people with disabilities that has reflected greater understanding of the individual's needs and rights, and this has been supported by new legislation outlawing discrimination. There is an increasing belief that people with disabilities should be allowed to develop to their maximum potential, and this includes the area of sexuality and reproduction. However, there is still some way to go towards enlightening society and altering perceptions as research still shows that people without disabilities will accept those with disabilities as friends and employees but they are still less likely to accept them as sexual or marriage partners. Interestingly, however, young people with physical disability only are as sexually experienced as their able-bodied peers. It seems that those who have cognitive impairment are more likely to be disadvantaged in the area of developing sexual relationships.

Psychosocial maturation

The process of maturing includes

- attaining a body that is capable of reproducing
- achieving independence in self-care tasks
- managing a range of complex emotions
- developing independent thought and problem solving
- developing and maintaining intimate relationships.

The process may be impaired by the young person's physical limitations and learning disability, but also by intentional or unintentional social isolation. Teenagers with a disability have fewer social opportunities than their healthy peers, often because a high degree of adult supervision is required and they are therefore less able to use social opportunities independently when they arise. Parents and carers may be at risk of infantilizing the young people with disabilities because of their continuing self-care needs. Young people with disabilities can therefore have fewer opportunities to learn about social behaviour, relationships and sex from their peers than able-bodied young people, for whom peer knowledge is still a very important source of information

Developing independence is an important part of growing up, and parents and carers sometimes need persuading to 'let their young person go'. Young people with disabilities should be allowed opportunities to develop their social independence via stays in respite care, school residential trips and social outings to the cinema or bowling with their peers. Some may be capable of socializing using texting and social network sites, and this should be encouraged as long as the young person is adequately protected and capable of understanding the risks and their own limitations.

Sex education

Sex education is an important educational tool that is presented in schools in the context of family life, loving relationships and respect for others. It forms part of the programme of personal and social development, rather than just sex education. Emphasis is placed on the development of relationships: distinguishing family from friends, friends from strangers, and what sort of bodily contact is considered acceptable. This is particularly important since these children are at risk of sexual exploitation by parents and caregivers, mainly because of their immature understanding and extended need for intimate physical care.

Children with disabilities may not have words to describe their body parts and sexual organs. This may impair their ability to communicate their needs and also make them vulnerable to abuse (see Chapter 61). Providing an appropriate vocabulary is important and forms part of training packages covering puberty and sexuality in young people with disabilities (see 'Further reading').

The task of informing children and young people still largely rests with parents, but teachers and other caregivers involved in the everyday care of the young person play a very important role in providing factual biological knowledge and practical advice on such subjects as menstrual hygiene and masturbation as a private activity. Paediatricians can help in opening discussions about issues in this area from early on to reduce the taboo and to provide accurate information. It is helpful, for instance, for parents to know that the self-stimulatory behaviour seen in their 17-year-old son who functions at the level of a 3-year-old is developmentally appropriate, as masturbation is accepted as a normal toddler behaviour. It is important to emphasize that the practical advice given should be sensible and within the law at all times.

Teaching sex education requires repeated and empathic instruction at an appropriate developmental age for each child. Some information may be taught in groups, but more individual attention will be required than for children without disabilities undergoing sex education. Excellent training packages are available for the purpose (see 'Further reading') and toys, pictures, videos and role-playing may be used to enhance the young person's understanding. Topics to be covered include

- normal pubertal development and body parts
- personal care and hygiene
- sexual expression and behaviour – public and privately appropriate
- contraception
- sexually transmitted infections
- sexual orientation.

Key messages regarding the onset of puberty and sex education

- Most learning-disabled children enter puberty at around the same age as their typically developing peers.
- Precocious puberty is more likely to be flagged up by parents than pubertal delay because of anxiety about early sexual development and menstruation.
- Investigations may be required to assess pubertal status and ascertain a reason for advance or delay; however, intervention is rarely required.
- The sexual needs of young people with disabilities are currently more recognized than they used to be. Sex education is an integral part of the curriculum and is delivered by parents and teachers, often individually at the young person's developmental level. Openness is to be encouraged to reduce taboo.

Further reading

Albanese A, Hopper NW (2007) Suppression of menstruation in adolescents with severe learning disabilities. *Arch Dis Child* 92: 629–32. http://dx.doi.org/10.1136/adc.2007.115709

Butler GE, Beadle EA (2007) Manipulating growth and puberty in those with severe disability: when is it justified? *Arch Dis Child* 92: 567–8. http://dx.doi.org/10.1136/adc.2007.116327

Cheng MM, Udry JR (2002) Sexual behaviours of physically disabled adolescents in the United States. *J Adolesc Health* 31: 48–58. http://dx.doi.org/10.1016/S1054–139X(01)00400–1

Children's Learning Disability Nursing Team, Leeds (2009) *Puberty and Sexuality in Children and Young People with a Learning Disability*. Available at: www.leedscommunityhealthcare.nhs.uk/what_we_do/children_and_family_services/childrens_learning_disability_nursing_team_cldnt/ (accessed 7 November 2012).

Contact a Family (no date) *Growing Up, Sex and Relationships: A Booklet to Support Parents of Young Disabled People*. Available at: www.cafamily.org.uk/pdfs/GrowingUpParents.pdf (accessed 25 November 2012).

De Loach CP (1994) Attitudes toward disability: impact on sexual development and forging of intimate relationships. *J Appl Rehabil Couns* 25: 18–25.

Evans AL, McKinlay I (1989) Sex education and the severely mentally retarded child. *Dev Med Child Neurol* 31: 98–101. http://dx.doi.org/10.1111/j.1469–8749.1989.tb08417.x

Lopponen T, Saukkonen A-L, Serlo W et al. (1996) Accelerated pubertal development in patients with shunted hydrocephalus. *Arch Dis Child* 74: 490–6. http://dx.doi.org/10.1136/adc.74.6.490

Murphy N, Elias ER (2006) Sexuality of children and adolescents with developmental disabilities. *Paediatrics* 118: 398–403. http://dx.doi.org/10.1542/peds.2006–1115

Proos LA, Dahl M, Ahlsten G, Tuvemo T, Gustafsson J (1996) Increased perinatal intracranial pressure and prediction of early puberty in girls with myelomeningocele. *Arch Dis Child* 75: 42–5. http://dx.doi.org/10.1136/adc.75.1.42

Other resources

TSL Education Limited (2010) Special Schools – Sex and Relationship Education. Video presented by David Stewart, Head Teacher, Shepherd School, Nottingham. Available at: www.tes.co.uk/teaching-resource/Special-Schools-Sex-and-Relationship-Education-6045905/ (accessed 7 November 2012).

61
Child abuse

David Cundall and Gillian Robinson

> **Learning objectives**
>
> - To understand that children with disabilities are more vulnerable to abuse.
> - To be able to identify risk factors and key markers for abuse.
> - To be able to write clear reports for children who are in the care system, so that accurate information can accompany the child.

The spectrum that we traditionally think of as abuse needs to be wider in the context of disability. The wider spectrum of abuse in children with disabilities includes:

- Feeding a child with an unsafe swallow and aspiration.
- Refusing to accept that the child has a disability.
- Totally unrealistic expectations of the child.
- Parents who understandably but unwisely protect their children from experiences that they would enjoy.
- Parents who embark on some unconventional treatments and therapies that range from harmless to unpleasant and dangerous.
- Insisting on walking and extensive physiotherapy programmes when the child would have greater participation as a wheelchair user.
- Rejecting signing and insisting on a purely oral approach for the profoundly deaf child, and conversely for deaf parents to insist that their hearing child only learns signing.

In these situations working with social services is useful, though no formal child protection proceedings are likely to be needed.

Prevalence

The evidence base for demonstrating abuse in the disabled population is weak because of the limited number of studies. There are also difficulties in defining what is abuse and also what is disability. Despite these problems, the existing evidence (Govindshenoy and Spencer 2007) shows that all types of abuse are more common in children with disabilities.

- Neglect: odds ratio 1.8 to 3.7.
- Physical abuse: odds ratio 1.6 to 3.9.
- Sexual abuse: odds ratio 2.2 to 3.14.

Risk factors

Child factors (Table 61.1)

Table 61.1 Child risk factors for abuse

Difficulty	Reason	Prevention
Behavioural or emotional	Outbursts can lead to inappropriate restraint	Appropriate behaviour management strategies
Communication	Frustration and misunderstanding between adult and child	All carers understand child's level of communication
Communication	Difficulty in describing abuse	Encourage words that would help
Learning difficulties	Difficulty in understanding appropriate behaviour and difficulty with communication	Appropriate sex and relationships education
	Wanting to be liked by others, being part of peer group	
Sensory impairments	More difficult to describe abuse and abuser if hearing or vision impaired	Facilitate communication as much as possible
Mobility difficulties	Unable to remove themselves from abusive situations	
Requiring toileting and/or changing by caregivers	Increased opportunities for sexual abuse	Implementation of good safeguarding practice in all situations
Multiple impairments	All of the above	

Family factors

Families of children with disability are under additional stress for the following reasons:

- their role as a carer as well as a parent (e.g. medications, feeding regimes, appointments)
- financial pressures
- the need for increased supervision
- limited social and community support
- lack of sufficient respite or breaks in childcare responsibilities
- the above factors leading to increase rates of marital discord with the potential for domestic violence
- drug and alcohol misuse
- parental mental health difficulties.

Community factors

The more people there are involved in care of an individual child, the greater the risk of all forms of abuse including sexual abuse. This is particularly true for children who need help with their hygiene needs.

Physical abuse

Children with neuromotor disabilities have fewer skin injuries with decreasing mobility. Therefore, skin injuries in this population which are unusual by their number, appearance or distribution should raise suspicion of physical abuse. Bruising that is not over a bony structure is more worrying, in particular bruising to the ears, neck, anterior chest and genitalia. Children using particular equipment, such as knee blocks with wheelchairs or splints, may sustain some bruising to certain areas which should be easily recognizable. These accidental bruises are often over the feet, knees and thighs. Asking about equipment use and seeing the equipment in use usually helps in determining whether the equipment could have caused the bruising.

Fractures

No study has been done comparing rates of fracture in children with and without disabilities. Fractures in children with limited mobility should raise concerns. It is important to note that immobility, steroids and antiepileptic drugs can lead to osteopenia and, therefore, decrease the level of trauma required to lead to fracture. Painless fractures occur in children with spina bifida and spinal cord injury.

Neglect

Neglect is difficult to define in a healthy child and this is more so than for a child with a disability. This is probably the most common form of abuse in children with disabilities; however, it is under-recognized.

Markers

- A child with ingrained dirt in skin creases, nails, and so on
- Inappropriate clothing
- Poor growth/failure to thrive
- An always hungry child
- Many missed appointments
- Untreated medical problems
- Infestations
- Missed immunizations
- Poor or absent dental care
- Attachment difficulties.

Sexual abuse

Children with disabilities may not have the language to express what has happened during the abuse. Sexual abuse may occur without symptoms.

Markers

- Sexualized behaviour
- A change in behaviour including persistent anger
- Wetting or soiling when previously clean
- Vaginal or rectal bleeding
- Vaginal discharge/sexually transmitted disease (including hepatitis B)
- Pregnancy.

Emotional abuse

Diagnosing emotional abuse is always challenging, and this is more so in children with disabilities. Behaviours which raise concern include

- changes in behaviour or unusual behaviours, including soiling and smearing for which there is no explanation
- unusual behaviours for the child's functional age
- dissociation
- deliberate self-harm and self-injurious behaviours.

Assessing a child for possible abuse

When assessing a child for possible abuse ensure that there is a multiagency approach.

- A careful history should be taken from the child and the different carers.
  - Ask about behaviour and sleep.
  - Ask about the family, their strengths and difficulties.
  - Check about immunizations.
- Carry out a full examination removing all the child's clothes.
  - Comment on the observed relationship between the child and carer.
  - Include growth parameters.
  - Look for signs of cleanliness, infestation and dental health.
  - Document the size and site and photograph any injuries.
- Investigation:
  - Have a low threshold for radiographs if the child is immobile and has communication difficulties.
  - Remember to screen for sexually transmitted diseases with urine for gonococcus and a nucleic acid amplification test for chlamydia, and low vaginal and, if possible, cervical swabs for abnormal flora when there are concerns about sexual abuse. Also consider blood borne virus screening: syphilis, hepatitis B and C and HIV.
- Interpretation:
  - Do the injuries seen fit with the history given?
  - Take into account the likely effect of the disability in this presentation. For example, unusual and/or unexplained bruising in an immobile child or an active autistic child who has difficulties in appreciation of danger.

Prevention strategies

- Training of carers, teaching staff and social care workers and family court staff so that they are aware of abuse as a specific issue in children with disabilities.
- Medical staff being aware of different patterns of injury that raise suspicions of abuse.
- Medical review should identify family factors that could lead to increased stress. Look for possible solutions including behaviour management strategies, respite care and support for the carer.

Advocate for appropriate support services for families in local and national service reviews.

Reference

Govindshenoy M, Spencer N (2007) Abuse of the disabled child: a systematic review of population-based studies. *Child Care Health Dev* 33: 552–8. http://dx.doi.org/10.1111/j.1365–2214.2006.00693.x

Further reading

National Collaborating Centre for Women's and Children's Health (2009) *When to Suspect Child Maltreatment*: Commissioned by the National Institute for Health and Clinical Excellence. Available at: http://www.nice.org.uk/nicemedia/live/12183/44954/44954.pdf (accessed 7 November 2012).

Royal College of Paediatrics and Child Health (2006) *Child Protection Companion*. Available at: http://www.rcpch.ac.uk/sites/default/files/asset_library/Health%20Services/ChildProtCompL.pdf (accessed 7 November 2012).

Websites

NSPCC Child Protection Research Briefing Neglect (2007): www.nspcc.org.uk/inform/research/briefings/childneglect_wda48222.html

Welsh Child Protection Systematic Review Group: www.core-info.cardiff.ac.uk

62
Life-shortening conditions and planning for the end of life

Toni Wolff and Anne M Kelly

Learning objectives

- To understand the importance of Emergency Health Care Plans (EHCPs) and how to prepare one with a young person and his or her family.
- To learn how to approach end of life care planning for children and young people with disabilities.

Introduction

Children with a disability may have life-shortening or life-threatening conditions. Some children will have a degenerative condition which will inevitably lead to death in childhood. Other children with severe non-progressive disability will be at risk of life-threatening events such as apnoeas, life-threatening chest infections or airway obstruction. When life-threatening emergencies can be predicted there needs to be a written EHCP, including the personal resuscitation plan, agreed in advance with the family, and held by the family.

When death in childhood is a probability the family (and sometimes the child or young person themselves) need information and support to consider their choices regarding end of life care. However, these discussions are very difficult to initiate. The development of an EHCP with the young person and family can be a useful way to start the discussions about potential life-threatening events and the appropriate care options.

Case vignette

Sharon is a 14-year-old female with severe bilateral cerebral palsy and epilepsy. She has had frequent admissions over the last year with prolonged seizures and chest infections. She presents unwell with severe breathlessness and reduced oxygen saturation after a prolonged seizure and probable aspiration. Her mother insists, 'Everything should be done'. There have been some 'end of life' discussions but a written plan has not been agreed. The acute paediatric team decide to ventilate and transfer her to the paediatric intensive care unit (PICU). Sharon becomes more unwell with increasing ventilator requirement over the next 3 days. Her mother initially refuses to accept that Sharon has developed incurable lung problems but changes her mind after discussion with an experienced PICU consultant. Sharon is transferred to the local children's hospice, where she is extubated and dies shortly afterwards.

More children like Sharon are surviving into young adulthood because of advances in medical care and particularly as a result of technological advances such as gastrostomy feeding and home-assisted ventilation. However, many of these children will die in childhood and there needs to be sensitive and timely discussions with their families about the child's prognosis and the most appropriate care when life-threatening situations arise.

National guidance in this area

The Association for Children's Palliative Care (ACT) care pathway, standard 5, states that 'Every child and family should be helped to decide on an end of life plan and should be provided with care and support to achieve this as closely as possible' (ACT 2004: 24).

* Recent General Medical Council guidance advises doctors to avoid making assumptions about patient choices at the end of life and provides information on the legal framework.
* The National Service Framework for children and young people recommends prospective discussions about end of life decisions. Children and parents should be involved and supported in making choices and care decisions, involving a written specific end of life care plan, including resuscitation choices.

Predicting when a child may die is very difficult. Children with life-threatening disability may be stable for years before experiencing a sudden acute deterioration; others may follow a more predictable pattern of gradual deterioration with increasing frequency of hospital admissions with failure to return to the preadmission level of health. It is not so important to accurately predict the timing of the child's final illness as to start discussions about the possibility of death and the choices available.

It is already accepted practice in paediatric oncology that the needs of the child and his or her family will be better served if the concept of palliative care is introduced at the time of diagnosis if the prognosis is uncertain. This approach is now being encouraged in managing children with non-malignant life-shortening or life-threatening conditions whose life expectancy may be very variable, as long as it is acknowledged that such discussions do not preclude the possibility of offering life-prolonging or curative therapies at a later date, should they become available. This allows

- greater attention to be focused on the child's quality of life at an earlier stage
- more openness with siblings and the rest of family who are included in the discussions
- more choice and control for parents over the response to acute events
- better emotional adjustment at the time of the child's death.

There is, however, evidence that in spite of all the guidance and encouragement to start discussions with families earlier and prepare written plans, this is still not happening for many children. They may present 'collapsed' in the emergency department prompting confusion about the best course of action. Discussions about the intensity of intervention may be fraught at the time of an acute deterioration, with carers feeling they are suddenly confronted with making a choice between the standard approach to resuscitation ('everything to be done') or an alternative approach with 'nothing being done', as seen in their eyes. Alternatively, there may be a brief discussion and a standard approach towards resuscitation may be taken because of the time pressures and lack of preparation of parents for this scenario. This may lead to inappropriate interventions and use of resources without benefit to the child.

What are the barriers to early planning?

- Reluctance on the part of the child's lead paediatrician to raise the issue.
- Difficulty predicting the end of the child's life.
- Parent or carer fears and avoidance of discussions.

The Emergency Health Care Plan approach to end of life planning

It is much easier for the paediatrician to raise discussions with the family about appropriate interventions in potentially life-threatening situations when drawing up with them a family-held EHCP than it is to start talking about an 'end of life' plan. An EHCP is always a positive plan communicating the best care for this particular child.

Case vignette

Gavin is 9 years old. He has late infantile Batten disease and is nearing the end of his life. He has generally increased muscle tone, with frequent seizures and spasms. He cannot sit without support, nor reach for objects. His oromotor control is poor and his cough is weak. He has been in hospital twice in the last 3 months with prolonged chest infections. His paediatrician meets with his parents together with his community nurse in a specially extended outpatient appointment. Gavin's parents know his diagnosis and that this is a life-shortening condition.

They discuss the fact that Gavin will have more chest infections and that these will be increasingly difficult for him to recover from. They discuss the benefits and burdens of different treatment options and agree that Gavin should continue to have intravenous treatment for chest infections but not invasive ventilation. A more intensive secretion clearance programme will be given on a regular basis to help to keep him well for longer in between infections. They agree that if Gavin stops breathing or his heart stops beating it would be best to cuddle him and allow him to die peacefully, preferably at home. These plans were then documented in the family-held EHCP (see Appendix XV). The community children's nurse went on to explore the family's wishes and choices to further develop the end of life plans.

Components and principles of Emergency Health Care Plans

The Council for Disabled Children has been working with the Royal College of Paediatrics and Child Health on core principles and guidance for developing EHCPs. These are briefly summarized below, but further information, leaflets and EHCP templates are available at www.councilfordisabledchildren.org.uk.

- Plans need to
  - be easily recognized by staff and carers, follow a standard format and be readily accessible in an emergency
  - be prepared in partnership with families, based on the principle that they advise the best medical care for the child
  - be dated and regularly reviewed and
  - incorporate a system for storage, distribution and version control.
- Plans must contain
  - background information – the diagnosis/medical condition
  - symptoms/signs the child shows indicating a deterioration
  - clear instructions on what to do in an emergency
  - who to call for support, with phone numbers
  - a clear statement on the front page about the agreed level of resuscitation if the emergency is life-threatening, that is a personal resuscitation plan (helpful for paramedical and emergency department staff, who will not have prior knowledge of the child) and additional information about the preferred place of care/death.

- **If there is disagreement between carers and medical staff about what is in the child's best interests**
  - a second opinion should be obtained
  - a compromise position may be possible
  - it may be possible to defer a decision as further time may make the situation clearer
  - discussion at the local clinical ethics committee may be helpful
  - if all efforts at mediation fail, then legal advice should be sought, and in the last resort the decision may need to be put before the courts.
- **Opportunities for open discussions about EHCPs include the following**
  - the first life-threatening episode such as a chest infection requiring intensive care
  - obvious general deterioration in the child's condition
  - the child starting care in a new setting such as a nursery or short-break service
  - the death of another child known to the family with a similar condition.

Discussions with the family should follow the same general principles as for breaking news (see Right from the Start template, available at www.scope.org.uk/rfts), with both parents present if possible, in a quiet room where interruptions are prevented, with enough time available to listen to their views. Parents often do not want to talk in front of their child, but may need help later to discuss it with their child and obtain their views. It is good practice to have one other person present to support the parents, such as the child's community nurse or keyworker.

As in all emotionally difficult conversations, the doctor needs to first explore the parents' understanding of the situation and then listen to their views. The paediatrician and parents then discuss what emergency events may occur and what will be the best management for the child. Sometimes parents are ahead of professionals and will be quite clear that they do not want intrusive interventions. Others may have avoided the issue and will fear talking about it, as they believe it will hasten the child's end and they would rather not contemplate this.

Discussions often need to be conducted over several meetings, and the doctor must have the time to listen and share information and opinions honestly and sensitively, but clearly. The plan needs to take into account the practical support that will be available to the child and family, particularly for care outside the hospital. The plan developed needs to keep the best interests of the child at its heart. It is neither about protecting health resources nor about endorsing parents' wishes if these are unreasonable. If an agreement on best care cannot be reached, then this should be acknowledged and the plan written up to this point with the intention to return to it at a later date. If the child deteriorates in the meantime, then discussions should continue between the acute team, community team if available, and parents before a course of action can be agreed.

The EHCP is only one part of the 'end of life' plan. The child and family need help to explore and consider documenting their choices regarding

- the preferred place of death and who will be present
- care of the body, organ/tissue donation, postmortem
- how to make keepsakes and memories
- funeral plans.

There are now numerous examples of end of life planning tools that have been developed and are being used by different clinical teams across the UK, for example the Wishes Document below. Others are available at www.togetherforshortlives.org.uk. All have been developed with the intention of communicating the best care plan for the child that has been agreed in advance by parents with the paediatrician who knows the child well. All plans acknowledge that although the agreement is written and signed by health staff and parents, *it is not legally binding*. Parents may withdraw their consent or change their minds about specific interventions at any time and their wishes must be respected. In these situations, emergency staff, as always, have the responsibility of acting in the best interests of the child taking into account all the information available to them.

Family-held EHCPs and end of life plans are invaluable in supporting communication with the local child death review team, particularly when a child dies suddenly outside the hospital and activation of the rapid response team is being considered.

The Wishes Document

The Wishes Document (Table 62.1) considers the wishes of the child and family at the various stages of the child's life and death.

Table 62.1 The Wishes Document

	Child	Family	Others: friends/school
Wishes during life	e.g. special holiday	e.g. family holiday	e.g. fund raising
Plans for when your child becomes unwell	e.g. treatment options	e.g. what may happen	e.g. visiting
Acute life-threatening event	e.g. preferred place of care	e.g. treatment options	
After death	e.g. funeral preferences	e.g. spiritual and cultural wishes	

Bereavement

When a child dies, families usually still need support from the team who cared for their child in life. The following are recognized stages of grief, but people do not always experience all of them or pass through them in a linear fashion:

- shock and disbelief at the loss
- feelings of anger and guilt
- intense sadness and yearning for the child
- acceptance and recovery.

Bereaved parents often need reassurance that the powerful emotions they are feeling are natural and to be expected. Different family members will grieve differently and support should be provided for each person according to their individual needs. Families are usually best supported in their bereavement by a familiar member of their child's team.

Parents should be offered an appointment with the lead paediatrician to discuss any questions they may have a few weeks after their child has died. Referral to a specialist bereavement support service should be considered if a parent is showing no signs of beginning to return to normal functioning by 6 months after their child's death. It is particularly concerning if they are ruminating on a particular issue.

Key messages

- There are increasing numbers of children with severe disability and life-shortening conditions who are at risk of acute clinical deteriorations and require an EHCP.
- Most of these children still, unfortunately, die in hospital, often on a PICU, without end of life choices having been discussed with the family.
- All paediatricians involved in providing a neurodisability service have a duty to undertake end of life planning with families at an opportune time and not just prior to death.
- Open and timely discussions about what may happen and what is the best care empowers families and reduces their fears and regrets when facing their child's death.

Reference

ACT (Association for Children's Palliative Care) (2004) *Integrated Multi-agency Care Pathways for Children with Life-threatening and Life-limiting Conditions.* Available at: http://www.knowledge.scot.nhs.uk/media/CLT/ResourceUploads/11895/act_pathway.pdf (accessed 7 November 2012).

Further reading

Brook L, Hain R (2008) Predicting death in children. *Arch Dis Child* 93: 1067–70. http://dx.doi.org/10.1136/adc.2007.127332

Brook L, Gallagher R, Curran A (2008) A plan for living and a plan for dying: advanced care planning for children. *Arch Dis Child* 2008; 93 (Suppl.): A61–6.

Fraser J, Harris N, Berringer AJ, Prescott H, Finlay F (2010) Advanced care planning in children with life-limiting conditions – the Wishes Document. *Arch Dis Child* 95: 79–82. http://dx.doi.org/10.1136/adc.2009.160051

General Medical Council (2010) *Treatment and Care Towards the End of Life: Good Practice in Decision-Making.* Available at: http://www.gmc-uk.org/End_of_life.pdf_32486688.pdf (accessed 7 November 2012).

Heckford EJ, Beringer A (2011) Child and family wishes: a case note review of end of life care planning for children with life limiting conditions. *Arch Dis Child* 96: A80. http://dx.doi.org/10.1136/adc.2011.212563.187

RCPCH (2004) *Withholding or Withdrawing Life Sustaining Treatment in Children: A Framework for Practice.* 2nd edition. Available at: www.rcpch.ac.uk/what-we-do/rcpch-publications/publications-list-title/publications-list-title (Accessed 5 December 2012).

Sutherland R, Hearn J, Baum D et al. *(*1993) Definitions in paediatric palliative care. *Health Trends* 25: 148–50.

Together for Short Lives (2011) *A Parent's Guide: Making Critical Care Choices for Your Child*. Available at: http://www.togetherforshortlives.org.uk/assets/0000/1081/A_parent_s_guide_to_critical_care_choices.pdf (accessed 7 November 2012).

Wolff A, Browne J (2011) Organizing end of life care: parallel planning. *Paediatr Child Health* 21: 378–84. http://dx.doi.org/10.1016/j.paed.2011.04.007

Wolff A, Browne J, Whitehouse WP (2011) Personal resuscitation plans and end of life planning for children with disability and life-limiting/life-threatening conditions. *Arch Dis Child Educ Pract Ed* 96: 42–8. http://dx.doi.org/10.1136/adc.2010.185272

Websites

Bliss: making critical care decisions for your baby: www.bliss.org.uk

Emergency Health Care Plans 2012: www.councilfordisabledchildren.org.uk/ehp

Section 15

Appendices

Appendix I

Normal developmental milestones in motor skills

Age	Gross motor	Fine motor
Birth–3mo	Primitive reflexes Head control by 3mo Prone – on forearms	Palmar grasp reflex Hands closed Hand regard
3–6mo	Primitive reflexes disappear Chin to chest on pull to sit Prone weight on extended arms	Hands open (3mo) Perceives distance Reaches for object (5mo)
6–9mo	Establish protective reflexes Sits independently (mean 8mo)	Palmar grasp Transfers object hand to hand
9–12mo	Sits and pivots Crawls Pulls to stand	Approaches with index finger (9mo) Pincer grasp (10mo)
12–18mo	Walks (mean 15mo) Crawls up stairs	Mature grasp of larger object, e.g. cube Marks on paper Able to give brick on request
18mo–2y	Squats to pick up object Rides on toy pushed along by feet	Scribbles on paper Can build tower of two or three bricks
2–3y	Runs Jumps	Circular scribble and later copies circle Horizontal and vertical lines Can build tower of six or seven bricks
3–4y	Stands briefly on one foot Pedals tricycle Climbs play equipment Throws overarm	Copies a cross Draws a man – three parts Bricks – tower of nine and train
4–5y	Goes upstairs – reciprocal feet Learns to hop Catches a ball	Copies a square – 4y Writes first name Makes a bridge Uses scissors
5–7y	Learns to ride bike Learns to swim Increasing competence at ball skills	Copies a triangle – 5y, diamond – 6y; Completes a clock – 7y Writes first and last name Letter reversal common (10% at 7y)
7–11y	Starts to have interest in team games	Draws two interlocking diamonds Cursive handwriting
11y plus	Co-ordination approaches adult level Increasing competence at team sports Increasing competence playing musical instruments	

Appendix II

Normal developmental milestones in communication

Age	Comprehension	Expression
Birth–3mo	Stills to certain sounds	Coos at mother, beginnings of reciprocal sound-making Different cries for different needs
3–6mo	Turns head to sound Comforted by carer's voice	Laughs, grunts, chuckles Copies sounds and facial expressions Early turn taking with sound making Coos – vowel sounds
6–9mo	Initiates physical contact Turns head to familiar voices	Eye contact followed by looking at object – referential looking Vocalizes to get attention Babble vowel sounds, later 'ba', 'da'
9–12mo	Understands word in context, e.g. shoes, bath, no, bye-bye Responds to name	Vocalizations and facial expression to communicate Imitates sounds and also babbles Points to request
12–18mo	Points to three body parts Identifies objects by sound, e.g. telephone Carries out simple instructions with gesture	Two or three words with meaning Makes symbolic noises, e.g. 'brum' Makes animal noises Vocalizes vowels and consonants
18mo–2y	Understands many single words Gives familiar objects on request Recognizes pictures of familiar people/objects	Jargons 6–20 words (18mo) Echoes keywords from adult speech Tries to sing
2–3y	Understands sentences *with* two keywords – where's *dolly's nose*? Understands and uses verbs Follows simple repetitive story	Two words together minimum 50 words+ Requests as well as names items
3–4y	Three words together Speech understandable by familiar adults Knows colours	Short sentences – 3+ words Personal pronouns, e.g. I, mine Asks what and why Can tell you their name
4–5y	Understands concepts of size	Speech understandable to all Counts to 10 Able to tell a story Vocabulary 2000 words
5–7y	Knows day and months of birthday Knows the alphabet Uses appropriate tense	13 000 words with meaning
7–11 years	Can read to themselves	Can tell complex story Likes to tell jokes Able to write stories of increasing complexity
11y plus	Increasing complexity of punctuation	Increasing sophistication of language Able to express ideas clearly in writing

Appendix III

Normal developmental milestones in cognitive skills

Age	Skill	Example
Birth–3mo	Reflex activity	Sucking and grasping
3–6mo	Able to regard object Recognizes carer	Hand regard, interest in mirrors later
6–9mo	Manipulates objects	Happier with carer than stranger Shakes rattle
9–12mo	Actions take on an intentional purpose Object permanence	Banging two bricks together when shown Searching for the hidden or fallen object Simple interactive games – peekaboo
12–18mo	More than one way to do things Starts to understand objects' function Starts to understand pictures	Move to get, or pull the string Will use simple pretend play, e.g. phone Cause and effect toys towards 18mo Looks at pictures in books
18months–2y	Starts to be able to solve simple problems – if objects present	Cause and effect toys Simple insert puzzles
2–3y	Solve more complex problems, but the object needs to be present Progression of imaginative sills	Simple puzzles Colour match Cardboard box is a house Small world play
3–4y	Gains basic understanding of concepts	Group by colour, size, etc. Count by rote Likes being read stories
4–5y	Develops early language and maths skills	Phonic letter sounds and early words Can write name Counts with meaning Knows shape names
5–7y	Develops logical thought Develops principle of conservation Understands reversal of operations	Simple addition and later subtraction By 7y counts in tens, twos and fives Amount of liquid same in different containers e.g. 3+4=7 and therefore 7−4=3
7–11y	Able to start to solve the problems they can see Able to read and write fluently	How to make a bridge from planks and blocks Cursive script – capitals, full stops and later question marks, speech marks, apostrophe
11y plus	Logical sequences Abstract solutions and hypotheses Abstract thought	Predicts next in a sequence, e.g. 2, 4, 8, 16 More dissolved as the solution is warmer What should your friend buy for the disco Algebra

Appendix IV

Normal developmental milestones – emotional and social development

	Emotional	*Social*
Birth–3mo	Expresses emotions – delight, distress	Smiles at face
3–6mo	Recognizes mother figure	
6–9mo	Responds to emotions of others as perceived by facial expressions	Finger feeds
9–12mo	Specific attachment to mother figure Wary of strangers Deliberately seeks attention	Waves bye-bye Claps hands Puts out arm when dressing
12–18mo	Becomes aware that they are separate to others including mother Uses behaviour interact with others Separation anxiety at most severe	Use spoon – inaccurate Drinks from cup Casting
18mo–2y	Starts to have temper tantrums	Skilled use of spoon Stops casting Stops mouthing
2–3y	Can show warmth of affection Recognizes some emotions – happy, sad More happy in routine. May have rituals Temper tantrums continue!	Puts on shoes and socks May be toilet trained Plays alongside other children
3–4y	Wants to please Concerned about other children Recognizes more emotions – pride, guilt	Toilet trained – needs help with wiping Plays with other children Undresses and dresses Washes and dries hands
4–5y	Can at times be self-willed and bossy Likes to do things for themselves Interested in exploring sex differences Difficulty separating fantasy/reality	Wipes own bottom Eats with a knife and fork Dresses – unsupervised
5–7y	Expresses emotions freely and openly Understands about fantasy/reality Frequent but brief quarrels with friends Initially does not know rules, e.g. stealing	Ties shoelaces Bathes without assistance Aware of stranger danger Has a best friend
7–11y	Refrains from asking questions that might embarrass others Able to control feelings, e.g. angry, hurt Pride in accomplishments	Can safely cross road Understands money Understands about time
11y plus	Develops independence from family Develops personal identity Emotionally labile Susceptible to peer pressure	Initially falls out with friends Able to plan dependent activities Able to make a meal

Appendix V

Problem-orientated medical record

FAMILY HISTORY	*UNIT NO:*		
	SURNAME: (block letters)		
	FIRST NAMES:		
	CHECKLIST FOR QUALITY OF PAEDIATRIC NEURODISABILITY CARE		

Nr.	Item	Date/ confirmation	Outcome/ comment
1	Diagnosis explained to parents		
2	Hearing assessment		
3	Visual assessment		
4	Psychological assessment		
5	Speech and language assessment		
6	Physiotherapy assessment		
7	Occupational therapy assessment		
8	Play therapy assessment		
9	Dietitian		
10	Dental advice		
11	Neurology opinion		
12	Genetic referral		
13	Dental advice		
14	Education notified		
15	Educational provision		
16	Benefits/Family Fund		
17	Contact a Family Support Groups		
18	Voluntary agencies		
19	Other clinics attended		

Left column labels:

Underlying diagnosis

Areas of functional difficulty

Secondary medical problems

Medical investigations (year of result)

FBC	....
U&Es	....
LFTs	....
TFTs	....
CPK	....
Lactate	....
Urine metabolic	....
CGH array	....
Chromosomes	....
Fragile X	....
DNA	....
EEG	....
MRI/CT	....

Year					
School					
Function					
Mobility					
Hand					
Vision					
Hearing					
Speech					
Behaviour					
IQ					
Feeding					
Toileting					
Washing					
Dressing					
Tech support					
Self protection					
Equipment					
Adaptations					

Appendix VI

Child development team report

Assessment date:	
Draft report issued on: (for parental comments)	
Final report issued on:	

Child's information

Child's name:	Date of birth:
Parent/guardian name(s):	Child's age on date of assessment
Address:	NHS no: Hospital no:

The following people were involved in your child's assessment:

	Name	*Contact information*
Parent(s)/carer(s)		
Specialist health visitor		
Paediatrician		
Speech and language therapist		
Clinical psychologist		
Occupational therapist		
Educational psychologist		

Family information

Names, and for the children dates of birth of all family members.
Also important figures who support the family, who the therapy team may meet, e.g. grandparents or childminder.

Professionals involved

This should include childminders, nursery or school.

Parental concern

These are gathered prior to the assessment and the assessment and report should aim to address these.

Background information

Birth history
Health in early childhood
Development

Assessment

Age on assessment
General presentation and attention
Communication

- Symbolic and pretend play
- Comprehension
- Expressive language and vocalizations
- Feeding

General learning abilities
Motor skills
Self-care

Summary and recommendations

- *The child's underlying medical diagnosis, which is explained.*
- *The child's current function – strengths and areas for development.*
- *The family strengths.*

Plan

- *Further medical management – investigations and treatments.*
- *Therapy plan with initial goals, set in discussion with the family.*
- *Family support plan – include benefits advice and information for the family.*
- *For liaison and support with education.*
- *Review date.*

Signature	
Signed on behalf of the child development team	Date

Circulation to:

Note

The whole of this report should be comprehensible to a lay person.

Appendix VII

School report

INFORMATION FROM SCHOOL

Name of child: _____ Date of birth:_____
School: _____
Class teacher: _____
Head of Year (high school): _____
Special educational needs coordinator: _____
Form completed by: _____Date:_____

What are the main difficulties (if any) for this child, as you see them?

What are the main strengths?

What is the child's current level of attainment (national curriculum level)

Reading	
Writing	
Mathematics	
Science	

Please tick to indicate if any of the following are in place for this child:

Individual educational plan ❑
Individual behaviour plan ❑
Any additional funding ❑ and level of funding ....

Please tick to indicate if any of the following have been involved with this child:

	CURRENTLY	PREVIOUSLY	NAME OF WORKER
Educational psychologist	❑	❑	....
Speech and language therapist	❑	❑	....
Other (please specify role)	❑	❑	....

Does this child receive any other special help? Please specify, e.g. small group work, pastoral programme, speech and language therapy, etc.

At present, how does this child compare with peers on the following?

	Poor	*Fair*	*Good*	*Excellent*
Attendance record				
Self-esteem				
Relationships with other children				
Relationships with adult staff				
Response to rules and discipline				
Behaving at playtime				
Home–school relationship				

Please could you write down any evidence you have of difficulties in the following areas

Score: 0=no concerns; 1=some concerns; 2=major concerns

	Communication	
Eye contact		0 1 2
Use of gestures		0 1 2
Ability to initiate and sustain a conversation		0 1 2
Understands if others hurt or upset		0 1 2
	Friendships/peer relationships	
Developing friendships		0 1 2
Maintaining friendships		0 1 2
Difficulties with bullying		0 1 2
Age range of friends similar or different to own		0 1 2
	Attention and concentration	
Butting into others' conversations		0 1 2
Ability to complete a piece of work		0 1 2
Ability to listen to instructions		0 1 2
Noisy in play/work		0 1 2
Excessive or inappropriate talking		0 1 2
Fidgeting/squirming or general activity level		0 1 2
	Coordination	
Number of accidents		0 1 2
Ball skills		0 1 2
Organization		0 1 2
Dressing and undressing		0 1 2
Pencil skills/writing		0 1 2
	Unusual behaviours	
Repeated actions		0 1 2
Unusual interests		0 1 2
Behaviour more difficult if routine changed		0 1 2
Difficulties with imaginative play		0 1 2
Outbursts		0 1 2

Thank you for your help, please return to _____ at _____

Appendix VIII

SPECIAL EDUCATIONAL NEEDS STATUTORY ASSESSMENT MEDICAL REPORT

CHILD

Surname: Forename:

Date of birth: Gender:

Address:

School/nursery:

MEDICAL CARE NEEDS

MEDICAL AND DEVELOPMENTAL DIAGNOSIS:

Child's diagnoses should be explained so that a lay person can understand the implications of this diagnosis in terms of the child's educational need.

MEDICATIONS AND TREATMENT:

This should include information about medications that are prescribed, and what they are used to treat.

EMERGENCY ACTION PLAN:

Plan should be included for any expected urgent medical situation (e.g. seizure, blocked ventriculoperitoneal shunt).

SPECIAL PRECAUTIONS OR RESTRICTIONS:

POSSIBLE IMPACT OF MEDICAL OR DEVELOPMENTAL DIAGNOSIS ON EDUCATIONAL PROVISION:

DEVELOPMENTAL BACKGROUND:

FUNCTIONAL PROFILE OF THE CHILD

Highlight if additional reports are needed (e.g. physiotherapy or speech and language therapy).

GENERAL PHYSICAL HEALTH:

VISION:

Should be formally assessed.

HEARING:

Should be formally assessed.

MOBILITY:

POSITIONING AND SEATING:

HAND FUNCTION:

COMMUNICATION AND LANGUAGE:

PERSONAL CARE, E.G. DRESSING/UNDRESSING:

CONTINENCE:

FEEDING:

BEHAVIOUR:

IS ADDITIONAL SUPERVISION REQUIRED:

Yes

SPECIAL RESOURCES

Will the child require adaptations to school organization: Yes/No
Will the child require adaptations to the setting/school site to enable access? Yes/No

MEDICAL EQUIPMENT:

SCHOOL TRANSPORT:

REVIEW PLANS: (DELETE WHERE APPROPRIATE)

Name of examining doctor: ....

Signature: ....

Designation: .... Date: ....

Appendix IX

School treatment plan for health emergencies (epilepsy example)

HEALTH CARE PLAN FOR A PUPIL WITH

Name:

Date of birth:

School:

Class:

Photo

Medical background

XXXX has epilepsy. She takes regular medication to help control her seizures.
Describe the different seizure types.
e.g. During a tonic–clonic seizure XXXX falls to the ground with jerking of all four limbs.
Afterwards she will be sleepy.

An emergency for the pupil

A tonic–clonic seizure lasting more than 5 minutes.

Action to be taken

1 Place in recovery position.
2 Duration of seizure.

3   Inform the parents.
4   If seizure lasts more than 5 minutes give XXXX (state dose in both mg and in ml) and route treatment to be given.

Location of medication

Contact telephone numbers

Family contact 1	telephone number
Family contact 2	telephone number
Consultant paediatrician	telephone number

Healthcare plan review date

Copies of healthcare plan held by

School
Parents
School nurse

Medication to be administered

Please note, it is parents' responsibility to keep the school up to date with medical information and to provide medication which is within its expiry date.

Signed: **Parent**   **Date**

                   Doctor   **Date**

Appendix X

Antecedents, Behaviour, Consequencess (ABC) recording chart

Date and time	Antecedents	Behaviour	Consequences
	What was happening just before the behaviour occurred? Did anything happen a bit earlier that might have upset the child?	Describe exactly what happened	What happened as a result of the behaviour?

Appendix XI

Sleep questionnaire

Name	DOB
Address 1	School/nursery
Address 2	
Telephone no.	Family health visitor
GP	Sleep practitioner
Referred by	Date

Household arrangements

	Name	*Age*	*Occupation/shift pattern*
Mother			
Father/partner			
Siblings	*Name*	*Age*	*School/sleep problems*
Other house-hold members			

Family history

Family health and well-being	
Factors contributing to family stress	

Child's history

Health	
Underlying diagnosis	
Present health	Pain Gastro-oesophageal reflux Cough Sleep apnoea
Present medication	
Present functioning	
Motor	
Comprehension	Situational understanding Objects of reverence Single words Short sentences
Expression	Behaviour Taking by hand Pointing Single words Short sentences
Night-time continence	In nappies and leak In nappies and dry Frequent wetting Occasional wetting Dry

Family life

Do you use babysitting or childminding services for your child?	
Does the problem stop you from going out or interfere with your social life?	
Does everyone in the family agree about and follow the same management plan for tackling the sleep problem?	
Has the sleep problem caused a problem for or caused complaints from your neighbours, e.g. because of noise, etc.?	
Permission to contact general practitioner/health visitor	

Bedtime and night routine

Where does the child sleep?

Any other address	Bed/cot	Own room	Shares room with	Shares bed with
Environmental features:	TV	Noise	Computer	Night Light
Sleep associations:	Blanket	Toy	Dummy	Other

Who cares for child in the day (list all)
Daytime routine

Who performs bedtime routine?	
Going to bed process	
Night sleep pattern/reason for any awakenings and how managed by carers. Any sleep-associated phenomenon like snoring, restless legs, head banging, night terrors, nightmares, teeth grinding, etc?	

Comments and observation:

Signed

Date

Appendix XII

Sleep diary

Name:

DOB:

Health professional:

Date started:

Day	pm							Mid night				am											Mid day		pm				
	6	7	8	9	10	11	12	1	2	3	4	5	6	7	8	9	10	11	12	1	2	3	4	5
⇨ Mon																								
Tue																								
Wed																								
Thu																								
Fri																								
Sat																								
Sun																								

Use arrows and text in line below to indicate any events which affected sleep, e.g. bed wetting, nightmare, etc.

Key: Asleep   Crying

Please choose your own colour keys for other activities, e.g. playing, etc.

Appendix XIII

Sleep log

Sleep Log

Name: JOHNNY NOKIP   **DOB** 20.06.2006   **Health Professional** AIMEE DOZE

Date started: 19.05.2008

Day	pm					Mid night	am											Mid day	pm					
	6	7	8	9	10	11	12	1	2	3	4	5	6	7	8	9	10	11	12	1	2	3	4	5
Mon																								
Tue																								
Wed																								
Thu																								
Fri																								
Sat																								
Sun																								

Notes on chart:
- Mon: "woke up screaming"
- Tue: "woke up frightened + screaming"
- Thu: "Screaming + frightened"
- Sun: "screaming + frightened"

Use arrows to indicate falling asleep (arrow pointing down) and waking up (arrow pointing up)
Write text in line below to indicate any events which affected sleep e.g. bed wetting, nightmare etc

Key:

| | Asleep | | Crying | | Feeding | | Playing | | Watching TV. |

Please choose your own colour keys for other activities e.g. playing, etc.

Appendix XIV

Disclosing difficult news to families

Practice checklist

What to check before starting

Room: • Private place • Comfortable room • Appropriate set-up for disclosure • Engaged sign • Room available for family afterwards • Availability of tissues, water, tea/coffee	Person communicating news: • Right notes/results • Right person (skills/seniority) • Sufficient time • Mobile/pagers switched off/handed over
Family: • Both parents present • Infant/child with parents	Interpreter: • Offer interpreter for either parent • Do not use family member/friend • Written translated information (request interpreter)
Team: • Agreed team plan for family support • Second professional for support/ assistance • Minimum number of people possible	Information and support: • Contact number of designated member • Written information/summary/useful, websites/support group contacts • Follow-up appointment date

How to communicate news

INTRODUCTION

- Ensure the room is set-up to be able to give eye contact to parents.
- Introduce everybody and acknowledge the child.
- Make arrangements for keeping children occupied.
- A separate session may be helpful for older child.

THE NEWS

- Use simple, understandable, non-judgemental, non-medical language.
- Check existing knowledge and concerns.
- Face-to-face verbal information.
- Active listening, body language. Be empathic, sensitive and honest.
- Use child's name and 'child first' language, e.g. 'babies with Turner's syndrome' rather than 'Turner syndrome babies'.
- Realistic messages given with hope. Not worst possible scenario but range of possible outcomes with probabilities.
- Avoid future predictions.
- Look for distress and/or anger. Acknowledge feelings. Remain calm. Stop and provide time for composure.
- Check understanding.
- Acknowledge concerns and uncertainties. Outline management plan and time frames.

CONCLUSION

- Give written information including information about support groups.
- Outline management plan and time frames.
- Disclosure advice for parents: advise them to provide honest and simple explanations. Offer to speak to other family members.

After communication completed

- Access to same room for family
- Support from team member if family to stay on.
- Good information handover to any team taking over care.
- Contact professionals involved and who can help.
- Debriefing.

Appendix XV

Emergency health care or resuscitation plan for a child/young person

Date plan created:

1.

> Name: Gavin Jones
> Hosp. no.:
> NHS no.:
> DOB: 18.09.2002
> Address:

2. Background

> Gavin has late infantile Batten's disease which is a life-limiting condition.
> He is at risk of prolonged seizures and life-threatening chest infections.
> Gavin has problems managing his respiratory secretions. He has a suction machine available at all times and home oxygen for chest infections.

3. Resuscitation plan

3.1 IN THE EVENT OF A SUDDEN COLLAPSE WITH RESPIRATORY AND/OR CARDIAC ARREST:

> Gavin may have airway obstruction due to secretions.

1. Comfort and support Gavin and his family or carers.
2. Reposition Gavin to open the airway. A nasopharyngeal airway may help.
3. Use suction to clear upper airway of secretions.
4. Give oxygen for comfort via face mask/nasal cannulae.

5. Give mouth to mouth/bag and mask ventilation – five inflation breaths.
6. More invasive resuscitation is not appropriate.
7. It is not appropriate to attempt resuscitation from a cardiac arrest.

3.2 GAVIN IS AT RISK OF GENERALIZED TONIC–CLONIC SEIZURES:

Rescue anticonvulsant medication for generalized tonic–clonic seizures lasting longer than 5 minutes is:
buccal midazolam – 10mg (1ml).

Name: Gavin Jones
Hosp. no.:
NHS no.:
DOB 18.09.2002
Address:

3.3 TRANSFER TO

Paediatric emergency department.
However, preferred place of death is home.

Ambulance staff can call ahead to alert receiving staff that child has a specific resuscitation plan.

3.4 WHO TO CALL (WITH PHONE NUMBERS)

If in hospital

Emergency paediatric medical team.

If at home

999 ambulance and community nurses on mobile telephone no.

If in school or short break unit

999 ambulance and parents on mobile telephone no.

3.5 COMMUNITYLAN HAS BEEN DISCUSSED WITH   BOTH PARENTS

3.6. THIS PLAN DOES NOT EXPIRE BUT WILL BE REVIEWED AS THE CHILD'S CONDITION CHANGES.

The patient or parent/guardian can change their mind about any of these options at any time.

3.7. CONSULTANT'S AGREEMENT

I support this Emergency Care/Personal Resuscitation Plan
Name and signature

.... date

3.8. PARENT OR GUARDIAN'S AGREEMENT

I have discussed and support this Emergency Care/Personal Resuscitation Plan
Name and signature

.... date

Name: Gavin Jones
Hosp. no.:
NHS no.:
DOB: 18.09.2002
Address:

4. Emergency care plan

4.1

Gavin is at risk of life-threatening chest infections. He will have increased effort of breathing, increased and green secretions. He may have fever.
Gavin is already taking prophylactic azithromycin 3 days per week.

1. Comfort and support Gavin and his family or carers.
2. Airway management, including oral/nasopharyngeal airway if it helps.
3. Oxygen for comfort via face mask/nasal cannulae.
4. Start oral antibiotics. Gavin's parents keep antibiotics at home.
5. Increase secretion clearance measures with support from community respiratory physiotherapist.
6. Consider admission for intravenous treatment if no improvement after 48 hours or if deteriorating rapidly and distressed.
7. Endotracheal intubation and invasive ventilation would not be appropriate.

4.2 TRANSFER TO

Paediatric emergency department.

4.3 WHO TO CALL IN THE EVENT OF A GRADUAL DETERIORATION

If at home:

GP and community nursing team on mobile.

If in school or short break unit:

Parents on mobile telephone no.

4.4 AMBULANCE DIRECTIVE IN PLACE

YES

Name: Gavin Jones
Hosp. no.:
NHS no.:
DOB: 18.09.2002
Address:

5. *Copies of this plan are held by*

Parents/guardian ☑ at home address

With patient at all times ☑ contact details:

School ☑ contact details:

Short break unit ☑ contact details:

Hospital notes ☑ contact details:

Community notes ☐ contact details:

Community nurses ☑ contact details:

GP ☑ contact details:

C/o parents as above
C/o school nurse School
Dr A Smith Paediatric Department Hospital
Manager Community Hospital
Manager Community Nursing Team
C/o Dr Valley Practice

Index

Notes

Page numbers in *italics* refer to material in figures, whilst numbers in **bold** refer to material in tables. *vs.* indicates a comparison or differential diagnosis.

The following abbreviations are used:

ADHD, attention-deficit–hyperactivity disorder; ASD, autism spectrum disorder; HIV, human immunodeficiency virus.